THE HISTORY OF AMERICAN NURSING

Edited by
Susan Reverby, Wellesley College

A GARLAND SERIES

HOSPITALS, DISPENSARIES AND NURSING

Edited by John S. Billings
& Henry M. Hurd

GARLAND PUBLISHING, INC.
NEW YORK • LONDON
1984

For a complete list of the titles in this series see the final pages of this volume.

This facsimile was made from a copy in the Sterling Library of Yale University.

Library of Congress Cataloging in Publication Data

International Congress of Charities, Correction, and
      Philanthropy 1893 : Chicago, Ill.)
      Hospitals, dispensaries, and nursing.

   (The History of American nursing)
   "Papers and discussions . . . of section III of the
International Congress of Charities, Correction, and
Philanthropy, which was held in Chicago, from June 12 to 17,
1893"—P.
   Reprint. Originally published: Baltimore : Johns Hopkins
Press, 1894.
   Includes index.
   1. Hospitals—Congresses.   2. Nursing—
Congresses.   3. Nursing—Study and teaching—
Congresses.   4. First aid in illness and injury—
Congresses.   5. Dispensaries—Congresses.   I. Billings,
John Shaw, 1838–1913.   II. Hurd, Henry M. (Henry Miles),
1843–1927.   III. Title.   IV. Series.
RA961.I6   1893   362.1′1   83-49145
ISBN 0-8240-6502-6 (alk. paper)

The volumes in this series are printed on acid-free, 250-year-life paper.

Printed in the United States of America

HOSPITALS

DISPENSARIES

AND

NURSING

PAPERS AND DISCUSSIONS IN THE INTERNATIONAL CONGRESS OF
CHARITIES, CORRECTION AND PHILANTHROPY, SECTION
III, CHICAGO, JUNE 12TH TO 17TH, 1893

EDITED BY

JOHN S. BILLINGS, M. D.
HENRY M. HURD, M. D.

BALTIMORE
THE JOHNS HOPKINS PRESS

LONDON
THE SCIENTIFIC PRESS, LIMITED
428 Strand, W. C.

1894

THE FRIEDENWALD CO., PRINTERS,
BALTIMORE.

INTERNATIONAL CONGRESS OF CHARITIES, CORRECTION AND PHILANTHROPY.

SECTION III.

The Hospital Care of the Sick, Training of Nurses, Dispensary Work, and First Aid to the Injured.

Honorary Chairman:

MR. HENRY C. BURDETT,
London, Eng.

Honorary Vice-Chairman:

LIEUTENANT-COLONEL J. LANE NOTTER, M. A., M. D.,
Surgeon-Major British Army, Netley, Eng.

Chairman:

JOHN S. BILLINGS, M. D., LL. D. Edin. and Harv., D. C. L. Oxon.
Surgeon U. S. A., Washington, D. C.

Secretary:

HENRY M. HURD, M. D.,
Superintendent, The Johns Hopkins Hospital, Baltimore, Md.

NURSING SUBSECTION.

Honorary Chairman:

MISS AMY HUGHES,
Superintendent of the Metropolitan and National Nursing Association, London, Eng.

Honorary Vice-Chairmen:

MISS E. P. DAVIS,
Superintendent of the University of Pennsylvania Hospital, Philadelphia, Pa.

MISS IRENE SUTLIFFE,
Directress of Nurses, New York Hospital, New York.

Chairman:

MISS ISABEL A. HAMPTON,
Superintendent of Nurses and Principal of Training School, The Johns Hopkins Hospital, Baltimore, Md.

Secretary:

MISS EMMA CAMERON,
Assistant Superintendent Illinois Training School for Nurses, Chicago, Ill.

PRELIMINARY NOTICE.

The papers and discussions herewith presented constitute the transactions of Section III of the International Congress of Charities, Correction and Philanthropy, which was held in Chicago, from June 12 to 17, 1893, under the auspices of the World's Congress Auxiliary of the World's Columbian Exposition. On Wednesday, June 14th, Section III, through its chairman, Dr. John S. Billings, of Washington, had charge of one of the general sessions of the Congress, at which time papers were presented by the chairman on the "Relations of Hospitals to Public Health"; by Lord Cathcart, of London, on the "Medical Charities of the English Metropolis"; by Miss Isabel A. Hampton, of Baltimore, on "Educational Standards for Nurses"; by Mr. Henry C. Burdett, of London, on "Hospital Finance and Method of Keeping Accounts," and by Lieut.-Col. J. Lane Notter, Professor of Military Hygiene, Army Medical School, Netley, on the "Applicability of Hygiene to the Conditions of Modern Warfare."

Sectional meetings were also held, at which papers were presented as follows:

Monday, June 12, 2 p. m. (Nursing Subsection included).

Organization of the Section.
"The Trustee of the Hospital," Mr. Richard Wood, Philadelphia.
"The Relation of Training Schools to Hospitals," Miss L. L. Dock, Baltimore.
"The Relation of the Medical Staff to the Governing Bodies in Hospitals," Dr. Edward Cowles, Somerville, Mass.
"Hospital Administration," Dr. H. Merke, Director Krankenhaus Moabit, Berlin.
"The Relation of Hospitals to Medical Education," Dr. Henry M. Hurd, Baltimore.

Tuesday, June 13, 10.30 a. m.
"Hospital Accounts and Methods of Bookkeeping," Mr. James R. Lathrop, New York.
"On Paying Patients in Hospitals," Dr. H. M. Lyman, Chicago.

"Paris Free and Paying Hospitals," Drs. Alan Herbert and W. Douglas Hogg, Paris.

"Isolating Wards and Hospitals for Infectious Diseases," Dr. G. H. M. Rowe, Boston.

"Dispensaries Historically and Locally Considered," Mr. Charles C. Savage, New York.

Tuesday, June 13, 2 p. m.

"On the Utility, Peculiarities and Special Needs of Hospitals for Children," Dr. William Wallis Ord, London.

"Ueber Militärlazarethe," Dr. Grossheim, German Army.

"Naval Hospitals," Dr. James D. Gatewood, Surgeon, U. S. Navy.

"The Marine Hospital Service," Dr. G. W. Stoner, Baltimore.

"Detention Hospitals for the Insane," Dr. Matthew D. Field, New York.

"Hospital Plans" (illustrated by Stereopticon Views), Dr. L. S. Pilcher, Brooklyn.

"Cottage Hospitals," Mr. Francis Vacher, Birkenhead, England.

"The Construction of Maternity Hospitals," Dr. B. C. Hirst, Philadelphia.

"Hospitals for Infectious Diseases," Dr. C. F. M. Pistor, Geheimer Medicinal-Rath, Berlin.

"Isolation Wards and Hospitals for Contagious Diseases," Dr. Alan Herbert and Dr. W. Douglas Hogg, Paris.

Thursday, June 15, 10.30 a. m. (Nursing Subsection included).

"French Training Schools," Dr. Leon Le Fort, Paris.

"Systems of Hospital Nursing in Amsterdam," Dr. Edouard Stumpf, Amsterdam.

"Nurses' Homes," Miss K. L. Lett, Chicago.

"Hospital for Contagious and Infectious Diseases," Dr. M. L. Davis, Lancaster, Pa.

"A Description of the proposed new Laundry of the University of Pennsylvania Hospital," Dr. A. C. Abbott, Philadelphia.

"Diet Kitchens in Hospitals," Dr. H. B. Stehman, Chicago.

"Hospital Dietaries," Miss M. A. Boland, Baltimore.

Friday, June 16, 10 a. m.

"First Help in Hemorrhage," Prof. von Esmarch, Germany.

"First Aid to the Injured and how it should be Taught," Dr. Henry G. Beyer, Surgeon, U. S. Navy.

"First Aid to the Injured from the Military Standpoint," Dr. Charles Smart, Surgeon, U. S. Army.

"Organization of First Aid to the Wounded in Paris," Drs. Alan Herbert and W. Douglas Hogg, Paris.

"The Ambulance System of New York," Mr. George P. Ludlam, New York.

"An Easy Method of Bedmaking and Improved Stretcher for Hospital and Military Use," Dr. E. D. Worthington, Sherbrooke, Quebec.

"A Short Sketch of the Chilian Hospitals," Dr. Luis Asta-Buruaga, Valparaiso.

" Hospital Saturday and Sunday," Mr. Frederick F. Cook, New York.

Descriptions were also presented of the Montreal General Hospital ; the Roosevelt Hospital, N. Y.; the Johns Hopkins Hospital, Baltimore, and the Royal Victoria Hospital, Montreal, which were ordered to be published.

The sessions and papers of the Subsection on the Training of Nurses were as follows :

June 13, 10.30 a. m.

"Trained Nursing in Berlin," Fräulein Luise Fahrmann, Berlin, Germany.

"La Source Normal Evangelical School of Independent Nurses for the Sick at Lausanne, Switzerland," Dr. Charles Krafft.

"Nursing Work of the Religious Orders of the Roman Catholic Church," Cardinal Gibbons.

" The Education of Nurses in the Catholic Religious Orders of Germany," Sanitätsrath Dr. Köllen, Berlin.

"Nursing in Scotland," Miss Rachel Frances Lumsden, Aberdeen.

" The Work of Deaconesses in Germany."

" Training Schools in America," Miss Irene Sutliffe, New York.

" Proper Organization of Training Schools in America," Miss Louise Darche, New York.

" Nurses as Heads of Hospitals," Miss E. P. Davis, Philadelphia.

June 14, 2 p. m.

"Needs for an American Nurses' Association," Miss Edith Draper, Chicago.

"The Royal National Pension Fund for Nurses," Miss Gordon, London.

"Alumnæ Associations for Nurses," Miss Isabel McIsaac, Chicago.

".District Nursing in England," Mrs. Dacre Craven, London.

" The Work of the Queen's Institute," Miss A. Hughes, London.

" District Nursing in America," Miss C. E. Somerville, Lawrence, Mass.

" Missionary Nursing in Japan and China," Miss L. Richards, Boston, Mass.

June 16, 10.30 a. m.

"Children's Hospitals," Miss Rogers, Washington, D. C.

" Obstetric Nursing," Miss Pope, Washington, D. C.

"Midwifery as a Profession for Women," Mrs. Henry Smith, London.

" The Nursing of the Insane," Miss May, Rochester, N. Y.

June 17, 3 p. m.

" Association for the Training of Attendants," Mrs. D. H. Kinney, Boston, Mass.

"The Instruction of the Sisters of the Red Cross," Dr. Goering, Bremen, Germany.

"Training Schools for Small Hospitals," Miss M. Greenwood, Cincinnati, Ohio.

"The London Hospital Nurses' Home," Miss Eva C. E. Lückes, London.

There were also presented, as part of the work of the Congress, through Baroness Burdett-Coutts, papers from Florence Nightingale, the Hon. Mrs. Stuart Wortley and Miss Louisa Twining.

TABLE OF CONTENTS.

III.—NURSING OF THE SICK.

IV.—DISPENSARIES.

V.—First Aid to the Injured.

VI.—Hospital Saturday and Sunday.

ILLUSTRATIONS.

I.

GENERAL SESSION.

THE RELATIONS OF HOSPITALS TO PUBLIC HEALTH.

By John S. Billings, M. D.

Address as Chairman of the Section.

The business of this Section relates to co-operative means for the care of those suffering from disease or injury, more especially of recent origin, excluding, for the most part, those forms of brain abnormity, or disease connected with what are known as insanity and idiocy, and also those forms of chronic and incurable disability which are not amenable to medical and surgical treatment.

Primarily, hospital aid was intended and provided solely for the benefit of the poor—of those who were unable to obtain, at their own expense or by their own efforts, proper care in case of sickness ; but its field of work has been steadily extending ; it now has relations with the interests of almost every class of the community, and its results have greatly modified the methods of treatment of many forms of disease among the well-to-do classes as well as among the poor.

It is largely by hospital organization and work that skilled physicians, surgeons and nurses are provided for the public ; and in the absence of hospitals, their proper and complete training is practically impossible.

Each succeeding year more people resort to hospitals and dispensaries for treatment, and this is especially the case in the United States. Forty years ago the number of hospital beds in our cities was very small in proportion to the population, when compared with the amount of such accommodation in the countries of Western Europe, and the demand for such accommodation was also small. People did not go to hospitals if they could help it ; it was believed that surgical operations and labor cases did not result so well in hospitals as they did in the homes of the people, even when these homes were very small and not especially well ordered. Hospitals were for sick paupers, and we did not have many paupers in comparison with European countries. The war of 1861–65, and the great influx of immigrants, have produced many changes in public opinion upon these points.

The war taught us how to build and manage hospitals, so as to greatly lessen the evils which had previously been connected with them, and it also made the great mass of the people familiar with the appearance of, and work in, hospitals, as they had never been before. Not only the tens of thousands of men who were treated in the great war hospitals in those days, but the hundreds of thousands of visitors, the parents, children, sisters and friends of these men, were thus educated, and they were educated not merely by what they saw and heard, but by what they did or tried to do to help make the patients more comfortable, by the work of the Sanitary and Christian Commissions, by the formation of local associations for giving aid and relief, and by becoming accustomed to the methods and results of voluntary co-operation in matters of this kind.

Since the close of the war the formation of training schools for nurses in many of the large hospitals has been an additional means of interesting the public in the work, and of keeping it informed as to the progress made in securing the safety and comfort of the inmates. With the increase of knowledge about hospitals and their capabilities has come an increased demand upon them for accommodation for persons in comfortable circumstances, who are affected with diseases which can be better treated in them than in private houses ; in other words, for private rooms for pay patients, especially those requiring surgical operations or suffering from certain forms of nervous diseases ; and from this class of persons and their friends the demand is now relatively greater in the United States than it is in Europe.

During the last thirty years the demand for free beds in the public wards has also greatly increased, owing in part to a relative increase in the number of the very poor in our large cities, and in part to the immigration of large numbers of people accustomed in their former homes to seek public aid and hospital relief in case of sickness, and bringing with them this habit, which extends to others by force of example.

The increase in free dispensary work, or out-patient relief, as it is sometimes called, has been even greater than that in free hospital beds, or in-patient relief, in our large cities, and the number of people who are not paupers who apply to these dispensaries for free treatment, although they are able to pay reasonable fees if required to do so, is becoming so large as to constitute a serious problem in hospital and dispensary management with us, as it does in London and other large European cities.

As the health of a community depends on the health of the individuals who compose it, it is evident that there may be important relations between hospital aid in all its aspects and the public health, and it is to some of these relations that I desire briefly to call your attention.

The importance of hospitals for certain forms of contagious and infectious disease, as a means of preventing the spread of such diseases, would appear to be almost self-evident, yet very few cities in this country are provided with them. If there is a city " pest house," as it is commonly called, it is the relic of a smallpox outbreak, and is usually empty and uncared for, located in some desolate suburb, the grounds overgrown with weeds, and the building itself corresponding in appearance to the ideas to which its name naturally gives rise.

We have several papers before the Section on the subject of hospitals for infectious disease, and it is, therefore, unnecessary for me to say anything about the plans and arrangements for such institutions, which will, no doubt, be fully discussed in the Section meetings; but there is one point with regard to them to which I will briefly refer, namely, the question as to whether they should, or should not, be entirely free to all persons, no matter whether they are able to pay for the accommodation provided or not. It is urged by the majority of English health officers that the isolation of a case of infectious disease in a special hospital provided by the sanitary authorities for that purpose is not, in most cases, any special benefit to or favor conferred upon the person so treated; that it is done, and made compulsory, for the benefit of the community and not of the individual, and that the community should, therefore, bear the cost. It appears to me that this is true with regard to necessary cost, and to that only. It is not only permissible, but desirable, that such an hospital should be able to furnish a private room, a special nurse, and other extra accommodations, when demanded, as they would be if such hospitals were made use of by well-to-do people, and the party receiving such extra service and accommodation should pay for it.

To make such hospitals really useful in preventing the spread of disease there should be the least possible delay and formality in admitting cases. If a child affected with scarlet fever or diphtheria is brought to the door and the medical officer recognizes it to be such, it should be admitted at once, without waiting to send for a permit from some official, and the general rule should be that a certificate from any competent physician that the person is suffering from such a disease as the hospital is intended for should be a sufficient warrant for his admission.

The increasing use of hospitals and free dispensaries to which I have referred is one of the signs of the socialistic tendency of the age, of the increasing tendency to subordinate the individual to the community in attempting to equalize the burdens and pleasures of mankind. If the process be carried a little further we might come to something like the scheme suggested by Mr. Havelock Ellis, in his recent book entitled " The Nationalization of Health." This is to the effect that hospitals of the future are not to be charitable or voluntary institutions, but are all to be under national control, to be supplied from national funds, and to be free to every one. The country is to be covered with a network of such hospitals, each having a large medical staff, including all sorts of specialists paid by the state. Private practitioners are no longer to be relied upon for medical attendance to the public,; it is supposed that they would only be consulted for minor and comparatively trivial ailments; the greater part of the work is to be done by medical officials. Private charity and individual philanthropy are no longer to be relied upon or encouraged; the whole business is to be done by machinery; health is to be equalized among the people. All hospitals are to be placed on the footing of hospitals for contagious diseases, and, with their medical staffs, are to become a part of a greater national bureau for the prevention of disease. As it is to the interest of a medical officer of the army and navy to prevent, as far as possible, the occurrence of disease among the command to which he is assigned, in order that he may have as little as possible to do in the way of treatment, so it is supposed that these other medical officials will be active, zealous and efficient agents in prescribing and enforcing state and municipal sanitation.

Two hundred and fifty years ago Sir Thomas Browne said that he counted this world not an inn but an hospital, a place not to live but to die in, and perhaps the plan I have outlined, when fully carried out, will make many men of his way of thinking. I do not myself think that this scheme will be carried out, but the present tendency is in that direction ; hospital aid will be more and more resorted to in coming years; there will be an increasing demand on the part of the constituted authorities, representing the majority of the people, for state or municipal supervision of what are at present private charities, upon grounds similar to those stated by Mr. Ellis, and it is important for us to recognize these facts and tendencies, whether we approve of them or not. I myself am of the opinion that hospitals supported by voluntary contributions confer quite as much benefit upon those who contribute the funds as upon those who are treated in them. If, however, there is to be public and official supervision of all free hospitals and dispensaries, should not these be in closer relation with and contribute more to the public health service of the cities in which they are placed than is the case at present? Even the city hospitals, those that are supported entirely by municipal funds, do not, as a rule, have any special connection with the city health departments, but are under entirely different management. They report the deaths which occur in them, and sometimes the cases of certain forms of contagious disease which are treated in them, but little more. As to the voluntary hospitals and dispensaries that are supported from private funds, they make the same sort of reports and nothing more. But if my view of the tendencies of the age is correct, the time is not far distant when the health office of a city will have a daily record, not only of all deaths, but of all cases of disease treated free in any hospital or dispensary in the city, with specifications of name, age, sex, color, place of residence, nature of disease and mode of final disposal. I need hardly comment on the value of such a record, both as an immediate emergency guide for the health officer and as a basis for statistical investigation of the healthfulness of different parts of the city.

I have already indicated the important relations to public health held by hospitals in their function of aiding in the training of physicians and nurses, and this is a point which should be constantly borne in mind in attempts to compare the efficiency and economy of different hospitals, or of the same hospital at different times. The teaching hospitals not only do the best work in the treatment of patients, who are more carefully examined and more scrupulously cared for in them than they are in non-teaching institutions, but they furnish the doctors and nurses required by the people in their own homes, and the quality of their work in this respect merits more scrutiny on the part of the public than it has heretofore received.

No doubt it would be a new idea to our mayors and municipal authorities if they were told that they are, to a considerable extent, responsible for the quality of teaching and the standard for graduation in those medical schools which obtain their facilities for clinical instruction in the hospitals supported by the city; yet it is the truth, since they have it in their power to enforce almost any standard of medical education which they choose to favor.

The tendency in this country is, however, towards the regulation of standards of medical education by the state, and some curious questions of jurisdiction will arise if a state should undertake to prescribe the conditions under which instruction in practical medicine and nursing shall be given in the hospitals of its several municipalities.

At present our best medical schools are desirous of having hospitals of their own, or at all events, hospitals in which they can control the appointments of the attending and resident medical staff, since, otherwise, the selection of some of their clinical teachers may be made by those who have no interest in, or responsibility for, the work of the school. For the same reason the establishment of a large general hospital by private endowment presents a strong inducement to the establishment of a medical school closely connected with it and under the same control; in fact such an hospital without a medical school and nurses' training school is only doing a part of the work which is rightfully expected and demanded of such an institution.

To a limited extent this obligation to promote the public health by increasing and diffusing knowledge as to the causes, nature and best methods of prevention or treatment of disease, rests also upon special hospitals, including those for the insane, and no such hospital can be considered as doing its complete and best work if it is not contributing to the training of physicians and nurses.

With the present rapid concentration of population in cities, the demand for hospital accommodation will steadily increase, and so also will the demand for municipal regulation of dwellings in their sanitary aspects, for increase of facilities for limiting the spread of contagious and infectious disease, and for skilled supervision of food supplies. All these things are more or less correlated, and they should be studied together.

It does not seem probable that any millennium will thus be produced, or that nature's methods of eliminating the idle, the vicious and the unfit by diminishing birth-rates and increased death-rates will be either rendered unnecessary or done away with by advances in medicine or in sanitation; but whether this be true or not, it is clearly the duty of those who have knowledge, means and opportunities, to investigate these matters carefully, and to do all that they can to lessen the sufferings and sorrows of those who are unable to help themselves.

THE MEDICAL CHARITIES OF THE ENGLISH METROPOLIS.

By Lord Cathcart, a Member of the Lords' Committee.[1]

Lord Bacon reminds us in his Chapter of Innovations, " It were well therefore that men in their innovations would follow the example of Time itself, which indeed innovateth greatly but quietly, and by degrees scarce to be perceived "; and that wise and witty Lord concludes with a reference to the Scripture; this passage so quoted shall

[1] *The Lords' Committee on Hospitals—The Order of Reference.* Metropolitan Hospitals, &c.—*Moved* [April 28, 1890] That a Select Committee be appointed to inquire with regard to all hospitals and provident and other public dispensaries and charitable institutions within the Metropolitan area, for the care and treatment of the sick poor, which possess real property or invested personal property, in the nature of endowment of a permanent or temporary nature ; and to receive, if the Committee think fit, evidence tendered by the authorities of voluntary institutions for like purposes or, with their consent, in relation to such institutions : And further, to inquire and report what amount of accommodation for the sick is provided by rate, and as to the management thereof ; and that the witnesses before the said Select Committee be examined on oath ; *agreed to* (The Lord Sandhurst) :

That the following Lords be named of the Committee :

Lord Archbishop of Canterbury.	Lord Saye and Sele.
Earl Cadogan (*Lord Privy Seal*).	Lord Clifford of Chudleigh.
Earl Winchilsea and Nottingham.	Lord Sandhurst.
Earl Lauderdale.	Lord Fermanagh (*Earl Erne*).
Earl Spencer.	Lord Lamington.
Earl Cathcart.	Lord Sudley (*Earl Arran*).
Earl Kimberly.	Lord Monkswell.
Lord Zouche of Haryngworth.	Lord Thring.

be the keynote of that which, by your favor, is now to follow. The text runs thus: "That we make a stand upon the ancient way, and then look about us and discover what is the straight and right way, and so walk in it." [1]

The medical charities of the English metropolis, and in regard to them the House of Lords' inquiry and reports of the years 1890, 1891 and 1892, are the subject on which I have now the honor to address you; and craving your kind indulgence, I would premise that the limited time apportioned permits me to touch the fringe only of a vast subject, and my present essay must be considered merely as an introductory chapter or preface to three large official volumes [2] exhaustive of the subject, and which volumes, I confidently submit, would amply repay the study of that noble army of kindred professional and lay humanitarians on both sides of the Atlantic —generous rivals—whose benevolent labors in the truly Samaritan direction now in question excite our appreciation and admiration.

It is truly British "to make a stand upon the ancient way and then look about us." In the heart of Old London, near which are situated the greater number of our Metropolitan Hospitals, a long succession of pregnant centuries seem spectrally to tumble over and jostle each other in the narrow streets—bygone centuries that have left many traces in the most busy and commercially frequented streets by ever-varying architecture—buildings, often like English laws and customs, the admirable constructions of our common ancestors. London, especially Old London, with crooked lanes and narrow alleys and beetle-browed houses, is nowhere spick and span and laid out symmetrically and mathematically in rectilinear blocks like American cities, and notably like your own vast and beautiful Chicago. In Greater London we have also to deplore that there is a wide and darksome gulf to be bridged between west and east, between the mansions of the rich and the dwellings of the poor—that East End, much of which is a cheerless region where squalor and unloveliness walk hand-in-hand; where, actuated by the passion of pity, kind hearts are exercised in the endeavor to bring to healthy lives sunshine, change, variety, happiness; and where for the sick and

---

[1] Jer. vi. 16.

[2] Reports, vol. i., Evidence, 1890, 5s.; Vol. ii., Evidence, 1891, 6s. 7d.; Vol. iii., 1892, 2s. 7d., Summary. Conclusions, particulars of every Metropolitan Hospital in tabular form. There is also an index analysis of the Evidence to accompany vols. i. and ii., price 1s. each index.

injured poor the London Hospital, as afterwards I shall have the pleasure of showing you, is very quietly doing a very grand and greatly appreciated work.

Of the London hospitals generally it may be said, with apparently inadequate structures and means, great and truly admirable work is being done. And praise be to God, this noble work is alike Jew and Gentile : no regard is had to either race or creed, the only qualifications being but too apparent—namely, medical need, necessity, and adversity.

We, indeed, in old England "make a stand upon the ancient way" : the London hospitals originate in monastic charity. St. Bartholomew's, the greatest of the English medical charitable institutions, was founded A. D. 1183 by Rahere, who also founded the adjacent Priory of the same name : the hospital, nominally under the Priory, was from the first virtually independent—not an almshouse, but a hospital for the sick. William Harvey, a small man with black hair, the immortal author of "Exercitatio de Motu Cordis et Sanguinis," a record of the greatest of the discoveries of physiology, was physician here for thirty-four years, 1609–1643. Some rules drawn up by him are to this day in full force : amongst other things his charge recites, "You shall prescribe such medicines only as should doe the poor good without regard to the pecuniary interests of the apothecary." St. Thomas's Hospital was originally founded in 1213 by the Prior of Bermondsey as an almonry ; purchased at the Reformation by the City of London, it was converted into a hospital for the sick ; rebuilt in 1871 in seven blocks, it was considered the model hospital for the world, until you, in generous rivalry, constructed your still more perfect Johns Hopkins Hospital at Baltimore. One word more on this curious subject of historical origins ; the Lock Hospital for venereal diseases—perhaps, having regard to the welfare of the general population, the most important of the London special hospitals—derives its name from the French "loques " = rags, lint applied to sores ; it was originally and from very early times a lazar-house, a spital for leprous people, known in 1437 as " Le Lokes." [1]

The Lords' inquiry was instituted in consequence of a most influentially signed petition, amongst others signed by sixteen hundred representative London medical men, 35 per cent of the medical

[1] See *London, Past and Present,* 3 vols. Wheatley and Cunningham. London : John Murray. 1891.

profession of the Metropolis. The concluding paragraph of the petition runs thus: "Your petitioners, for reasons set forth at length, pray your right honorable House to appoint a Select Committee to make inquiry in regard to the financial and general management and the common organization of medical institutions, endowed and voluntary, and in regard to the administration of poor-law institutions for the aid of the sick in the Metropolis, and to make recommendations."

On the motion of Lord Sandhurst, a Select Committee of fifteen was appointed on April 28, 1890—"a strong committee"; that is to say, a committee largely composed of experts or of persons having wide experience in the conduct of affairs. Such committees have plenary powers to call for all persons and papers, the evidence is taken on oath, witnesses are examined and re-examined—virtually cross-examined—to any extent that may appear necessary; and—this is most important in any inquiry—the witnesses, however outspoken, are by privilege absolutely safeguarded.

Lord Sandhurst was throughout in the chair of the committee, and he was the mainspring of the whole inquiry. A man in the prime of life, subject as fully as any one to all the distractions of business and society, I may mention him as an example of the devotion evinced by laymen in the working of our medical charities. As chairman of the Middlesex Hospital, I believe, when the political party to which he is attached is not in power, and he is consequently free from official duty, he visits the charitable institution he admirably administers almost every day of every week.

In the several reports of the committee, full and most detailed information is virtually given either by reported parole evidence, or by schedules of queries with replies in regard to every institution in "Greater London" for the relief of the sick poor. These institutions are (1) charitable, and (2) provided under the poor-law. They may further be classified as follows:

General hospitals, with and without schools.

Special hospitals.

Dispensaries, provident, part pay, charitable, and poor-law.

Poor-law infirmaries, and

Hospitals for infectious cases under the Metropolitan Asylums Board.

Roughly estimated, at the commencement of the inquiry the committee was to contemplate some 24,000 beds, with 122,000 in-patients to occupy them for one year, the out-patients treated during that period being 1,585,381.[1] Of old, a witch's prayer was said to be read backwards—a course in such case perhaps objectionable enough, but as regards the hospital committee reports, I venture to recommend this method of evil origin as the most convenient, and with your permission in my further observations I propose to follow it. Namely, read the general conclusions of the committee, in vol. iii. ; then where most interested refer back to the summary of evidence, which in turn will refer the reader retrogressively to the evidence given *in extenso* in the first and second volumes. I propose to myself, then, in this paper to follow henceforth this simple and, I hope, exact method—namely, to run rapidly through the conclusions arrived at and recommendations made by the committee, and which, so far as they go, have my full concurrence ; condensing these conclusions as honestly as I can under the various heads; and afterwards under these respective heads giving you in a friendly manner and concise form my own candid impressions and views on those salient and practical points which I think will most interest my practical and experienced audience.

Endowed Hospitals.

The three great endowed hospitals, St. Bartholomew's, St. Thomas's, and Guy's, might have an improved system of management; regret is expressed by the committee that in St. Thomas's and Guy's, from want of funds, some beds are vacant and others let.

On this I need only observe that, amongst others, the late Dr. Steele, of Guy's, an excellent and most experienced witness, told the committee that all hospitals are best administered by weekly boards —this system so strengthens the hands of the immediate hospital authority. The drainage of St. Bartholomew's was found by the committee to be very defective. As a consequence, I am glad to see by the newspapers, this crying evil has been remedied by reconstruction at a cost of some 16,000*l*. Here is the last account of a year's work at St. Bartholomew's :

5953 in-patients, 16,143 out-patients, and 142,745 casualty patients, were treated there during last year. In addition 1775 women were attended in confinement, of whom 6 died. The total number of children born was 1802, including 60 twins. During the year a large number of patients were relieved from the Samaritan Fund on

---

[1] See Appendix to this paper.

their discharge from the hospital, and 936 patients were sent to convalescent homes.

Much that I have to say under other heads will equally apply to the endowed hospitals; so, with the observation that the most economical administration is often the most efficient administration, and that, in my opinion, it is wonderful how institutions living from hand to mouth hold their own with those largely endowed, I pass on to consider the

General Hospitals.

The committee observes that the eight general hospitals with medical schools, supported virtually by voluntary contributions, are, according to the evidence, well administered on a nearly uniform system. Individuality should be maintained; generous rivalry tends to medical and administrative efficiency. The committee desires to remove exclusive London diploma restrictions, and would throw open hospital appointments, as at St. Mary's Hospital, to all suitable graduates. There appears to be an omission in the conclusions of the committee which I do not think was intended, for eight general hospitals without schools are worthy of honorable mention. The committee notes the enormous amount of work carefully done by unpaid boards of managers.

I now proceed to give you my own views, which naturally fall under these heads: A few general observations; the patient, the public, and the practitioner; ending by an example—a little sketch of the poor, very poor districts effectually ministered to by the London Hospital.

A general hospital with us takes all manner of diseases except certain highly infectious complaints which are treated in the rate-supported asylums. Proper hospital work was well defined in the evidence; it is to lodge and cure or relieve bad and necessitous cases. These general hospitals are characterized by kindness to the living and decent reverence for the dead; on this latter point especially, the kindness to the living being obvious, we made strict inquiry. Entire publicity is happily of the essence of our voluntary hospital system; that publicity, in my opinion, is sadly wanting in the rate-supported infirmaries. I am justified in thinking they could not stand the test voluntary hospitals are submitted to, for it is in the interest of subscribers and others to see that their money is well spent. It is an axiom, then, that the officers of institutions which exist by the charity of the public should have nothing to conceal. It were well to ponder over the following suggestive observation: no conceivable Government could undertake for a day the commissariat of our vast English metropolis; any such attempt to feed and otherwise supply from four to five millions of people would utterly break down. So in regard to the proportionate sick: only the free co-operation of the voluntary and rate-supported hospitals can hopefully undertake to cover, even inadequately, the vast and daily increasing field for hospital requirements that opens out before us.

That patients come faster—much faster—than money is the universal experience. Very humble, very poor persons find their way into the voluntary hospitals, but lower depths are still dredged for the poor-law infirmaries. I fear in the nature of things, moribund cases in London stand a bad chance or no chance of being taken into a voluntary hospital (please bear in mind my previous definition —proper hospital work is to "cure or relieve"; Dr. Steele, of Guy's, estimated that two-thirds of the patients came from the neighborhood of the hospital). In most hospitals, mercifully, anæsthetics are administered outside the operating theater. The very cleverly managed Charing Cross Hospital has a reception ward always ready for accidents, so that the general wards during the night are undisturbed. There is also in that hospital a well-arranged mortuary chapel—a thoughtful gift—into which bodies are removed from the dead-house when the friends of the deceased visit the hospital. In every case we found very proper arrangements were made in relation to the dead, and every consideration shown for the feelings of their friends. Patients as a rule are very grateful, and nurses are often worried by the grateful tender of unacceptable and unpermitted little presents. The patients have no objection to clinical instruction; their sense of self-importance is gratified by notice and publicity. A patient, it is said, has four values: as a worker he is valuable to the community; he is necessary for purposes of medical instruction; as a case he is professionally interesting; and should a well-to-do patient be improperly admitted to the hospital, the general practitioner is interested by reason of the loss of possible fees. The immediate problem is how to harmonize these various interests. Again and again this essential question will arise, and will continue to arise. How to limit voluntary hospital charity to the worthy—that is to say, to the indigent?

Public opinion, with us, no doubt desires to reform hospital administration and adjust the claims of poverty, so that the charities shall not foster pauperism; of this more hereafter when we reach the out-patient department. Meanwhile it may be well to note certain facts pretty well established by the evidence.

High authorities who have studied abroad, and compared home with foreign institutions, are not in favor, as a general system, of State-paid hospitals. In all voluntary hospitals there should be, under the weekly board, a resident official, with full authority. It is desirable to maintain a chain of responsibility, avoiding anything like divided authority; I think I heard even the phrase "a benevolent despotism." The sanitary zone is important—that is, an aerial space all round each hospital, which with us does not invariably exist.

The difference between beds and occupied beds is 25 per cent.; apart from beds vacant from want of funds or patients, there must be a working margin of from 10 to 12 per cent. In any great emergency I should fear a breakdown in our voluntary system; working under extreme high pressure, there must be overcrowding—necessity knows no law. Miss Nightingale [1] goes fully into the question of the space per bed on the plan required for efficient nursing. The Middlesex, an old building, has 88 square feet per bed; St. George's, 69 square feet; the new St. Thomas's has 112, which is considered sufficient. Teak, or hard wood floors, dry rubbed and polished, are everywhere being substituted for deal planking and wet swabbing.

Sanitation and Listerism have wonderfully reduced hospital mortality; public opinion should insist on a plan of the hospital drains kept up to date and exposed to public view. Fire arrangements should be studied and concerted with the admirable Metropolitan Fire Brigade. There is usually a properly constructed furnace for the cremation of such nasty things as cannot be taken by the drains. Newspaper reporters should be invited and encouraged to attend all general meetings.

The Samaritan funds are kept separately, and usually well administered. St. George's Hospital is a good example of management in this respect; even the families of patients are sometimes visited and helped. In all hospitals it is frequently necessary to burn the whole of the clothes of a patient, and consequently on discharge a new fit-out must be provided. In some hospitals the friends of the patients are expected to provide or pay for tea, sugar and butter; but where, owing to extreme poverty, this is impossible there is usually a supply from the Samaritan fund. One general hospital, with 179 occupied beds, calculated that for all the patients a free

[1] *Report*, vol. i. p. 607. "On the Nursing Service of Hospitals."

supply of tea, sugar and butter would cost 400*l.* a year. I always ask in a hospital to taste the beef tea ; its quality is not a bad test of management.

The question was constantly asked of hospital authorities, what do you do in infectious cases, such as smallpox and scarlet fever? and the constant reply was—"Wire for an ambulance and it comes at once." This is the latest account of the ambulance service in London : At a meeting of the Sanitary Inspectors' Association, it was explained that there were two principal voluntary services—namely, the St. John's Ambulance Association and the Hospitals Association. With respect to the first, the system of training men and women had been extended throughout the kingdom, and, indeed, over many parts of the world. Members were deputed to go on ambulance duty on public occasions like the Lord Mayor's Show. In 1891 the associations were supported by donations and subscriptions to the extent of 4000*l.*, by sales of shares 8000*l.*, fees for removal of patients by the invalid transport corps about 1500*l.*, or a total income of about 13,500*l.* The annual expenditure was about 10,500*l.* The association had recently established an invalid transport corps for the convenience of sick and injured persons (infectious cases excepted).

The Hospitals Association had proved a valuable adjunct to the ambulance system. By that association 2101 cases had been removed in three years. The Metropolitan Asylums Board's removals by ambulance had doubled those of any previous year, the number being about 32,000.[1]

We now come to the hospital medical officer.

This comprehensive question was asked : In regard to what has been called martyrdom of hospital appointments it is argued that you eminent medical men have used these general hospital appointments as a ladder by which to climb to fame, and that thereby you derive benefit, and that if any eminent man wants to give up his hospital appointment there are six other eminent medical men ready to take that appointment ? *Answer.*—That is quite probable.

Question.—And that to a large extent is the view of your profession ? *Answer.*—That is quite probable.

Notwithstanding, say I, all honor to the army of professional men who so nobly bear the heat and burden of the day. Medical educational interests must to some extent militate against the reform of hospital abuse by well-to-do patients ; necessarily medical men are more interested in cases than in the social fitness of the patients.

[1] The *Times*, April 10, 1893.

The London Hospital is in the midst of the poor and for the poor —the docks, the river side, Spitalfields, and other very poor districts —purely and simply the poor man's hospital. The expenditure last year was 60,000*l.* 10,070 in-patients and nearly 113,000 out-patients were treated during the year. The nursing staff is 250. Go there on visiting day—say Sunday afternoon—you find it swarming with visitors; little satisfied groups round most of the beds. There is no question at all—these visitors in fustian and frieze are socially of the right sort—they believe in this hospital, of which they are very proud. Applying the same test in the West-end of London, I confess I have had my misgivings; patients in shirts and shifts are much alike, but not so the friends—broadcloth and silk, top hats and gum-flower bonnets are in such cases sad tell-tales, suggesting now and then even a bank account and a check-book. Hear the late Mr. Montagu Williams, Q. C.,[1] magistrate of Worship Street and Thames Police Courts, well and honorably known as the " Poor Man's Magistrate"; his impressions are quite consistent with the evidence taken by the Lords' committee. The London Hospital, says Mr. Williams, is full of variety—a greater variety of people than in any other—a mass of suffering humanity representing nearly every nationality on earth. There is not another hospital in England— not in the world—so well conducted. I have visited at all hours to take dying depositions and for other objects, and consequently I am well able to judge. Seven hundred and seventy-six beds can be made up. Two wards are endowed for Jews, with separate kitchens and cooks, kosher meat and unleavened bread ; the Passover is celebrated and all Jewish rites are strictly observed. The nurses are Christians, and the often Yiddish-speaking patients, with wonderful powers of dumb-show, will take medicine from no other hands ; but the Christian nurses dare not touch the dead—so soon as the breath of life flutters to depart there instantly appears the Jewish "watcher." The nurses as a body, says Mr. Montagu Williams, are amiable, patient, and gentle. In the London Hospital we have an admirable example of the maximum of good and efficient work effected with a minimum of expenditure.

Convalescent Homes.

The committee says the accommodation for convalescents in detached homes and otherwise is deficient; this causes one or other of two evils—premature discharge or hospital congestion; besides,

---

[1] *Round London.* London : 1892.

patients would often recover more rapidly if sent into the country. To this I have only to add that we were told the patients much prefer the seaside.

Out-patients.

On the questions of out-patients and dispensaries, much evidence was taken by the committee. The out-patients' departments are open day and night for the relief of the poor; as regards medical education they are of essential importance. They are available, and private medical practitioners, whilst retaining their patient, should more fully avail themselves of out-patient departments for consultative purposes. These charities are not abused to any serious extent. When doubt arises, a patient should be called upon to establish a *primâ facie* case for charitable relief. Each out-patient attends on the average about three times. The committee do not attach undue importance to statements as to the reduction, owing to the unpaid work of the hospitals, of the fees of medical practitioners. It is obvious there must be some tendencey in that direction. But in London, with its heterogeneous and migratory population, there are above the pauper line very many persons who, owing to continued illness, a numerous family, or otherwise, are quite unable to pay for medical assistance.

Upon this I beg you to observe that there are out-patients and out-patients; in other words, there is invariably a sifting process, and the trifling and more numerous cases are called casuals, cut fingers and that sort of thing, which are attended to once for all.

Out-patients in their original inception naturally arose from in-patients, and to relieve hospital congestion—" You may go home, but let us see you occasionally ; we should be glad to know how you get on "; or, " Your wound will require to be dressed every second day "; and so on—this is the little seed which has produced an enormous tree. Some hospitals limit new cases to fifteen medical and fifteen surgical patients a day, but even then hard cases are allowed to make bad law. Often—too often—the medical man administering an out-patient department sees it is not medicine that is wanted but a basin of soup.

Sir Andrew Clark, the President of the College of Physicians, every word of whose evidence should be carefully studied, for it is as weighty in substance as it is admirable in style, told the committee " that to close the out-patient departments of the hospitals would be the greatest public calamity, and disastrous to the art of medicine." After an eloquent account of how medicine is or should be taught, Sir Andrew added: " In the hospital wards disease is seen in its later stages, in the out-patient department in its inception." Sir Andrew said, as his own experience at the London Hospital, he could, in the out-patient department, see three or four hundred people in an afternoon.

Overlapping is where a patient may go from place to place, from voluntary to poor-law institutions, or otherwise—say, for example, for some particular treatment or appliance; there was evidence in regard to this evil against which it is difficult to guard.

The medical profession, like other learned professions, is overstocked; and in London competition is probably much more severe between medical men and medical men than between medical men and the out-patient departments of the voluntary medical charities. Private adventure dispensaries, for example, are set up in poor districts; say an altogether unscrupulous qualified medical man runs several of these dispensaries under cover of his own name, and employs unqualified assistants; medical fees in that district are immediately reduced almost to a vanishing-point. An out-patient department, however, well managed, is a social test in itself; crowds, long waits, unpleasant neighbors, crying and irritating children. There is also some little risk of looking in with one complaint and coming out again with another.

No man in England is so high an authority on the condition of the people of East London as Mr. Charles Booth; his arbitrary division of the people is " poor " and " very poor." " By ' poor,' " he says, " I mean a bare income, such as 18s. to 20s. for a moderate family ; by ' very poor,' those who fall below this standard. With my ' poor ' it is a struggle, while the ' very poor ' live in a state of chronic want." The evidence taken by the committee shows the wage limit alone is as a test absolutely fallacious ; this limit is an element only in the general consideration of a case for voluntary medical relief.

Is voluntary medical relief a first step to pauperism ?—this crucial question now stares us in the face. This question, like many others, must be answered relatively. No doubt forty years ago there was a very strong and honorable feeling of independence in the country, and which largely, but in lesser degree, prevailed in the town—a feeling well expressed by the poet:[1]

[1] Hood.

> No parish money, or loaf,
> No pauper badges for me ;
> A son of the soil, by right of toil,
> Entitled to my fee.
> No alms I ask—give me my task ;
> Here are the arm, the leg,
> The strength, the sinews of a man,
> To work and not to beg.

This once fine rural population, by agricultural distress, is now more and more driven in upon the towns to further congest already existing congestion. Modern legislation—I state facts, I do not desire to question policy, but to state facts, when I say that our legislation has tended and tends to rub off sensibilities; the receipt of poor-law medical relief does not disqualify for the parliamentary franchise, elementary education is free, we propose to limit the hours of adult labor ; again, we have the slavery of trade unions—abnormal upheavals of unskilled labor—starving strong men with their pockets full of pawn-tickets reluctantly fighting for weeks for an intangible punctilio, and they themselves with their wives and children rattling begging boxes under everybody's nose. When I consider all these and other like things in their due proportions and relations, I am not of opinion that appreciably voluntary medical charity with us is a first step towards pauperizing the community.

The Distribution of Hospitals,

in the opinion of the committee, is no doubt faulty ; this is owing to the extraordinary growth of the population. On this I need only observe that the poor dislike dislocation and separation from their friends, but a poor man will often pass several hospitals to reach one for which, for some reason or another, he has a preference.

Medical Education,

in the opinion of the committee, would be promoted by the affiliation of the London medical schools to a teaching university. The presence of students in the poor-law infirmaries would be stimulating as regards the medical officers by reason of the observation and criticism which is brought to bear on diagnosis and treatment.

It is of the essence of clinical teaching that where the beds are, there are the professors and students gathered together. The entrance examination of the medical student is of great importance ; he should be well grounded in ordinary knowledge. Under a very recent regulation, students before registration may now present themselves for examination in chemistry, physics and biology. Mr. Pickwick's friends, the " Bob Sawyer," " Ben Allen," and " Jack Hopkins " types of medical student, are happily extinct; all the deans of schools reported the conduct of the students of our day as exemplary. Many of the hospitals have a students' club, a valuable institution, which keeps the young men together, and where they can dine and pass their spare time in a homely and comfortable manner. Medical students now do not " walk the hospitals" only; they render very valuable and most devoted and charitable services. I should like to say a great deal about the clever young medical ladies, but must refer the curious to the reports of the evidence. Suffice it to say they are honorably mentioned ; they are not any of them frightened by the sight of blood, and they are not predisposed to think of love when it is their duty to diagnose or to dispense. Mrs. Blackwell, M. D., of New York, was the first medical woman to register in England ; this was in 1858 ; following Mrs. Blackwell came Miss Garrett, now Mrs. Garrett Anderson. Medically-disposed ladies could not do better than refer to the ample evidence with which Mrs. Garrett Anderson, M. D., favored their lordships ; Dean of the London Medical School for Women, this eminent lady is with us the recognized head of the female branch of her profession. There are now forty-five medical women practitioners in London.

Special Hospitals.

The committee concludes, as to their use and abuse, that the marked hostility of the medical profession in regard to them arises from the fact that numerous small hospitals have been instituted by certain medical men, with a view only to their own advancement, leading to waste of money and the deception of the public. There are, however, exceptions ; for instance, hospitals for children and the Lock hospitals have special claims for favorable consideration. Lock cases, owing to the character of the diseases (venereal) and the patients, should be separately treated. Patients in a highly contagious condition discharge themselves on such occasions as race meetings ; there should be a power of detention.

I would observe that honorable mention should be made, amongst others, of the Seaman's Hospital, late the good ship " Dreadnought "; this institution down the river is exactly what its name implies, and

is simply invaluable. These special hospitals, which in their nature
and by comparison are very costly, have been called private-adventure
hospitals, but the term is resented by some specialists : the public
little recognize how medicine is now specialized. The committee
was told, as an argument in favor of special hospitals, that it was to
the Samaritan Hospital we owe the opportunities given to Sir
Spencer Wells of doing work which throughout the world is famous ;
it was said at that time by a surgeon of a general hospital, in regard
to these now common abdominal operations, that failure, followed by
death, deserved to be treated as manslaughter. It is noteworthy
that special hospitals are largely supported by wealthy persons who,
in a medical sense, have specially suffered ; specialty is, of course,
Adam Smith's division of labor, but the general hospitals now have
special wards.

Cordially concurring as I do with the general conclusions arrived
at by my colleagues, I feel it my duty now to entreat more especial
attention to the evidence *in extenso* given in regard to Lock diseases. You will please bear in mind that in England the late Contagious Diseases Act and its repeal, and the policy or otherwise of
that repeal, is still a burning political or religio-political question. I
append my own conclusions on the subject, premising that no value
should be attributed to my view except in so far as it is consistent
with and duly reflects the evidence.

The Lock Hospital, as regards the general welfare of the population, is undoubtedly the most important of all the special hospitals,
and yet it lives from hand to mouth, and even now is in debt. The
London Hospital and St. Bartholomew's have Lock wards ; separation is obviously essential in these highly contagious and most offensive primary Lock cases. There is, without question, in the medical
charities of London, a disposition to minimize the treatment of these
cases ; the Lock Hospital receives Lock cases from most of the
general hospitals, as well as from workhouse infirmaries. The out-
patient department of the Lock Hospital does valuable work which, in
a pecuniary sense, is by the male out-patients themselves gratefully
and tangibly acknowledged. Gummatous disease, a tertiary and
non-contagious condition, somewhat similar to cancerous disease,
may be found in all the general hospitals ; many young persons
suffering from allied and inherited skin and other affections which,
until recent years, were not recognized as of syphilitic origin, are
also treated in the general hospitals and elsewhere. Numerous

infantile and congenital cases are usually relegated to the hospitals for children. There is, unquestionably, amongst the general population, a considerable syphilitic taint. It is in evidence that on occasions such as the Derby race week, abandoned women in a highly contagious condition not only discharge themselves from the Lock Hospital, but they induce other women in a like condition to leave with them. Taking all the female patients, 31 per cent, and of prostitutes 43 per cent, leave the hospital in a condition to spread contagion; the question of detention naturally arises, but unless the Contagious Diseases Acts were in some form revived, detention in a voluntary hospital would tend to discourage and deter applicants for treatment; one witness well observed, "We are a hospital, not a prison." The evidence shows the existence of an actuating feeling that in Lock cases the sinner should suffer for the sin, and that such cases are not fit objects for public charity; enlightenment and self-interest, not to speak of humanity, should dispel any such mistaken notion; not only are virtuous women, innocent children, and unborn babes frequently victims, but the physical welfare of the whole population of the country is more or less involved. In the words of the secretary, words which are almost pathetic, "It is obvious on the face of it that the Lock Hospital is such a difficult charity to beg for."

That excellent English medical paper the "Lancet," I found a valuable and trustworthy assistant during the whole of the inquiry. A leading article[1] well treated the Lock question in the sense I have endeavored to suggest; it pointed to the importance of such cases as objects for study. Harlots, it is said, should not be left to suffer and infect; a man eaten up with syphilis is certainly an object of charity; and lastly attention was called to the Great Exemplar, strangely forgotten during a heated controversy;—the Great Physician " healed all manner of sickness and all manner of disease."

The medical superintendent of Marylebone Infirmary answered thus:[2]

Question.—These poor wretched people (suffering from venereal disease) simply rot at home in their own dens?

Answer.—They do rot—it is quite a true expression. I had a man the other day who had not had anybody by him for a fortnight, a mass of sores; he was found out by a policeman. The Lock refuge for women, crippled as it is for want of funds, is the blessed

[1] July 5, 1890.   [2] *Report*, vol. ii., p. 642.

means of rescuing and socially restoring many an unfortunate—there is always with us the " one more unfortunate! "

Oh ! it was pitiful !
In a whole city full,
Home she had none.

Hospital Accounts.

The conclusions of the committee refer to the important matter of the desirable uniformity of hospital accounts, the object being, for purposes of comparison, a reliable estimate of the cost per bed. A mass of interesting evidence bearing on this subject was taken, and every probability now points to a satisfactory understanding for common action.

I wish to call attention to the appendix of the third Report of the committee. There will be found at length the " Index of Classification," on which uniformity of system must greatly hinge ; with this index before him each hospital accountant can without difficulty dissect, post, and narrate uniformly. The cost per bed as the unit is of course the best standard of comparison. To arrive at the actual cost per bed there must be as well a common understanding as to the deduction to be made on account of each out-patient—it would be costly to keep a separate out-patient dispensary account. A complete system is now being worked out by a committee of hospital secretaries; dating from 1872, the original conception of this excellent system is due to one who has done so much for the hospitals of the world, to Mr. Henry C. Burdett.

In regard to uniformity of accounts, and the essential importance of that uniformity, the sum of the whole matter is that everything on earth is relative, and all criticism depends on comparison.

Nursing.

The subject of hospital nursing mentioned in the conclusions of the committee is very fully dealt with in the evidence reported. The committee note with satisfaction that the health of the nurses in London is good. The thorough training of a nurse should occupy at least three years.

I dare not rush in where angels might fear to tread; that is to say, the evidence taken in regard to the nurses and nursing is exhaustive —it is too voluminous to be treated adequately in this paper. I venture consequently, referring to the Reports, to indicate only its general tendency. The general position of the hospital nurse has been greatly improved of late years, and that improvement is progressive—better messing, where possible, comfortable single rooms apart from the wards, more holidays and hours off duty, and consideration duly given to pay and superannuation.

I have had the pleasure of making the personal acquaintance of many of the very able matrons of the great London hospitals, and, knowing them, I am not at all surprised that under such guidance the hospital nursing generally should be excellent. These ladies rejoice in their time-honored title of matron=mother, which exactly describes what their position is and should be. The matrons, or some of them, deprecated the use of such pretentious and misleading appellations as " lady superior " and " lady superintendent."

Miss Florence Nightingale is the founder of our nursing system, and with reverence I always picture her to myself as a saint with a nimbus. She found the " Sairey Gamp and Betsey Prig " school of nursing, and replaced that old effete school with active, trained, cheerful, two-steps-at-a-time-up-a-stairway young women. Miss Nightingale's " Suggestions for improving the nursing service of hospitals, and the method of training nurses for the sick poor," will be found in the first volume of the Report, p. 602.

An interesting paper on nurses, by Mr. Burdett, will also be found in the second Report of the committee, p. 808.

Miss Isla Stewart, matron of St. Bartholomew's Hospital, wrote[1] a paper on hospital nursing, from which, fully recognizing the justice of her observations, I now cite. The " ministering angel " point of view is imaginary; there is no more self-sacrifice in a hospital than out of it. The nurses are not pale-faced, pious, and overworked, but a merry set of hard-working women, who eat, sleep, and enjoy with zest any pleasure that comes in their way. They gossip and grumble, but are kindly, being generally intelligent, yet rarely intellectual. Towards the world the nurse is a woman desiring independence; towards the hospital her relations are purely commercial ; towards the patients the nurse is a paid attendant, bound to attend to their comfort and well-doing. Sentiment, often the salt of existence, is a factor more or less in the pleasure derived during a hospital career, but sentiment is a personal affair. Desire for independence, distaste for idleness, and the high standard required in scholastic teachers, drive the upper classes into nursing. Qualifying examinations discourage hospital nurses of limited education. Nursing for

[1] *Murray's Magazine*, August, 1890.

livelihood and independence, coupled with a high motive and sympathy, forms a class from which comes the high estimation in which nursing is held, and supplies all the best matrons, sisters and nurses. Please understand that "sister" simply means the head nurse of a ward ; religious nursing sisterhoods have been tried in the London general hospitals and failed, chiefly, I think, owing to divided authority leading to want of subordination. At present there is but one survival, and that sisterhood finds head nurses of wards only ; all the other nurses are purely secular and handicapped, perhaps unjustly, because they can never in that hospital rise to be head nurses or ward sisters, the legitimate object of a nurse's ambition.

To continue, Miss Stewart goes on to say that nursing is a happy life where there is a medical school ; interests, variety, all the science of the day, together with a freedom not usually enjoyed by single women in home life. Hospital life for women is rarely demoralizing ; views enlarge, natures expand, the details of sorrow and sin widen nature without leaving a stain. Take, for example, the case of a ward sister confided in by her patients, and the trusted colleague of her medical officer ; this is happiness indeed.

The position of the hospital nurse has been touchingly summed by another clever writer :[1]—" To avoid being mawkish and sentimental, and in the swing of reaction, we nurses are apt to treat the patients in hospitals as mere material ; but if one realizes that the occupant of each bed is a human soul with its own rights and its own reserves—if one takes the trouble to knock at the door, in fact, and ask admission instead of leaping over the wall—life becomes pretty intense, a good deal gets crowded into a very few hours."

Poor-Law Infirmaries,

according to the conclusions of the committee, are well-managed institutions that require extension, as there is still an objectionable necessity for treating the sick poor in the sick wards of workhouses. These infirmaries have been established since the year 1867.

I find Dr. Bridges, the Government medical inspector of these poor-law institutions, well puts their conception thus :—Formerly there existed *no* separate provision for chronic diseases amongst the destitute. They were "warehoused" in workhouses. Then Miss Louisa Twining began her work, and was succeeded by the " Lancet " Commission and the Act of 1867. Gradually the infirmary system

[1] Mona Maclean, *Medical Student.* London : Blackwood, 1893.

was built up, after a separate struggle with the Board of Guardians in each Union. The underlying principle was adequate indoor relief. So gradual had the growth been that the medical profession were only just beginning to realize what had been done. If it had been less gradual, the ratepayers would have rebelled. That was a lesson of caution and patience in making further improvements. My friend Mr. Albert Pell, a great authority on matters relating to the poor and poor laws, gives this definition:—The qualification for admission to a hospital is disease; to a poor-law infirmary destitution—I should say destitution together with disease. The evidence of Miss Louisa Twining, given before the committee, is very interesting: this lady is vastly respected, having done for poor-law medical and other institutions, and following in her footsteps, very much that which Miss Nightingale has done for hospitals and nursing in general. Of the poor-law infirmaries, fourteen are on the pavilion system. Chronic cases are sent to the infirmaries from the general hospitals, and these institutions are full of chronic cases of great educational interest. Publicity and increased medical visitation would, in my opinion, be most desirable. The committee was told that the interests and reputations of eminent medical men will maintain the general hospitals with schools; otherwise—and it would be calamitous—there would be a danger of the poor-law infirmaries swallowing up the voluntary hospitals. The committee was plainly told that " the feeling of degradation in regard to a taint of pauperism is dying out." One witness said further that he was told by a poor-law medical officer that he was in the habit of urging the poor to go into the infirmary, calling it the parish hospital; another medical man said he did not care how much a poor man's sensibility was rubbed off—from a medical point of view the thing is to cure. The evidence shows that the tendency within the infirmaries is to keep as much as possible out of sight and out of mind the ugly and repellent words " poor law " and " pauper."

The fever hospitals of the Metropolitan Asylums Board differ from the poor-law infirmaries, inasmuch as they take infectious diseases without regard to pauperism; these fever hospitals are working at high pressure, as will be seen by the following account, the last issued by the board.

The chairman presented his annual report, which stated that during last year 13,093 scarlet-fever patients were received in the hospitals, an increase of 6556 over any previous year. During the year 46,074 cases of infectious disease were notified to the board, as against 26,522 in the previous year. The expenditure during the past year exceeded that of 1891 by 177,964*l.*, which is attributed to the fact that 96,000*l.* was expended on the provision of temporary accommodation for the large number of patients by the erection of wooden buildings and furnishing them, and also on the erection and fitting up of the new hospital at Tottenham.

It is most satisfactory to find that quite recently clinical instruction in the fever asylums has been provided for under rules laid down by the Royal College of Physicians.

The Hospital Saturday and Sunday Funds

are mentioned in the conclusions of the committee, and the objects of these funds, and their methods of administration, are fully explained in the reports.

The Sunday fund, now known throughout the world, is no doubt a valuable distributor for the busy and modest donor; and considering the turn-over in London is nearly 42,000*l.*, the costs of collection and administration are on a scale of exemplary moderation. The Sunday-fund administration has promoted and prepared the way for desirable uniformity in hospital accounts, it has established to some extent a standard of efficiency, and hence it has appreciably invited and assisted wholesome comparison and criticism. And last, but not least, the Sunday fund limits on one Sunday at least the unholy war and strife of otherwise irreconcilable religious creeds and sects.

The Saturday fund, which is of a self-helpful nature, a penny-a-week working man's fund, does not appear to gain much ground in London; the workshops in competition with the churches are nowhere. Let us hope this unfortunate state of affairs arises chiefly from want of knowledge and management. I am sure the working man is not lacking in appreciation and good will, and where, in combination, he does subscribe liberally, as in the case of a sick club, there is a very natural desire for a *quid pro quo* in the shape of so-called letters of admission. I would like to point out that one great underlying principle seems invariably to affect these funds in question, and all others of a like nature; it is this: Experience tends to show that the amount of money available for religious and philanthropic purposes bears a fixed and definite proportion to the national income.

Co-operation.

The committee observes with regret the absence of any cordial and actuating desire for co-operation as between the various medical charities. On this point the valuable evidence, in the second volume of the Report, of Mr. Charles Stewart Loch, the Secretary of the Charity Organization Society, will well repay careful study.

A Proposed Central Board.

The committee in the last paragraph of the various conclusions contemplates and propounds a scheme for a central board, the essential principle of which should be free co-operation. There is a table of suggested grouping of hospitals for purposes of representation on the central board. One great object of such board should be to secure the inter-co-operation of medical charity, and the co-operation of medical with general charity.

It is satisfactory to observe that Mr. Burdett, in his comprehensive hospital annual for this year, tells us that a committee has been formed to consider the desirability or otherwise of creating a central board as suggested by the Lords' committee, and there is good reason to hope that a working and popular scheme may be arrived at. Another and very important work by the same author, "The Hospitals and Asylums of the World," is in many respects complimentary to the reports of the Lords' committee. Mr. Burdett gave valuable evidence before the committee, which evidence, in its entirety, I commend to those interested in hospital management.

The general hospitals in London, the three endowed hospitals excepted, subsist mainly on legacies and windfall donations; annual subscriptions usually do not suffice to pay wages, leaving nothing from this source for maintenance and administration.

Lastly, we are brought to this conclusion of the committee—in my opinion the most important outcome of the whole inquiry. It should always be borne in mind that the establishment of poor-law infirmaries and rate-supported fever asylums under the Metropolitan Poor Law Act of 1867 has, in great measure, altered the relations between the poor and the hospitals, and everything associated with medical charity ; and the committee cannot shut its eyes to the possibility that, if some organization—a central board—such as that recommended is not adopted, a time may come when it will be necessary for voluntary hospitals to have recourse either to government aid or municipal subvention.

Let me say, in conclusion, I am not, as regards my paper, in any sense a volunteer. I prepared this unworthy introduction to the Reports of the Lords' Committee on Hospitals at the desire of Dr. Billings, the distinguished chairman of your Chicago section on hospitals. I am far from wishing, even in the most remote degree, to appear didactic—I have a list of your own grand medical institutions before me ; if in America you excel in many things, or indeed in all things, I should from a feeling of common humanity, not to speak of our kinship, heartily rejoice. I would, however, remind you at least of one common interest, of one bond of union—the ever-illustrious surgeon of St. George's Hospital ; his memory commands our keenest interests, our warmest sympathies. This is the centenary of John Hunter, the greatest name inscribed in those noble annals which together form the fame-breeding history of scientific medicine.

Hunter died on October 16, 1793, in Leicester Square, having been taken suddenly ill on the morning of that day at St. George's Hospital. It was said of him at the time of his death, and the saying is true to our day :[1]

" The profession has lost in him one of its principal pillars and ornaments, and mankind may lament in him one of their best benefactors. The ardor and success with which he cultivated natural knowledge and philosophy, and rendered them subservient to his profession, had deservedly raised him to the first name. The monument of industry and genius which he has left behind will best speak his praise and call for the gratitude of this and future ages."

John Hunter became one of the most brilliant of the fixed stars of our national genius, " not so much by his contributions to the stock of human knowledge, which in themselves were colossal, as by his opening up a line of investigation which was entirely original, and by his marking out in the clearest way the paths which all future investigators must tread who desire to decipher the problems of life, disease and death."

It was well said the other day at Oxford[2] that medicine is one of the noblest of sciences ; that sober, absolute and positive science of medicine is but another name for works of mercy—the relief of human suffering in its most overwhelming form. The idea was further suggested—but the phraseology is my own—that the next generation of medical men will be fully occupied in considering how doth the little busy bacillus improve each dark and shining hour.

Vast problems rapidly expand with a dense population such as that of Greater London ; certain I am " we must make a stand on the ancient way," relying as heretofore on the truly Anglo-Saxon combination of private and public means. Reform, let us hope, will be on

[1] *The Oracle* of October 18, 1793.   [2] Lord Salisbury.

many lines, blending and harmonizing in the grand result. I have sometimes thought that I may personally have pushed inquiry to the extreme verge of conventionality ; if I have erred, I humbly make amends when I say that I have no prejudices. I have been trained from boyhood to evidence ; and as the result of this widely extended inquiry now in question, allowing for the imperfections which so clog all human affairs, knowing well that all things of earth are of the earth earthy, I have yet notwithstanding everything that is good and appreciatory to testify as regards the great voluntary medical charities of the English Metropolis.

APPENDIX.

The following summary was laid before the Committee at its first meeting :

HOSPITAL AND DISPENSARY ACCOMMODATION OF ALL KINDS IN THE METROPOLIS, WITH TOTALS OF IN- AND OUT-PATIENTS : INCOME AND EXPENDITURF.

	1	2	3	4	5	6	7
	No. of beds.	No. of occupied beds.	In-patients in one year.	Out-patients in one year.	Total expenditure.	Total income.	Difference between total expenditure and total income.
General Hospitals with Schools (11)	4,525	3,398	44,364	551,663	£ 389,499	£ 356,894	£ — 32,605
General Hospitals without Schools (8)	747	420	5,684	107,151	41,577	40,147	— 1,430
Special Hospitals (67)	3,616	2,553	26,850	398,038	244,691	254,669	+ 9,978
Free Dispensaries (26)	..	..	..	162,219	21,257	19,254	— 2,003
Part-pay Dispensaries (13)	..	..	..	102,302	9,710	8,996	— 714
Provident Dispensaries (35)	..	..	..	125,674	16,287	16,298	+ 11
Poor-law Infirmaries and Sick Asylums (27)	11,905	9,639	38,556	..	336,205	336,205	..
Poor-law Dispensaries (44)	..	..	..	114,983	19,984	19.984	..
Surgical Apparatus Societies	..	..	..	23,351	..	15,717	..
Hospitals for Infectious Diseases (8)	2,766	1,820	6,593	..	129,313	129,313	..
Totals	23,559	17.830	122,047	1,585,381	1,208,523	1,197,477	..

EDUCATIONAL STANDARDS FOR NURSES.

ISABEL A. HAMPTON,

Superintendent of Nurses and Principal of the Training School, The Johns Hopkins Hospital.

While fully appreciating the honor done me by our Chairman, it has not been without much hesitancy that I have undertaken to express my views upon so important and complex a subject as " The standards of education for nurses." The subject is important because it deals with the problems of health and disease, of life and death. It is complex because so many diverse factors and interests must be taken into consideration. The social problems of human misery and suffering and how best to alleviate them have been wonderfully worked out since the days when Charles Dickens first began to exert the power of his genius upon the mind of the public in order to bring it to an active sense of its responsibility in such matters, and perhaps in no branch of philanthropy has the change been so marked as in the care of the sick of all classes in all countries. And when we consider the few years which have elapsed since the modern system of nursing has been introduced, and contrast the present conditions with those which formerly prevailed, we might at first sight perhaps be excused if we regarded our present methods with some complacency instead of all the time struggling to find room or ground for improvement. But with progress going on in every branch around us, are we alone to stand still?

The present history of hospitals in America shows that the hospital nursing is with few exceptions already being done by the members of regularly organized schools for nurses, and that where such schools do not exist steps are being taken for establishing them. Next, we find that the demand for trained nurses is steadily on the increase for cases of sickness in private families, and what is still more important, that district nursing is being introduced into almost every large city in the country. Then, too, missionary boards are requiring that their women for foreign work shall prepare themselves by receiving a course of training in nursing. Lastly, when we see that women are beginning to look upon a thorough knowledge of nursing as an essential groundwork for their medical education, we cannot but be convinced that training schools for nurses and trained nurses are established facts—important factors in hospitals, in houses, and for the community at large.

In considering the standard of education requisite for such workers we have to consider (1) the kind and quality of the work required, and (2) the order of woman necessary to meet such requirements.

In the daily routine of a hospital, with its variety of patients, the work of a nurse, even while herself receiving instruction, is not without its immediate results. The hospital is her workshop in which she must serve an apprenticeship, and from the day she enters it the preservation of human life and the alleviation of human suffering are to some extent delivered into her hands. Can a woman, in any other kind of work which she may choose for herself, find a higher ideal or a graver responsibility? Where human life and health are concerned, what shall we term "the little things"?

Again, in the progress that medical science is making she has her allotted part to perform. To be sure she is only the handmaid of that great and beautiful science in whose temple she may only serve in minor parts, but none the less is it her duty to endeavor to grasp the import of its teachings, that she may fulfil wisely her share. It requires, for instance, more than mechanical skill on the part of a nurse to follow the preparations for an antiseptic operation, full of significance as it is in every detail, and the saying that "dust is danger" must have a bacteriologically practical application in her mind. Nor can just any one appreciate the full meaning of the physician when he says "the nursing will be half the battle in this case." For the simple performance of nursing work such knowledge is requisite, but when the wider duties of either head-nurse in a hospital or principal of a school for nurses are assumed, where one must not only know, but be capable of imparting that knowledge to others, then the responsibilities become proportionately greater.

Turning from hospitals to consider the requirements for this work elsewhere, we find that nursing in private families and district nursing among the poor in their homes are the two great fields in which the nurse will be principally occupied. Here she is frequently even more closely identified as the physician's lieutenant, for whereas in a hospital a doctor is usually within ready call to render either advice or assistance, on the other hand in private practice her knowledge and skill in the absence of the physician must be depended upon in critical illnesses or unlooked-for complications until his aid may be secured. To this part of the work in particular may be applied the following words taken from a physician's address dealing with the relation of the nurse's work to that of the physician: "The hands of a nurse are the physician's hands lengthened out to minister to the sick. Her watchful presence at the bedside is a trained vigilance supplementing and perfecting his watchful care; her knowledge of his patient's condition an essential element in the diagnosis of disease; her management of the patient, the practical side of medical science. If she fails to appreciate her duties, the physician fails in the same degree to bring aid to his patient."

In district nursing we are confronted with conditions which require the highest order of work, but the actual nursing of the patient is the least part of what her work and influence should be among the class which the nurse will meet with. To this branch of nursing no more appropriate name can be given than "instructive nursing," for educational in the best sense of the word it should be.

Realizing, then, the kind and quality of the work to be done, we pass on to the consideration of the order of woman required to perform such duties, and those of us who have had much experience with nurses, and know all we would have them to be, and how much they really must be, as the various classes of women pass in review before our mental vision, will be inclined to agree with the writer of a letter which came to me a short time since. After asking me to recommend a head-nurse for a hospital, and enumerating at length the qualities she must possess to be successful, he concluded with the words, "In short, we require an intelligent saint." The idea still prevails in many minds that almost any kind of a woman will do to nurse the sick, and that the woman who has made a failure of life in every other particular may as a last resource undertake this work. After many years of continuous work among patients and nurses, I am convinced that a woman, to become a trained nurse, should have exceptional qualifications. She must be strong mentally, morally, and physically, and to do thorough work she must have infinite tact, which is another name for common sense. She should be as one of the women of the Queen's Gardens in Ruskin's *Sesame and Lilies*, or such an one as Olive Schriner describes when she says, "A woman who does woman's work needs a many-sided, multiform culture; the heights and depths of human life must not be beyond her vision; she must have knowledge of men and things in many states, a wide catholicity of sympathy, the strength that springs from knowledge and the magnanimity that springs from strength." Only in so far as the women of our training schools attain to this standard will the institutions and communities in which they labor feel and show forth the influence of that "sweet ordering, arrangement and decision" that are woman's chief prerogatives. What class of women have the same practical privileges of learning the means to be used for the prevention of disease or of realizing their importance? Who then is so competent or who has greater opportunities for daily practising these than herself, and teaching them to others? And intelligent she ought and must be to do this wisely; otherwise she is a mere machine, performing mechanically the task before her, not knowing why or caring for what it all means, and the public loses thereby the services of one who should be valuable in showing them something at least of the beauty of the laws of hygiene and their application, and who can fortify her teaching with scientific facts.

Let us then consider (1) what is the present standard for the trained nurse, (2) what are her educational advantages, and (3) in what ways is she deficient?

The object of schools for nurses is primarily to secure to the hospital a fairly reliable corps of nurses; and it is in order to insure a continuous source of supply that such schools are established and certain inducements are offered to women to become pupils in them. These inducements are set forth in the circulars of general information published by each school. But when one compares these circulars, the teaching methods of no two schools will be found to be alike, all varying according to the demands of the various institutions and their several authorities. Each school is a law unto itself. Nothing in the way of unity of ideas or of general principles to govern all exists, and no effort towards establishing and maintaining a general standard for all has ever been attempted. Some institutions consider that a two years course of instruction is essential; others place it at a year and a half; and others again at a year. In England a few schools insist upon three years. The hours of daily work also differ widely, some requiring from their pupils nine hours a day of active service; others as high as twelve and thirteen hours. The theoretical instruction is usually not included in the nine hours work, and it is difficult to speak definitely upon this subject, as the length of such a course, the subjects and the extent to which they are taught are again dependent upon the opinion upon this matter of the governing body of each particular school. We also find no general rule governing the special attainments or degree of education required from the women who present themselves as candidates. On the contrary, a woman who has been refused by or dismissed from one school for lack of education, dishonorable conduct, inefficiency, etc., frequently gains admittance into another, where the authorities have not so high, if any, standard required from those whom they accept. But notwithstanding all these differences, each woman who graduates from any of these schools usually has a document with the high-sounding name of diploma presented to her, and henceforth she is known as a "trained nurse," which in nowise indicates what amount of knowledge or fitness she really does bring to her work. In fact it is no unusual occurrence for schools to graduate nurses whom they at once, when relieved from their presence in the hospital, refuse to recommend or sustain in their work.

A "trained nurse" may mean then anything, everything, or next to nothing, and with this state of affairs the results are far from what they should be, and public criticism is frequently justly severe upon our shortcomings, or else is content with superficiality where like meets like. This criticism falls both upon the woman herself and upon the institution which she represents. Sometimes the one only, in others both deserve censure. Can a woman be expected to give properly a hypodermic injection to a patient if her school has never taught her how this is to be done? The school and not the nurse is to be blamed for her ignorance in such a case. Or again, abscesses may follow such injections unless the nurse has been taught the practical significance of antisepsis. Or again, can she be expected to have at her fingers' ends the principles and practice of invalid dietary when she has never been practically taught such a thing? And when a really capable woman realizes that she does not know enough to do her work sufficiently well to honorably receive the full com-pensation of a skilled nurse, and that she is not worthy of such res-ponsibility, and if she is willing to give up more time and labor to go once more into a hospital where she may be really taught what she wants to know, where shall we find one capable school willing to take her? For we wish to mould our own fresh material, not being Michael Angelos to make Davids out of others' failures. Sadly frequent, too, are these requests made to the authorities of our larger schools, and in most instances they are the fruits of the systems prevailing in our smaller hospitals and sanatoriums. Such places are legitimate enough in their way, and indeed many are very

necessary, still the mere fact that they are hospitals in nowise justifies
them in establishing training schools for the sake of economy, and
accepting as their pupils women who, perfectly ignorant of what they
need, go to them and give up a year or two years of precious time,
and then find that their education has been thoroughly inadequate
to enable them to fulfil what is afterwards required of them. We
cannot but feel that a real injustice is often done in such cases. If
the nurse had gone into such a hospital as a philanthropist it
would be different, but she went there for the purpose of acquiring
a certain kind of education. Again, these small hospitals, not
having the same number to select from as the larger schools, are
apt, and in fact do take women who, not being intellectually capable
of comprehending the high calling into which they have been
admitted, tend to lower the standard to which we are striving to
attain. As an instance of such small hospitals which have come to
my notice while writing on this subject, I have in my mind one, the
superintendent of which informed me that their hospital contained
30 beds and that they had a training school of 11 nurses. But
the most pernicious of small hospitals is the specialty hospital or
private sanatorium, which owes its existence solely to the desire of
the owner to make money for himself, and in which a training school
is organized for the sake of securing cheap nursing, with an utter
disregard for the interests of the women employed. One doctor
who owns such a hospital with 25 beds has 16 nurses, who are given
a two years' course in this particular specialty, but four of these
nurses are actually sent to his private patients at $25 per week, this
money going to the hospital, while the nurse receives $16 per month.

This brings us to the question of the advisability of sending nurses
out of the hospital into families during the second year of their training. It is true that such a procedure materially assists in the maintenance of the hospital, and to some institutions it is very necessary,
but is it exactly what should be done in the best interests of the
education of the nurse? The majority of schools make the statement
in their general circular that they reserve the right to send their
pupils out to private duty during their second year, in order to help
to meet the expense of their maintenance and education. This may
have been all well and good in the earlier schools when hospitals
were not so numerous in the land and when the question of supporting them was a more serious difficulty than now. The additional expense of maintaining a school was not to be thought of,

and it was thus necessary to appropriate some of the pupils' time towards providing an income. But now that wealthy philanthropists and societies are erecting hospitals of all kinds, they should see to it that the question of maintaining a nursing corps is provided for, instead of expecting the nurses to do philanthropic work by earning money to support the hospital at the sacrifice of their own education. As a matter of fact the services rendered by a good training school to a hospital are sufficient to warrant the expenses incurred by the school, for in any case a certain amount of work has to be performed, and for those who do it the hospital would be obliged to provide board and lodging or the equivalent in money besides the regular wages. Under what other system then could an equally efficient class of workers be secured in the same systematic way, giving a full nine hours service daily and receiving financially less than the ward maids? It is understood that the equivalent is to be made up by the education given. Is it not then a most serious responsibility on the part of such hospitals or training schools to see that the education is made as complete as possible?

After much practical experience, I maintain that no such course of education can be thoroughly given in one year, but yet I find that very many schools limit their didactic teaching to the first year and make the second year's work of a purely practical nature and divide it between hospital work and private duty. It is absolutely necessary that class work and lectures should be carried on through the second year as well, and if this is done, then private nursing outside of the hospital is out of the question, as such interruptions would seriously interfere with any systematic teaching. I also hold that it is necessary to have the pupil under the daily observation and criticism of her teachers. This is impossible if she leaves the hospital for private duty, and one of two things must be true, viz: either she is as yet unfit to be entrusted to do her work without some supervision, or else, if she is really capable of doing this work in the second year she should not be held by the school at all. In the latter case, why not make the term of pupilage only one year and graduate her? There is another side to this question, that of justice to the patient, but as this does not really come under the head of the standards we are just now discussing we will pass it by.

It may seem that I find little that is good in the system at present followed in our training schools. I am far from wishing to disparage pioneer efforts, but I would maintain that now that our oldest school in America has attained to its majority, we can no longer fall back upon the plea that our art is still in its infancy. Our founders achieved well and nobly, but it surely was not intended that we should work on forever on the old lines. There are plenty of problems to work out, and schools for nurses are capable of much finer work than has yet been done, if we to whose hands the work is now entrusted are willing to take a broad and comprehensive view of the subject. The principal of a school for nurses performs the least part of her duty, and throws away many of her privileges, if she is content to confine herself to the limitations of her own particular school. She must look into and go abroad among other schools, and teach her nurses to do the same, recognizing what is good in others and being ever ready to adopt any improvement. There is so much that we can learn from each other, and sooner or later we must also recognize the fact that we are all trained nurses, and that until something of a common standard is reached the imperfections of the few must be borne by all. Briefly, then, some of our chief aims should be to bring about a spirit of unity among the various schools, and to establish a standard of education upon which we may all be judged. This of necessity must be based upon the opinions of no individual mind or committee, but upon the consensus of the impartial judgments of many really experienced in the requirements for such work; for in this way alone can we command a thoroughness of work and a selection of women that we cannot now boast of. In doing this, the first step should be to bring about in all our schools, as far as possible, a uniform system of instruction, so that the requirements for graduation should be about the same in each. We might well lengthen the course of instruction in training schools to three years, with eight hours a day of practical work. This would relieve the hospital and school of having to deal with so much new material at so frequent intervals. It would then be possible to select our nurses much more carefully than can sometimes be done, for it happens at times that vacancies occur which must be filled without waiting for the right candidates to present themselves, and it would insure far better results by securing to the hospital nurses with more practical experience.

A school naturally divides itself into two classes, the quite competent and those who are fairly competent. The first division is apt, bright, intelligent, and readily taught, and at the end of the second year one is unwilling to part with them just yet, seeing in them the superintendents and good hospital workers of the future, to whom the opportunity should be given of developing their executive ability. Then the incompetent ones are dull and slow of comprehension, and they require to be taught over and again, and at the end of two years glimmerings of the fact that they are beginning to be really interested in the work for the work's sake may be discovered, and one is very loth to let them go until the interest becomes a reality, and so for them really the third year is needed before they may be safely trusted to their own devices.

The three years' course would also tend to exclude the purely commercial woman, who enters the school, and gets through the course with as little exertion to herself as possible, only seeing in everything she does future dollars and cents, and never working for the love of her work. With this length of course it would be possible to make a better subdivision of the pupils into classes, so that every member could receive her practical teaching, her class teaching and lectures according to her grade in the school and her individual ability. There should be stated times for entrance into the school, and the teaching year should be divided according to the academic terms usually adopted in our public schools and colleges. To compel a class of students to attempt to listen to a lecture on a hot July night is barbarous. The summer months should be reserved for vacations and practical nursing only. In short, the educational atmosphere should be encouraged and developed in every way possible. Even the name of "Nurses' Home" should be changed to "Nurses' School," as the accepted term "Home," as applied to institutions, has no educational significance. And the title of the teacher should be Principal of the School, as well as Superintendent of Nurses. In this third year those who are capable should be made head-nurses, or some direct responsibility should be laid upon them, and those who wish to fit themselves for teachers in other schools should have the opportunity of acting as assistants to the principal of the school, to learn the clerical and administrative duties of such positions. In this way a class of two might be under her instruction for a year at a time, their positions being those of senior and junior assistants, with a moderate salary attached. Unfortunately, few women get these opportunities, and the majority are forced to assume the charge of training schools with no equipment for the work further than that they have been able to acquire as head-nurses; and the hospital, school, and often the new superintendent herself suffer accordingly while she is gaining the necessary experience. In fact a Normal School for preparing women for such posts is quite as necessary as those established for other kinds of teachers.

The eight-hour system will also be advisable, for the reasons that the health of the nurses will not bear the strain of a three years' course with longer hours; besides, is it not poor economy and mistaken judgment for a country to sacrifice the health of one class of people in trying to restore that of others?

Then it would do away with the continual breaks in the day's work caused by the half-day and two hours recreation system, and if a systematical course of theoretical teaching is entered upon, shorter hours of practical work are absolutely necessary, as the overpowering physical weariness following a long day's work makes mental effort out of the question, and to require tired-out women to attend evening lectures after nine hours of physical exertion, and the mental excitement attendant upon hospital work, is little short of tyranny. And this mental development is necessary for the best results in the work if we would command the services of an intelligent class of women.

In considering standards of education for nurses we must not overlook the smaller hospitals, cottage hospitals, etc., for they have their work to do as well as the large institutions, but that they are in no position to offer adequate teaching or experience to a woman who would become a thorough nurse is very evident.

How then can we meet the problem of supplying good nursing, and at the same time making good nurses? It can only be met by the larger schools entering into arrangements with the smaller schools to supplement their teaching. This plan, of course, would require that the standard of women and of education should be the same, and the teaching on practically the same basis, while the head-nurses of the smaller schools must be thoroughly competent women. In a city where distances are not too great, one school may successfully undertake the care of two or three hospitals. For instance, a children's hospital may better be associated with a general training school, and the same holds good with a hospital dealing with obstetrics, or with any other special branch. As for private sanatoriums owned by private individuals, the nursing should unquestionably be done by salaried nurses who have graduated from some reputable school.

A final word as to the practical qualifications which should be required of women who present themselves as candidates to be taught nursing. A good practical English education should be insisted upon. By this is meant that the candidate should come up to the standard required to pass the final examinations in the best high schools in the country, special stress being laid upon her ability to express herself either in writing or orally with quickness and accuracy. Her knowledge of arithmetic should be of an eminently practical nature and so that she can readily deal with problems involving fractions, percentage, bookkeeping, etc. This much is absolutely necessary. Of course more than this is desirable, as no other study develops the reasoning powers in the same practical way, and women who do not possess any education in arithmetic beyond the few simple rules, simply applied, are at once placed in a disadvantageous position upon entering upon their work in a modern hospital. Of course, if she has in addition a knowledge of languages and a broad general reading, the candidate is all the better prepared for undertaking and obtaining success in her career as a nurse.

Aside from this mental equipment there are other qualifications of a practical nature that should be insisted upon. Every woman before entering upon hospital work should be a thoroughly trained housekeeper. Practical household economy should be a part of her *home education*, for in hospital wards the nurses are the stewards, the caretakers of the hospital property, and upon their thrift and careful ordering must depend the economical outlay of the hospital funds. I cannot dwell upon this practical household economy with too great emphasis, for experience has shown me to a painful extent how this branch of woman's work is neglected or superficially understood by so many women in all ranks of life. A total lack of or appreciation for the principles that govern such work will inevitably be followed by a deficiency in thoroughness and system. In the nurse should be found evidences of this practical knowledge; it should be seen in the way she cares for her own room, her personal appearance, and in the order and system which attends any work to which she puts her hand, and her knowledge of the value of the articles she has to work with should be shown by the way she cares for them. But too often, alas! training schools are obliged to not only teach in two short years all that pertains to nursing, but try as well to teach the first principles, at least, of domestic science, and much valuable time is spent in doing this that should really be given to nursing. When a graduate nurse goes into a private family and earns the just reproach of being extravagant and careless in the care of property, and when the details of her work are without finish, the blame should be put down to her early home training and not to her training as a nurse.

Time does not permit me to more than touch upon some of the most glaring defects in our system of nursing and to outline very briefly some changes that might be of general advantage, but I trust that sufficient has been said to arouse interest enough among hospital and training school workers to induce them to persevere in working out the problems, the solution of which will give us more united work and a more uniform standard of education for all who are to go out into the world as trained nurses; for only from institutions in which the head, the heart and the hand are trained to work together in harmony can come forth the true nurse.

HOSPITAL FINANCE AND METHOD OF KEEPING ACCOUNTS.

Mr. Henry C. Burdett, of London, England, then made the following remarks upon Hospital Finances and the Methods of Keeping Accounts:

"Finance is the keystone of the arch upon which all institutions stand. Its condition is the test of sound management, without which it is certain that we should be much better off without than with our institutions. The subject of finance may be treated from the income side, bringing out very forcibly the differences and the advantages and disadvantages of the various systems prevailing in different countries. But I must leave this side of the question untouched, and, in these remarks, will deal only with expenditure.

It has been stated as an axiom that the best hospital administration aims "to cure the greatest number of patients with the smallest number of beds, in the shortest time, at the least expense." This may be good economy, but in hospitals the principle may be carried too far. At my first visit to Chicago, in 1882, I found its largest hospital in such a condition that I felt I must do as I did on a similar occasion in Dublin,—return to my country with sealed lips; because I believe that if a correct and literal account had been given of the condition of affairs which I found in it, it would have staggered this city, and it certainly would have astonished others.

It is quite wrong for any institution to endeavor to treat at any time more patients than it has adequate provision for. I have seen in one of our largest hospitals in England two wards, managed by different physicians—one admirably administered, and the other overcrowded, with a bad atmosphere and suffering patients. The physician who controlled the crowded ward had a kind heart, as it was said, while the other physician was more strict in his management, and would accept no more patients than could be properly cared for. It appears to me that kind-heartedness which introduced extra beds into wards intended to contain a certain number calculated for the best interests of the patients, is a form of kindness from which the world has suffered too much.

It has been stated that it is impossible that different hospitals shall prepare and publish accounts upon a uniform basis. All I can say to this is that if, after eighteen hundred years of Christianity, we have not yet become able to devise a fairly uniform system which will be accepted by intelligent men and women as a reasonable method of statement of accounts, the experience of these eighteen centuries has been to very little purpose. I have found, in discussing this question for individual institutions, that the administrators did not find it very difficult to accept a system which would give uniformity and require very little change in their present methods of accounts. The following appears to me to be the best system for hospital accounts. Every report should contain :

(1). An Income and Expenditure Account, containing a detailed statement of the receipts and expenditures under classified heads.

(2). An Invested Property Account, showing all the property of the institution, the various securities held, and the income derived therefrom.

(3). A Balance Sheet.

(4). A Special Appeal Account. This should show all the money received as the result of appeals or personal canvassing, apart from old subscriptions, the Hospital Sunday and Saturday Funds, and other regular and assured sources of income. It should also show every item of expenditure connected with the issue of these appeals, including advertisements, salaries, commissions, printing, stationery, postage, and every other item of the kind. Such an account enables any governor to keep an eye upon the management, and to ascertain if the efforts put forth are adequate to the purpose, and if they combine the minimum of expenditure with the maximum of results.

If there are any special funds. such as a Samaritan Fund, a Convalescent Fund, a Chaplain's Fund and so forth, a separate statement should appear in the report in each case.

Turning now to the books which it is desirable to keep, I may deal with them under two heads.

I. *Receipts.*—These should include: 1. a Cash Book; 2. a Cash Analysis Book; 3. a Subscriber's Register; 4. a Legacy Book; and 5. an Invested Property and Rent Book.

The Cash Analysis Book will contain, under their proper heads, every item of receipt throughout the year, and the total of each column, *i. e.* donations, subscriptions, investments, and so forth, should agree with the total given in the published accounts, as well as with totals given at the end of the lists of subscriptions, donations, legacies, and invested property, published in the report. This is easily arranged by having two columns in the report, one showing the amount of former subscriptions and donations received from individuals, and the other, amounts received from each during the past twelve months.

II. *Expenditure.*—The books required to keep a correct account of the expenditure of public institutions are: 1. The Analysis Journals; 2. a Journal; 3. a Ledger; 4. a Wages Book; and 5. Petty Cash Books,—one, at least, for the secretary, and one for the matron or lady superintendent.

I must confess that during the last twenty years I have at times made large demands upon the patience, kindness and good will of the officers of various hospitals throughout the country. I have often troubled them with inquiries and requests for the filling up of various forms, involving the expenditure of a considerable amount of time and labor and the exercise of no little patience and care. I am happy to take this opportunity to publicly thank the whole body of hospital officials for their generous co-operation and courtesy. I have, of course, always been ready to assist anybody with information of facts when application has been made to me, and so I am proud to think a feeling of confidence has grown up between myself and the officials which enables us to trust and help each other to an extent which I believe has been fruitful in results to the benefit of the charities in which we are so greatly interested. I should like to make some definite return for all the kindness I have received. Many of the inquiries and most of the returns would have been unnecessary had the accounts, of the larger institutions at any rate, been kept upon something like an identical plan. Unfortunately, where the managers have endeavored to follow a particular form of accounts they have naturally adopted their own method of classification, and so the attempt has largely failed to accomplish what is desired.   For instance, it is a common thing to find alcohol, *i. e.*, wine and malt liquors, placed in one report under " Provisions "; in another, under " Surgery and Dispensary"; and, in a third, under a separate heading of its own.   Very many other items are treated in an equal variety of ways, and so the reports are most difficult to analyze, and it is almost impossible for any one, even with the largest experience and knowledge, to compare the expenditure of one institution with that of another upon an identical basis. I have, therefore, thought that I might make some little return for the kindness I have received if I published a glossary as an appendix to the system of accounts which I am about to explain to you, and the heads of which I have already given.   I have this glossary here on the table before me. It has been compiled with commendable diligence by Mr. Michelli, the secretary of the Seaman's Hospital of Greenwich, and I hope that in the course of the evening some of you will put it to the test, by asking through the Chairman under what head particular items are to be classified.   I have also arranged that leaves from the various books, together with this glossary, and a brief explanation of the system, shall be given in the forthcoming edition of the Hospital Annual, so that persons who are interested in the matter may be able to study them at leisure, and, if they please, to alter their system of accounts, and so obviate the necessity for many, if not for all, the inquiries so frequently addressed to them under existing circumstances.   Such a general system of accounts, if generally adopted, must tend to secure to the officials no small amount of comfort and advantage.

Finally, I may say that I have prepared an analysis of the accounts of all the chief hospitals throughout the country upon an identical basis, the whole of which will appear in the Annual."

Mr. Burdett explained his system of accounts, illustrating his remarks by reference to large diagrams of the various books.

THE APPLICABILITY OF HYGIENE TO THE CONDITIONS OF MODERN WARFARE.

BY LIEUT.-COLONEL J. LANE NOTTER, M. A., M. D.,

Army Medical Staff; Professor of Military Hygiene, at the Army Medical School, Netley.

I offer no apology for bringing forward this subject, for since 1860 England has practically been annually engaged in some form of military expedition or other in various parts of the globe, and has in consequence gained an experience in practical sanitation in war unequaled by any other country. I venture, as the representative of that army, to bring forward some considerations as to how far, consistent with the exigencies of modern methods and conditions of warfare, the general principles of hygiene can be applied with a view to mitigating, if not obviating, much of the disease and suffering incidental to military operations; at the same time not losing sight of the fact, that notwithstanding the greatest efforts the hygienic ideals of peace-time are impossible of attainment during a period of war.

Inasmuch as the *raison d'être* of the existence of a standing army at all is essentially the drilling, training and preparation of the individual soldier for purposes of war, we find that the very first care is the proper selection of troops, and in making this selection we find these factors prominently asserting themselves: they are size, weight and age of the men.

The consideration of these factors is essentially one for peace-time, and a nation having once committed herself to war has no choice left in dealing with these matters, but every available man must be utilized for military service, regardless of temperament, age or any other consideration.

While the hygienic bearings of military life are fairly simple in peace-time, the moment war breaks out we find the conditions alter materially, in fact so much so that all hard-and-fast rules or preconceived ideas as to the attainment of a perfectly hygienic mode of life by an army in the field are practically impossible. To state this briefly, the only hygienic methods possible are those which the circumstances of time and place admit of. We must use what we can get, taking care, however, to arrange the work and condition of labor which the individual has to perform as much as possible in accordance with our hygienic ideal. Being in a state of war, this will naturally be difficult to state in its entirety.

Food and Drink.—The feeding of large masses of men in the field will need to be conducted on the same dietetic principles as the feeding of similar multitudes in peace-time. The main points on which this will differ will be absence of regularity and difficulty of supply; the former must necessarily be subordinate to military exigencies, but the importance of regularity in feeding should never be lost sight of.

As to the nature of the supply, in the present day of excellent methods of preservation of food-stuffs, little difficulty is likely to arise, provided the transport arrangements are adequate. The maintenance of a regimental supply-unit would seem to be preferable to the larger one by brigades. In fact, to adequately carry out a proper supply the regimental unit should be rigidly adhered to. It should also be clearly understood that the emergency ration is purely a supplementary one, and in no case ought to be reckoned as a part of the ordinary field ration.

As concerns the supply of drink to an army in the field, water must necessarily form the staple element. With an advancing column systematic filtration is impossible. Reliance will have to be placed on simply boiling the water before filling the water-bottles. When this cannot be done, the only safeguard will be that of selecting the purest supply possible. Men should be taught the danger likely to follow on drinking water the source of which is unknown, unless this has been previously boiled. If a filter is to be employed at all, some form of the Chamberland-Pasteur seems to be the best; but as yet no form at once portable and easily used has come under my notice. All medical officers are unanimous in condemning the issue of alcohol as a ration in the field. The only form in which it is admissible is in the form of light red wines, which are best taken when freely diluted with water. The consensus of opinion on this point is so unanimous that further reference need not be made here.

Preventable Diseases.

Within the scope of this paper it is impossible to deal with the many diseases incidental to warfare. Briefly stated, those which most frequently render men non-effective are diarrhœa, malaria, heatstroke, and footsoreness. These are all more or less preventable.

Diarrhœa.—In the field, diarrhœa is a disease which is early met with, consequent on a change of food and chill. It has occurred in every expedition, and is frequently followed by enteric fever; the passage of the one disease into the more severe being rapid, and increasing as the age of the men composing the force diminishes, the younger men suffering the most. In camps and on the march the latrines should be kept in a perfectly sanitary state, and as disinfectants are not always available, they should be dug deep and narrow, and covered in with six inches clean earth daily, the same trench not being used for many days in succession. Men suffering from diarrhœa which does not yield in a day or two to simple remedies should be passed on to the field hospitals for further treatment.

Malaria.—As regards malaria, little can be done on service to make a temporary site in a malarious country healthy. Any form of subsoil drainage is impossible, and the rule should be not to occupy such positions longer than actual necessity obliges. With the rapidity of movement incidental to modern methods of warfare, men will seldom remain sufficiently long in one place to undertake work of any permanent character. The securing of an ample supply of food ; the avoidance of chill, damp clothes, night air, and with the issue of an early morning ration of coffee or cocoa, with biscuit, is about all we can do. For operations in malarious countries the selection of troops is one of importance, for there is no "seasoning " process against paludal fevers ; on the contrary, one attack, in place of conferring immunity, predisposes to another. The prophylactic use of quinine has not been followed with any success under the circumstances mentioned.

Heatstroke.—Heatstroke is a thoroughly preventable disease; it occurs in two forms, by direct solar heat, and by the effect of a heated atmosphere independent of the sun's rays. Against the result of direct solar heat a proper protection for the head and body is necessary. Marches should not be undertaken in the tropics when the sun's rays are vertically over the head; the morning or evening is the time indicated. If military necessity demands it, it is better that men should march at night than that they should be exposed to the risks incidental to a mid-day march; but the fatigue which this occasions should not be lost sight of, nor the inconvenience of reaching a camping-ground or bivouac in the night and darkness.

On the march the most open order must be maintained. If the ranks close up, the temperature in the ranks rises and the air around the men becomes loaded with organic impurity.

The men should march at ease, with as great freedom of movement as possible; their coats, etc., open, and weights they have to carry as far as possible reduced to a minimum. This lessens the mechanical work which they have to do and thus fatigue is lessened. Halts should be frequent and sufficient, and every advantage taken of any shade.

Some of the symptoms of heatstroke may also be caused by the reflected rays of the sun through the orbit when the optic nerve is exposed to direct rays of light.

In the tropics neutral-tinted glasses are frequently worn, and the sense of relief and coolness experienced by the wearers tells the advantage their use affords. They were found effective in the form of goggles in the Egyptian campaign of 1882 as protection against glare, heat and sand, and thus in warding off ophthalmia.

If racial prejudices could be overcome there is no doubt that the headdress worn by Asiatics would be of immense advantage to Europeans when fighting in the tropics, as it affords a coolness and protection which the present helmet fails to secure.

To guard against the effects of indirect heat the most open order in camp must be maintained, and when tents are used, only those with double flies should be sanctioned for the tropics. The lining should be of a pale blue color, as used in the Sepoys' tents in India. Men should not occupy the tents at night unless the country is a malarious one, and even then a very slight covering will afford protection against malaria. Overcrowding is one of the most constant and most dangerous factors in the production of heatstroke.

On the march the early symptoms of heatstroke should be watched for and timely aid afforded. The staggering gait, the flushed countenance, abnormally frequent micturition and the absence of perspiration, should at once demand the attention of the surgeon and timely aid be afforded.

Footsoreness.—Footsoreness is one of the most troublesome ailments the surgeon is called upon to treat on the line of march. The initial hardness of the leather used in the military boot is the cause of much suffering. Once the boot is moulded to the shape of the foot it does not press unduly, and as regards wear excels any other; but this is a comparatively slow process. Greater pliability of the material should be aimed at, as well as greater care in fitting the foot. The heels should be low and flat, as these have an important influence on the rhythm, which in its turn influences the rate of speed and lessens fatigue.

Camps.

In war any theoretical ideas of the site for a camp must be abandoned and advantage taken of any position which presents itself. So, too, as regards tents. The advancing army in any future European war must be prepared to bivouac where military exigencies require it to halt, and so far as we at present foresee, the transport available will not be more than equal to providing provisions and ammunition for those in front, and removing to the lines of communication or to the base the sick and wounded of the force. On this account some sort of light shelter tent which can be readily adjusted seems indispensable : one to be carried between every two men, the parts being interchangeable. It might also be made so as to afford protection against rain, if worn as in the German army in the form of a " poncho."

As regards sanitation, it is useless to attempt much. There are, however, two points which should claim the personal attention of the surgeon, and these are :

1. The nature of the shelter provided.
2. The disposal of excreta.

So long as men are on the march and are not provided with tents, density of population on a given area matters little, but when, however, tents are occupied, this becomes an important factor. Whether in tents or in civil buildings, any overcrowding is soon followed by disease, and the best efforts of the military surgeon should be directed to mitigating this error.

The best kind of a tent is still a desideratum, but the chief points to be aimed at are to secure adequate protection from the weather, a free movement and interchange of air, a double fly for tents when campaigning in the tropics, that the tent should be as light as possible, and should not be of too conspicuous a color.

In malarious countries the soil under the tent should be beaten down as far as possible, so as to prevent exhalations from the ground and to keep the tent floor impermeable. Temporary drainage should also be secured.

Camp Latrines.—Camp latrines should be placed to leeward of the tents and at least fifty to one hundred yards distant. The trenches should be deep rather than wide, so that the surface exposed to the sun and air may be as small as possible. If the camp is for more or less permanent occupation the trenches may be four or five feet deep, small quantities of soil being added daily and the trench filled in when within two feet of the surface.   For merely temporary use all trenches should be one foot wide, one foot deep, with a space of one foot between each line, the trench to be filled in when six inches from the surface.

Trenches are only suitable for men in perfect health.   For those suffering from slight diarrhœa or dysentery it is no easy matter for men to get up, say, six or eight times in the night and to grope their way to one of these trenches, or to avoid falling into it if they succeed in their expedition.   A man suddenly attacked with illness could not do it; a lazy man would not do it if he could find a handier place near by : both might be excused for refusing to go, say, one hundred yards away, under a burning sun, during tropical rain, or with a thermometer at or below zero Fahrenheit.

A latrine barrow would obviate most of the inconvenience, the body made of a sort of box, suspended on an iron bar springing from the wheel-axle.   Such a movable latrine could be easily placed in the most convenient situation and emptied as often as necessary ; it could be wheeled off to a safe distance and brought back after cleaning and disinfection.   No one knows, except they have experience of it, what labor and anxiety this question of latrines gives.   Fevers have been the scourge of armies, and of all armies that become stationary for a short time.   Why ?   Because of this great latrine difficulty.   To take over houses or civil buildings and to use the common privies or water-closets, such as exist in continental towns, would be simply to invite the spread of enteric fever, cholera, etc., and to avoid the risk which is always present I most strongly advocate some system such as I have very briefly sketched out here.

First Aid.

In war, with the modern arms of precision and the vast size of continental armies, it is impossible to have an adequate "first aid." The medical services in all armies are undermanned, and even in peace-time it is difficult to find surgeons for the work to be done. The cost of medical service is so large in proportion to its strength that it is hopeless to expect any increase of that strength.   The problem then is, how can we best utilize what now exists for meeting the exigencies of war ?

In the British army the Army Medical Staff is divided into two branches, executive and administrative.   In the former, all wars have shown the officers to be fully competent for the discharge of their duties; the failure, if failure there has been, has happened in the administrative grade. In war it is not difficult to obtain a number of surgeons well up in their professional work; but what it is almost impossible to form at a short notice is a body of officers thoroughly trained in army medical organization according to existing regulations; men of good administrative ability, having a full comprehension of the urgent necessities which spring from modern warfare, and with a knowledge how to apply the available medical assistance as effectively as practicable whenever and wherever it is most imperatively required.

To obtain this there should be a large extension of the system of personal responsibility, so that the mind may be trained on a larger basis, that medical officers in peace-time should have more independence and deal within their province with questions of greater magnitude. The defects in the past have been largely in the direction of a want of independence on the part of the medical department. They have always been fettered by being dependent upon other corps for material. No medical department can ever be thoroughly efficient which has not actual and absolute control over all elements essential to its successful working.

Owing to the large numbers likely to be engaged in future wars, large numbers are likely to be placed *hors de combat* within a short time. The best system of first aid must necessarily be unable to deal adequately with such numbers. There is need for the public to recognize this fact and so to avoid any outburst of hysterical clamor. If nations will make war they must pay the penalty.

Disposal of the Dead.

The disposal of the dead on the battlefield is a sanitary question of the first importance. In any future war it must be impossible to resort to burial as a means of disposal, and it is useless to waste time in discussing the best disinfectants to use. Incineration, as practiced at Sedan, by pouring tar on the bodies and then setting fire to the pile, was a demoralizing and futile process. Burial alone means labor, and labor can ill be spared or expended in this direction in war. Civilized armies are bound, not only in their own interests but of those who inhabit the districts close to the scene of action, to dispose of their dead so that they shall be no nuisance. Cremation seems the only satisfactory solution of the difficulty. It disinfects the soil and air, it is speedy, and has no demoralizing effect on the *morale* of men ; it renders the immediate neighborhood healthy for the sick and wounded ; it does not defile the ground ; in a word, it is cheap and effective and satisfies every sanitary requirement, and it is hoped that this method, which has already made some considerable progress among the community at large, will in all future wars be put into practice, and that the old plan of burial will give place to cremation as the only safe method for disposing of the bodies of those who fall on the field of battle.

II.

SECTIONAL MEETINGS.

THE TRUSTEE OF THE HOSPITAL.

By Richard Wood,

President Board of Trustees, University of Pennsylvania Hospital.

He who passes by a hospital and regards it with a casual eye may
only think of it as a place of pain and suffering, and quicken his pace
with a shudder.   But if, as he looks, its ambulance perchance deliver
at the door some prostrate wretch, and if pity prompt him to follow
the pale form to the receiving ward, he will observe with what kind
and careful scrutiny the patient is regarded by the young resident
physician ; how every immediate necessity is promptly ministered
to ; how the case is quickly scanned, recorded, placed in its appropriate ward and diagnosed by the skilled medical practitioner or
surgeon of the visiting medical staff.   Having observed the unfortunate one thus brought under hospital treatment, he will follow its
processes, will notice their regulated flow from due authority of
director or superintendent, will note the daily visit of physicians-in-
chief, the hourly watchfulness of doctors in charge, the constant
tending of nurses, neat and attentive, the use of clinical thermometer,
their relief of the person, the giving of ordered diet and medicines,
the hot applications, the cool, moist bandage, the bath of ice, the
sterilized knife, the antiseptic dressing.   He will note the art, skill,
precision that runs through all.   This art and skill (if the hospital
be a teaching one) he will see being taught to groups of students
at the bedside, or in process of transmission to other hundreds
circling above the clinic bed on the rising benches of the lecture-
room.   After observing these remedial processes he will give an eye
to the hospital building ; to its spaciousness, clean walls and floors,
voidness of odor, equable temperature, perfect ventilation, to its
large, tidy kitchen and busy laundry.   In its office he will find
careful records of the nativity, residence, conditions of life and

disease of patients, of numbers received, of cured, benefited or dead. These records, and the sight of convalescents lounging on rolling chairs in the corridors, will assure him that a good chance of return to strength and vigor awaits the poor wretch upon the stretcher whom he followed from the ambulance to the hospital. But more than a return to outer air will he find provided for in the ministrations of the hospital. He will see by the bedside the ministers of religion consoling the sick and praying for the dying, and upon the day of worship will hear in the wards or the chapel songs and praises offered to the Author and Disposer of All. The hospital will have become to him a place intent with earnest action and holy thought—a place whereon might fitly rest the foot of the ladder the patriarch beheld, while angels "ascending and descending" bore the blessings of the life that is, and of the life that is to be. Never again will he pass a hospital with a casual eye or a fearful tread, for he has learned to know it to be a tree of life, the leaves whereof are "for the healing of the nations."

But our supposed visitor, however much he may have observed the hospital and become infused with its movement, will not have seen that which gives direction to the movement and force to its action. He will not have detected the unseen agent which brings the hospital into relation with its surroundings, and gathers together the vital forces that quicken and sustain its life; he will not have seen the root of the tree; he will not have seen the governing body of the hospital —its Board of Trustees.

When any competent authority decides a mass of suffering to require organization for its relief, and that a hospital must be founded, it needs also to decide how to govern the hospital. Hospitals are commonly founded by authority of governments, national or municipal, by church authority, by universities and medical schools, and by bodies of charitable people. Military and naval hospitals are commonly placed under the administration of the respective medical national service. A single officer may be in sole charge of a great hospital. During the late rebellion in the United States the President of this Congress commanded the largest military hospital in this country—the Satterlee, in Philadelphia. National civic hospitals, of which there are several on the continent of Europe, are controlled by civic authorities and sometimes cared for by high personages. When calling in 1887 at one of the most charming and best appointed hospitals in Berlin, I was told it received a daily visit from the Empress Augusta of Germany.

But government hospitals, cared for by state authority and supported by the public purse, do not most concern a Congress of the charities of the world. A very minor number of all hospitals are national, and these do not satisfy the innate charitable sense of mankind so fully as others which depend upon the personal aid of large numbers of people.

There must be certain unlikenesses between the boards of hospitals organized upon foundations of differing character. The board which controls the hospital of a great city almshouse will contain more politicians than the trustees of a church hospital, and this in turn more clergymen than the management of a hospital founded by a medical school or by a body of charitable citizens.

There will probably be differences also in modes of administration. A hospital which is also a great school of medicine and nursing, will demand higher intelligence and executive ability in its chief officer than a simple infirmary. Indeed, few positions require more tact, skill, and special knowledge. Such a hospital must be equipped with a larger and more varied staff of physicians, both resident and chief, and a greater number of well-trained nurses and of nurses undergoing instruction.

The purposes of the administration of different hospitals will also vary. However much care, for example, be given to sick paupers, it will not be quite of the same kind bestowed upon patients who pay $15 to $40 per week for private rooms.

The differences in the *personnel* of the governing boards of hospitals and the variation in their aims produce diverse methods of procedure and conduct of affairs.

It may be permitted to me, as a citizen of Philadelphia, to select four of her chief hospitals as examples of their respective classes, viz., the Philadelphia Hospital, the Pennsylvania Hospital, the Hospital of the Protestant Episcopal Church in Philadelphia, and the Hospital of the University of Pennsylvania. Nor let it be, by this Congress, thought unfitting to set forth examples from Philadelphia. We meet to celebrate the discovery of a New World. Of this New World, Philadelphia, beyond all others, is the Historical City, the home of the Continental Congress and of Washington; the spot whereon was brought into form and being the idea of constitutional federated liberty, which is the type of modern republican life, and which caught from the pious founders of Pennsylvania the thought that all men are equal before the law in person and in conscience.

Not alone to republican life, but to all life, however governed and organized, to men everywhere has Philadelphia presented an unique and precious example; an example that should not be lost to a Congress inspired by charity. Her founder was the Columbus of a new civic polity—a polity resting on charity. And every subsequent explorer along all the coast and capes, along all the lines and turning-points of polity has but sought what William Penn realized, the ideal and prayer of humanity—peace. Unarmed, her inhabitants came among savages and dwelt with them without thought of harm. Nature seemed to sympathize with the affections of men.

> The winds with wonder whist,
> Smoothly the waters kiss'd,
> Whisp'ring new joys to the mild ocean,
> Who now hath quite forgot to rave,
> While birds of calm sit brooding on the charmèd wave.

Life proceeded in this vein for seventy years. The Philadelphians freely shared with all honest men the blessings which it brought. Multitudes came to partake of them, and with the multitudes came the light of common day and common life, and with these a great almshouse infirmary—the Philadelphia Hospital.

The Philadelphia Hospital.

This hospital is the oldest in America, save the Hotel Dieu of Montreal and perhaps some Mexican hospitals. It has become famous in several particulars. In it poetry makes Evangeline find her dying lover. In it probably originated the gratuitous giving of professional service in the public institutions of America—a questionable good. In it originated the clinical instruction of this country in obstetrics. In it Doctor Gerhard in 1836 first clearly established the distinction between typhus and typhoid fever, and also reduced the mortality of *mania a potu* 50 per cent by a new treatment. Its staff has been enriched by the famous names of Doctors Physick, Chapman, Hodge, Pancoast, Agnew, and Gross. Its great copper roof, by an act that outdid the carrying away the gates of Gaza by Samson, has, by one of its political superintendents, been stolen and put into his pocket, a feat accomplished by substituting for the copper a tin roof, selling the former as old metal and pocketing several thousand dollars by the trick; this and like performances finally providing the superintendent with free lodging in jail.

It has also became a very great hospital. Speaking in round numbers, it treats annually 10,000 cases, a tenth of whom are insane. From its earliest days (with some intermissions) instruction in the arts of healing has been given in it. In 1845 its amphitheater was the most capacious and finely arranged in the country, and capable of seating from seven to eight hundred persons, "and for over sixty years it had been continuously" (I quote the words of Doctor D. Hayes Agnew) "the great clinic school of the country, annually opening its exhaustless treasures of disease to crowds of educated, zealous inquirers after medical knowledge." In this year an untoward event brought all this magnificent instruction to a close.

Let us inquire what was this event, and examine of what sort was the governing body of the Hospital that abolished this great clinical school. From and after 1781 the almshouse and its infirmary (the Philadelphia Hospital) were under the direction of the guardians of the poor of the city of Philadelphia. These guardians from 1803 to 1854 were a body of thirty or more, elected directly by the popular vote of the corporation of the city of Philadelphia and of the corporations of the adjacent districts or liberties. They were therefore directly subject to the changes of political sentiment and the scheming of the lower orders of politicians, and little stability and permanence could be expected in their plans and systems. It is therefore not a little remarkable that they permitted the administration of the Hospital to rest for so many years in the hands of a medical board, composed of gentlemen who acted as volunteers, without pay, and therefore in some sense in a spirit of independence. This striking fact can be most easily accounted for by the eminent character of these gentlemen.

Indications of restlessness with the medical board are not wanting in the history of the guardians. Trouble culminated on June 30, 1845. The resident physicians were boarded at the table of the steward. On this day at dinner a cockroach, attempting to run across the table, was indecorously smashed upon it. Thereupon the residents demanded to be transferred to the table of the matron. Their demand was refused; they resigned unanimously, and were dismissed. The medical board tried to adjust differences and failed. The guardians determined to abolish the board—a board "composed of the ablest men in their various departments on the continent." Thus were the doors of the Philadelphia Hospital, as a school of instruction, sealed for nine years. Its government was placed in the hands of a chief resident physician with three consultants.

In 1854 the city and adjacent districts were consolidated. The guardians were reduced in number, but still elected by direct popular vote. Many abuses seem to have existed during the administration of the board thus elected. It has passed into familiar speech and printed history as the " board of buzzards."

In 1859 the board of guardians was purged by the Legislature of Pennsylvania. It was reduced to nine members, three appointed by the district court, three by the court of common pleas, and three by the common council of Philadelphia, one every year for three years, and in case of vacancy the appointing powers were to fill such vacancy. The new board consisted of the most respectable and intelligent gentlemen in the community. They rescued the Hospital from the vortex of politics, dispensed with the office of chief resident, and re-established the control of the medical board. As a result its mortality diminished 25 per cent, and it again became " the great clinical school of the country." Government by this board continued twelve years.

In 1871 the Legislature increased the board to twelve members, who were to be appointed entirely by city councils and none by the courts. Political influence became much stronger than in the previous board,—the theft of the copper roof was accomplished, but the fame of " the buzzards " was not attained.

In 1887 the Legislature reorganized the whole government of the city of Philadelphia by an act known as the Bullitt Bill. This act removed from popular election the members of various executive boards managing public affairs, and gave the power of appointing these boards to the mayor of the city. The idea was that the members of these boards would feel responsibility more keenly when directed to one man, than when diffused among a multitude of voters, and that the people could better hold the mayor responsible for good government than the members of a score of boards.

It seemed that a case had arisen in which concentration of power in the hands of one man would work advantage to the people. The guardians of the poor were therefore abolished and a department of the city government created entitled the department of charities and correction. It consists of a president and four directors, appointed by the mayor and subject to removal by him. These gentlemen are practically out of the range of politics. They are a very intelligent and devoted body, who work without compensation. They weekly inspect the Almshouse and the Hospital and maintain

them in a very creditable condition. Their annual expenditure for
these purposes is about $700,000. They appoint the superintendent,
nurses, and all subordinate officers; also the 42 doctors who now
compose the medical board of the Hospital, and the corps of resident
physicians numbering 16, the latter under civil service rules. Their
medical, surgical and nursing service is of a high order, and there
are no stray cockroaches to threaten the existence of a magnificent
clinic.

Passing from the Almshouse Infirmary of the city we come to
consider

The Pennsylvania Hospital.

This hospital was founded in 1751, largely through the efforts of
the celebrated Benjamin Franklin. It was designed to be the hospital of the province of Pennsylvania,—"for the relief of the sick
poor and the care of lunaticks." "The increase of poor diseased
foreigners and others, settled in the distant parts of this province,
where regular advice and assistance cannot be procured, but at an
expense that neither they nor their township can afford," is among
the reasons given for establishing it.

The opening words of the preamble to the act authorizing the
hospital, "Whereas the saving and restoring useful and laborious
members to a community is a work of public service, and the relief
of the sick poor is not only an act of humanity, but a religious duty,"
have a curious likeness to the kindly and shrewd nature of the author
of Poor Richard's Almanac. It is as if it were said, the state ought
to aid to restore the sick to health because it is humane to do so,
and because, when in health, they can pay taxes or work for others
who so pay. In these thoughts lie the germs of state aid to
hospitals.

The act incorporated the contributors of the Pennsylvania Hospital
and permitted any one to be a member who contributed £10. It
authorized the contributors to elect twelve managers and a treasurer;
to make laws for the hospital, provided they be not repugnant to the
laws of England, and to hold real estate of a yearly value of £1000;
and it also ordered the provincial treasurer to pay £2000 to the
contributors for the erection of a building whenever a like sum was
in hand as endowment. The board of managers still acts under the
original charter granted by the Provincial Assembly.

It has contained a long succession of men among the best and

noblest of the community, many of them descendants of the founders
of the commonwealth, or of those closely affiliated with them. There
has grown around this hospital and its board a sentiment which
touches on the romantic,—a sentiment composed largely of love
untouched by any fear of abuse of trust or misapplication of funds.

The board of managers conducts three large hospitals, one of 200
beds for the sick and two for the insane (one male and one female),
of a joint capacity of about 450 beds. Its yearly expenditure is
about $300,000, its income from endowment being about $60,000.
In the year it last reported upon there were treated in the hospital
for the sick 2170 patients, and its percentage of deaths (deducting
51 who died within 24 hours after entering) was 5.94. Its *per diem*
cost for each patient was $1.36. It has treated in all 128,000
patients, of whom 82,000 were cured and 21,000 improved.

The Pennsylvania Hospital was "one of the first, if not the first,
to adopt the enlightened" system of Pinel. One pure and distinguished man, Dr. Thomas S. Kirkbride, presided as officer-in-chief
over its two hospitals for the insane for 42 years. The managers meet
monthly. They are divided into twelve committees of two each, one
of which visits each of the hospitals once a week.

Among the various committees of this board is a medical committee, consisting of the president of the board and the three senior
members thereof, whose duty is to meet and confer with a similar
committee of the medical officers of the hospital, upon any subject
which they may wish to present to the board for its consideration
and approval; this committee reports to the board at its stated meetings any matters that have been before it, with its approval or disapproval as the case may be. This is a most important committee. It
touches the very core of the usefulness of the hospital. The care
with which it is constituted shows its importance to be appreciated.

"Unity of executive control means efficiency of management."
Hospitals form no exception to the rule "that those are best qualified to conduct a business successfully who are best acquainted with
its requirements."

The relation between the managers of a hospital and its medical
staff should be almost, though not quite, that of partnership: a partnership between those who best understand the material and business
questions to be dealt with, and those who are skilled in ailments and
remedies. It is a relation in which each side should carefully weigh
what the other thinks, and each should have a fair conception of the

value of the other's opinion. The managers should consult the staff, for example, on the construction of wards and matters of hygiene, and, speaking broadly, the staff should respect the views of the managers touching certain methods of medical and surgical practice.

The managers of the Pennsylvania Hospital have balanced these questions evenly, but have not shrunk from the responsibility of their position. They have not been men who would fail to urge even upon a renowned professor new methods of practice of acknowledged and proved value, and they have been known to forbid to a distinguished doctor the use of a fad to which he had become addicted,—I mean poulticing with earth.

A neglect of some of these simple thoughts has resulted in securing for the capital of France one of the most costly and least healthy of all recent monumental hospitals, as a careful authority tells us.

It need hardly be said that a large dispensary and a fine clinic have always been maintained by the Pennsylvania Hospital; to be a teacher in this clinic has been, and perhaps still is, to hold the blue ribbon of American clinics.

The Hospital of the Protestant Episcopal Church of Philadelphia

was chartered in 1851, for the declared charitable objects for which hospitals usually exist, and also " to provide the instruction and consolations of religion, according to the principles of the Protestant Episcopal Church, for those who are under the care of the institution."

Every person contributing at one time a sum not less than fifty dollars is entitled to vote at the annual election for managers. The board of managers consists of twenty-four communicants of the Protestant Episcopal Church in Philadelphia, one-third being clergymen, in addition to the bishop of the diocese, he being *ex officio* president of the board, which body, during a vacancy in the episcopate, is entitled to choose one of its own number president. The managers are chosen so that eight are subject to re-election every year. Seven members for ordinary business and thirteen for other affairs are a quorum. The treasurer is not a manager. The managers appoint each year a medical board, which takes entire medical care of the patients and control of the nurses and attendants.

The bishop of the diocese appoints a chaplain to celebrate divine worship in the chapel and to minister to the sick in the wards and at their homes. No other religious ministrations, more in accord with the conscience of the patient, are prohibited. Every business meeting of the board is opened with "collects from the book of common prayer, or a form of prayer provided by the Bishop."

The most prominent committee of the managers is that of arrangements and buildings. It is chosen by ballot and consists of not less than seven managers. Its duty is to take care of the Hospital building and grounds; also "to consider and take action subject to the order of the board, in regard to all matters affecting the management or interests of the Hospital"; provided no debts be incurred on contracts made without the previous sanction of the board.

The visiting committee of the board is composed of one clerical and two lay members, who each serve six weeks, except one of the two laymen chosen on the first committee of the year, who serves only four weeks, his place being supplied by a layman from the committee next in order. The term of service of this layman is six weeks. At the end of this term his place is supplied by a lay member of the following committee, and thus a connection is established between the committees throughout the official year.

This Hospital has been one of best repute in Philadelphia. It is a model among church hospitals. In 1892 the daily average of patients in its wards was 207, and 23,028 patients were treated in its dispensary. Its total cost of maintenance was $95,646.33. Its revenues are largely drawn from the numerous congregations of the Episcopalians of the diocese, and it is a favored recipient of the bounty, legacies and memorials of the rich men of that denomination.

The Hospital of the University of Pennsylvania

belongs to that University. It is not governed directly by the trustees thereof, but by a board of managers composed as follows: The provost of the University, *ex officio*; the director of the Hospital, *ex officio*; four of the trustees of the University; four of the medical faculty of the University; three of the medical alumni of the University; nine representatives of contributors; four representatives of the board of women visitors—twenty-six persons in all. There is also a board of twenty-four women visitors, four of whom are represented on the board of managers. These appointments are either made by, or subject to, the approval of the trustees of the University.

This organization is complex, but has preserved the control of the

Hospital in the University, and has also been found sufficiently elastic to interest the benevolent community in its support and several influential people in its management who have no other connection with the University.

Under this management the Hospital has obtained very satisfactory buildings, and endowments which yield $30,000 a year, and has been able to expend $80,000 per annum in maintenance. It treats over 1300 cases in its beds and about 8000 in its eleven dispensaries. It maintains an active training school for nurses, and affords bedside and clinical teaching to 800 medical students.

The distinctive features in this management are the majority of physicians in the board, and the large body of women visitors. Both seem good. The first secures a close relation between medical and business interests, giving to the former the preponderance which is fitting in the hospital of a medical school. Experience has proved women visitors invaluable in household affairs, in the training school and among the nurses. Their organic connection with the board of management has greatly facilitated internal good government and economy, and aided the general administration to attain its deservedly high repute.

What, that touches the Trustee of the Hospital, are we to learn from these four brief naratives? Mainly these things: that the door of a municipal hospital should not be ajar for a political trustee; that the faithful trustee gathers about himself general love and respect; that a trustee should be diligent and have much personal knowledge of the affairs he administers; that he should exercise good discretion in the appointment of medical officers, and should listen carefully to their views in much that concerns the business he conducts; that he should remember final responsibility rests upon himself, even in medical administration, and that he should not permit this to fall below standards of excellence approved and generally accepted; that he will find comfort and aid from associating women in his labors. Finally, we may learn how great sympathy and material support are at the command of the good trustee.

There is among the uninstructed a horror of the hospital. The ignorant imagine the sick there to be at the risk of untried remedies, to be the subject of experiment because poor and treated freely.

The trustee who promptly pays the bills of a hospital will have done something to dispel this illusion. Men appreciate the honest payment of bills, and confidence given for one reason spreads like a beautiful vine and envelops all.

The hospital deals with life and death, and its trustee should feel himself to rule and give direction in the constant presence of the Eternal, that all he does or permits to be done should be done painstakingly and with an honest conscience. So will he evoke the delicate sentiments of men, and command the generous forces charity places at the disposal of suffering.

This charity has been ever-existent. Though greatly developed by Christianity, it has other parentage as well. It is indeed true its strength has been most exhibited among modern Christian nations—that the hospital revenues of Great Britain and Ireland (for example) are £1,340,744/1/3—(this Congress should thank Henry C. Burdett for these figures)—but it is also true that remotest ages, that temples of Egypt, cities of Greece, certain emperors of Rome, that the Buddhist, the Saracen and the Crusader, the fire-worshiper and the Aztec, the Hun and the Frank and the Saxon, tell the tender story of love for and organized care of the sick.

DISCUSSION.

THE CHAIRMAN.—I will say that I saw this paper when it was in the rough, and my comment on it to Mr. Wood was that I thought his declaration that the trustees should have a say-so in the methods of medical and surgical treatment in the hospitals would be likely to produce some criticism, so far as I know anything of the nature of doctors who attend hospitals. Mr. Wood had it that in all methods of treatment the Board should have control, but after listening to me he interpolated the word "certain"; I said they might interfere in "certain" methods. It is a very responsible matter for trustees to interfere in such a matter, although—as Mr. Wood says—it has been done. A physician in one of the prominent hospitals in Philadelphia, a surgeon, acquired the idea that dressing wounds with fresh earth was the proper way to treat them, and he urged it in all kinds of wounds and all sorts of operations. Of course the trustees were right in preventing this, as we know. But how do the trustees know how to put their finger on and interfere, except by the information that they obtain from some other doctors? They do not get that information out of the depths of their internal consciousness, nor probably by studying up the latest records in bacteriology and surgery. Now, whenever you have one set of doctors coming to a board of trustees in order to explain to them that another set of doctors is doing wrong, or one particular doctor in the hospital is doing wrong, and asking the board of directors to interfere in that, I think you all can see that it is a very difficult task that they have undertaken. I do not think I should lay it down as a general rule, as Mr. Wood has done, that it is the duty of the Board to look after the practice of the doctors and keep them straight.

MR. C. C. SAVAGE, of New York.—As a trustee of a hospital, I want to ask one single question : Who is responsible for the care and management of the hospital ? The trustees or the physicians? If the trustees are responsible for it, then they must have supreme authority over it, and the doctors themselves must be subordinate to the trustees, otherwise we have confusion and lack of discipline. Now take the hospital with which I am connected, the Demilt Dispensary, where the physicians nominate the physicians to the board of trustees. We should not hesitate one moment if a doctor came before us that we did not approve, to reject him, even on the nomination of the medical board, and we sometimes take the liberty of changing the views of the medical board. I believe, sir, that the lay management of a hospital does most effective work, provided the board of trustees is not too large.

MR. ARTHUR RYERSON, of Chicago.—As president of a hospital, I am very much interested in the question of the duties of the trustee. I think there is one very clear principle that governs the whole thing : the government must be in the hands of a board of trustees, but having appointed a medical board, the only correct rule is to let the medical board run the medical affairs ; and so far as I am concerned, that is a position I have always taken.

Now there is another question in regard to this matter ; it is a much more practical question here in Chicago, and if any one can throw light on it I shall be very glad to get it, and that is this: " How to get a good, active board of trustees of a hospital, and after having gotten a board, how to get work out of them ? " I think you will find the great difficulty in Chicago is to get men of this kind ; our men are very busy, and it is almost impossible to get an active working board of trustees. I should like to have some of our friends from the East, particularly from Philadelphia, throw some light on this question. I know in Philadelphia they do not have so much trouble, and I should like to know how to get an active working board of trustees.

MR. H. C. BURDETT, of London.—I should like to say that there is no doubt that this question of the relations of the medical staff to the governing body is of the essence of the whole spirit upon which the administration of any great hospital is conducted. If these relations are not sound the whole institution must suffer, and ultimately fall into mismanagement. Now I began my experience in hospital administration before the days of trained nurses. In the hospital of which I was governor it used to be the common practice for the members of the medical staff who met in the wards, to go together into the nearest corner and hold a medical board meeting. While we found at that time, as representing the lay administration, great difficulty in getting proper discipline and proper attendance from the medical staff. And after, in these latter thirty years, considering this question very fully, and being acquainted with the systems in force in all countries, I have come to this conclusion, that it is desirable, as the last speaker said, that you shall have a medical board, and that all medical matters shall be relegated to that board. If the trustees, or the lay governing body, have medical questions to deal with, it is far wiser and better for them to send these questions to the medical board and to get the opinion of that medical board in writing, as a whole ; because if a medical man cannot stand and is not prepared to stand or fall by the judgment of his colleagues, it is perfectly certain that he is an undesirable member of any medical staff. On the other hand, there are no men and no class of workers in hospitals to whom the whole institution is more greatly indebted than to the medical board, and I think they are entitled to the independent position which an independent board gives, and I believe that to be the true solution of all the difficulties relating to the administration of a hospital. With a lay governing committee it must necessarily have a large medical staff.

On the question which the last speaker raised, viz., how are you to get a good board of management and to secure the individual attendance of that board, I have a word to say. It seems to me that the greatest and the most valuable gift which any man or woman can give to hospitals, or to any other public institution, is the gift of personal service, and I venture to say as a stranger in Chicago, and I hope in saying I shall give no offense, that this is a question for the churches; that if Chicago, with its ever-growing, increasing prosperity, finds that the doctrine of personal service is not yet popular among its citizens, I say it is the duty of the churches of this city to preach the privilege of personal service, to drive that privilege home into the heart of every man and woman in the city; because I know from my own experience, from the experience of one of your own millionaires, a great man, who is now dead, but who was a personal friend of my own, and who gave enormously to charity, who told me this—and it is a word that I wish might reach the heart of each man in Chicago—"I never knew what was the worth or the value of the privilege of money until I learned to give and to give largely to good objects." Now what better object can you have than to take an active part in the administration of a great medical charity? I do not think there is a better work in the world, and I hope that the difficulties you have here will be overcome. They are not confined to Chicago, unfortunately; we have the same difficulties in London. But still these difficulties are overcome, and there are institutions where there is an *esprit* which you can feel when you enter the doors, and where the privilege of personal service is a real living force, which every man and woman in that hospital or that institution feels and is moved by, and delights to serve under. That is the true spirit; and if once you could get that spirit anywhere—and until you get that spirit you should never rest—you will not have to lament a large board with small attendance, but you will have, as you have in many cities now, thank God, a competition in good works for the privilege of serving on your hospital boards, and for the privilege of giving a little of the time, which means money to every citizen, to the good work of administrating charity.

MR. C. C. SAVAGE, of New York.—The question was asked as to the way to get a good board. I believe the best way is to first avoid ex-officio members, although I am one myself; and second, to elect for a term rather than for life, and when any member of a board has ceased by reason of other duties or other interests to do his duty, drop him off from the board without regard to who or what he is. In other words, keep your board constantly fresh by new blood, and I believe in that way a hospital or any charitable institution can be maintained in vigor, and only in that way.

THE RELATIONS OF THE MEDICAL STAFF TO THE GOVERNING BODIES IN HOSPITALS.

BY EDWARD COWLES, M. D.,

Superintendent, McLean Hospital, Somerville, Mass.

In the organization of human society the strong and self-supporting must take care of the weak and dependent. Among the noblest motives of humanity is the love that protects the weakness of infancy, sickness, age and infirmity. In the same spirit the Christian world has built its hospitals out of the love of man for his fellow-men.

But the hospital is no longer almost solely the refuge and the hardship of the poor; it affords superior care in sickness for all. Modern science is so elaborating and refining its methods that many things are done for the cure of disease and the amelioration of human suffering which can be done only in hospitals. With more complexity of manipulation in the art of medicine, special conditions for its practice have become necessary. The training of women as nurses has aided largely in the attainment of better methods by the precision of nursing care.

It has come to pass, therefore, that the salient facts of the present time in the history of hospitals are, the building of many small hospitals, the appreciation of their value to every community, and their increasing influence in teaching the gospel of health. Every such hospital becomes for its locality a school of health; it is an educator of all who have to do with it; every physician is trained by it, and every woman is a better nurse. In the end, according to Havelock Ellis, every physician in the country should be attached to a hospital, and every person should be living within the district of an institution of health. It is safe to say that the time will come in our country when a local hospital, if only the smallest cottage that can be fitly used, will be accounted the need and demand of every thriving community, and that it will be supported by the people whom it serves. In the more complete national care of those interests in which the guardianship of life is concerned, these hospitals will become so many centers of sanitary control in a way never before possible. This means the increasing of the sum of human happinesss, and involves the highest physical, intellectual, and moral development of the nation.

It is the glory and the hope of modern philanthropy that it is learning the principle of prevention, and to know that moral weakness, sin and crime are so largely maladies which spring from bodily ill-being. We know that the initial conditions of diseases of mind and morals, as of diseases of the body, are often caused by offenses against the laws of health. Knowledge of the causation of disease, which teaches the means of prevention, is the most helpful aid to the social economist, whose doctrine is that public health is public wealth. In a broader socialism it is the highest philanthropy that promotes a general knowledge of the laws of life which must be obeyed to cure both physical and moral ills. We are sharing in our time in a wonderful awakening, in which there are the strongest forces at work in the union of science and philanthropy.

The hospital has always been regarded as embodying the spirit of the Good Samaritan. It is an Hôtel Dieu, and its administrative care has been held as a sacred trust. In the present uplifting of hospital work toward its larger sphere, those who maintain the existence of the hospital and have the keeping of the greater interests now centered in it are charged with a greater and more sacred trust.

The relations (to the hospital and to each other) of the sick, the greater public, and those who govern, administer, and serve in it, are very complex. Important among these are the relations of the medical staff to the governing body. But these are conditioned by a proper conception of the hospital—its character as an institution. Its usefulness depends upon a proper organization, in which certain fundamental principles should be supreme which form the natural laws of such institutions. Departures from these principles become inherent weaknesses that are obstructive of usefulness, or mar the harmony without which the best work cannot be done. Upon the basis of a sound organization, the various elements fall into their natural places and are easily co-ordinated. For these reasons the hospital has a vital character of its own, and for the present purpose it is needful to consider three elements prominent in such institutions:—1, the hospital itself; 2, the governing body; and 3, the medical staff.

1. The hospital itself. The business of managing a hospital is the same, in principle, in a small hospital as in a large one. It has to be learned like any other special business, and governing bodies need the knowledge that comes only by experience. Hence the importance of correct principles. It is easy to go on when the beginning is

right, but difficult to change a faulty system once established. These many new hospitals now building are practically, in many cases, new ventures by inexperienced organizers of such work. For every new one a compilation of by-laws and rules is made from those of existing hospitals, with the inherent faults. It is often that new ideas are added that seem expedient but end in trouble and disappointment. There are two primary sources from which trouble and failure are likely to come. These are either faults of the system, which even good people cannot get on with; or faults of individuals under a good system. It has been known to happen that when the organization is correct and individuals are at fault, the governors have tried to remedy matters by changing both the individuals and the system. Faulty systems sometimes seem to work well, but that is only a proof of exceptional goodness of individuals; it is often at the cost of trials and sacrifices of faithful hospital officers whose lives are hard enough at the best.

A fundamental principle is that the benefits of the hospital belong to the greater public, of which the sick who are immediately concerned are the representatives. It is through the work done for them that the great principle of preventive medicine gains its results. A sound administration of hospital work promotes the greatest good of the greatest number. This indeed is the function of the hospital as a health station and a school of health. Every opportunity, consistent with the first duty to the sick, for the improvement of professional knowledge and skill of physician and nurse should be utilized for the advancement of the greatest good. But the interest of the sick man, who intrusts himself to the keeping of the hospital, is still paramount; any interest, personal or otherwise, that conflicts with this primary principle must be subordinated to it. This applies to all hospitals, whether those largely endowed, with histories of great work done, as by pure charities, or the many newer and smaller ones that must be supported largely by those who use them; or those attached to medical schools for the use of clinical teaching; or corporate institutions for patients of the private class.

The business of the hospital should yield as its product the greatest remedial good that can be gained from the investment made in it of capital and service. This means the furnishing of the best available service for the sick, and that it is legitimate to improve the skill and value of that service for the larger benefit of humanity.

The hospital, as a place for the conducting of its business, is also the habitation of its beneficiaries and of those who do its work. It has, as a fundamental principle, an integral character,—a precisely defined individuality. It has a peculiarity not commonly recognized: while it conducts a *business*, it is the *home* of those who live in it. It exists as a family and as an organic unit in the social order. As a social unit, its inner life, in its order and discipline, should be complete within itself, and have a properly respected head, on the basis of thé family principle.

The management of a hospital is often likened to a business, such as that of a manufactory or a mercantile house. It is more than that by having a different human element in it; the special work of the hospital is done by a family, and should be governed with due regard for its domestic unity. The competent head of the household should have training and capacity for conducting the business, and have sole charge of all administrative affairs, under the direction of the governing body.

2. The governing body has its attitude to the hospital plainly indicated by the two general principles above stated. It has the responsibility of medical and other appointments, which should have due regard to the special prerogatives of family headship. It fixes responsibility definitely upon the superintendent by requiring of him the selection and nomination of all his assistants; to hold him responsible for all that happens he should have a fair chance to protect his responsibility. This is the true principle; and then if there is failure it is the fault of the individual and the remedy is plain. The functions of the governing body are *legislative*, in making proper regulations and maintaining them through an executive head or agent; they are *judicial*, in cases of appeal from those exercising its delegated authority; and there are the functions relating to the *subsistence of the hospital.*

The governing body of any hospital is solely responsible for the presence of any patient admitted to its keeping, whether "free" or "private." It is responsible for his proper care and for his discharge at a fitting time, in all of which it may act upon the recommendation and advice of the medical staff. It is responsible for affording all the requisite conditions, appliances, instruments and service to the best of its ability. Failure in efficiency, as of instruments or nurses, who are virtually skilled instruments, are administrative faults, and should be referred to the executive disciplinary head.

In direct relation to the medical staff, the governing body has the special duty of not only providing the best available professional service for the sick in its keeping, but of so enlisting the continuance of that service as to promote the increase of the skill that is only gained by experience. The governing body should also seek to enhance the benefits of this service to the sick by any other legitimate means that lead to scientific advancement in medicine and surgery.

In the interests of the sick and of promoting in the largest way the efficiency of the hospital, the trustees may properly stimulate that interest in the work, on the part of the medical staff, that tends to the increase of its zeal and efficiency. Here is to be applied the principle of conservation of values. In accordance with a fundamental law in the social order in the struggle for existence, every individual should have a wholesome sense of duty to fulfil his personal obligations to those having claims upon him. His charity should not begin at the hospital nor be given solely there. The laborer is worthy of his hire. Fortunately for the hospital and its governing body, it is incidental to professional service in it that such service increases the skill of the physician, and has a reflex value to him in increase of reputation and the productive power of his labor. This is good for the hospital, for himself, and for the betterment of his usefulness to society at large.

The governing bodies in hospitals have been finding increasing difficulty in the questions arising from the necessity of accommodating the principle just stated to the traditions of the charitable institutions in their keeping. These difficulties have been formulated in the " pay-patient " question, and are being solved in many directions by a change of policy in this matter.

This question is on the issue as to whether it is equitable for self-supporting people to be treated in hospitals upon payment for board and nursing care, and make no compensation for the professional service as they would do in their private homes. This recent period in the evolution of hospitals will doubtless be reviewed as one of transition. There is now forthcoming the evidence that appears to throw light upon the obscurity as to the equities of this troublesome question. It is not to be expected, perhaps, that governing bodies can yet see quite clearly the way to properly adjust all the interests involved, however legitimate each may seem. But the new conditions must be studied as they arise, for they appear to be leading by their very force as facts to a solution of the problem.

The great institutions in the large cities, with their splendid endow-ments, honorable records and traditions as pure charities, are coming to hold an exceptional position, by the minority of their number, in the now rapidly lengthening list of hospitals.

It is to be said for the great hospitals that they make a large return to the medical staff for the professional service rendered, and that appointments to such service are sought by men of the highest ability, and are accounted as having a definite and well-defined value. The conditions are such that all concerned, including the greater public, are benefited by the association, as has been set forth already. But the discussion of the question for its present bearing is best directed to the conditions of the new order of hos-pitals,—those that are being built to meet the wide-spreading sense of their value, and are developing in the profession at large the special skill that modern medicine and surgery require for the common need.

It can hardly be questioned, in the new status of hospitals, that their common use by self-supporting people demands a proper co-ordination of the interests of patients, hospital, and physicians alike, on the broad principle that equity in the exchange of values most soundly promotes human progress. It is interesting to note that the facts as they stand appear to be illustrating the law of social evolution that mutual interests finally adjust themselves on an equita-ble basis. The common arrangement in many of these smaller hos-pitals is that the leading local physicians are appointed to the staff for attendance upon hospital beneficiaries, but that any reputable medical man of the town has the privilege of attending private cases. Thus comes quite nearly true, in that locality, Havelock Ellis's dictum that every physician in the country should be attached to a hospital. Many among the larger towns and smaller cities in New England could be cited in proof of this.

Now there are a number of obvious truths to be noted in these circumstances, omitting for the moment the philanthropic motives in the exercise of which the medical profession takes reasonable pride. The governing body in such a hospital distributes the privilege of attending the sick as generally as possible, its special obligations to beneficiaries being fulfilled by appointment of the best service for them. All these privileges are generally acceptable to physicians. There is no clinical teaching, and little addition to local professional reputation, from the appointment alone. A physician will treat a private patient in the hospital whom he could not afford to send there and deprive himself of a fair *honorarium.* The hospital needs all the board money from such patients it can get, to aid in its support. The patient gets superior attendance in the hospital. In fact, the more the hospital is used in this way, the better it is for everybody. It is exactly for this reason that all are agreed, in every community, that a hospital is a good thing; and it is found to be comparatively easy to have one, now that there are trained women for the managing and nursing.

It seems perfectly evident that these things all tend to bring it to pass that serious medical and surgical and contagious cases will be treated commonly in local hospitals. It seems equally obvious that the " pure charity " principle, applied to every such hospital, would be adverse to this new and natural movement in the direction of higher sanitation and prevention. It is by the recognition of the rule of equity in the exchange of values, in compensation for service rendered, that these governing bodies are in an important way promoting the growth of these hospitals. The more valuable the hospital service can be made to the physician, the better he can afford to educate himself to a fitness of qualification for it ; the more completely the " pure charity " principle is carried out, the fewer hospitals, or the less the physician can afford the increasing cost of acquiring his profession.

The discussion of this principle of the conservation of values may be left here with the question as to how far it is reasonable, in the broadest view of the interests of human progress, to apply it to the great charitable institutions.

3. The medical staff may now be considered as to its relations to the governing body in a hospital. Its environment being so fully defined in the foregoing discussion, its place in the matter is easily found.

The medical staff does its duty to humanity as its special honor, in contributing out of what it has to give, its share of service for the common weal. The physician visits the hospital, prescribes and directs, and applies his skilled manipulations. He responds to the call of the governing body, with advice to the best of his knowledge, in all that touches the welfare of the sick ; but whatever control he exercises in certain special details, it is delegated authority, and the responsibility for all executive acts rests upon the trustees, whose prerogatives must therefore be respected. Every patient, " free " or "private," is a part of the hospital household, and all failures in executing the physicians' prescriptions and the like are administrative faults, and should be referred to the executive disciplinary head.

The physician may give his services to the suffering poor ; he may seek at the hands of the governing body, service in a hospital which is a pure charity, and accept as equivalent the reflex benefits to himself (and future patients) of experience and increase in skill and reputation; or the opportunity for clinical teaching which may be justly claimed of every hospital beneficiary when not harmful ; or in the new order of hospital work, the physician may equitably receive compensation from those whose ability it is, and pride it should be to make fair return for value received.

These principles, essential to a sound organization, will guide to a proper adjustment of the relations of the medical staff to the hospital and to its governing body.

UEBER DIE VERWALTUNG VON KRANKENHÄUSERN.

H. MERKE,

Verwaltungs-Director des städtischen Krankenhauses Moabit, Berlin.

" Das Wohl des Kranken ist das höchste Gesetz," so sollte, in geringer Abänderung eines bekannten Ausspruchs, das Motto lauten, das über dem Eingang eines Krankenhauses zu prangen hätte, um anzudeuten, dass von diesem Gesichtswinkel aus alle Einrichtungen, die ein Krankenhaus aufweist und alle Massnahmen, die in einem solchen, in welcher Richtung auch immer getroffen werden, betrachtet und auf ihre Güte hin geprüft werden müssen.

Nach zwei Seiten hin bekundet sich nun vornehmlich die Sorge für das Wohl des Kranken im Krankenhause und zwar einmal in Bezug auf die directe Pflege desselben, wie sie in seiner Wartung und Behandlung zu Tage tritt—also die rein ärztliche Thätigkeit— das andere Mal mehr indirect durch die Fürsorge für alle die Einrichtungen und Veranstaltungen, die nothwendig sind, um den vielseitigen Bedürfnissen eines Krankenhauses, die doch schliesslich immer wieder nur im letzten Grunde dem einzelnen Kranken zu Gute kommen, Rechnung zu tragen—und hier setzt die Verwaltung des Krankenhauses ein.

Gross sind die Aufgaben, die der ärztlichen Thätigkeit, wenn
irgend sonst, grade im Krankenhause gestellt sind, gross aber auch
und eine volle Menschenkraft in Anspruch nehmend diejenigen, die
der Verwaltung in demselben harren. Denn wenn hier auf der einen
Seite mit der Fürsorge für das Wohl der Kranken weise Sparsamkeit
gepaart sein muss, die es verhindert, die vorhandenen Mittel für
Unnöthiges und Unzweckmässiges zu verwenden, so muss anderseits
auch grade eine umsichtige Verwaltung danach streben, alle Fortschritte und Errungenschaften der Technik wie der Hygiene für ihr
Gebiet nutzbar zu machen, d. h. den immer weiteren Ausbau des-
jenigen Theils der Gesundheitslehre anzubahnen, den wir die
Hygiene des Krankenhauses nennen.

Sind es doch fast alle Zweige der Verwaltung, in denen diese
letztere ihre Thätigkeit entfaltet: nicht minder in der Nahrungsmit-
telversorgung, hier Hand in Hand gehend mit den Forderungen des
Arztes, die Krankenverpflegung betreffend, wie in der Desinfection
und dem Wäschereibetriebe, wo sie die Gefahr der Weiterverbreit-
ung und Uebertragung von Ansteckungsstoffen vorzubeugen hat, in
der gesundheitsmässigen Beheizung und Lüftung der Krankenräume
sowohl, wie der Arbeitsräume, in denen das Arbeitspersonal beschäf-
tigt wird.

Allein es handelt sich bei der Verwaltung eines grösseren Civil-
krankenhauses—und auf ein solches beziehen sich die folgenden
Ausführungen hauptsächlich, während sie die Militairhospitäler sowie
die dem medicinischen Unterricht ausschliesslich dienenden Kliniken
ausser Acht lassen,—es handelt sich also bei der Verwaltung eines
derartigen Krankenhauses nicht allein um die bisher aufgeführten
Gesichtspunkte, die ich, weil wie mir scheint bisher zu wenig berück-
sichtigt, absichtlich in den Vordergrund gestellt habe, sondern ebenso
massgebend ist die richtige Organisation der Verwaltung, die es
ermöglicht, dass bei dem ganzen grossen Betriebe einer Anstalt ein
Zusammenstoss von Sonderinteressen vermieden wird, die einzelnen ausführenden Organe, sowohl von ärztlicher wie von beamteter
Seite, gleichmässig zusammenarbeiten und so das Interesse der
Anstalt wie das der Kranken nach jeder Richtung hin gewahrt wird.

Wohl lassen sich allgemeine Grundsätze für eine derartige Organisation aufstellen, die stricte Durchführung derselben jedoch in
jedem Einzelfalle zu verlangen, wäre, wie jeder Schematismus,
grundfalsch, denn diese Organisation muss sich richten nach den
lokalen Verhältnissen, der Grösse, der Bauart und den besonderen

Zwecken der einzelnen Anstalten. Hier das jedesmal richtige zu treffen ist jedenfalls eine der Hauptaufgaben einer gut geleiteten Verwaltung.

Dieses vorausgeschickt, tritt nun zunächst die Frage entgegen, wer an der Spitze der Verwaltung einer solchen grösseren Anstalt stehen soll, eine Frage die heute noch, wie vor Jahren, wenigstens bei uns in Deutschland immer eine brennende ist und deren Beantwortung, je nach der Stellungnahme, ja fast möchte man sagen, nach dem Stande des mit der Lösung dieser Frage Beschäftigten, im heterogensten Sinne ausgefallen ist. Hie Arzt, hie Verwaltungsbeamter, so lautete und lautet noch heut das Feldgeschrei, sobald dieser Gegenstand zur Discussion steht.

Betrachten wir, bevor wir uns über die vorliegende Frage äussern, wie Staat und Gemeinde sich derselben gegenüber bisher verhalten haben, so finden wir, dass man die Lösung derselben auf vier verschiedenen Wegen versucht hat: man betraute entweder eine aus Mitgliedern der vorgesetzten Behörde bestehende Commission mit der eigentlichen Administration und liess die Kassen und Oeconomiesachen, sowie die Bureaugeschäfte von einzelnen Beamten, die eine untergeordnete Stellung einnahmen, bearbeiten, während die Aerzte einfach auf die Behandlung der Kranken angewiesen waren, oder man stellte einen Arzt oder einen Verwaltungsbeamten an die Spitze der gesammten Anstalt, oder man theilte die Leitung des Krankenhauses zwischen einem Verwaltungsbeamten und einem auch mehreren Aerzten, die einander coordinirt waren.

Von dem ersteren Modus der Verwaltung des Krankenhauses durch eine Commission, ist man wohl überall zurückgekommen und zwar mit vollem Recht; denn ein erspriessliches Wirken, ein freudiges Schaffen, eine volle Hingabe an die Aufgaben einer Krankenhausverwaltung ist dort nicht zu erwarten, wo fast jede persönliche Initiation gehemmt wird und wo die Prüfung der in einem Krankenhause stets neu auftauchenden Bedürfnisse in den Händen von Personen liegt, die, dem eigentlichen Krankenhauswesen mehr oder weniger fernstehend, naturgemäss ein geringeres Verständniss für dieselben besitzen, ganz abgesehen davon, dass durch eine derartige Einrichtung die ganze Verwaltung eine ungemein schwerfällige wird.

Die zweite Modalität, die Stellung eines Arztes an die Spitze der Gesammt-Verwaltung eines Krankenhauses, ist an verschiedenen grösseren Krankenhäusern durchgeführt und erfreut sich speciell in ärztlichen Kreisen einer grossen Beliebtheit. Unser Urtheil hierüber, wie über den dritten Modus, einem Verwaltungsbeamten allein die Gesammtverwaltung eines Krankenhauses anzuvertrauen, werden wir weiter unten angeben. Was endlich die Theilung der Verwaltung zwischen einen Verwaltungsbeamten und einem Arzte betrifft, so hat dieses Princip in Berlin beispeilsweise sowohl bei dem Königlichen Charité Krankenhause, wie in den 3 Städtischen allgemeinen Krankenhäusern Anwendung gefunden in der Weise, dass dem Verwaltungs-Director mehr die Leitung der eigentlichen administrativen Angelegenheiten, den ärztlichen Directoren (im Charité Krankenhause ist nur ein ärztlicher Director vorhanden, während in den Krankenhäusern der Stadt Berlin je zwei, und zwar einer für die innere, der andere für die chirurgische Station angestellt sind) speciell die Vertretung der ärztlichen Interessen obliegt.

Von vorn herein müsste es als das Natürlichste erscheinen, dass in einem Krankenhause ein Arzt an der Spitze der Anstalt steht; handelt es sich ja doch um ein Haus für Kranke, und deren nächste Bedürfnisse kennt und versteht naturgemäss am besten der Arzt. Dies Raisonnement ist richtig, sofern es sich unmittelbar um den Kranken selbst und dessen Wartung, Pflege u. s. w. handelt; hier soll und muss dem Arzt vollständig freie Hand gelassen werden, hier darf kein Fremder, kein Laie, und wäre sein sontiges Wissen und Können auch noch so gross, störend eingreifen wollen.

Anders aber gestaltet sich die Sachlage, wenn es sich um die grosse Menge alles dessen handelt, was zwar nicht unmittelbar zu dem Kranken und seiner Pflege in Beziehung steht, aber doch alle die Vorkehrungen und Einrichtungen in sich begreift, die nöthig sind, um für das Wohl des Kranken nach jeder Richtung hin ausgiebig Sorge tragen zu können, d. h. um die eigentliche Verwaltung.

Bereits im Eingange dieser Besprechung haben wir kurz die Aufgaben, welche der Verwaltung eines Krankenhauses zufallen, gestreift und wollen an dieser Stelle, wo die Frage zur Entscheidung steht, wer die Verwaltung des Krankenhauses führen soll, noch einmal auf dieselbe zurückkommen.

Betrachten wir noch einmal kurz die Aufgaben, welche der Verwaltung eines Krankenhauses zufallen.

Sie hat in jeder Beziehung das Interesse der Anstalt zu wahren und dasselbe nach aussen hin zu vertreten. Sie hat darauf zu achten, dass die allereigentlichste Bestimmung eines Krankenhauses für das Wohl der Kranken zu sorgen und Alles aufzubieten, was zur Pflege und Wiederherstellung derselben nothwendig ist, nie aus

falscher Sparsamkeit ausser Acht gelassen wird. Sie ist ferner verant-
wortlich der vorgesetzten Behörde für die richtige Führung der
nothwendigen Bücher und Acten, sowie für eine zweckentsprechende
Finanzwirthschaft in der Anstalt. Hier hat sie veraltete Verwaltungs-
maximen zu beseitigen, den Geschäftsgang nach Möglichkeit zu
vereinfachen, für aüsserste Klarheit und Uebersicht Sorge zu tragen.

Hierzu kommt die Beaufsichtigung des wirthschaftlichen Betriebes
der Anstalt in der Oekonomie sowohl wie im Wäschereibetriebe,
auf die wir im Speciellen noch am Schluss dieser Abhandlung
zurückkommen werden. Ferner ist es Aufgabe der Verwaltung, die
bestehenden hygienischen Einrichtungen voll auszunutzen, nicht vor-
handene zu schaffen, fehlerhafte zu vervollkommnen.

Wie sie aus der wissenschaftlichen Forschung die Nutzanwendung
für die Praxis ziehen soll, so wird sie auf ihrem Gebiet durch scharfe
Beobachtung neue Fragen aufwerfen, deren Beantwortung wieder der
Wissenschaft zufällt, ein Wechselverkehr, der beiden Theilen zu
Gute kommt.

Treten wir nun der Frage näher, ob ein Arzt ausschliesslich der
Leiter eines Krankenhauses sein soll, so müssen wir auf Grund der
obigen Auseinandersetzungen dieselbe verneinen.

Die reinen Verwaltungsangelegenheiten liegen dem Arzte, seinem
ganzen Bildungsgange entsprechend, vollständig fern, nirgends hatte
er in seiner Vorbildung Gelegenheit, sich mit ihnen zu beschäftigen,
tiefer in sie einzudringen, ein Verständniss für dieselben zu gewinnen. Ein neues Feld, das ihm vollständig fremd ist, und dessen
Studium Zeit und Mühe voraussetzt, müsste er bearbeiten, werthvolle
eigene Errungenschaften in seiner Wissenschaft für das Gemeinde-
wohl ungenützt lassen und das Alles zu dem einzigen Zweck, um im
günstigsten Falle annährend auf diesem Felde das zu leisten, was ein
Anderer, der das Verwaltungsfach zu seinem Beruf gewählt hat,
ohne sonderliche Mühe schafft. Soll man wirklich eine wissenschaft-
liche Capacität auf dem Gebiete der Medicin dieser Wissenschaft
entreissen, nur um aus ihr einen mittelmässigen Verwaltungs-Be-
amten zu machen? Ich meine nein!

Die zweite Frage würde lauten, ob es sich empfielt, einen Verwaltungsbeamten an die Spitze eines Krankenhauses zu stellen.
Auch hiergegen würden wir uns erklären, da durch eine derartige
Einrichtung besonders bei den Aerzten nur zu häufig der Glaube
hervorgerufen wird, als würden, bei einer scheinbaren Collision der
ärztlichen Interessen mit denen der Verwaltung, erstere den letzteren

hintenangesetzt. Es hat zudem stets etwas Missliches für sich, wenn in einem Krankenhause der Arzt unter einem Nichtarzte fungiren muss.

Ich würde deshalb dafür plaidiren, dass die Leitung eines Krankenhauses einem ärztlichen Director und einem diesem coordinirten Verwaltungsdirector zu übertragen ist. Freilich sind an den letzteren ganz besondere Anforderungen zu stellen.

Zunächst genügt es durchaus noch nicht, dass derselbe in irgend einer anderen Verwaltung Tüchtiges geleistet hat, um ihn für einen derartigen Posten als besonders geeignet erscheinen zu lassen, vielmehr muss der Nachweis gefordert werden, dass er ausserdem bereits in gleichen Anstalten sich diejenige Summe von Kenntnissen und Erfahrungen angeeignet hat, die vorhanden sein muss, um in diesem eigenartigen Verwaltungsfach erspriessliches leisten zu können. Ferner muss er unbedingt auf dem Gebiet der Hygiene, und speciell der Krankenhaushygiene, gut durchgebildet sein, da bezügliche Fragen, wie wir oben auseinander gesetzt haben, fast täglich in der verschiedensten Form und Richtung an ihn herantreten.

Der Preussische Minister für das Unterrichtswesen hat erst neuerdings wieder in Anlehnung an einen früheren Erlass die Behörden aufgefordert, geeignete Beamte aus den einzelnen Ressorts auf längere Zeit zu beurlauben, um ihnen die Möglichkeit zu geben, sich an einem der verschiedenen hygienischen Institute, wie sie bereits die Mehrzahl unserer Universitäten besitzt, in dieser Wissenschaft wenigstens allgemeine Kenntnisse zu erwerben; ebenso muss auch von einem Beamten, der die Leitung eines Krankenhauses übernehmen soll, eine genauere Kenntniss derjenigen Zweige der Hygiene, die speciell auf das Krankenhauswesen Bezug haben und auf die wir oben bereits hingewiesen haben, gefordert werden. Man könnte hier den Einwurf erheben, dass es genüge, wenn der ärztliche Leiter der Anstalt die nöthigen hygienischen Kenntnisse besitzt und dass auf ihn in dieser Beziehung recurrirt werden könnte, allein, dem ist entgegenzuhalten, dass auch in rein wirthschaftlichen und technischen Fragen, in denen der Arzt in der Natur der Sache noch nicht so bewandert sein kann, wie der Verwaltungsbeamte, mehr und mehr die hygienische Seite derselben, und zwar mit Recht, in den Vordergrund tritt und dass auch hierin der Beamte auf Grund einer entsprechenden hygienischen Vorbildung im Stande sein muss, selbstständig zu urtheilen und Verbesserungen zu schaffen.

Mit einem solchen Maass von Kenntnissen ausgerüstet, wird es dem Verwaltungsbeamten nicht schwer fallen, bei dem ihm coordinirten ärztlichen Leiter der Anstalt sowohl, wie bei dem übrigen ärztlichen Personal sich diejenige Achtung zu erwerben, die unbedingt nothwendig ist, um gemeinsam und in gegenseitiger Unterstützung im Interesse des Krankenhauses, d. h. im Interesse der Kranken zu schaffen und zu wirken.

Die vorsteheden Ausführungen beziehen sich, wie bereits erwähnt, auf grössere staatliche oder communale Krankenhäuser, für die Krankenhäuser kleinerer Gemeinden, die gewöhnlich nur über 30–50 Betten verfügen, mögen dieselben nicht in jeder Beziehung zutreffend sein; insbesondere wird man hier schon aus Sparsamkeitsrücksichten in der Regel die Leitung der Anstalt in die Hände des behandelnden Arztes legen, was bei der geringen räumlichen Ausdehnung solcher Krankenhäuser, der nur auf das Nothwendigste sich beschränkenden, häufig recht primitiven Einrichtungen und dem leichteren Ueberblick über dieselben auch als ausreichend erscheinen muss. Immerhin sollte hier wenigstens der Verpflegung der Kranken, die für gewöhnlich in den Händen eines Oberwärters ruht, sowohl von Seiten des Arztes wie der zuständigen Behörde ganz besondere Aufmerksamkeit gewidmet werden.

Wenn ich bisher bei dem Thema über die Verwaltung von Krankenhäusern die Personenfrage berührt habe, so geschah dies, abgesehen von ihrer Bedeutung an und für sich, auch besonders einem mir persönlich geäusserten Wunsche entsprechend ; ich will nun noch versuchen, wenigstens einige Zweige der Verwaltungsthätigkeit kurz zu besprechen, eine eingehendere Behandlung verbietet die kurzbemessene Zeit.

Ein wichtiges Hülfsmittel bei der Krankenbehandlung bildet bekanntlich eine gut geregelte *Verpflegung* der Kranken. Die Entscheidung darüber, welche Speisen dem Patienten in den einzelnen Krankheitsstadien zuträglich sind, welche nicht, liegt in den Händen des behandelnden Arztes, die Sorge für gute Beschaffenheit und richtige Zubereitungsweise in denen der Verwaltung. In den Berliner städtischen Krankenhäusern sind fast vollständing übereinstimmende Diätvorschriften gegeben, nach denen die Verpflegung der Kranken, sowie des Personals etc. zu geschehen hat, und von denen ein Exemplar in der Anlage a hier beigefügt ist.

Ohne auf die Einzelheiten der Verpflegung selbst näher einzugehen, möchte ich hier eins der wichtigsten Nahrungsmittel, das Fleisch, herausgreifen und über die Art und Weise der Beschaffung desselben, sowie seiner Aufbewahrung und Verarbeitung in Dauerform, wie sie in unseren Krankenhäusern geübt wird, und, wie ich sie aus langjähriger Erfahrung heraus als bewährt empfehlen kann, berichten. Die Lieferung für den Fleischbedarf des Krankenhauses wird in einer engeren Submission, die unter den ersten en gros Schlächtern des Centralviehhofes, von denen bekannt ist, dass sie nur Thiere erster Qualität schlachten, ausgeschrieben wird, gewöhnlich an den billigst Liefernden vergeben. Die Vorschriften über die Qualität des zu liefernden Fleisches, sowie über die Auswahl u. s. w. der einzelnen Fleischstücke finden sich in der beiliegenden Anlage b. niedergelegt. Die Controle darüber, dass das Fleisch in vorgeschriebener Güte geliefert wird, führt der von der Stadt Berlin angestellte Director der städtischen Fleischschau auf dem städtischen Central Vieh- und Schlachthof resp. sein Vertreter, der aus der Zahl der dort fungirenden Thierärzte gewählt wird. Jedes zur Lieferung für das Krankenhaus bestimmte Thier wird einem dieser Herren lebend vorgeführt und zunächst untersucht und begutachtet, nicht entsprechendes sofort zurückgewiesen, darauf unter seiner Controle geschlachtet und, falls es nach nochmaliger Untersuchung der einzelnen Theile den vorgeschriebenen Bedingungen entspricht, von dem controlirenden Director resp. seinem Stellvertreter gestempelt und ausserdem mit einer den Stempel des Krankenhauses tragenden Plombe versehen. Durch diese Einrichtung wird die Verwaltung, soweit dies überhaupt möglich ist, vor einer Uebervortheilung von Seiten des Lieferanten geschützt.

Zertheilung des gelieferten Fleisches, sowie Verarbeitung desselben zu Schinken, Wurst u. dergl. besorgt ein im Dienste des Krankenhauses stehender Fleischer; sämmtliche Fleischwaaren, die hier consumirt werden, werden von diesem Fleischer hergestellt, Nichts von auswärtigen Lieferanten bezogen. Dieser Beschaffungsmodus bietet, abgesehen von den pecuniären Vortheilen, die der Anstalt aus ihm erwachsen, die *Garantie, dass nur gesundes Fleisch in guter Qualität zur Wurstfabrikation etc.* zur Verwendung kommt, dass also auch das hergestellte Fabrikat von ausgezeichneter Beschaffenheit ist.

Frisch geschlachtetes Fleisch eignet sich bekanntlich nicht zur sofortigen Verwendung bei der Speisenbereitung, da es in diesem Zustande gekocht oder gebraten hart und zäh wird, man muss dasselbe vielmehr einige (6–8) Tage liegen lassen, ehe man es verbraucht.

Für diesen Zweck sind Aufbewahrungsräume nöthig, sogenannte Fleischkammern, in denen es die entsprechende Zeit hindurch verwahrt wird. Von der richtigen Construction dieser Aufbewahrungsräume hängt es wesentlich ab, dass das Fleisch vor dem Verderben geschützt und in seiner Qualität nicht verschlechtert wird und es muss deshalb grade in grossen Anstalten, wo grosse Fleischmengen vorräthig zu halten sind, ein grosser Werth auf die zweckentsprechende Einrichtung dieser Kammern gelegt werden. Eins der besten Conservirungsmittel für Fleisch ist die Kälte und zwar in Form fortwährend zugeführter kalter, aber auch möglichst trokner Luft; es wird indess nur wenig Krankenhäuser geben, die sich den Luxus einer Kaltluftmaschine leisten können und das directe Einbringen von Eis in die Vorrathskammern schützt nicht vor dem sogenannten Beschlagen und Schmierigwerden des Fleisches, d. h. vor der Ansiedelung und schnellen Verbreitung von Schimmelpilzen auf der Oberfläche, wodurch eine Entwerthung desselben herbeigeführt wird. Am besten conservirt man das Fleisch, ohne der Aufstellung mehr oder minder kostspieliger Apparate benöthigt zu sein, nach unseren Erfahrungen in Räumen mit unausgesetzter Luftcirculation, die am einfachsten durch Offenhalten der mit Drahtgaze versehenen Fenster und Anbringung entsprechend grossen angeheizten Absaugeschloten erzielt wird. Wände, Decken und Fussböden müssen so gehalten sein, dass sie leicht abgewaschen, desinficirt und die letzteren direct entwässert werden können. In diesen Räumen werden die Fleischtheile einzeln, so dass sie sich nicht berühren und in Folge dessen von allen Seiten von der Luft umspült werden, aufgehängt. Es ist ferner nöthig, alle frische Schnittflächen, sowie alle feuchte Oberflächen des Fleisches sofort mit reinen trockenen Leinentüchern abzutrocknen, um keine feuchten Nährböden für die Ansiedelung von Mikroorganismen zu schaffen; die zum Trockenreiben des Fleisches benutzten Tücher, sind vorher durch Dampf zu sterilisiren und nach jedesmaliger Verwendung zu reinigen.

Ein unerlässliches Erforderniss für jedes Krankenhaus, das immer noch nicht genügend gewürdigt wird, ist das Vorhandensein von genügend grossen zweckentsprechend angelegten und eingerichteten *Desinfectionsvorkehrungen* zum Desinficiren der Krankenwäsche sowohl, wie der von den Kranken mitgebrachten Kleidungsstücke (*auf die speciell ein ganz besonderer Werth gelegt werden muss*) und der im Krankenhause benutzten Anzüge. Leider findet man auch heute noch selbst in neuerbauten grossen Krankenhäusern, wie

beispielsweise biz vor Kurzem in dem neuen allgemeinen Krankenhause der Stadt Hamburg in Eppendorf zu diesem Zweck Heiss-
luftapparate, obwohl doch längst durch Robert Koch's grundlegende
Versuche, die zum grössten Theil in unserem Krankenhause angestellt wurden, die Unwirksamkeit dieser Art der Desinfection festgestellt ist. Als bestes und sicherstes Desinfectionsmittel für
Effecten ist strömender Wasserdampf von mindestens 100° Celsius
Temperatur anzusehen und nur solche Apparate, in denen dieser
zur Anwendung kommt, sollten zur Desinfection benutzt werden.
Die bauliche Anlage soll derartig gehalten sein, dass eine vollständige
Trennung der zu desinficirenden Gegenstände von den desinficirten
durchführbar ist. Der leichteren und billigeren Dampfbeschaffung
wegen ist es zweckmässig, sie in unmittelbarer Nähe des Kessel-
hauses zu errichten.

Die Desinfection des Verbandmaterials geschieht in kleineren Apparaten ebenfalls unter Verwendung strömenden Wasserdampfes von
mindestens 100° Celsius, die am zweckmässigsten in der chirurgischen
Abtheilung aufgestellt sind.

Zur Desinfection von Se- und Excreten, haben sich bei uns Koch-
apparate bewährt, die sich in einem der Vorräume jedes Kranken-
saales resp. Pavillons befinden und in denen, bevor man sie den
allgemeinen Canalisationsanlagen zuführt, die Excremente sowohl,
wie der Inhalt der Spei- und Uringläser abgekocht werden.

Was schliesslich den Wäschereibetrieb im Krankenhause betrifft,
so muss in erster Linie dafür gesorgt werden, dass das mit der
Wäsche beschäftigte Personal vor Ansteckung geschützt und durch
die bei dem Kochen der Wäsche sich entwickelnden Wasserdämpfe
nicht übermässig belästigt wird. Das erstere geschieht wie oben
besprochen, durch eine vorhergehende gründliche Desinfection der
Wäsche im Desinfectionsapparate; die Belästigung durch Wasserdämpfe vermeidet man durch Benutzung hoher continuirlich mit vor-
gewärmter frischer Luft versorgter Waschräume, die durch ange-
heizte Schlote gut und schnell entlüftet werden können. Am
empfehlenswerthesten ist der Betrieb mit Maschinen, wie er jetzt
wohl auch überall durchgeführt wird. Das Trocknen der Wäsche
in stark erwärmten Räumen während der kälteren Jahreszeit ist als
ungemein schädigend auf die Gesundheit der dabei beschäftigten
Personen wirkend, was ich aus eigener Erfahrung bestätigen kann,
gänzlich zu verwerfen; an Stelle dessen sind Trockenmaschinen
(nicht Tirvirs, Schieber zum Herausziehen, welche unnütz Platz

wegnehmen und durch ausströmende Wärme das Bedienungs-Personal belästigen) in denen bei sehr reger Ventilation bei ca. 35° R. getrocknet wird, zu beschaffen.

Ich habe in dem Vorstehenden nur vereinzelte Punkte aus dem grossen Gebiete der Krankenhausverwaltung cursorisch streifen können, möge das Wenige, was ich geboten und das, zunächst an einheimische deutsche Verhältnisse anknüpfend und auf diese Bezug nehmend, schliesslich wohl auch für ausländische zu verwerthen ist, freundliche Aufnahme finden, mögen auch speziell die kurze Besprechung einiger Zweige der Krankenhaus-Hygiene Anregung geben, sich mehr und mehr mit dieser letzteren zu beschäftigen und zu ihrem weiteren Ausbau beizutragen.

THE RELATION OF TRAINING SCHOOLS TO HOSPITALS.

By Miss L. L. Dock,

Assistant Superintendent of Nurses, The Johns Hopkins Hospital, Baltimore, Md.

The establishment of training schools in America dates back only twenty-one years, and the entire modern system of trained nursing, beginning with the foundation of Kaiserswerth in 1827, is not yet sixty years old, Hospitals, on the other hand, have existed for hundreds of years. In this, the present day, training schools are numbered by the score, and each year sees new ones opened, as one hospital after another falls into line and issues its circular announcing that "arrangements have been made to provide two years training to women desirous of learning the art of caring for the sick." Did the hospital, then, call the training school into existence? Strangely enough, it did not, though the two seem now so fundamentally united. The training school idea did not originate within the hospital, but was grafted upon it by the efforts of a few inspired ones outside, who saw the terrible need of the sick, who knew the inadequacy of the care they received, and who bravely knocked at the hospital doors, first closed, but gradually opening more and more widely.

The mutual need of one for the other was not, at the outset, equally felt by both. The hospital was absolutely necessary to the school; the school was *not* necessary to the hospital, according to the crude and ignorant idea of what was sufficient for the sick, under which hospitals had been mismanaged for centuries. Good nursing is indeed necessary for the best results and for the fully perfected work of the hospital, and it was to this truth that different honored members of the medical profession bore witness long before the time when the half unwilling hospital accepted the training school on sufferance. The first attitude of the school was, therefore, that of an applicant, and its work experimental. After a few years trial it has so well proved itself that the hospital is now the one to hold out inducements, and the consequent growth of the school has been so phenomenally rapid as to give rise on the one hand to congratulations, and on the other to the question: is it built on a strong foundation?

A study of the present conditions existing between hospitals and training schools is at first sight dispiriting. In their relations to each other may be discovered a formlessness, a lack of tradition, an adoption of hasty and tentative methods, and an acceptance of imperfect results, for which the training school is often blamed, though much of the fault lies with the hospital. But discouragement over this state of things, though natural, need not be severe, when we remember that the hospital has had hundreds of years in which to develop, while the training school has had but little over half a century. Medicine is old, while nursing, though one of the most ancient of occupations, is the very youngest of professions. Moreover, on closer observation of what seems at first a heterogeneous mass, there may be seen in it elements of order and strength and permanence. There are three points of view from which the relation of the school to the hospital should be considered. The first shows an outline of the material and financial connection between the two, and considers the value of the school as an economic factor in the history of the hospital. The second sees the school as a moral force. The third faces the responsibility of the hospital to the school, and the way in which the school meets the demands of the hospital.

The training schools of America may be broadly separated, as to their outward form, into two classes: those which are an integral part of the hospital, and those which are independently organized and attached to the hospital by contract. The first is quite the larger class, and in it, with but few exceptions, are found the schools established by those hospitals in which, from their general characteristics, one would naturally expect to find expression to some degree of the reforming spirit of the times; the private and endowed hospital, church, college, or university; and a small number of municipal hospitals.

The independently organized schools were the pioneers. First in the line of advance, they most triumphantly illustrate the moral force at work in the development, still rudimentary, of nursing. These are the schools which, by the courage and goodness of women preeminently, have been affixed to those hospitals that need them most and want them least—the city or county hospitals, where local politics grow at the expense of the neglected sick poor—in all ugliness, contemptuous of disinterested work, and hating to be interfered with. Individual ability and determination alone have made it possible to force the purifying influence of the training school into these places; for it may be safely asserted that in no instance has the political element of any municipal hospital ever voluntarily introduced reform into the nursing, or yielded to it save on irresistible pressure brought to bear from outside by those who had no political capital to make, who feared no one, and who were determined to succeed.

No stronger contrast could be shown than that between typical schools of these two classes: the one established by an enlightened and humanitarian hospital—a peaceful existence secured to it; the other a pioneer—its position insecure, its history full of exciting vicissitudes. In the one instance may be found union in an almost complete degree. There may be identity of interests and of aims; a recognition of mutual benefits; a sense of mutual obligation; a reciprocal feeling of personal pride, admiration and attachment. The other is an example of the "incorporated union," which Gladstone declares can never become perfect. The training school attached to the political hospital can never truly become one with it until in the evolution of the civic virtues local politics either change their nature or are removed from the field.

The standard and aims of the school are absurdities to the hospital controlled by politics; the methods and tone of the hospital are odious to the school. From first to last its history is one of struggle and strenuous effort to obtain decent conditions, to resist degradation, and to do good work in the face of obstructions and difficulties always great and sometimes enormous. At the same time the line must be drawn with prudence, for it is in the power of the hospital to terminate its agreement, or to make conditions such that it is impossible for the school to continue its work. Such a course annihilates the training school, and shows the bare hardness of the fact, once stated, that it is not necessary to the life, only to the improvement of the hospital. This possible destruction of the school is not an imaginary catastrophe; on the contrary it has occurred in more than one instance. As, however, not all political hospitals, even the most unscrupulous, are immediately likely to overthrow their training schools, and as not all private hospitals realize the ideal, there are some advantages claimed by the independent school over the others. For one thing, it is possible for it to become (as one of our largest schools is at this moment) self-supporting; always a more dignified position than that of being supported, and to be so recognized. Moreover, it is free to live its own life, uninfluenced by what may be cramped and mean in that of the hospital, and to develop unhindered in whatever lines of progress may open up to it. But among those which are the personal property of hospitals of illiberal and narrow policy, what half-dead training schools we see! their scope and possibilities closely repressed, their educational advantages selfishly restricted, their outlook limited and their influence a drag. How easily are the rightful claims of the school then sacrificed for the benefit of the hospital, and how difficult to defend themselves against injustice and even oppression when the relation is only that of owner and property. But beyond all this, the independent school has this advantage over the other, that the very isolation and difficulty of its work brings out and strengthens in it those hardy virtues, endurance, frugality, self-denial, and courage, which are not easily cultivated in a softer atmosphere.

Of the internal dissensions that sometimes mar the relations of the training school and hospital, there are, broadly speaking, two sources: one is a weak government of the school itself; the other is the failure to separate clearly the medical and the nursing provinces.

The wide-spread want of a sound conception of the idea of discipline is a direct cause of some of the most unsatisfactory conditions existing between hospital and school. The most blurred and wavering lines in the whole structure are directly traceable to this fundamental weakness. It is perhaps natural enough that the women who enter the schools should have rudimentary ideas on the subject, but it might reasonably be expected that this imperfection should not be found in those who undertake to govern them ; yet it is unquestionably true that in the experience of most schools there have come times when it was vividly realized that boards of directors, women's committees, and even the medical staff themselves, though all strong on discipline as a theory, are as broken reeds when the practical question comes up of maintaining it at the cost of some difficulty. The organization of a training school is and must be military. It is not and cannot be democratic. Absolute and unquestioning obedience must be the foundation of the nurse's work, and to this end complete subordination of the individual to the work as a whole is as necessary for her as for the soldier. This can only be attained by a systematic grading of rank, a clear, definite chain of responsibility, and one sole source of authority, transmitted in a straight line, not scattered about through boards and committees, but concentrated in the head of the school as their representative and delegate. They cannot represent themselves ; they cannot do her work, nor exert her influence. She must do this herself, and there is no danger of making her an autocrat if they will consistently maintain their own just and true position, that of wise advisers, or judges if need be. Most unsound is the policy of the hospital which habitually interferes in the affairs of the school ; and the most undignified expression of weakness of this kind is that which gathers up from women in training, who have not yet proved their merit, opinions, information, or complaints upon school or hospital matters.

Leaving out of sight the dishonorable element in this practice, it is at once evident that all discipline must be at an end if authority is thus handed over to the ranks ; yet this fatal short-sightedness has hampered the work of more than one school.

To say that there are any lines on which the medical profession may not control the nursing world may sound revolutionary. It is not so. On the contrary, in the clear perception of what those lines are rests the only security for future order and harmony of action. It may be claimed that if the military idea is the basis of the school, the members of the medical profession being undoubtedly the superior officers, should properly control the school throughout its entire course, and even in its internal management, and that the whole subject of the teaching, training and discipline of nurses should be at the discretion of medicine. This might hold good except for one simple yet radical point of difference. The private soldier in the ranks and the officer in command have the same profession. The officer is also a soldier and knows every detail of the common soldier's work and life. The nurse and the physician have different professions. The doctor is not a nurse, and only now and then is one found who fairly comprehends the actual matter-of-fact realities of the training school. On this fundamental difference rests the claim of the school to be ruled, as an educative and disciplinary body, by those of its own origin. For another reason the separation of the medical power from training school affairs should be rigidly enforced, and that is the destructive effect of personal influence on the idea of duty. In hospitals about us may be seen the results of giving the hospital staff any practical hold over the school. What, for instance, is the consequence of allowing young internes to choose their own undergraduate head-nurses? The standard of the work is at once lowered by the introduction of the personal element. The pupil nurses are exposed to the temptation of seeking the favor of individuals. Partizan cliques invariably form, whose self-interest may be directly opposed to the best interests of the hospital and its nursing work ; and promotion on a true merit-basis is utterly and at once impossible. In the struggle against influences of this kind the school is likely to be unjustly condemned by the hospital as troublesome. Arbitrary, insubordinate, its head as the natural enemy of the medical staff; a false position into which, by unfairness and jealousy, she is sometimes ungenerously forced.

On one field only does the school properly come under the command of the medical profession, and that is in the direct care of the sick. Here indeed the command is absolute. The whole purpose of the school centers around this point, and the pride of the well-drilled nurse is to make this service perfect.

Now for the first time in the history of medical science can its orders be carried out faithfully, fully, and at all hours. The uselessness of expecting such obedience from even intelligent persons who have not been trained is well illustrated by the remark of a lady of position and education, concerning the orders given her by the physician for her child's diet. " I shall do just half of what the doctor said," she observed, " as I always make a discount for each doctor's own particular fad."

This obedience to orders, founded on principle and animated by an intelligent interest, is the dominant characteristic of the new system of nursing, and is the secret of its success in its professional work. Without it the most desirable and charming qualities would be useless to the nurse; but with it, the value of her practical work to the hospital is at once and widely demonstrated.

There is much evidence to show that the material prosperity of the hospital is largely due to the work of the training school. To just what extent this is true would perhaps be impossible to say, for where a dawning rationalism in medicine, antisepsis in surgery, a growing intelligence of public opinion, and trained nursing are contemporaneous, each stimulating and being stimulated by the others, no one could candidly ascribe results to one isolated influence. Yet, whether it be only a coincidence or not, in this country, at least, a definite impetus and advance in hospital work dates from the foundation of trained nursing. The testimony received from over forty hospitals is unanimous on this point, not one exception having been met with. "Our results are better both in medicine and surgery," they say; "the work of our hospital has extended in every direction. There is a marked diminution of the popular dread of hospitals. Private patients come in greater numbers, and many ascribe their willingness to enter to the presence of the nurses. The difference in the general comfort and happiness of the patients alone would be enough, if there were nothing more, to secure the gratitude of the hospital to the school, while the difference in the death-rate marks an era in the treatment of the sick."

To illustrate these general statements, the experience of two small hospitals, selected at random, may be cited. One, a hospital for children, had for years under the old regime the character of an orphan's home. Thirty or forty little ones with chronic diseases collected in it; acute or serious cases were rare; operations infrequent; public interest was languid. Within three years after the introduction of trained nursing, the medical staff and general management being unchanged, new wards were built, an operating room was added, and an active service of acute medical and surgical cases kept 80 beds constantly filled and constantly changing. The other is a hospital for gynecological and obstetrical patients. In former times only those applied who had no other resource, and half the beds were empty. The nursing was reformed. A few years after the change the statistics showed in one year 38 operations and 143 births; the same number of years after the change, 144 operations and 257 births. Such facts show the practical value of the school in a strong light, and tend to modify the statement sometimes made by hospital boards that the school is an expensive luxury. The difference

made in the value of the hospital as a field for clinical medicine is
alone sufficient to repay the debt of the school.   The actual cost of
the school is not always easy to demonstrate.   Hospitals supporting
their own schools do not as a rule keep separate accounts, and the
only definite statistics to be found are those of the independent
schools, which receive so much from the hospital for services
rendered.   The old plan of nursing cost much less than the new.
Nurses were paid from $12 to $20 a month ; two or three were considered enough for 30 or 40 patients, for as they could do but little,
but little was expected of them.   Their lodgings were in any spare
corner of the hospital, and their table was coarse and cheap.   But in
the race of competition this economical system had to be given up
for one that would give better results, and the hospitals had to consider the practical question of how to get their nursing done.   To
secure graduate work would be at this stage an impossibility.   The
supply is not sufficient; moreover, the graduate who receives on an
average of $20 a week at private duty, naturally will not toil for an
hospital for a smaller sum, unless some inducement is offered, such
as a position of responsibility, or further training in the line of some
specialty.   Even leaving the money out of the question, it would be
precarious to attempt the nursing of a general hospital, or even a
ward, with graduates, for their different methods would produce
irregularity and unevenness in the work, and their independence of
the hospital would permit untimely changes and general insecurity.
The training school offers the hospital the most practicable way out
of the difficulty.   The expenses are undoubtedly large in comparison,
for while the actual sum paid monthly to the pupils as an allowance
is, per capita, smaller than that paid the old-time nurses, yet the
number necessary to do the work according to a revised standard is
fully three times as large.   Moreover, comfortable and healthful surroundings and proper food are now understood to be necessary provisions to make for nurses, and finally, some expense must be
incurred for theoretical instruction, so that the whole difference in
cost may be roughly estimated as about 1 to 5.   Nevertheless this
plan offers the hospital distinct advantages.   The training school is
a flexible instrument, and though more expensive than the old
method, is less so than graduate nursing would be.   The promise
of an education secures a steady supply of intelligent women, thus
eliminating all uncertainty on that score.   The discipline and strict
subordination of the school make it possible for the hospital to exact

from it an amount of work which it would be quite impossible to demand from women over whom it had no special hold; while the chain of responsibility and the careful supervision of the school secure an average quality of work as good, if not even better than that which would be obtained from nurses working merely as employees.

Practically, then, the hospital secures nursing for $12 a month on its pay-roll, which at its market value would bring at least $15 a week, while the living expenses are little or no greater in the one case than in the other, the cost of lectures and educational appliances being the only additional outlay in the support of the undergraduate school. There are those hospitals which, in the desire to economize, find ways of minimizing cost at the expense of the school. The outlay for teaching purposes is cut down, and the number of nurses reduced by giving to each the longest possible hours of duty. Yet in comparison with hospitals and training schools in other countries, it is gratifying to find how much more generous a spirit is, on the whole, shown in those of our own country. Among the foremost there are comparatively few, and among the most prominent only one or two, that make their nurses a source of revenue by working them outside. The returns on this point are imperfect, yet are sufficient to show there are many small hospitals compelled by actual poverty to bring in an income from private duty, and others where poverty is less evident and where the school is evidently founded on a mercenary basis; while among those that are larger, yet still not in the front rank, one reports earnings covering one-eighth of its expenses; two earn two-thirds each; three earn one-half each; while two schools report earnings which cover almost the entire cost of their maintenance and tuition. In other words, these different schools bring in incomes varying from $300 to $5000 and $6000 a year. In the two latter cases it is quite evident that the schools, besides giving the hospitals an amount and quality of work which the hospitals could not possibly secure if they had to pay for it, really support themselves and pay for their own tuition at the same time—a rather remarkable arrangement, one must confess, and one which the hospital surveys with the utmost complacency, keeping the school in the meantime in an attitude of the strictest subserviency, as though the hospital were the benefactor and the school the grateful recipient of benefits. A survey, then, of the whole subject compels one to believe that financially the school is not the debtor of the hospital. Although it is costly, yet its economic value is not measured by the dollars spent upon it. Its part in building up or adding to the prestige of the hospital is not computed and paid for, yet it is vast, and has a definite money value in the returns of the hospital.

Of all the attributes of the school its moral strength is the most easily demonstrable, and its reformatory work is the part of its whole work in which it can most securely stand on its own merits. Other forces may seek to divide with it the diminished death-rate and better results in medicine and surgery, but the changes wrought in the moral atmosphere of the once foul old hospitals we have all known of are peculiarly and entirely its own. Those who know the internal affairs of institutions are aware that people outside can form no idea of what conditions formerly existed within the walls of, say, some great city hospital where the city paupers were collected. The misery of the neglected sick was one thing, the depravity and moral degradation another. The one could be described; the other was indescribable. The badness was worse, even, than the sufferings of the sick, for they ended with death. No nurse who has had some such hospital service could ever tell all of her experience, yet she has gone in and worked through many such places, and they can never again return to what they were before. In these old hospitals the medical profession labored unselfishly over the diseases of the body; ministers of the church passed in and out and strove with souls; charitable women brought flowers and food and a temporary cheerfulness, but degraded and vile they remained throughout until the youth, strength and energy of the training school assailed them and, by coming to live among them, transformed them. "This place used to be like hell," said an old hospital patient to the newly established nurse, "but now it is like heaven."

Even among hospitals of the better class have been found many where, under an outward appearance of decorum, there was rampant a coarse vulgarity, or an utter lack of principle, or a spirit of tyranny, from the highest to the lowest. These have presented the most difficult and delicate tasks of regeneration, for such evils are subtle, resistant, and well organized. Many battles have been fought by the training schools against all these hostile forces; battles of which few people will ever know. Many victories have been gained, each one of which makes the future easier and more promising. Many nurses have laid down their health, or their lives, in such struggles, as uncomplainingly as the soldier in time of war.

The last division of my subject, the responsibility of the hospital to the training school, and the way in which the school meets the demands of the hospital, will be so forcibly treated in another paper that it is not necessary to take it up here. It will be shown that the whole responsibility of the hospital is to give the school a thoroughly good education and time in which to assimilate it. It will be shown that the shortcomings of the school are largely due to imperfect preparatory training, and to the crowding of work and study into the short period of two years time. With a fuller comprehension on the part of the hospital of the real work and the actual purposes and the aims of the training school, and with renewed patience and energy on the part of the school, there will gradually die away that mistrust on the one hand, and something like aggressiveness on the other, which have marked the relative relations of many hospitals and schools, and which are already beginning to disappear. In the cordial co-operation of the future, as outlined in the paper mentioned, lies the hope of those who are working toward what they know to be the possibilities of nursing.

DISCUSSION.

MISS LETT, of Chicago: In regard to the trouble between the training schools and the hospitals, I think that the matter of discipline is not clearly understood by the hospital authorities, although, as Miss Dock says, theoretically they are willing to preach it but they do not care to practice it. And then I think a good deal of trouble may come by the selection of a head of a training school. They do not take sufficient trouble to get those of experience. To overcome that difficulty, the period of training in our training schools ought to be longer than two years; it ought to be prolonged to at least two and a half years.

MISS DARCHE, of New York: I merely wish to say that I think the paper is conclusive about matters of discipline. There is only one way to settle that, and that is the authorities should put at the head of the training department some one they have confidence in. If they have not confidence in her, remove her, but let her have the management of matters of discipline in her department. It seems to me that would settle the whole matter; if they have not confidence in the head, remove her.

DR. HURD, of Baltimore: I am very much of the opinion that there is really no division of interest between the hospital and the training school, and I deprecate myself the statement on the part of any one that there is. , The only object of the hospital is to take care of the sick; the only reason of the existence of the training school is to furnish a proper training in taking care of the sick; there really can be no opposition in the ends which both the hospital and the training school have in view. I have always regarded it most unfortunate that the original training schools were outside the hospitals, and that one of those training schools still regards itself as a municipality outside of the hospital, with full authority to criticize hospital methods, and to complain of them without making any special effort to better them. The attitude of that school has constantly been inimical to the hospital with which it is connected. I believe there should be the greatest identity of interest between the hospital and the training school; the hospital ought not to ask anything unreasonable of the school, and the school ought not to ask anything unreasonable of the hospital. My own view is this, that the great difficulty has been in not giving enough authority to the superintendent of the nurses' training school. I believe it is the duty of the hospital authorities to make no mistake in selecting the superintendent of nurses; and when selected, she should have their heartiest co-operation. Allow her to carry out her own plans and ideas; let her select and discipline her nurses, and make her responsible for the well-being of the school. If she proves to be not the right person, get another; but do not allow the board of trustees of the hospital to interfere in the internal management of the training school. For my own part, I believe that the hospital and the training school should constantly work together, that nothing can hurt the training school without hurting the hospital, and that nothing can help the school which injures the hospital; and that training school and hospital should go on together.

The CHAIRMAN: I will simply say that if the superintendent of the training school is perfect, knowing her own business, and having full power of discipline, and is a lady of tact and education, the whole business must necessarily be left entirely to her; that such a woman never does have any particular trouble. But I say that such women are extremely rare, just as men who are qualified to take charge of and command a big establishment are extremely rare. The difficulty comes not with getting your theoretical set of rules and regulations giving the superintendent of nurses full authority, but it comes sometimes when she finds it necessary to discipline some nurse who is perhaps attractive in manner and ways, and who is particularly satisfactory to some of the trustees or to some of the medical staff; that nurse appeals—she has been treated with great injustice—and the appeal comes to people who do not know anything about the matter.

In my capacity as director of a hospital I have that sort of appeal come to me sometimes; occasionally, once in a while, I think—twice, perhaps, I thought—they were a little hard; but nevertheless the rule of the superintendent of the training school goes with me. And if that is not satisfactory, why then we must get another superintendent.

THE RELATION OF HOSPITALS TO MEDICAL EDUCATION.

By Henry M. Hurd, M. D.,

Superintendent of The Johns Hopkins Hospital, Baltimore, Md.

It is not my purpose to argue the duty of hospitals to promote medical teaching. They have always contributed to it, and always will, in an increasing degree, as medical education becomes better organized and more efficient. The hospital, whether avowedly so or not, has always been a school of medicine, sometimes to the few who were attending physicians, resident physicians or internes, and sometimes, and now, I am glad to say, more often, to those who are pursuing medical studies. The relation of hospitals to medical education has been reciprocal for good. Medical teaching has improved hospital work, and hospital work, on the other hand, has improved medical teaching. Neither can exist without the other. It is my purpose in this brief paper to point out methods whereby hospitals can best subserve medical teaching, and to emphasize the duty of promoting it. A hospital which does not contribute to the advancement of medical knowledge, by bringing the results of its investigations and experience to the training of medical students, in the plastic stage of their education, fails to attain its highest good or to surround itself with the brightest investigators. The duty being apparent, to point out the best method of attaining the desired end must be the sole object of the present inquiry.

1. *Pathological Institutes.*—First in importance I would place the organization of a good pathological institute in connection with every

hospital. By this I mean much more than an autopsy room and a museum for the preservation of morbid specimens. These are valuable, but their work is not of prime importance compared with what may be accomplished by systematic investigations in all branches of pathological study. Facilities should be afforded for the study of every morbid product. There should be opportunities for systematic bacteriological examination of pus, serous effusions, the products of inflammation, the bodily secretions and excretions, false membranes, new growths and the like. The diagnosis of diphtheria and of follicular tonsillitis, for example, should here be made by cultures, coverslip preparations and the microscope. The different forms of peritonitis should be differentiated similarly. The effusions of pleurisy should be studied bacteriologically to determine the presence or absence of the tubercle bacillus. Malarial fever should be differentiated from other forms of continued fever by the presence of the plasmodium. The micrococcus lanceolatus, otherwise known as the pneumococcus, should be searched for in pneumonia and cerebrospinal meningitis. Such studies are impossible unless rooms are provided, specially fitted up with apparatus, instruments and trained observers constantly at hand for the purpose. These studies give a definiteness to diagnosis by excluding possible diseases of other origin, and certainty to prognosis.

The microscopic study of tumors and new growths while an operation is in progress and before its completion is of equal value. Three examples drawn from actual occurrences in a Baltimore hospital will serve to make my meaning clearer. A patient with a suspicious abdominal tumor, presumably malignant, had submitted to an exploratory operation, and a frozen section while she was on the operating table, and before the operation was completed, showed the growth to be tubercular in character. The cavity of the abdomen was drained and washed out with a sterilized salt solution, and the patient made a good recovery. A second patient seemed to be suffering from a simple abscess of the breast, but a bacteriological examination of the contents of the abscess cavity showed that the inflammation was tubercular in character, and led to the examination of the surrounding tissues, which were found to be filled with tubercle bacilli. A radical operation for the removal of these diseased tissues then followed, and a condition was found present which justified a grave prognosis. In another case a culture made during a severe abdominal operation subsequently showed that a chronic peritonitis had been caused by a virulent streptococcus, and led immediately to the isolation and separate nursing of the patient to prevent the infection of the ward. Such instances are of daily occurrence, and the wisdom of these expert examinations is fully established by repeated experience.

In dressings, also, subsequent to surgical operations, similar sources of infection are revealed by bacteriological examinations, and the communication of infection to other patients may be prevented by the knowledge thus acquired. This work, while of prime importance, ought not to impede the true work of a pathological laboratory, which is to study the origin, course and effects of disease upon every organ of the human body. Every large hospital ought to have a paid pathologist whose whole time should be given to this form of study, and he should be provided with a sufficient number of assistants to do this work thoroughly. Diseased tissues and organs should be examined in gross at the autopsy table, and afterwards the material should be studied in frozen sections and by hardened specimens. Cultures should also be made post mortem of all products of inflammation, to determine their precise character. These studies clear up obscure diagnoses and lead to the more successful treatment of other cases.

2. *Clinical Laboratories.*—Every hospital ought also to have a clinical laboratory for blood examination, urinary analysis, the examination of the stomach contents, and the examination of feces and sputum. The blood should be examined as a matter of routine in all forms of wasting disease. The value of the methods of Ehrlich in the different forms of leukæmia is attested daily by practical observation. The differentiation of malarial from typhoid or other forms of continued fever is frequently only possible when the plasmodium has been demonstrated in the blood. The importance of a bacteriological examination of cholera-stools for the presence of the comma bacillus has been recently demonstrated in the late cholera epidemic in Europe. The equal importance of searching dysenteric stools for the presence of amœbæ coli has been demonstrated many times in the clinical laboratory of the Johns Hopkins Hospital during the past year. Abscesses in the liver and lungs and one jaw abscess have thus been shown to be dependent upon this protozoan. The confusion which exists in the profession to-day regarding malarial hæmaturia can only be cleared up by similar expert examinations. In such clinical laboratories syphilis often needs to be differentiated from

tuberculosis by the microscope. In skin affections also, like urticaria, favus, the different forms of dermatitis, tinea versicolor and tuberculosis need to be similarly studied. The presence of the otomycosis aspergillus in ear affections can only be definitely shown by the microscope. The tetanus bacillus, the streptococcus of erysipelas, the staphylococcus of suppuration, and the pneumococcus of pneumonia and meningitis should also be similarly demonstrated when present. In no other manner can medical education be made definite and thorough. The day of theories and brilliant hypotheses to account for many of these diseases is past, and demonstration ought to replace them.

3. *Operating Rooms.*—Every hospital of any size, and especially a hospital to which medical students have access, should have surgical operating rooms arranged for carrying out a perfect surgical technique. Here should be consistent and constant efforts to reduce the dangers to patients from the infection of wounds to the minimum. These operating rooms should be object-lessons in thorough surgical cleanliness. There should be apparatus for hand disinfection and facilities for scrubbing and cleansing the hands. Every step in the technique of antiseptic surgery should be carefully prescribed and followed. It is now evident that infection of wounds does not come through the air or from atmospheric conditions, but rather from actual contact. Pus-producing germs gain access to wounds at the hands of the operator or his assistants, or by infected instruments or ligatures, or through infected skin-stitches, or by subsequent dressings. Hence it is of the utmost importance that the technique pursued in every hospital operating room be thorough and consistent to the end, that every person may know the reason of the procedures adopted. Students and physicians should be trained to appreciate understandingly what is harmful and to be avoided, and what is harmless and permissible. It may be asserted, with confidence of no successful contradiction, that in the technique of many surgeons unnecessary precautions are frequently taken, and necessary precautions are as frequently omitted, from a lack of adequate knowledge of the true sources of infection. These can only be adequately taught by bacteriological methods. Ligatures, instruments, bandages, and all forms of dressings, should be sterilized in such a way as to meet every bacteriological requirement. Cultures taken from the first dressings made subsequent to an operation should not grow upon any form of culture media. Experiments which have been made in wound infec-

tion have clearly demonstrated its sources, and its methods of prevention. Each operating room should be as carefully arranged to carry out antiseptic precautions as the laboratory of the bacteriologist. More than this may also be asserted. Every operating room ought to pursue careful and systematic experiments upon hand disinfection. No one believes that an ideal excellence has yet been attained. These fruitful experiments are alone possible in large operating rooms, with frequent operations and abundant facilities for carrying on the work thoroughly. It is most gratifying to call to your attention the fact that two large operating rooms have lately been constructed in New York with every facility for this systematic work. If they contribute, as they undoubtedly will, to the simplification and perfection of surgical technique, their erection will fully justify the outlay, large as it may seem to the unthinking critic.

4. *Photographic Rooms.*—An equally important part of the educational outfit of a general hospital should be a well constructed and well arranged room for photography. Here medical men should be trained to do photographic work in the various departments of hospital service. Each man should be taught the manipulation of cameras and photographic plates, and should learn methods of developing, printing, enlarging, etc. Photo-micrography has proven a very disappointing branch of photography. A poor drawing which accurately portrays what the observer sees is generally much to be preferred to the most finely finished micro-photograph with its blotches of color and flattened surface. Not so, however, with what may be termed gross medical photography. Its field of usefulness is apparently limitless. Many surgical conditions should be photographed upon the spot, even while an operation is in progress. The rapidity and accuracy with which newly discovered or newly recognized forms of disease have been made known to the medical public are well shown by the disease known as acromegaly. Although this disease was first differentiated and described by Marie in 1886, its peculiar facies became at once familiar to physicians throughout the world by the excellent photographic reproductions which were distributed, and to-day it is easily recognized wherever found, by medical men who have never been shown a case. In a similar manner cases of myxœdema and the various forms of paralysis have been accurately portrayed, to the great advantage of the student of medicine. Photographs of skin diseases, deformities, muscular atrophies and hypertrophies, ulcers, tumors, aneurisms, surgical

operations, surgical methods and surgical dressings, portray these conditions much more clearly and satisfactorily than pages of description. In many instances these representations are sufficient to enable the observer who has not seen the case, to confirm the diagnosis.

5. *Charts and Graphic Representations, Histories.*—Allied to photography are the various forms of charts and graphic representations. These should be made with absolute accuracy and regularity, and should form permanent records in the hospital. The same is true of medical histories, which ought to be made up daily, at the bedside. Such medical histories should be classified, indexed, catalogued, and rendered accessible, so that any fact of medical interest may be referred to at a moment's notice. There should be a medical staff large enough to do this work thoroughly well. The influence of these careful records upon medical knowledge can hardly be estimated; their greater influence in training medical men who are connected with hospitals to habits of careful, painstaking, exhaustive observation and faithful records of the same is undeniable.

6. *Dispensary Work.*—The position of carefully conducted medical work in dispensaries or departments for out-patients, in training medical men, is well recognized. The patients who present themselves for treatment at these clinics more nearly represent the patients with whom physicians come into daily contact than ordinary hospital patients. Hence the same necessity in dispensary practice of training students in habits of quick, accurate and thorough diagnosis and of painstaking records of the clinical facts which are obtained. Clinical methods and clinical records ought to be as systematic and complete in the dispensary as in the hospital. The facilities afforded by a dispensary for the study of physical diagnosis are, if anything, more valuable than those of a hospital. The same is true of the opportunity for learning the methods of diagnosis in minor surgery and the application of the ordinary surgical dressings. Practical work in the diagnosis and treatment of diseases of women is here feasible and, under competent supervision, often proves most valuable. The opportunities for studying the specialties of medical practice are also of extreme value and should be utilized regularly. Every department of a dispensary ought to be under competent expert medical supervision, and all branches should be so conducted as to promote the training of students. The practical difficulty in many dispensaries is that the clinical material is not properly utilized.

7. *Libraries, Reading Rooms, Societies and Journal Clubs.*—
Every hospital should foster a good medical library and a reading
room filled with the best and latest medical periodicals, and all
members of the staff should be expected to use them and should
have time to do so. In most hospitals the medical men are sadly
overworked, and through a superabundance of routine work lose all
time, and too often all inclination, for medical reading or study. The
advantages of a medical society and of a journal club are too obvious
to require more than a mere brief mention. These organizations
should exist in the staff of every large hospital.

8. *Medical Staff.*—A careful consideration of the subject leads me
to urge that all large hospitals be furnished with an increased medical
staff, and that the terms of service of a portion at least of the medical
men be considerably increased. It is evident to all who have watched
hospital work that the usual term of service, extending over a period
of 12, 16 or 18 months, brings active young men fresh from medical
schools into hospitals, to send them out to give place to other inexperienced young men about the time they are fitted to do independent
work. The hospital consequently suffers from the mistakes which
they make while they are receiving training, and by an inexorable
rule loses their services as soon as they are fairly well-trained to do
efficient and fruitful work. This difficulty would be removed if
arrangements could be made to give all fourth-year medical students
routine hospital duties under competent supervision. This would
train them in practical work to such an extent that when they assumed
hospital appointments they would be fitted to undertake independent
work, and could supervise the work of other fourth-year men wisely.
In each department of hospital service a chief resident should be
appointed whose term of service should extend over a period of at
least three years. This would enable him to fit himself thoroughly
for giving instruction to all assistant resident physicians and to wisely
direct their work. Such service is possible in European hospitals,
and if a similar service could be inaugurated in the leading hospitals
of this country it would mark a decided advance in hospital work.

In conclusion, I would urge the duty upon every hospital of doing
every branch of hospital work as well and as thoroughly as it can
possibly be done. If philanthropy recognizes it to be a duty to care
for the sick poor and to minister to their comfort by convenient,
well-appointed, well-ventilated and well-warmed apartments, the
same duty demands that their medical care shall be equally thor-

ough, painstaking and scientific. The best should be constantly striven for, and nothing but the best should satisfy those who are charged with their care. Every hospital should be an object-lesson in the proper care of the sick. It should demonstrate the best methods of medicine, surgery and gynecology, the most approved nursing, the best cooking for invalids and their kindest care.

DISCUSSION.

MR. BURDETT, of London.—I should like to say that I think it is very important that we should have a paper of this kind read this session. It is important because it clearly lays down and brings out clearly to the non-technical mind the reason why the cost of administering hospitals tends steadily to increase, and what those who give to hospitals really get back in return for their money. A man is very often amazed by the demands which are constantly made for more and more money, especially for buildings, and I do think that Dr. Hurd's paper will fulfil a very useful purpose, and I hope it will be printed and widely circulated among hospitals.

I should like to say further that those who are interested in seeing the result of what Dr. Hurd has referred to should certainly go to the hospital at the World's Fair. It is situated between the Fine Arts Building and the Government Building of the United States, and you will find there objects of the greatest interest to everybody who is connected with hospitals. And speaking as a practical man, and one who has visited most exhibitions during the past twenty years, I venture to say fearlessly that the exhibit in that building is the most valuable, as I believe it to be the most interesting, to scientific visitors to this city during the Fair. Dr. Billings has had a great deal to do with that exhibit, and you will see there illustrated in the most interesting manner the action of photography, and all the other appliances relating to bacteriology and the sciences which now are included in the study of medicine. I certainly do hope that many of you will go there because I believe it will give you great pleasure.

I also wish to say in reference to Dr. Cowles' paper that I believe the relations of the medical staff to hospitals must ultimately be altered materially. I attribute the great difference in the expenditure of hospitals largely to the fact that at the present time the medical staff gives gratuitous service. I hope to see the day when every medical man will be paid for the services he renders to our hospitals, and I believe with the advent of that alteration will come the enforcement of true economy, and something like a uniformity of cost in hospitals of the same class. It would confer an immense justice on the younger members of the medical profession, and I believe if you will pay the doctors to-morrow that the actual expenses of the hospital—and I am speaking as one who has worked for a great many years—would tend to be rather less than more than it is at present.

HOSPITAL ACCOUNTS AND METHODS OF BOOK-KEEPING.

By James R. Lathrop,

Superintendent of the Roosevelt Hospital, New York.

Having been requested by the Secretary of this Section of the International Congress to prepare a paper upon " Hospital Accounts and Methods of Book-keeping," I propose to comply with that request by placing before you, in as brief a manner as consistent with an intelligent showing, the methods in that direction which, after years of experience, have been found most satisfactory in the Roosevelt Hospital, of which I am Superintendent.

It will be my aim to make mention of those books which may be regarded as needful in any well organized hospital, and to illustrate the use of them by sketches submitted with this paper. The books may be enumerated thus:—

Class A.

Those which relate to Patients.

1st. A book entitled "Admission of Patients," containing a printed form of questions to be asked of each patient by the entry clerk and usually referred to as the "History on Admission." The information comprised in the form is:—

Date...................... ....
Name and Address ....
Ward ....Age ....Birthplace........ ....
Occupation.............. ....Civil Condition......... ....
Parentage...........How long in U. S.........How long in City ....

How admitted ....
Apparent ailment when admitted ....
Name and Address of Friends ....
Had Patient Valuables ....*Left*..... .... *in office* ....
Examined by Dr. ....
Discharged ....
Diagnosis at Discharge ....

2d. A register entitled "Admissions and Discharges," not alphabetically but chronologically arranged, and designed for recording
daily changes in detail, each admission and each discharge in numerical order from the date of the opening of the hospital; for example,
the first patient received into the Roosevelt hospital on the occasion
of its opening, Nov. 2, 1871, was numbered 1. The first patient discharged was also numbered 1, although the two were not identical.
In other words, the number 1 did not necessarily mean the same
patient. On the first of this month the admissions had reached a
total of 40,368, while 40,222 represented the number discharged.
Subtracting the one from the other showed the admissions to have
been 146 more than the discharges. That difference represented the
number actually remaining in the hospital on June 1st.

3d. A book entitled "Register of Patients," alphabetically arranged,
and written up daily from slips of admission and bedside cards which
accompany patients to the wards when admitted and are returned to
the office upon their discharge. The cards contain the following
items of information :—

Ward, (to which patient belongs) ....
Division, (with which connected—Medical, Surgical, or Gyneco-
    logical) ....
Name of Patient ....
Age .... *Birthplace* ....
Civil condition, (married or single) ....
Parentage .... *Occupation* ....
Years in U. S. .... *Years in City* ....

The cards are signed by the entry clerk in the name of the Superintendent when patients are sent to the wards, and when discharged
are signed by the House Physician, Surgeon, or Gynecologist, who
then records thereon the diagnosis and information as to whether
the patient had been discharged "Cured," "Improved," "Not

Improved" or " Dead." These cards furnish the means for "closing the accounts" of patients on the " Register of Patients." This book is designed, primarily, for use in readily ascertaining the presence of patients in the hospital at time of inquiry or at a prior date.

4th. A book entitled " Record of Rejected Patients," whose application for admission has, for any reason, been refused. The information therein recorded is :—

Date of Application ....

No.............(in order of application each month—thus showing how many persons have been refused admission during the month).

Name and Residence, (of applicant) ....

By whom recommended........................... ....

Date of examination ....

Where examined, (whether at the hospital or elsewhere).............

By whom examined, (what physician or surgeon)........ ....

Diagnosis. ....

Disposition of case, (that is, why rejected; whether because of lack of room or for the reason that the applicant's malady did not come within the scope of the work of the hospital, and where referred.) ....

5th. A book entitled "Daily Record," containing a census of patients in the hospital. This is written up in the entry clerk's office—the information being gained from returns made by the nurse or orderly in charge of each ward. If the returns do not agree with the number shown to be in the hospital by deducting from the number representing the last admission that number representing the last discharge (as illustrated in my reference to the book entitled " Admissions and Discharges,") an investigation is instituted to account for the difference.

6th. A book entitled " Statistics for the Annual Report." This is a record showing the nationality and sex of the discharged patients. It is written up at least once a month. The course of procedure is very simple. There are forty lines on each page of the book of discharges ; each line represents a case ; first ascertain the number of males and then of females ; the sum of both must be forty ; then learn the number of males of each nationality represented and again the number of females ; the sum of all the nationalities of both sexes must be forty. The results are tabulated in this book (" Statistics for the Annual Report") and at the end of the year are footed up, this quickly giving the desired information. In a hospital where the changes are numerous such a book is very helpful.

7th. A book entitled "Receipt Book for Effects," belonging to deceased patients and designed to show, by the signature of receiver, to whom delivered. This book is kept by the entry clerk. In another book a record is kept of valuables deposited by patients on admission.

CLASS B.

Those which relate to Officers and Employees.

1st. A book entitled "List of Officers and Employees," an alphabetical register in which the signatures of the employed are taken (at the time of their engagement) to a printed contract at the head of each page, reading:

"Contract: I, the undersigned, accept the terms herein mentioned, agree to do faithfully the work assigned to me, and to conform to all rules of the Hospital while in its employment; and it is distinctly understood and agreed, that whether I am paid by the day, week, month or year, my engagement is to terminate upon notice by the Superintendent that my services are no longer required; and, upon payment being made to me for the actual time of service rendered, I agree to accept and receipt for the same in full consideration for all demands against said institution. The Hospital reserves the right to deduct for absence from whatever cause."

In this book, in addition to the signatures of the employed, appear the following items of information:—

Name, (written by the clerk)................. ....

Employment, (to which assigned)................................. ....

By whom recommended... ....

Date of employment ....

Salary or Wages. ....

Left, (date) *and cause*.......(to be recorded by the Superintendent).

The value of this book consists not only in having the signature of the employed to a very definite contract, but in preserving such information with respect to the nature of the employment, time of service and cause of leaving as to enable a superintendent to return an intelligent answer to any inquiry made concerning a former employee, or to refresh his own memory in the event of an application for re-employment.

2d. A " Pay Roll " of officers and employees, classified by departments—employees in each department being grouped together, and the signature of each being taken when receiving pay for services rendered. At the top of each page is a printed heading reading: " We, whose signatures are hereunto subscribed, severally acknowledge to have received the sum set opposite our respective names, being wages in full for the time specified." Opposite each name are two columns, of which one is used to record the number of the employee in the particular department in which he is engaged, and the other to indicate the total number of employees in the hospital. This information is utilized at the end of every year in determining the daily average number of employees throughout the year. In this class of books I may refer to one entitled " Record of Attendance of Visiting Staff." It is designed to show the hour of arrival and departure of the physician or surgeon on duty in each division of the hospital during the successive days of the year. One line is devoted to each day. If any one of the three divisions of the hospital is not visited by a member of the visiting staff, the fact becomes apparent to the visiting member of the board of trustees, who may invite an explanation.

Class C.

Those which relate to the Purchase of Supplies.

1st. The " Order Book," in which are recorded, in duplicate, all orders given for supplies—one, the stub, being retained for future reference, and the other delivered, over the signature of the Superintendent, to the dealer, who, by a foot-note, is enjoined to supply a bill with every article furnished, and to furnish no article except upon the order of the Superintendent.

2d. A book entitled " Account of Supplies and Materials Received," in which are recorded all invoices of goods received, their receipt having first been certified to by the head of the department for which the goods are intended. The headings in this book are:—

Remarks......................... ....
Articles, with quantity and cost..
From whom purchased ....
Dealers' Ledger folio............(indicating the page therein on which the date and amount of an invoice may be found).

3d. A book entitled "The Dealers' Ledger," posted from the register just described, and in which are written the names of the dealers and the amounts of their invoices.

These records render it possible to file the invoices when audited, paid and receipted, the " Dealers' Ledger " and "Account of Supplies and Materials Received " being available for reference whenever it becomes desirable to learn the source of supplies and the prices paid for them.   They are only books of memorandum and should not be confounded with the General Ledger of the hospital.

4th. A book in which are recorded the minutes of the weekly visiting committee of the board of trustees ; an important duty of that committee being to audit the dealers' bills and monthly pay-roll, presented by the Superintendent for approval before payment.   They also inspect the weekly reports of patients admitted and discharged, and attend to such other matters as are brought to their notice.

5th. A book containing drafts upon the treasurer for the sum of the audited bills, and signed by the weekly visiting committee referred to.

CLASS D.

Those which relate to the receipt and payment of moneys.

1st. A book of blank forms of "Receipts," with stub, used for acknowledging the receipt of money paid for the board of patients.

2d. A Petty Cash Book, in which an entry is made of all moneys received and paid out at the hospital.

3d. A Cash Book, in which weekly entry is made, in a classified form, of the receipts and expenditures recorded daily in the Petty Cash Book.

4th. A Patients' Ledger, which is really part of the General Ledger, but, for convenience, is bound under separate cover.   In it credit entries are made from the Cash Book to the individual accounts of patients, of such sums of money as are received from them for board.   In this book debit entries are also made from the Cash Book, for any sums that have been refunded because of their discharge before the expiration of the time for which board has been paid. The accounts in this book are balanced by entries, from the Journal, of charges there made for board during the actual time of stay in the hospital.

5th. The "Journal."   This is the book of original entry for :—

1st. Recording all hospital expenses paid by the treasurer.

2d. Recording the weekly total of petty expenditures, appearing in detail in the Cash Book. The money is drawn for the same from the treasurer in gross sums by draft of the visiting committee.

3d. Charging the individual accounts of paying patients with board, etc.

4th. Charging " Board Account," by a single entry, with the total amount received from paying patients during each week, and crediting " Paying Patients' Account" with the same, the details appearing in the Cash Book.

5th. Charging Paying Patients' Account monthly, by a single entry, with the total amount refunded to paying patients discharged before the expiration of the period for which they had paid board in advance, and crediting " Board Account" with the same, the details appearing upon the Cash Book.

6th. The " Ledger." This book contains all general accounts other than dealers' and those of individual paying patients.

7th. A book entitled the " Expense Book." The trustees of the Roosevelt Hospital regard this as one of the most valuable books of its kind for their use kept at the institution, for the reason that it affords an opportunity for an analytical comparison of the expenses of the hospital, monthly as well as annually, the expenditures under each head being so classified as to facilitate ready comparison. It has therefore seemed to me best to illustrate its use by making my sketch of this book a complete transcript from the record of the original for the past year.

In presenting these sketches with the accompanying explanations, I wish to say that superiority over methods employed by other institutions is not claimed for them. They are representative of the system followed at the Roosevelt Hospital, and are the outgrowth of my own experience there and elsewhere. My one motive in accepting the invitation to treat this subject was a desire to be helpful to new institutions confronted with the necessity of adopting a plan of bookkeeping which would be adequate to their needs. This must be my excuse for the minuteness of detail which you may have remarked. The most I could hope for, in the case of the older institutions, was that some modification of their present system might be suggested by a consideration of the varied list presented.

The following memoranda and specimen pages are appended to give those who desire them definite details for guidance in ordering similar books or forms.

Class A, No. 1. See page 106. Binding, cloth sides, leather back and corners. Size, 250 leaves or 500 pages, each 10½x7½ inches. 2 blanks to each page.

No. 2. Admissions and Discharges. See page 107. ⎫
No. 3. Register of Patients. See page 107. ⎪ Forms on
No. 4. Record of Rejected Patients. See page 108. ⎬ pages
No. 5. Daily Record. See page 108. ⎪ 115-118.
No. 6. Statistics for Annual Report. See page 108. ⎭

No. 7. Receipt Book for Effects. See page 109. Binding, three-quarter board, marble-paper sides, roan back and ends. Size, 200 leaves; printed one side; one form of receipt, each 3¾x8 inches.

CLASS B, No. 1. List of Officers and Employees. See page 109. Binding, full sheep. Size, 150 leaves or 300 pages, 12½x10¾. Indexed throughout, or from front to back.

No. 2. Pay Roll. See page 110. Binding, full cloth with duck cover. Size, 100 leaves or 200 pages, each 14½x12½.

No. 3. Record of Attendance of Medical Staff. See page 110.

CLASS C, No. 1. Order Book. See page 110. Binding, cloth sides, leather back and corners. Size, 200 leaves, printed on one side, two blanks to each page, with duplicates as stubs for retained copies of orders; each page 12x10½ inches.

No. 2. Account of Supplies and Materials Received. See page 110. Binding, cloth sides, leather back and corners. Size, 250 leaves or 500 pages, 12½x10¾ inches.

No. 3. The Dealers' Ledger. See page 111. Binding, extra full sheep. Size, 250 leaves or 500 pages, 12½x10¾ inches.

No. 4. Minutes of Visiting Committee. See page 111. Binding, full sheep, with duck cover. Size, 200 leaves or 400 pages, 11½x9 inches.

No. 5. Draft Book. See page 111. Binding, cloth sides, leather back and corners. Size, 200 leaves, printed one side, 5 drafts to each page, 16¼x13½ inches. Drafts perforated, and drafts and stubs numbered in duplicate from 1 to 1000.

CLASS D, No. 1. Receipts. See page 111. Binding, full duck. Size, 150 leaves or 300 pages, each 12x9¾ inches, four blank receipts to a leaf, with endorsement on back of each as follows: "Payment for board and treatment must be made for four weeks in advance.

The amount of two weeks' board at the rate agreed upon will be retained in every case, though the patient remain a less time in the Hospital."

No. 2. Petty Cash Book. See page 111. Binding, full red leather. Size, 150 leaves or 300 pages, each 9¾x6⅞ inches.

No. 3. Cash Book. See page 111. Binding, extra sheep, with duck cover. Size, 250 leaves or 500 pages, each 15½x10½ inches.

No. 4. Paying Patients' Ledger. See page 111. Binding, extra sheep, duck cover. Size, 250 leaves or 500 pages, each 15½x10½ inches, ruled for four accounts on each page.

No. 5. Journal. See page 111. Binding, extra sheep, duck cover. Size, 250 leaves or 500 pages, each 15½x10½ inches.

No. 6. Ledger. See page 112. Binding, extra sheep with duck cover. Size, 250 leaves or 500 pages, each 15½x10½, ruled for one account to each page.

No. 7. Expense Book. See page 112.

ROOSEVELT HOSPITAL.

DAILY RECORD OF PATIENTS ADMITTED AND DISCHARGED.

..................189

ADMITTED.													DISCHARGED.						
No.	Name.	Civil condition.	Class.	Ward.	Date.	No.	Name.	Class.	Age.	Birthplace.	Ward.	Admitted.	Discharged.	Condition.	Disease.	Remarks.

Binding, full sheep, with duck cover.   Size, 100 leaves or 200 pages, each 17¾ inches high by 11½ inches across.

REGISTER OF PATIENTS.

Ward.	Name of Patient.	Class.	Relatives or Friends.	Birthplace.	Occupation.	Age.	ADMITTED.		Disease.	DISCHARGED.		
							Month.	Day.		Month.	Day.	Condition.

Binding, full sheep with duck cover. Size, 150 leaves or 300 pages, each 17⅛ inches high by 15⅜ inches across. Indexed throughout, or from front to back.

RECORD OF REJECTED PATIENTS.

Date of Application.	No.	Name and Residence.	By whom Recommended.	Date of Examination.	Where Examined.	By whom Examined.	Diagnosis.	Why Rejected.	Where Referred.

Binding, cloth sides, leather back and corners. Size, 180 leaves or 360 pages, each 15¾ inches high, and 11¾ inches across.

DAILY RECORD.

Ward.	No. Patients, Medical.		No. Patients, Surgical.		No. Patients, Gynæcological.	Total.	Admitted.			Discharged.			Remarks.
	M.	F.	M.	F.	F.		M.	S.	G.	M.	S.	G.	
1.													
2.													
3.													
4.													
5.													
6.													
Pr. Fl.													

Binding, cloth sides, leather back and corners. Size, 200 leaves or 400 pages, each 5¾ inches high by 9¾ inches across.

STATISTICS FOR THE ANNUAL REPORT   FOR THE YEAR ENDING DEC. 31, 18

	American.		Irish.		German.		English and Scotch.		French.		Scandi-navian.		Italian.		Swiss.		Spanish.		Sclaves.		Belgian and Dutch.		Austrian.		Poles.		Russian.		West Indies.		South American and Cuba.	
	M.	F.	M.	F.	M.	F.	M.	F.	M.	F.	M.	F.	M.	F.	M.	F.	M.	F.	M.	F.	M.	F.	M.	F.	M.	F.	M.	F.	M.	F.	M.	F.
Males.																																
Females.																																
Discharge Book Folio.																																

Binding, full sheep, leather corners.   Size, 100 leaves or 200 pages, each 15¾ inches high by 9¼ inches across.

Record of Attendance of Visiting Staff.

1892.

| | MEDICAL DIVISION. | | | SURGICAL DIVISION. | | | GYNÆCOLOGICAL DIVISION. | | |
| | | Hour of | | | Hour of | | | Hour of | |
Date.	Name.	Arrival.	Departure.	Name.	Arrival.	Departure.	Name.	Arrival.	Departure.
January 1									
" 2									
" 3									

Binding, extra sheep. Size, 100 leaves or 200 pages, each 13½ inches high by 13¾ inches across. The left-hand column on opposite pages containing the days of the month, printed in chronological order. The book complete covers a period of eight years.

DISCUSSION.

MR. BURDETT, of London : I shall have to speak on this subject to-morrow, therefore I will not say much about it in the Section, but I should like to say this. As far as I am able to follow the paper, which is necessarily very technical and very difficult to follow, I do not see any account of a subscription register among the numerous books which Mr. Lathrop gave us at some length. Now there is a good deal of attention paid to another book, and that is the ledger for paying patients, and I only rise here now on this point to say how grateful and thankful I am to the United States that they, in a new country, and having to build new institutions, founded the hospitals on the principle that every man shall have held sacred to him the right of contributing anything which he can afford to his maintenance in the institution. There is nothing doing more injury to the old countries of the world than the continuous, ever-increasing amount of free medical relief which is being given in our medical institutions. I am confident that the out-patient department is the portal to pauperism. It is there that people begin to learn that they can get something for nothing, and they are not ashamed of doing it. From there they pass into the in-patient department, where they get great benefits and large expenditures upon them, without any effort on their part, without being required to defray any part of the cost of the treatment and maintenance. Finally, if they should be in a surgical ward or have an appliance of any kind, they are positively given that apparatus without any attempt on their part to give one penny of the cost. Now the evils attending free medical relief are, as I said before, most momentous, they are disastrous and destructive of all the principles of independence ; and whereas I would be the first to advocate the fullest and fairest and largest amount of help to men or women who are unable to provide it for themselves, I do, as I said before, thank the United States that in this country at any rate, to-day, the first thing an applicant for medical relief is made acquainted with is the fact that he is entitled to the privilege of paying what he can toward the cost of that relief.

There is one word of warning I would like to utter. I was in New York last week and I visited some of the hospitals there, and I found at least in one of them the truth of the statement made by Professor Peabody yesterday, that where there are philanthropists and where there is a vast amount of money to be distributed, there comes the danger to the individual citizen, because the amount of funds in one of those hospitals is so large that I am told (and I verified it by the figures) that the tendency there is to increase the free beds and to decrease the paying beds. Now that increase is being made without proper and adequate and full inquiry, so far as my investigations went; and I do certainly hope that the administrators of the great American hospitals will set their faces like a rock against the development of free beds, until they are perfectly certain that in any large population where this subject comes up for discussion those free beds are absolutely necessary to provide for those who cannot in any way or to any extent provide for themselves; otherwise we shall see that our anchor, the anchor of hope of the United States, is gradually slipping. And what will become of us in the Old World I don't know, except we arrive at this stage, that everybody will get free medical relief; because it has grown from 1870, when we had one in three, till 1880, when we had one in two of the whole population who got free medical relief; and according to the last figures, one in every one and a half of the population now receives this free medical relief. I do therefore hope that looking at this question in its widest bearings, from a single point of view, you will be proud of this system; that you will let nothing interfere with it, or tend to break it down, and that your basis shall be: "Show us that you require free medical relief and you shall have it; but you must prove the necessity before we offer, nay, before we will ever attempt to thrust upon you this free gift, which, though a gift, may tend to weaken your moral fiber and thereby lessen your uses and privileges as a citizen."

MR. C. C. SAVAGE, of New York: This question which Mr. Burdett has raised in regard to free beds is one of the most vital questions affecting the whole hospital discipline. As far as New York is concerned, our private hospitals are supposed to be pay hospitals, but ninety per cent. are really free. Any one who looks at the subject knows that that ought not to be so. I fully agree with Mr. Burdett on that point. But how to effect a remedy is a matter which has not yet been solved. And what income should a patient have in health to entitle him to a free bed? Some sum might be adopted as a guide; shall it be an income of ten dollars a week or fifteen dollars a week? Then again comes up the question, whether he has a wife and children dependent on him or not. All these questions come up, and we find it almost impracticable, if not quite so, to lay down any rule which shall govern the free beds. The tendency

is with us, Mr. Burdett, as it is with you, to increase rather than to
diminish free beds. If some method could be devised by which
more pay patients should be received in our hospitals, or more money
received from those who are now free patients, we should undoubtedly uphold the moral stamina of the patient, and relieve the hospital of the great burden of their support.

MR. BURDETT: I should like to say that I don't think, from our
experience, you can work the weekly wage at all ; but I do think
this: if you give a patient the privilege of paying, and force home
your principle, which is the kernel of the whole question, that a man is
expected to pay, at any rate a minimum sum, you fix a minimum
charge and you will usually get it. The cottage hospitals, of which
there are now six hundred in England, have grown up in the rural
districts, where the population have lower wages than anywhere
else ; there the patients pay half a dollar a week at least, most pay a
dollar and a quarter, and we find in that way the people are always
cheerfully willing to pay this ; very many pay much more. The
best way is not to strike a wage limit, but to deal with each case ;
and that can be done by the superintendent or the board of visitors,
who examine these cases, and say : " Well, you must prove to us that
you require free relief, or you won't get it ; you must at any rate pay
the minimum charge."

The CHAIRMAN: There is no hospital which publishes statistics of
its patients and its results in such a way as to be comparable with
other hospitals, for the reason that no hospital gives the figures in
groups of ages. In making up a life table, or in collating vital
statistics, we want to know the number of persons of each of certain
age groups, as from 20 to 25 years, that have been in a hospital for
a given time ; then the number of deaths that take place out of that
number. Now some hospitals give us the number of deaths by years
of age, but they do not give us the age groupings of the patients
who do not die, and hence the data for calculation of ratios are
wanting. In my judgment, a record of a hospital should be summed
up once a month, the number of patients, with distinction of sex, and
the number of patients in each group of years. It is impossible to
compare statistics of mortality of different hospitals, or of different
methods of treatment, unless you know the ages of the patients
treated. One of the best things that could be done for scientific
medicine and vital statistics in this country would be, in all our old
hospitals and asylums for the insane, to go over the old records and

take out the data of all patients by quinquennial age periods, and the deaths in the same way, and so get them into a shape in which they would be comparable.

Lt.-Col. J. LANE NOTTER, of England: I should like to add to your remarks, Mr. Chairman, how very important this question of statistics is in England. We found that comparison was almost impossible until we attempted this method of age grouping. Take for instance consumption: in what ages does this disease occur? Now this is most important with reference to factory legislation. In factories, where large numbers of young people are exposed to humidity and the atmospheric conditions which are found in workshops, it is especially liable to develop. By getting these groups of ages we can tell the average lifetime that these people are likely to last, and we can take such preventive measures as have been taken lately in England in order to minimize the evil attending working in such factories. Age grouping of hospital statistics has a much larger bearing than at first appears upon sight, because it gives an insight into the causes of mortality; it aids us in taking these preventive measures which reduce the causes of disease, and enables the statistician to point out what is the saving in life and the probable mitigation of the number of deaths which occur in the early period of life and among people engaged in unhealthy trades of all kinds.

In military life we have also found it of the greatest advantage; not only is the age group given, but the actual numbers furnishing the sick are given. We can tell easily enough whether the younger men or the older men living in a tropical country, under the same conditions, suffer most. It really is an important point, and well worth the attention of those who have the charge of hospital accounts and books.

DR. HURD: I asked Mr. Lathrop to prepare this paper because I was extremely anxious that all hospital workers throughout the country should see the forms in use at Roosevelt Hospital, where I think the system of business methods is exceptionally good. I think in this country, especially in smaller hospitals, a great and increasing difficulty has always been the lack of business methods. I learned of a hospital the other day in a city of 250,000 to 300,000 inhabitants, where a new superintendent had gone into office and found a fine hospital disorganized in every department. The matron bought what she felt like buying, and the engineer and superintendent of nurses bought likewise. Each one of the resident physicians ordered drugs and supplies by telephone, without any regard to what might have been ordered by any one else; and the result was that a score of people in that institution were buying supplies without authority, without system, by telephone, and by word of mouth, until the expenses of the hospital were such as to frighten the contributors. The situation required a very determined stand on the part of the superintendent, who had the satisfaction of cutting down the expenses of the hospital very materially, by introducing a systematic method of purchase and a strict responsibility for all payments. He informed me he found it necessary to take stringent measures to make the change, and in several instances to require those who ordered goods to pay for them. One officer, in fact, felt so much aggrieved by the limitation of his prerogative that he resigned; he could not endure to be in an institution where he could not buy what he pleased. For these reasons I am extremely anxious that these forms should be followed in smaller hospitals, in order to insure the economical expenditure of hospital money.

MR. C. C. SAVAGE: If there are any superintendents or trustees of hospitals present, I would call their attention especially to the Expense Account Book. I know an Expense Account Book is of great value in comparing what has been purchased and its cost from time to time. It has to me a wonderful value in that line. I think every trustee would find it so by experience.

ON PAYING PATIENTS IN HOSPITALS.

BY HENRY M. LYMAN, A. M., M. D.,

One of the Attending Physicians to The Presbyterian Hospital in Chicago, Ills.

As an example of the experiment of requiring payment for hospital service, I desire to relate the experience of The Presbyterian Hospital in Chicago. This hospital was erected under the auspices of the Presbyterian churches in this city, at a cost of about one quarter of a million dollars. It furnishes accommodation for two hundred and twenty-five patients. Its staff of officials and employees resident in the building consists of a Superintendent, who is a physician, six interne physicians and surgeons, forty-three nurses furnished by the Illinois Training School for Nurses, and seventy-three subordinate servants, making a total of one hundred and twenty-three persons actively engaged in the hospital. The nurses, however, do not sleep in the building. At night the day nurses retire to their rooms at the Illinois Training School, a short distance from the hospital, and their places are occupied by the night nurses, who, in their turn, leave the building in the morning. The medical and surgical service of the hospital is in the hands of a visiting staff of physicians and surgeons who reside in the city. Any patient who desires such an arrangement can employ any reputable physician or surgeon to attend him in the hospital, even though not connected with the hospital staff. This privilege has thus far worked without friction; and it is often a great convenience for an outside physician or surgeon to avail himself of the advantages of hospital nursing and attendance while caring for a patient who otherwise would have been relegated to the imperfect installation of a private house or a hotel.

At the outset of their undertaking the directors of The Presbyterian Hospital resolved that so far as possible they would seek to avoid everything that tends to pauperize the community. It is, believed that the great County Hospital affords sufficient accommodation for the really indigent poor of the city and county. It is, therefore, understood that patients who seek admission to the Presbyterian Hospital must pay for the services there rendered. If unable to pay, they must have payment made for them by some one else. Medical and surgical attendance must also be paid for, just as if the patient were in his own house or in a hotel. As a matter of fact, however, the members of the medical staff are exceedingly lenient in this matter and have never exacted payment from any patients who were in straitened circumstances. In this arrangement the members of the medical staff deal with the patients very much as they would treat similar individuals in their *clientele* outside of the hospital. Thus far the experiment has proved very successful and satisfactory.

Returning now to the subject of hospital finance alone, it appears that during the year that ended March 31, 1893, the daily average number of patients under treatment was one hundred and eighty. The total annual expense of the hospital during that period was $83,447.15. The daily cost per patient was $1.27, making the weekly cost per patient $8.89. This sum, therefore, represents the unit of hospital charges. But since many patients require much more than the bare necessaries of hospital accommodation, the charges are graduated in such a way as to afford different degrees of accommodation and outlay. The weekly charge is, accordingly, graduated from three dollars to twenty dollars per week. During the year ending March 31, 1893, the weekly charges were as follows: Free to 843 patients; $3 to 27 patients; $5 to 77 patients; $6 to 154 patients; $7 to 87 patients; $8 to 527 patients; $10 to 249 patients; $12 to 136 patients; $15 to 160 patients; $20 to 39 patients.

The amount of money received from these patients reached the sum of $58,751.54, leaving a deficit of $24,695.61. Of this, $19,500 are made up to the hospital by the income from endowments furnished by charitable individuals and by different churches that contribute yearly gifts for the maintenance of free beds. These contributors are permitted to designate patients who shall be the recipients of their charity, and in this way many of the city churches provide hospital care for their indigent members. In this way provision is made for sixty-five free beds each year, and the income from this source, amounting to $19,500 during the year ending March 31, 1893, added to the income from patients who paid their own way, makes a total of $78,251.54, leaving an actual deficit of only $5195.61. This sum is finally liquidated by the benevolent contributions of the different Presbyterian churches in Chicago.

By the method thus outlined, it is evident that the hospital is actually on an almost self-supporting basis. Were it not for the large number of patients in the so-called "free beds," from which the income is less than the actual cost of maintenance, the hospital could easily be made self-supporting, so great is the number of patients who would gladly pay full price for the privilege of admission. It is true that the cost of the original installment, its enlargement, and extraordinary repairs, is left out of view in these estimates, consequently the fact remains that the Presbyterian Hospital of Chicago, with all its high endeavor to avoid the semblance of pauperizing its constituency, is none the less a monument of charitable purpose and action. No patient enters its doors unless he pays or has payment made for him, according to the services rendered; yet no one does make and very few can make any adequate pecuniary return for the use of the immense investment of capital and good-will that is represented by this noble charity.

DISCUSSION.

MR. SAVAGE, of New York.—You have an expense for repairs, I suppose? How do you meet that?

DR. LYMAN.—The expense is met out of this income; that is included in the general expense, all these things are included in the general outgo of eighty-three thousand dollars. The building is not included in that; a new building when needed will have to be provided for by gift.

A DELEGATE.—Are there not individual endowments as well as the endowments of the churches?

DR. LYMAN.—There are some; I should have said there have been some.

MR. RYERSON, of Chicago.—I am very glad to hear Dr. Lyman's speech, because it is a subject I have always taken a great interest in and given a great deal of thought to. The institution I have the honor to preside over is an old institution, that is, old for this city, probably the oldest charity in this city, and we have been met there, in this question of pay patients, with the feeling, that I think is gradually becoming more common, that a hospital was not necessarily an institution of charity. Now I think there is a great deal of truth in what Dr. Lyman has said, that you may do a man just as much harm by pauperizing him when he is ill as by doing it when he is well; and in sort of an intuitive way I have come around to see it myself. I think I began in my past experience with the idea that a hospital is necessarily a charitable free institution, and an institution like St. Luke's Hospital, which I represent, which has grown up gradually, and was not begun in the scientific way that the Presbyterian Hospital was, has difficulty in meeting this question, and I should like if possible to have some light thrown on these difficulties now. At the time St. Luke's was begun, the County Hospital, with its splendid provision for charitable work, was not in existence, and therefore the public looked to institutions like St. Luke's for help. Consequently, when I first became identified with the hospital I found a feeling very largely prevailing among the friends supporting the hospital, that we were in some way violating our pledge to the public by taking pay patients, and it has been a great difficulty with me. I hope in some way this paper of Dr. Lyman's will be made public, because I think that the public ought to know that just as much good is sometimes done by an institution which does not attempt to pauperize a man because he is ill, but regulates its charges by his condition ; that is the true scientific plan, I think. All I have ever done is to tell my superintendent to exercise his tact and his discretion in the matter, to get at the facts as best he may, and then regulate the charges according to the patient's circumstances. Of course we base our regular charges, as the Presbyterian Hospital does, upon the per diem cost.

Then another question. We have a large number of endowed beds, some by money left us and some by money given us, and I think as a rule we are able to take as many free patients as these endowments provide for ; but circumstances might arise when we would not be able to take as many free patients. If our income fell off in any other direction we could not receive such patients.

Then in what position do hospitals who have received endowments stand to those persons who have furnished such endowments ? I have known of cases where people who have subscribed some sum to the institution, take advantage of that position to send down to us their servants or dependents, and expect us to give them free medical service and care, and all at the expense of some imaginary account. Now that is a very embarrassing situation, and it is a situation that a hospital that is bound by these endowments is tied up by. It seems to me that you cannot attempt any fairer plan than this : I figure out my final income, and then earn enough money from my pay patients to come out square at the end of the year. That has been the plan that I have endeavored to go by.

DR. PILCHER, of Brooklyn.—I was hoping, as Dr. Lyman progressed with his account of their arrangements, inasmuch a I understood him to say that he is one of the attending physicians of the hospital, that he might give us some information as to the arrangements which are made by the paying patients of the hospital as to the remuneration paid to the attending staff; for I take it that just at this point there is an extremely important question involved in hospital management. It always has been the part of members of the medical profession to devote themselves personally to the care of unfortunates who are dependent upon charitable relief, as a part of their contribution to the great fund of charity. We are always ready to devote ourselves personally to the care of those people who are proper candidates for charitable relief, but as I understand it, in this institution there are at least two-thirds of the patients who are not proper candidates for charitable relief. I would like very much to know whether in this institution it is required of members of the staff who attend the charitable patients without pay, to also attend without pay the pay patients?

DR. LYMAN.—I will say with regard to that matter that the patients in the hospital can be classified into two classes, the productive patients and the unproductive; all those who pay or have paid for them a sum per week not exceeding eight dollars are considered unproductive patients, and they are attended, so far as medical and surgical attendance is concerned, gratuitously by the staff of the hospital. The productive patients are those who pay ten dollars or more per week; they are allowed to make such selection as they please as to attendance. We have a somewhat peculiar method of attendance in the Presbyterian Hospital that has so far worked very well indeed.

Persons who come to the hospital who come under the head of productive patients and are promised extra privileges in the way of room and attendance have also the privilege of selecting their medical and surgical attendant, and they are attended by the regular hospital staff or by any resident physician in the city or out whom they choose. With the matter of medical compensation the hospital management has nothing to do; it only knows that its patients who are unproductive will be attended by the hospital staff gratuitously, and that those who are productive will pay their own physicians and surgeons, just exactly as they pay their physicians and surgeons in their own home.

DR. PILCHER inquired whether any steps were taken to ascertain whether those who desired accommodation at eight dollars per week were able to pay more.

DR. LYMAN stated that it was understood a man did not go into the common wards unless he was obliged to.

DR. PILCHER.—That hardly answers the question. Human nature is perhaps the same all the world over, and there are doubtless men who are perfectly satisfied with the accommodations of the general ward who would be able to pay considerably more than that. The question is, are the common wards restricted to those who are not able to pay more than eight dollars a week?

DR. LYMAN.—No, I do not think there is any examination made as to the ability of the patient to pay more; the schedule of prices is presented to him and he selects.

DR. PILCHER.—It is quite apparent that an opportunity is here

presented for people to obtain gratuitous medical attention who would
be perfectly able to pay the proper fees.

MR. BURDETT.—I should like to say that it is a great pleasure to
me to meet a representative of the Presbyterian Hospital of Chicago.
I have been trying for years to ascertain how that institution is conducted, and I had come to the conclusion that possibly the books
were somewhat complicated, or there was some other reason why we
could not get some information. St. Luke's Hospital has always,
and even the Cook County Hospital has sent us tables for the purpose of comparison, and—as I shall have to point out to-morrow—
the work which we endeavor to do is done in the interest of all the
hospitals, not in the interest of any individual person at all. It is a
very considerable labor and considerable expense, and I do hope
that one result of this congress will be that instead of having one
hospital only of which we have any knowledge in Europe (because
that is the only institution that will supply even a report), that in
future years we shall be able to give a proper account of every hospital in Chicago. I only mention that by the way. I hope I may
say it without any offense at all; I am quite sure from the answers
given by the reader of the paper and the evident interest he takes in
hospitals that it will be his desire, as it is mine, that full justice shall
be done to every institution in Chicago by the authorities who are
responsible for supplying details.

Now in regard to the point at issue. The president of St. Luke's
has said that he has endeavored to build up a system of paying
patients. If you go through St. Luke's and examine the books, as I
did, you will find that the receipts from paying patients have gone
up and the receipts from churches have steadily gone *down*. Now
I venture to say (I speak quite freely and frankly) that this is a fact
which the people of Chicago should take very closely to heart. It is
a condition which is not worthy of the intelligence of a great city,
because I have gone most carefully into the system presented at St.
Luke's Hospital, and I find that every poor man is taken in freely,
and that every other man is allowed to come in and pay what he can.
This is the system in vogue at St. Luke's; I have personally verified
it; and I spent some two hours in going into it yesterday, and I
declare it is one of the best systems that a hospital can be conducted
on, and I believe it is the only safe system and satisfactory way in
which you can conduct a hospital. Now if this is so, what can we
say to the churches of this city who positively every year, as this

system is being improved, show less and less interest! It is a fearful, a most troublesome thing, and I do really hope that the newspapers of Chicago, which I find very interesting reading, from their lightness, will have a serious turn to-morrow morning, and that at any rate one editor in the city will find, say six lines which he can spare to this question in the leading column, considering its interest, its importance and its worth. I am afraid there is no reporter present; but I know by past experience in Chicago that even walls have ears; there is an editorial ear in some wall here and I hope it will take this seriously to heart. I notice they take great credit for exposing rogues; let them take credit for one day for exposing the fact that St. Luke's Hospital, situated in one of the poorest districts of the city, is doing a glorious work in the best possible way and the people of Chicago are every year turning their backs more and more upon it! Shame! Let this not be continued!

Now, sir, with reference to what you said with reference to the question of the medical staff; I am one of those who have come to this conclusion, that for the well-being of all the hospitals I would pay every medical man who gave any services whatever to any hospital, because I believe that the payment of the medical staff will represent a less sum than the eleemosynary system of relief which the great medical profession have given for so many years free.

I would say also that while I know nothing about the case of the Presbyterian Hospital, individually, I think it is quite possible that Dr. Lyman, in his desire to be fair and to state nothing beyond his own knowledge, did not do exact justice even to his own institution, because I find that while you have this system of paying patients in the general ward, you have also got a system of careful inquiry into the circumstances of the patient, as I found in St. Luke's Hospital, even in the wards themselves, where they had a case only recently of a man who came in and declared that he was unable to pay anything, and representing himself to be without means, he got relief; but it was discovered after he had been in the hospital several weeks that he had means, through seeing who came to him, and watching the man; and he was made to pay every single penny. So I think it is very probable that at the Presbyterian Hospital they have the same system. I believe they are continually on the watch to arrive at the facts, and if that is so, I venture to say, as a good friend and upholder of the medical profession, as a man who is immensely interested in the hospitals as well as in the profession, that they have the best security possible in these hospitals.

Mr. Ryerson.—I would like to say one thing about our medical men, and that is this, we do not allow any outside medical men to treat patients in our hospital. I have always found that medical men were perfectly satisfied to treat a few patients free, and not only to treat a few patients free, but frequently to treat free those patients who are able to pay hospitals eight or nine dollars and able to do no more, and to rely only on patients who are apparently able to pay say fifteen or twenty dollars a week or more for separate rooms, for the payment of fees. Of course they would not do that if every man was allowed to practice in the hospital, because that would limit their field.

The Chairman.—I am sorry that we have not time for further discussion on this matter, because there are one or two points, particularly the relation of medical men to paid patients in hospitals, that are important, and it would be interesting to bring out the different methods that are pursued in different hospitals. A hospital whose chief purpose is medical education, having a staff selected from the teachers in a medical school, and the members of that staff having the sole privilege of placing pay patients in the institution, or at all events having the first privilege, is quite different from a hospital having no connection with any training institution, relying mainly upon its resident physicians for its medical attendance, and which allows any physician to send in pay patients and to attend them. The relations between the hospital organization and the medical staff appear to me to be quite different in these two cases.

ISOLATING WARDS AND HOSPITALS FOR INFECTIOUS DISEASES.

By G. H. M. Rowe, M. D.,

Medical Superintendent of the Boston City Hospital.

The finding of the "Rosetta stone" unlocked the secret which the ages had thrown over Egyptian hieroglyphics. The discovery of the bacillus was the key to the mystery of the cause, development and spread of infectious diseases. The impossible became possible. The pathological laboratory has demonstrated that infection is a micro-organism whose characteristics are being gradually revealed, and, what is of greater importance, it has taught us the agents for its destruction.

The physical laboratory has not exhausted the limits of the power and usefulness of electricity, nor has the pathological laboratory yet worked out the full scope of infection in its multifarious and far-reaching destructiveness.

These investigations and the deductions from them will make the basis of future professional treatment and the management of infectious diseases, but the economic and social bearings of the problem demand study from other points of view. Time forbids a historical or statistical review, and I proceed at once to briefly work out a few hospital equations that are paramount in the management of infectious diseases.

This audience needs not to be told that on the first appearance of an infectious disease it should be immediately removed to a place of isolation, not only for its proper treatment, but for the protection of others. If the case appears in a home, probably an attempt will be made to isolate there, usually resulting in a separation that does not isolate. Epidemics are created by such futile attempts. Sanitary practice does not keep pace with sanitary knowledge. Not removing a person with an infectious disease to a hospital or some place securing absolute isolation, should be held as a punishable offense against society. Public health will never be assured till an enlightened popular sentiment co-operates to this end.

Every general or cottage hospital should have a suitable place to promptly isolate all cases of infection that may arise within its own walls. Infection, in this connection, includes not only eruptive fevers, but also all diseases liable to convey surgical infection. In recent years, whenever a general or well-appointed cottage hospital is built, a separate building is found among its resources for this purpose. But there are many pretentious hospitals having more than 100 beds for general medical and surgical diseases, founded twenty years ago, or even less, without such provision. The same is true not only in America but in England, even in London, owing to the original defective plan or want of the money necessary for the construction of such a building. There are scores of pretentious hospitals in the United States where provision for infectious cases cannot be found outside the buildings where such cases may arise. When an infected case appears, the usual policy is to temporize by placing it in some part of the building supposed to be less exposed than the ward where the case previously was assigned. This makeshift is never satisfactory, and if other persons escape, it is usually by a happy chance. No hospital of modern construction should for a moment hazard any compromise in providing proper isolation in a building for exclusive use of infectious cases. With such a building properly equipped, and with a suitable ratio of intelligent nurses whose hospital life is regulated by discreet and rational rules, the management of infection becomes somewhat easier. In wards having a score or less of patients suffering with a variety of infectious diseases, the regulations demand great exactness. The problem becomes yet more difficult when the wards number from forty to fifty such cases. In municipal hospitals having several hundred beds, many infectious cases, eliminated from the regular medical and surgical wards, must be provided for. This aggregates quite an array of infectious cases, in one ward for men, another for women. Besides the complication of infection requiring the greatest skill, these wards are generally attended by the Visiting and House Staff, who are likely to have duties in other parts of the hospital. The relations of these wards to other parts of the house in the matter of domestic service, supplies, clothing, laundry work, and the infinite number of minute adjustments, all combine to exact the most judicious and vigilant regime. Many cities or large towns of from 8000 to 15,000 inhabitants have cottage hospitals which are forced to meet the requirements of their communities. They cannot select their cases, where public opinion is not rightly educated on such matters, and the hospital is apt to condone harmful admissions, under the delusion of keeping peace. Medical science demonstrates that public welfare makes imperative special, isolating wards, not only in municipal but in cottage hospitals. This is more easily accomplished in hospitals that are private corporations, but is difficult in hospitals dependent on municipal appropriations.

There is a variety of practice about admitting to the wards connected with general hospitals, such infectious diseases as scarlet fever, diphtheria, measles, and the ordinary infectious diseases occasionally epidemic. But no hospital, either large or small, municipal, corporate, or cottage in its organization, should receive infectious fevers into its general wards. Is it absurd to state a rule so self-evident? I have frequently seen, in this country, a case of scarlet fever or diphtheria simply removed from the other children by putting it in a room by itself—a mere pretense of isolation, I have also seen in a prominent London hospital with a medical school attached, cases of scarlet fever and diphtheria in beds contiguous to those of patients with ordinary medical diseases. Exclude infectious diseases from all general hospitals, unless provided with separate special buildings for each disease. These wards should be absolutely isolated by distance, with separate service, both nursing and domestic ; and the physicians and surgeons in charge, as well as the house staff, should have no active connection with the general wards. Every precaution should be taken to render the care and treatment, if not absolutely, yet practically, independent, so as to reduce the possibility of carrying infection to other parts of the hospital. With obvious advantages, it is far from the ideal plan. The difficulties and dilemmas of infectious disease wards attached to a large hospital are so numerous that the wisest policy seems to forbid it, except as a relief for cases developing within its own walls. In large communities, the only system that is beyond criticism is to make for infectious diseases a separate establishment, independent and isolated. Bear in mind in this discussion that cholera, typhus fever and smallpox are excluded. Obviously, from their deadly nature, these must be treated each in a hospital specially devoted to its care, isolated in location as well as classification, although not necessarily under different boards of government. It is comparatively easy to lay down dictums indicating the best method, but pernicious conditions exist in many American cities which complicate the problem. It is a lamentable fact that the cities in this country possessing accommodations for infectious diseases among the poorer classes, to say nothing of the "well-to-do," can be counted on the fingers of one hand. To the best of my knowledge, Boston is the only *large* city where a hotel guest or a citizen in good circumstances can obtain suitable accommodations in a hospital, if he is ill with diphtheria, scarlet fever or smallpox. In most cities the better class of corporate general hospitals absolutely refuse him admission. He is referred to the health authorities. What then? Generally the resources at its disposal are merely barracks or old buildings, diverted to hospital purposes after being abandoned as unsuitable for uses less humane. I do not forget the numerous cottage hospitals with special isolating wards which have sprung up within the past fifteen years in our more thrifty and enterprising towns. This indicates a growing intelligence in medical matters, and the possible advance to separate buildings.

But it is in the larger municipalities where the proper accommodations are most deplorably lacking. The situation is the more humiliating, considering how many American cities and towns erect new and pretentious hospitals at almost needless expense, on the best modern lines, while little or no progress is made towards establishing isolation hospitals for the poor, to say nothing of buildings to which the better class would resort. We recognize the superior systems employed in European capitals, especially in Germany, and also in the health districts of Great Britain, notably the urban, sanitary districts.

Political methods, so rampant in municipalities, greatly affect sanitation and public health, and too often prove a stumbling-block to progress. The present rapid strides in scientific, educational and industrial affairs, and in public works, absorb so much energy and capital that public sanitation will wait indefinitely unless the medical profession employs Wendell Phillips' favorite weapon, "Agitate, agitate!" Optimists would fain believe that the trend of education, the truths of the laboratory, the altruistic spirit of the times, will eventually make clear to average intelligence the importance of having the proper means for stamping out the deadliest foe to public health. It is the duty of hospital workers and sanitarians not to cease forcing upon public authorities the necessity of intelligent action, until every municipality, through its public treasury, shall provide special hospitals always available for infectious diseases. Is it not the wisest policy to put such hospitals under the immediate control of the local board of health? They have so close a connection with other vital matters properly belonging to health boards that it conduces to unity of action to have the suppression of infection under one authority—a practice that obtains in Great Britain.

But what general plan shall be pursued for special infectious disease hospitals, say in a city of about 500,000 inhabitants, with a total requirement of perhaps 250 beds?

The first step is a site sufficiently large for liberal distribution of buildings, reasonably easy of access, and yet well isolated from sections thickly populated. In the present state of public opinion, if it is *not* easy of access, it defeats its own ends. Smallpox, like cholera and typhus, should be provided for in a hospital by itself, and the opinion of so eminent an authority as Dr. Thorne Thorne that a smallpox hospital should not be within a mile of an inhabited house is a wise and safe guide. As in Glasgow, smallpox might be cared for within the boundaries of an infectious group of buildings, but administered by itself and having no physical contact with the rest of the establishment. Other divisions should provide for the ordinary infectious diseases, each disease having its own buildings with divisions for each sex. Each building may be absolutely separate and yet be a component part of the whole. The group should have administration building, a domestic building, a service house containing the heating installation, laundry, mortuary, and a special home for nurses and the domestic service. Nurses, especially in infectious disease hospitals, should always be given quarters of their own in a building not occupied by patients, and of a quality to attract the class of women most desirable for hospital work.

The wards should be of moderate size, not to exceed thirty beds. The number of buildings for each disease should be sufficient to allow one building, so to speak, to "lie fallow" for renovation and disinfection. This reserve is a large factor in reducing the mortality in an infectious disease hospital. This generous installation of site, buildings and appointments, is not always practicable, either from the topography of a city, an available site, or the financial condition of a municipality. Such establishments, we are happy to say, do exist. The Belvidere Hospital for Infectious Diseases, in Glasgow, Scotland, is a most notable example. It covers 31 acres of land, and has 35 buildings with accommodations for infection usually prevalent in a large city. No better argument for isolation hospitals can be adduced than a rehearsal of the experience of the health authorities of Glasgow in changing the most unhealthy city in Great Britain, with the largest mortality, into a clean healthful city with a low death rate.

A more feasible but less perfect arrangement is a site in or near the thickly settled portions. Insure the best possible isolation by high walls and perfect administration. Provide separate administration and service buildings, give each disease and sex its own wards, and keep the ratio of beds to patients as liberal as possible. Such provisions, intelligently planned and wisely administered, will afford a powerful weapon to crush out infection. Liverpool, a city especially exposed to infection, has an admirable instance of a hospital of this class, and so eminent an authority as Mr. Henry C. Burdett assures us that "on the whole, this hospital may fairly be regarded as one of the best arranged infectious hospitals yet erected. Considering the restricted site, the arrangements are most satisfactory."

The opinion is gaining ground among hospital superintendents and sanitarians that large numbers of infectious cases cannot be treated to the best advantage under one roof without increasing the mortality rate. This has been demonstrated in hospitals and institutions devoted to the care of sick children. The ideal way to treat a case of acute highly infectious disease would be to have two rooms which the patient should occupy alternately for twelve hours, with proper safeguards in all the conditions of transfer. The same law of rotation, with a larger proportion of time, would be admirable for the occupancy of infectious disease wards. Many small, isolated buildings on one site yield better results than a few buildings of larger size on a restricted site. Increased cost is an objection to this. Unfortunately, public opinion, squeamish and short-sighted in public sanitation, backed by legislators ambitious for low tax rates, and cajoled by the always-sensitive taxpayer, is an effective and potent obstruction to the more intelligent methods.

Fire departments recognize that it is the first five minutes that count, so the first case of infection is the most important one to fight. Dr. Thorne Thorne has made the most exhaustive study ever attempted on infectious disease hospitals, and he instances scores of examples to show that epidemics have been crushed by having the means to isolate the first case. He insists that such buildings should be constructed in non-epidemic times, rather than under conditions of panic, and that immediate and permanent usefulness of hospitals is impaired by hurried erection.

In conclusion I am asked how the city of Boston ranks in the means for the suppression of infectious diseases.

Boston has possessed since 1877 a smallpox hospital for 50 ward patients, and six rooms for private paying patients. By the irony of fate, the last private patient was a well-known Boston poet. The hospital is half a mile from the nearest habitation, located on an excellent site, well appointed for its purpose as most cottage hospitals, which it resembles in external appearance. It is to-day, and has been every day during the last sixteen years, occupied by a man and his wife, both nurses experienced in the disease, and ready at all times to receive a patient. It has its special ambulance which can always be summoned by telephone, and a reserve of portable huts and protected nurses when many cases occur. Dr. McCollom, the city physician, confidently asserts that 150 small-pox patients can be properly provided for at forty-eight hours' notice. This again is a good illustration of Dr. Thorne's proposition, and the suppression of smallpox in Boston, and its very low mortality, through a long series of years, is an object-lesson worth heeding.

The Boston City Hospital has 480 beds distributed among eighteen wards, including a men's ward of ten rooms, each accommodating four cases either of erysipelas, cellulitis, pus in any form, or any uncleanly case arising within our own walls or from outside. There is also a ward containing twelve rooms, accommodating forty-eight women, which receives similar cases, including pelvic or puerperal septic cases.

The hospital also has two other wards, one for scarlet fever and one for diphtheria, each having thirty-two beds for both free and pay patients. These are separate buildings, built in 1886, of high cost construction, and in air supply, heating and ventilation, service rooms and special appointments, equal to the best of modern hospital wards; indeed, they are the most admirable of the hospital. In all respects they supply the same amount and quality of professional care, nursing and comforts afforded by any ward in the hospital, whether free or paying. The nursing is done by the nurses in the training school, and the seniors of the house staff are in turn isolated for attendance in the wards.

These wards are administered by the strictest regulations, and are practically isolated, but their proximity to the general wards imperils others, and proves the correctness of my proposition, that no wards designed for infectious fevers from without should be an integral part of a large general hospital. In spite of every safeguard, and after allowing for sources of infection from ward visitors and the dangers imminent to a hospital of 750 people, cases now and then *do* crop out that may fairly be attributed to the infectious fever wards. The labor involved in a large general hospital is always great and exacting. Ought it to be augmented by the strain of preventing the transmission of infection from special wards to the non-infectious wards?

During the last seven years, 752 cases of scarlet fever and 2227 cases of diphtheria have been treated in these wards. It has given a wide experience of the dangers of infectious disease wards on the grounds of a large general hospital, and teaches " how not to do it."

This unhappy condition, I am glad to say, will soon be remedied. After a repeated and persistent course of education imposed by the hospital management upon the city authorities, Boston is constructing a special hospital for infectious diseases, which I feel sure will be unrivaled in this country. The trustees already have $237,000 solely for this purpose. This, however, will not complete it, and

$140,000 additional has been promised in the next loan bill, making $377,000 for this special purpose. Contracts have been made for $203,000, and the buildings are well under way. Time forbids a description of them, but they are in the best lines of modern hospital construction, and intended for 250 patients, at a cost of about $1500 per bed. The plans and details are the result of much study by eminent authorities, and will give Boston a strong weapon for fighting infectious diseases. For the present it will be under the management of the Boston City Hospital, and will be administered in a manner equal, and we hope superior, to the general wards. The plan of these wards may be seen in the Boston City Hospital exhibit in the Anthropological Building.

In the May number of *The Forum* the learned president of this Section, in an article on municipal sanitation, asks this question: "Where is the place to which a lady living in a boarding-house or temporarily stopping at a hotel could take her child afflicted with scarlet fever?"

In Massachusetts, the cities of Boston, Cambridge and Newton all possess such accommodations. Three other hospitals in New England have isolation disease wards either under construction or projected. The isolating wards of the Boston City Hospital alone have private rooms for eighteen paying patients at $15, $20 and $25 per week. Their accommodations, treatment, nursing and general care, including diet, compare well with that usually given medical and surgical paying patients in first-class general hospitals.

Boston goes a step further. The hypothetical case of scarlet fever, and also any citizen, rich or poor, can have their clothing and all infected fabrics taken for purification to the new and well equipped sterilization house of the Board of Health, and returned, without charge.

Hospitals are only one part of the splendid enginery demanded for working out the extermination of infectious diseases. I cannot forbear calling attention to the collateral means. There must be efficient local boards of health, co-operating with state boards, all of which are controlled by a central national organization under the United States Government. The highest intelligence of expert sanitarians would thus penetrate all communities and concentrate action on a common foe.

GRUNDZÜGE FÜR BAU, EINRICHTUNG UND VERWALTUNG VON ABSONDERUNGSRÄUMEN UND SONDERKRANKENHÄUSERN FÜR ANSTECKENDE KRANKHEITEN.

FÜR DEN VOM 12. BIS 18. JUNI, 1893, IN CHICAGO STATTFINDENDEN INTERNATIONALEN WOHLFAHRTS-KONGRESS ENTWORFEN VON

DR. MORITZ PISTOR,

Geheimer Medizinalrath, vortragender Rath im Königlich Preussischen Ministerium der geistlichen, Unterrichts- und Medizinal-Angelegenheiten in Berlin.

Ordentliches Mitglied der Königlich Preussischen Wissenschaftlichen Deputation für das Medizinalwesen; ausserordentliches Mitglied des Kaiserlich deutschen Gesundheitsamtes.

Ehrenmitglied der Gesellschaft für öffentliche Gesundheitspflege in England; korrespondirendes Mitglied der Schlesischen Gesellschaft für vaterländische Kultur; korrespondirendes Mitglied der Königlich Belgischen Gesellschaft für öffentliche Gesundheitspflege.

Meine Damen und Herren! Der ehrenvollen Aufforderung des General-Stabsarztes der Vereinigten Staaten, Dr. John S. Billings, Vorsitzenden der III. Sektion für Krankenhauswesen, Ausbildung von Krankenpflegerinnen, unentgeltliche ambulatorische Krankenbehandlung und erste Hilfe für Verunglückte des internationalen Kongresses für Wohlthätigkeit, Gefängnisswesen und Wohlfahrts-Einrichtungen zu Chicago, dem Kongress meine Ansichten über Isolir-Räume und Isolir-Krankenhäuser für ansteckende Krankheiten vorzutragen, bin ich mit grosser Freude nachgekommen.

Nach den Statuten des Kongresses III Nro. 13, stehen mir nur 30 Minuten für die sehr umfangreiche Aufgabe zur Verfügung; ich werde mich bemühen, soweit möglich, in Kürze diejenigen Sätze zu fassen, welche mir für die Beurtheilung der Bedingungen zur Unterbringung von ansteckenden Kranken in gesonderten Räumen oder in Sonderkrankenhäusern nach den neuesten Anschauungen und Erfahrungen wichtig erscheinen, und bitte die Versammlung, ein etwaiges Ueberschreiten der vorgeschriebenen Zeit ebenso zu entschuldigen, wie mit Rücksicht auf die Kürze derselben das Zusammendrängen des Materials und eine etwa lückenhafte Behandlung desselben nachsichtig zu beurtheilen.

Einleitung.

Mitmenschen, die an ansteckenden Krankheiten litten, suchte man schon im grauen Alterthum von den Gesunden abzusondern; es sei nur an die Häuser für Aussätzige erinnert. Dieser Grundsatz hat sich erhalten und findet einen umfangreicheren Ausdruck in der Errichtung von Pesthäusern während des Mittelalters. Mehr und mehr hat im Laufe der Zeit die Ansicht sich befestigt, dass es für eine grössere Anzahl von ansteckenden Krankheiten im Interesse des Gemeinwohles erforderlich ist, die von solchen Krankheiten Befallenen von ihren Mitmenschen möglichst abzusondern, um der Verbreitung von übertragbaren Krankheiten mit Erfolg entgegentreten zu können. Heute sind alle Hygieniker darüber einig, dass in dieser Absonderung eines der wichtigsten Schutzmittel zur Beschränkung der Verbreitung infektiöser Krankheiten liegt. Darauf weisen auch die Gesetzgebungen aller Kulturländer hin, indem dieselben bald strenger, bald weniger streng die Unterbringung von an ansteckenden Krankheiten leidenden Personen, welche in der eigenen Wohnung nicht in genügender Weise abgesondert werden können, in Sonder-Krankenhäusern fordert. Wen die bezüglichen Bestimmungen für die einzelnen Länder interessiren, den verweise ich auf den trefflichen Bericht des Professor Dr. F. Felix auf dem VI. internationalen Kongress für Hygiene und Demographie zu Wien im Jahre 1887 "Ueber die Nothwendigkeit und Anlage von Isolir-Hospitälern," XV. Thema, Heft 15 der Referate.

Historisch sei noch bemerkt, dass 1746 in London das erste Blattern-Absonderungshaus errichtet worden ist; welches bis auf den heutigen Tag, wenn auch wesentlich erweitert und inszwischen räumlich verändert, fortbesteht.

Im Jahre 1802 wurde das London Fever Hospital, zunächst mit 18 Betten, ebenfalls aus freiwilligen Beiträgen hergestellt, in Gray's Inn eröffnet. Seither sind in allen Kulturstaaten Absonderungshäuser eingerichtet und in Amerika, Deutschland, Dänemark, England, Frankreich, Italien, Skandinavien in grösserer Anzahl in Betrieb gesetzt worden. Wie hoch sich die Zahl jener Häuser in den einzelnen Ländern zur Zeit beläuft anzugeben, ist mir nicht möglich.

Welche Kranken sind abzusondern?

Von Eintritt in die enger begrenzte Aufgabe ist noch die Frage zu erörtern, welche Kranken sollen abgesondert werden?

Allgemein wird verlangt, dass die an Cholera, Pocken, Fleckfieber, Gelbfieber und Pest Leidenden von anderen Kranken und Gesunden getrennt werden müssen. Ich kann nicht umhin hier im Gegensatz zu einzelnen Autoren darauf hinzuweisen, dass meines Erachtens Cholerakranke bei gehöriger Vorsicht allerseits sehr gut mit anderen Kranken zusammengelegt werden könnten, wenn nur zuverlässig dafür gesorgt wird, dass die Ausleerungen der Kranken von anderen Kranken fern gehalten werden. Der Umstand, dass die Cholera nur durch die Ausleerungen der Kranken nach den heutigen Anschauungen, sofern dieselben virulente Kommabazillen enthalten, übertragen wird, lässt eine Trennung dieser von anderen Kranken oder Gesunden überflüssig erscheinen. Ich für meine Person spreche mich dessenungeachtet für eine Isolirung von Cholerakranken in eigenen Räumen oder Häusern aus:

1, weil die Fernhaltung der Ausleerungen von anderen Kranken seitens des Pflegepersonals mir zweifelhaft bleibt, bei grossen Cholera-Epidemien wird man selten selbst in grösseren, geschweige denn in kleineren Ortschaften und auf dem Lande über ein auch nur annähernd zuverlässliches Pflegepersonal verfügen können;

2, weil der Anblick eines Cholerakranken ein so erschrecklicher ist, dass man denselben anderen Mitkranken ersparen soll.

Inwieweit die übrigen Infektionskrankheiten in Betracht zu ziehen seien, darüber gehen die Ansichten auch auseinander. Es dürfte indessen die Forderung wohl keinem ernsten Widerspruch von fachwissenschaftlicher Seite begegnen, das Diphtherie, sowie Scharlach-Kranke der Absonderung unterworfen werden. Einzelne Landesgesetzgebungen, zum Beispiel diejenige Englands, verlangen auch die Unterbringung der an Rose und Keuchhusten Erkrankten in Sonder-Krankenhäuser. Für Gebärhäuser muss die Absonderung der an Kindbettfieber leidenden Frauen von den übrigen Insassen unbedingt verlangt werden.

Dagegen scheint es mir zu weit zu gehen, wenn auch Masernkranke in Hospitälern und so weiter abgesondert werden sollen; für solche Kranke wird eine Absonderung wohl nur unter den ungünstigsten äusseren Verhältnissen zu fordern sein. Aehnliches gilt meiner Ansicht nach für den Keuchhusten.

Darmtyphus und Ruhr, welche lediglich durch die Ausleerungen verbreitet werden, bedürfen selbst im Falle einer grösseren Verbreitung und bei heftigen Erkrankungsformen keiner Absonderung, sobald für Unschädlichmachung und Beseitigung der Ausleerungen der Kranken in zuverlässlicher Weise Sorge getragen wird.

Unter allen Umständen wird man bei jeder Ueberführung von an den genannten Krankheiten leidenden Personen in ein Krankenhaus zwei Punkte nicht ausser Acht lassen dürfen:

1, das Gefühl der Angehörigen soweit das Gemeinwohl dies gestattet ist zu schonen, damit die Abneigung gegen die Verpflegung in öffentlichen Absonderungs-Einrichtungen bei der Bevölkerung nicht vermehrt wird;

2, durch zu weitgehende Forderungen tritt eine Erhöhung der öffentlichen Ausgaben ein, welche ebenfalls der Sache selbst leicht nachtheilig werden kann.

Art der Absonderung.

In welcher Weise soll nun die Absonderung stattfinden? Kann man vom Standpunkte der öffentlichen Gesundheitspflege fordern, dass jede Gemeinde, gleichviel ob gross oder klein, Absonderungsräume oder gar Absonderungs-Krankenhäuser für ansteckende Kranke der genannten Art schafft? Darauf dürfte zu bemerken sein, dass unter Umständen, zum Beispiel beim plötzlichen Auftreten von Cholera, beim Ausbruch von Fleckfieber, Pocken, Gelbfieber und Pest, unbedingt Absonderungsräume und sei es auch nur in Form von Zelten oder Einzelzimmern geschaffen werden müssen. Dass kleinere Gemeinden dauernd derartige Räume bereit stellen oder gar besondere Krankenhäuser für diesen Zweck errichten, kann nicht verlangt werden; es würde das eine finanzielle Belastung sein, die kleine Gemeindewesen nicht zu tragen vermögen. Wohl aber können und sollen Gemeinden von 50,000 Seelen und mehr derartige Einrichtungen schaffen, welche in gewöhnlichen Zeiten zur Aufnahme von an Scharlach, Diphtherie und so weiter Erkrankten benutzt werden können, beim Ausbruch der Landseuchen, Cholera, Pocken und so weiter geräumt, desinfizirt und für die Aufnahme der an der hereingebrochenen Epidemie Erkrankten hergerichtet werden. Sollte eine Ortschaft über 50,000 Seelen aus finanziellen Gründen ausser Stande sein, ein Sonderkrankenhaus zu errichten, so wird man sich damit begnügen müssen, bei dem vorhandenen allgemeinen Krankenhause Absonderungsräume, in Gestalt besonderer Zimmer, oder einer oder mehrerer Baracken, einzurichten. Städte von mehr als 100,000 Seelen und so grosse Gemeindeverbände deren einzelne Ortschaften nahe bei einander gelegen sind, können und müssen Absonderungs-Krankenhäuser einrichten.

Solche Häuser sollen niemals für eine zu grosse Anzahl von Betten vorgesehen sein und müssen entsprechend der Belegung, welche meines Erachtens 300 Betten nicht übersteigen sollte, genügend mit Ärzten und Pflegepersonal versorgt sein; wenn 50 und höchstens 70 Kranke auf einen Arzt und 2–3 Wärter zählen dürfen, dann wird denselben im Allgemeinen genügende Pflege zu Theil werden. Eine Anzahl von 100 Betten für einen Arzt erscheint schon etwas zu hoch gegriffen, weil Kranke solcher Art meist Arzt und Pflegepersonal sehr in Anspruch nehmen.

Wir wenden uns nun zunächst dem Bau von Absonderungshäusern zu, werden dann die Absonderungsräume in allgemeinen Krankenhäusern und zuletzt die beweglichen Baracken besprechen.

Bau von Sonder-Krankenhäusern und Sonder-Räumen.

Absonderungs-Krankenhäuser sollen, damit sie ihren Zweck erfüllen, fern von bewohnten Gebäuden, doch auch nicht zu fern von der Stadt errichtet werden. Man darf betreffs der Entfernung von menschlichen Wohnungen nicht zu ängstlich sein, wenn man die Beförderung von Kranken aus der Stadt in das Absonderungshaus nicht unendlich erschweren und damit die Absonderung selbst bei der Bevölkerung missbillig machen will. Es leidet der Kranke unter einem langen Transport im bequemsten Krankenwagen, und dadurch wird das berechtigte Gefühl der Angehörigen verletzt. Nach meinem Dafürhalten wird es genügen, wenn man Isolirhäuser in einer Entfernung von etwa 100 Metern von menschlichen Wohnungen anlegt und zwar, soweit es möglich ist, auf einem etwas erhöhten Gelände, welches den Winden freies Spiel gestattet, damit ein steter Luftwechsel auch um das Gebäude stattfinden kann. Eine grössere Entfernung von bewohnten Gebäuden kann abgesehen von Pesthäusern nur für Pockenhäuser in Betracht kommen. Für Cholera und Fleckfieber, sowie die sonst erwähnten ansteckenden Krankheiten ist bei einiger Aufmerksamkeit im Betriebe eine Uebertragung der Krankheitskeime in die Nachbarschaft lediglich durch die Luft nicht zu fürchten. Dafür muss allerdings Sorge getragen werden, dass zwischen dem Isolirhause und dem nahegelegenen zum Aufenthalt für Menschen dienenden Häusern keinerlei Personenverkehr stattfindet. Zur richtigen Würdigung der Ansteckungsgefahr muss man die Thatsache in Erwägung ziehen, dass Uebertragungen selbst der kontagiösesten Infectionskrankheit, des Fleckfiebers, in den allgemeinen Krankenhäusern, welche mit Absonderungsbaracken oder Absonderungszimmern versehen sind, bei der Häufigkeit dieses Verhältnisses verhältnissmässig selten in neuerer Zeit vorgekommen sind, seitdem man dafür mehr und mehr Sorge getragen hat, dass für die an Fleckfieber Erkrankten besonderes Pflege- und Dienstpersonal sowie eine eigene Verpflegungseinrichtung vorhanden ist. Der Personenverkehr dient stets der Uebertragung aller jener hier in Betracht kommenden Krankheiten in erster Linie.

Die Grösse des Baugrundstückes soll nach Ansicht vieler, besonders englischer Autoren so bemessen sein, dass auf jedes Krankenbett 200 Quadratmeter Grundstücksfläche entfallen. Ich verkenne gewiss die Berechtigung eines solchen Wunsches im gesundheitlichen Interesse zuletzt, kann aber die Besorgniss nicht unterdrücken, dass diese Forderung zu weit geht und deshalb selten erfüllt werden wird; es dürften 150 Quadratmeter Baufläche für jedes Bett ausreichen, um auch noch einen Garten für die Genesenden um das Hospital zu schaffen. Ist anzunehmen, dass in kurzer Zeit die Bevölkerung sich an dem in Frage kommenden Ort erheblich vermehren wird, dann empfiehlt es sich allerdings, eine grössere Grundfläche für jedes Bett in Aussicht zu nehmen, damit bei Zunahme der Bevölkerung baldmöglichst eine Erweiterung des Absonderungs-Lazarettes stattfinden kann.

Für ausgedehnte Gemeindewesen über 50,000 Seelen erscheint es trotz der voraussichtlich schnellen Bevölkerungszunahme kaum rathsam, dem etwaigen Bedürfniss durch Erweiterung *eines* Baues Rechnung zu tragen, vielmehr zweckentsprechender, in solchen Fällen die Anlage mehrerer excentrisch belegener Sonder-Krankenhäuser nach verschiedenen Stadtseiten ins Auge zu fassen, um einen zu weiten Transport der Erkrankten zu vermeiden.

Baugrund.

Soweit es die Verhältnisse gestatten, wird man einem trocknen, durchlässigen Untergrund, als Baugrund den Vorzug geben; ist man auf feuchtes Gelände angewiesen, so sind diejenigen Vorkehrungen zu treffen, welche für die Trockenlegung eines solchen Baugrundes durch Drainage, Isolirschichten in den Kellerräumen und dergleichen mehr erprobt sind. Diese jedem Sachverständigen bekannten Dinge hier bis ins Einzelne zu erörtern, halte ich nicht für erforderlich, da sie in nichts von den allgemeinen Vorschriften über Trockenlegung des Baugrundes für bewohnte Gebäude, insbesondere auch für allgemeine Krankenhäuser verschieden sind.

Auch über die Orientirung der einzelnen Gebäude erscheint mir eine besondere Auseinandersetzung überflüssig, man wird dieselbe nach den klimatischen und sonstigen Verhältnissen zu wählen haben. Wie bekannt, sind die Ansichten in dieser Beziehung getheilt; nach meinem Dafürhalten wird man in kalten Ländern die Krankenzimmer gegen Süden, bei gemässigtem Klima nach Osten und in heissen Gegenden nach Norden legen, um die Leidenden vor übermässig heissen Zimmern zu schützen. Das etwa lästige Sonnenlicht lässt sich durch Vorhänge von Stoff, Läden, Jalusien und dergleichen mehr abhalten, und Kälte durch zu rechter Zeit und in geeigneter Weise bewirkte Heizen bewältigen; von der Sonnenhitze durchglühete Zimmer sind bei selbst vorzüglichen Lüftungs-Einrichtungen schwer kühl und für den Kranken behaglich zu machen.

Dass die gesammte Anlage durch eine Umwährung begrenzt wird, dass der Garten mit hochstämmigen Bäumen zur Erzielung von Schatten besetzt wird, sei nur erwähnt.

Bei dem Bau einer derartigen Einrichtung ist darauf Rücksicht zu nehmen, dass die für das ärztliche und Pflegepersonal bestimmten Wohn- sowie die Wirthschaftsräume entweder in einem besonderen Gebäude untergebracht, oder aber durch eine abschliessende Wand von den Krankenräumen vollständig getrennt werden; wo es die Verhältnisse gestatten, sind auch die Wirthschaftsräume nicht mit den Wohnstätten unter einem Dach anzulegen, damit Ärzte und Pfleger nicht durch Küchenlärm und Küchendunst gestört und belästigt werden.

Bauart.

Was nun die Art der Ausführung im Allgemeinen anbelangt, so muss man unterscheiden zwischen der eingeschossigen und zweigeschossigen Baracke, einem Bau ohne Seiten-Korridor, vielfach auch in Holz oder Fachwerkbau ausgeführt, und dem massiven Pavillon oder Block mit Seiten-Korridor.

Ich gebe der eingeschossigen, in festem Material hergestellten Baracke vor allen anderen Einrichtungen für alle ansteckenden Krankheiten den Vorzug, weil diese Art des Baues besser wie jede andere eine vollständige Absonderung auch der einzelnen ansteckenden Krankheiten unter sich gestattet. Bei grösseren Anlagen kommt es doch wesentlich darauf an, dass die Kranken je nach der Art der Erkrankung in eigenen Räumen, welche lediglich solche Kranke aufnehmen, untergebracht werden. Nur im Nothfall kann es zugelassen werden, dass Kranke, welche an verschiedenen ansteckenden Krankheiten leiden, zusammengelegt werden; immer muss auch dann mit Vorsicht und Sorgfalt ausgewählt werden; so sind zum Beispiel Blattern- und Fleckfieberkranke stets zu isoliren, weil die Uebertragung dieser Krankheiten zu leicht stattfindet. Man wird daher darauf Bedacht nehmen müssen, für die in den einzelnen Ländern oder Landestheilen am häufigsten vorkommenden ansteckenden Krankheiten Einzelhäuser oder doch mindestens abgesonderte Einzelräume herzustellen. Wo, wie in Norddeutschland, Diphtherie und Scharlach niemals vollkommen verschwinden, wird man für diese Krankheiten je einen Sonderraum in grösseren Gemeindewesen herstellen; wo Fleck- und Rückfallfieber endemisch sind, in Ländern, in welchen die Pocken noch häufig verbreitet auftreten, sind Sonderhäuser für solche Kranke ein unabweisbares Erforderniss. Das schliesst nicht aus, dass diese Sonderhäuser, selbstredend nach gehöriger Reinigung, für andere Zwecke nach dem Erlöschen einer Epidemie benutzt werden können.

Die einzelnen Baracken oder Pavillons müssen in gehöriger Entfernung, mindestens 30 M. von einander und von Wohn- und Wirthschaftsgebäuden errichtet werden; ein solcher Abstand dürfte im Allgemeinen zur Verhütung von direkter Ueberführung von Infektionsträgern genügen. Lassen sich nach dem zu Gebote stehenden Baugrunde grössere Abstände erreichen, so kann dies nur günstig wirken. Die einzelnen Baulichkeiten sind unter sich, mit den Wohn- und Oekonomiegebäuden durch bedeckte, aber nicht von beiden Seiten geschlossene Gänge zu verbinden, um Ärzte, Pfleger und Bedienstete, insbesondere der Küche, sowie auch die Speisen beim Durchtragen zu den einzelnen Kranken-Abtheilungen gegen die Ungunst des Wetters zu schützen.

Für die zweigeschossige Baracke und den massiven, stets mehrgeschossigen Pavillon bleibt die Fundamentirung abgesehen von angemessener Verstärkung dieselbe, wie bei der eingeschossigen Baracke; die Gebäude sind unter allen Umständen zu unterkellern und wo es der Baugrund erfordert, in der Fundamentirung mit Isolirschichten zu versehen.

Wände.

Die Wände sind auch bei der eingeschossigen Baracke nur im Nothfall in Holzbau herzustellen; im Allgemeinen werden die Wände auch im Baracken-System jetzt in Stein oder anderem festen

Material aufgeführt. In neuester Zeit hat man Eisenkonstruktion gewählt, auch Gipsdielen zum Beispiel in der Krankenabtheilung des Instituts für Infektionskrankheiten in Berlin. Im Uebrigen können gute Backsteine, Moniermaterial und dergleichen mehr Verwendung finden.

Wesentlich bleibt für alle Konstruktionen, dass die Innenseite sämmtlicher Wände des Gebäudes durchweg, nicht allein in den Krankenräumen, möglichst glatt gehalten ist. Zu diesem Zweck kann man dieselben entweder mit mehreren Schichten Oelfarbe überziehen oder mit Mettlacher Fliesen bedecken, welche mit Porzellankitt gefugt sind, oder aber ganz und gar aus glasirten gebrannten Steinen aufbauen, deren Fugen wiederum durch Emaillefarbe oder Kitt gedeckt und glatt gemacht sind; so ist zum Beispiel die „New Royal Infirmary" zu Liverpool, eröffnet 1891, durchweg in Krankenräumen jeglicher Art, Korridoren, Kellern und Küchen gebaut.

Sind die Wände auf die eine oder andere Weise geglättet, so werden dadurch wie durch Vermeidung aller Ecken an dem Zusammenstossen der Wände unter einander mit der Decke und mit dem Fussboden Staubablagerungen thunlichst verhütet und lassen sich, wenn sie eingetreten sind, in leichtester Weise entfernen. Um die Ecken in den Räumen zu vermeiden, rundet man die Wände sowohl an der Stelle, wo sie mit dem Fussboden, als auch mit der Decke und unter sich zusammenstossen ab; statt der Ecken entstehen so ausgehöhlte glatte Kehlungen.

Ein Anstrich, der sich in dem Institut für Infektionskrankheiten bewährt hat, besteht aus einer starken Grundirung der Gipsdielenwände in Oelfarbe, auf welche dann Emaillefarbe in mehreren Schichten aufgetragen worden ist.

Fussboden.

Auch der 'Fussboden muss möglichst glatt sein. Zu diesem Zweck wird von der Mehrzahl der Autoren festgefugtes Eichen-Riemenparquett empfohlen. Felix und andere Autoren sprechen sich dagegen aus, weil die Fugen niemals so dicht seien, dass der Staub nicht einzudringen vermöge. In englischen Sonderkrankenhäusern wird das Bohnen eines solchen Fussbodens ebenso wie der Oelanstrich vermieden und der Boden möglichst häufig nass aufgewischt. Wenn man Holzfussboden überhaupt wählt, so scheint mir das

Vermeiden des Bohnens wenigstens nöthig, damit ein häufiges Aufnehmen des Staubes mit feuchten Tüchern stattfinden kann.

Um jenen Uebelständen von Grund aus zu begegnen, ist wiederholt vorgeschlagen und ausgeführt worden, die Herstellung des Fussbodens aus Terrazzo, Mettlacher Fliesen und dergleichen. In letzterem Falle ist die Kälte des Fussbodens nicht zu unterschätzen und wird man sich, um den Nachtheilen, welche daraus für die Kranken entstehen, vorzubeugen, entschliessen müssen, solche steinartigen Fussboden nur unter der Bedingung anzulegen, wenn derselbe durch Fussbodenheizung erwärmt werden kann; ein Punkt der indessen der reiflichen Ueberlegung nach den bisher gemachten Erfahrungen noch bedarf.

Grösse des Einzelbaues.

Was nun die Grösse der Baracke selbst anbelangt, so soll dieselbe für mindestens 10 Betten ausreichen, aber auch den Belagraum für 24 Betten nicht überschreiten. Es scheint nicht zweckmässig, eine noch grössere Anzahl Schwerkranker in einen Raum zu bringen und würde es nach meinem Dafürhalten, falls nicht der Kostenpunkt dabei in Frage kommt, sich immer empfehlen, höchstens 20 Kranke in einen Raum zu bringen.

Der für jedes Bett erforderliche Luftraum soll nach englischen Forderungen 60 Kubikmeter betragen, so dass also bei einer Höhe von $4\frac{1}{2}$ Metern nach Abzug von Ofen- und Nebenplätzen für jedes Bett ein Flächenraum von $13\frac{1}{2}$ Quadratmetern nöthig sein würde. Dabei verlangt Felix noch eine Lufterneuerung von 60 Kubikmetern in der Stunde. Englische Isolirhäuser gewähren bei reichlicher Lüftung sogar 70 Kubikmeter Raum (Fever Hospital in Leicester, Liverpool und Glasgow, sowie einzelne Absonderungshäuser in London). Wo es die Verhältnisse gestatten, kann es nur dankbar anerkannt und mit Freuden begrüsst werden, wenn dem Kranken ein reichlicher Kubikraum an Luft gewährt und letztere ausserdem oft erneuert wird. Es darf indessen nicht verkannt werden, dass die Forderungen von immer grösserem Luftraum für den einzelnen Kranken eine grosse finanzielle Belastung der Gemeinden bilden, und, wenn es gelingt, mit etwas weniger Kubikraum auszukommen und die Kranken durch reichliche Zuführung von frischer Luft dabei schadlos zu halten, so kann das für die gesammte Hospitalfrage nur günstige Folgen haben.

Lüftung.

In der Krankenabtheilung des Berliner Institutes für Infektionskrankheiten hat man sich genügt, für jedes Bett 40 Kubikmeter Luft zu gewähren, hierbei aber durch vortrefflich wirkende Entlüftungs-Vorrichtungen eine Lufterneuerung von 80 Kubikmetern für jedes Bett in der Stunde, noch bei niedrigster Temperatur der Aussenräume, erlangt.

Für die Entlüftung der Räume in der eingeschossigen und dem Dachstock der zweigeschossigen Baracke sorgen gegenüberliegende nicht zu kleine Fenster in Verbindung mit dem Dachreiter auf der First des Daches, welcher selbstverständlich so eingerichtet sein muss, dass die Kranken nicht durch Zugluft belästigt werden, in ausgiebigster Weise.

Neben dieser natürlichen Frischluftzuführung hat man fast überall zu künstlichen Unterstützungsmitteln gegriffen und die verschiedensten Methoden dabei zur Anwendung gebracht. Die besten Anlagen der Art sind stets mit der Heizung verbunden, so dass die zugeführte Menge frischer Luft nich kalt, sondern vorgewärmt, in die Krankenräume hineinkommt. Ich kann hier nicht auf die verschiedenen Lüftungsvorrichtungen näher eingehen, ohne die mir nach der Aufgabe und namentlich nach der zur Verfügung stehenden Zeit gesteckten Grenzen weit zu überschreiten, muss mich vielmehr auf die Äusserung beschränken, dass für Isolir-Spitäler und Isolirräumen nur die bewährtesten Lufterneuerungsanlagen genommen werden sollten; gerade in diesen Fällen ist eine zuverlässige Lufterneuerung das dringendste Erforderniss.

Dass man sich in England und Russland mit Vorliebe der einfachen Luftkammern bedient, dass in Deutschland das Pulsions-System verbunden mit der Heizung, vielfach in Anwendung kommt, die Meidingerschen und Böhmeschen Mantelöfen, sowie andere ähnliche Vorrichtungen ihre Verwendung gefunden haben, sei kurz erwähnt.

Das Dach sei leicht aber fest für jede ein- wie zweigeschossige Baracke. Der Dachreiter muss vorsichtig so konstruirt sein, dass durch denselben reichlich Luft zugeführt werden kann, aber die eindringende Luft nicht zu schnell in den Krankenraum hineingelangt; dies ist durch zweckmässige Anlage der Dachreiter und verstellbarer Luftklappen sehr gut zu erreichen.

Raumvertheilung, Nebenräume.

In jeder eingeschossigen, wie im Obergeschoss einer zweigeschossigen Baracke für 10 bis 20 Betten muss ausser dem Krankensaal ein Abort, ein Baderaum, ein Wärterzimmer, eine Theeküche und wo möglich ein oder zwei Räume für Einzelkranke oder für ansteckungsverdächtige Fälle, welche der Absonderung bedürfen, vorhanden sein. Die Abortvorrichtungen, welche je nach den Verhältnissen an Kanalisation und Wasserleitung anzuschliessen sind oder aber Tonnen- bezw. Kübel-System haben sollen, sind mit einer Einrichtung an geeigneter Stelle zu verbinden, welche bei bestimmten Krankheiten das Kochen gefährlicher Ausleerungen und damit die gründlichste Vernichtung von Krankheits-Keimen ermöglicht.

Die zu diesem Zwecke nach dem Vorgange der bei dem Auftreten der Cholera in Petersburg nach einem 1887 von Wassiljew gemachten Vorschlage von einem Herrn Sangalli getroffenen Einrichtungen sind auf Rudolph Virchow's Befürwortung von dem Verwaltungs-Direktor des Berliner städtischen Krankenhauses Moabit, Merke, 1892 in sehr einfacher Form modifizirt worden und haben sich wirksam erwiesen; Merke beschreibt seine Einrichtung in der Berliner Klinischen Wochenschrift, Jahrgang 1892, Nro. 38, etwa folgendermassen:

Statt des sonst vorhandenen Ausgusses für Wirthschaftswässer etc. neben dem Closet waren schon früher zwei nebeneinder liegende gusseiserne, innen emaillirte viereckige Becken angebracht worden, von denen das eine, für die Aufnahme der Excremente bestimmte bedeutend tiefer war, wie das daneben gelegene flachere. Beide communicirten durch einen zwischen dem Boden des flachen Beckens und der gemeinschaftlichen Scheidewand gelegenen Spalt mit einander, so dass Flüssigkeiten, die in das flache Becken gegossen wurden, durch diesen Spalt in das tiefer gelegene benachbarte abfliessen mussten. Letzteres hat in der Mitte seines Bodens eine grosse Abflussöffnung, die durch ein schweres Metallventil verschliessbar ist; das Ventil selbst ist durch eine den Rand des Beckens weit überragende runde Metallstange, die mit einem Handgriff versehen ist, leicht zum Zweck des Oeffnens zu heben. Ueber dem flachen Becken befinden sich Kalt- und Warmwasser-Auslasshähne.

In dieser Einrichtung waren bisher alle verdächtige Entleerungen der Kranken etc., auch im Sommer 1892 Cholera-Dejektionen, letztere unter Zusatz von Kalkmilch desinfizirt worden, bevor diese Substanzen in die Kanäle abgelassen wurden.

Um dieselbe Vorrichtung zum Kochen von Cholera-Excrementen brauchbar zu machen, wurde von der in jeder Baracke des städtischen Krankenhauses Moabit vorhandenen Dampfleitung ein Kupferrohr abgezweigt und in das tiefe Ausgussbecken so geleitet, dass es zweimal in Spiralwindungen auf dem Boden des Beckens um die Abflussöffnung herumgeführt wurde, während das Becken selbst durch einen abhebbaren Doppeldeckel oben verschlossen werden konnte. Folgendes Ergebniss wurde erzielt:

1. Das Kochen des im Becken vorhandenen Gemenges von Excrementen und Kalkwasser kommt je nach der Menge der vorhandenen Flüssigkeit mit Leichtigkeit in 4 bis 10 Minuten zu Stande;

2. die mit dem Kalkwasser gemengte Flüssigkeit schäumt beim Kochen sehr stark auf;

3. beim Kochen der Fäcalmassen mit Kalkwasser entwickelt sich ein penetranter, äusserst übler Geruch.

Das Abkochen der Fäcalien war somit erreicht, aber der dabei entstehende sehr üble Geruch musste vermieden oder beseitigt werden. Dies gelang durch Zusatz einer 5 prozentischen Lösung von übermangansaurem Kali statt der Kalkmilch zu den Dejektionen im Abflussbecken.

Für die beim Kochen sich entwickelnden Wasserdämpfe ist auf dem Ausgussbecken ein Abdunstrohr aufgesetzt, das über Dach geführt ist.

Bacteriologische Versuche haben ergeben, dass das Kochverfahren, welches selbstredend auch auf Typhus- und anderen Ausleerungen, sowie tuberkulöse Sputa Anwendung findet, alle Mikroben sicher vernichtet.

Ausserdem muss hier ein kleiner Desinfektionsapparat, bestehend in einem R. Koch'schen Topf, oder ein ähnliches gleich zuverlässiges Geräth vorhanden sein, welches alle Wäschestücke und sonstigen Gebrauchsgegenstände, die der Kranke besudelt oder benutzt hat, sei es ohne oder in Desinfektions-Flüssigkeit, aufnimmt.

Unsaubere Leib- wie Bettwäsche bringt man am einfachsten und besten in einen starken leinenen Beutel, welcher mit Desinfektionsflüssigkeit oder auch nur mit Wasser angefeuchtet ist, um jede Uebertragung der Krankheitsstoffe zu verhüten, befördert den gefüllten Beutel sofort in die Waschküche und in den Waschkessel mit siedendem Wasser, in welchem Beutel und Inhalt mindestens 30 Minuten gekocht werden. Auch hier muss der Grundsatz festge-

halten werden: Peinlichste Reinlichkeit und Entfernung aller
Schädlichkeiten sind überall und jeder Zeit die vorzüglichsten
Desinfektionsmittel.

Die Einrichtung von Fallröhren, welche innen mit Zinkblech,
Glas oder sonstigem glatten Material ausgefüttert und dazu bestimmt
sind, aus den Krankenräumen besudelte Wäsche und Verbandstücke
in untere Sammelräume zu führen kann ich für zweckmässig nicht
halten. Selbst bei grosser Reinlichkeit, die zur Zeit umfangreicher
Epidemien nicht immer aufrecht erhalten werden kann, ist hier die
Gefahr einer Festsetzung von Keimen sowohl im Schlot wie namentlich im Sammelraum nicht ausgeschlossen, und damit die Möglichkeit weiterer Verbreitung gegeben, wohingegen der Transport in
feuchten Beuteln eine Weiterschleppung der Keime vollständig verhindert, nebenbei sehr viel weniger kostspielig ist, wie jene Einrichtungen, welche leider auch in neuen Sonder-Krankenhäusern sich
hin und wieder noch finden.

Bei der zweigeschossigen Baracke ist die Decke des unteren
Raumes so fest herzustellen, dass Infektionsstoffe in den oberen
Raum nicht gelangen können; aus demselben Grunde ist die in den
Oberstock führende Treppe unmittelbar am Eingang des Gebäudes
in einem besonderen Treppenhause anzuordnen. Ist die ganze
Baracke nur für eine Infektionskrankheit bestimmt, so sind diese
Vorsichtsmassregeln nicht absolut nothwendig; da aber überall
Verhältnisse eintreten können, welche zur Belegung beider Geschosse
mit verschiedenen Kranken zwingen, so wird man gut thun, demge-
mäss jede zweigeschossige Baracke zu bauen. Auch aus diesem
Grunde empfiehlt es sich nicht, zweigeschossige Baracken und feste
Pavillons mit mehreren Geschossen für die Unterbringung ansteck-
ender Kranken einzurichten. Bei Pavillons wird man darauf sehen
müssen, dass niemals ein Mittelkorridor angeordnet wird, oder todte
Ecken entstehen, dass vielmehr nur Seitenkorridore mit reichlicher
Lüftung angelegt werden.

Erholungs- oder Tage-Räume.

Jeder Einzelbau, sei es nun Baracke mit einem oder zwei Geschossen oder Pavillon, wenn solcher beliebt wird, muss in jedem Geschoss
einen Erholungssaal für Genesende erhalten, so dass diejenigen,
welche nicht mehr an das Bett gebunden sind, sich frei bewegen
können, ohne die noch bettlägerigen Kranken zu stören; in diesem
Raume ist auch für Unterhaltung durch angemessene Lektüre und

harmlose Spiele zu sorgen. Ebenso ist für jedes Stockwerk oder
für jede Krankenabtheilung auf der Sonnenseite eine Veranda anzuordnen, damit die Kranken, welche den etwa vorhandenen Garten
noch nicht betreten können, oder falls ein solcher mangelt, doch die
so nöthige Gelegenheit des Aufenthalts in frischer Luft haben. Dass
ein Garten bei Sonderkrankenhäusern neben einer derartigen Einrichtung ein besonderer Vorzug ist, liegt auf der Hand.

Heizung.

Für jedes Gebäude eines Isolirspitals ist eine besondere Heizvor-
richtung anzulegen, damit nicht durch die Heizkanäle Fortführung
von Mikroben stattfinden kann. Um diese Forderung zu erfüllen,
sind die Baracken des Berliner Institutes für Infektionskrankheiten
mit Käuffer'schen Ventilationsmantelöfen versehen, welche bei guter
Beheizung der Krankenräume in Verbindung mit den aus Gipsdielen hergestellten Luftschloten zum Abführen der verdorbenen
Luft, wie schon bemerkt, einen sehr günstigen Luftwechsel bewirkt
haben.

Auch andere Mantelöfen gute Kachelöfen in Verbindung mit
Kaminen finden zweckmässige Verwendung, wenn nicht reichliche
Mittel zur Verfügung stehen und bei Isolirräumen an öffentlichen
Krankenhäusern, von welchen sogleich die Rede sein wird.

Desinfektions-Anstalt, Leichen- und Sektionshaus.

Weit und zwar nicht unter 40 Metern entfernt von der Gesammt-
anlage sollen die Desinfektionsanstalt und das Leichenhaus mit
dem Sektionszimmer in üblicher Weise angelegt sein.

Eine Desinfektionsanstalt für ein Sonderkrankenhaus ist derartig
einzurichten, dass diejenigen, welche mit den infizirten Gegenständen
zu schaffen haben, auch in der Lage sind, sich selbst hinterher durch
ein Bad reinigen zu können. In den Fever-Hospitals verschiedener
englischer Städte, so in Glasgow, Leicester, Liverpool, Leeds, London, habe ich 1891 eine meines Erachtens sehr zweckmässige Einrichtung gefunden. Der Desinfektionsapparat ist, wie in anderen
Ländern, in einem besonderen Gebäude aufgestellt, welches in einem
Vorraum der einen Seite die infizirten Gegenstände aufnimmt;
dieser Raum ist nur für die Bediensteten der Anstalt und Diejenigen
zugängig, welche kranke Angehörige zum Krankenhause oder infizirte Gegenstände gebracht haben. Von hier gelangt man durch
einen Gang in eine durch eine feste Mauer vollständig getrennte, neben

dem Aufnahmraum für die desinfizirten Effekten belegene Einrichtung zum Baden. Nachdem die begleitenden Angehörigen oder die Ueberbringer von infizirten Effekten ihre eigenen Kleidungsstücke abgelegt haben, treten sie durch diesen Gang in das Bad, reinigen sich sorgfältigst, warten noch einige Zeit in dem warm gehaltenen Raume und nehmen dann ihre desinfizirten Kleider aus dem Apparat durch eine nach aussen führende Thür zurück, durch welche die gebadeten Personen selbst die Anstalt verlassen. Ähnliche Einrichtungen finden sich jetzt auch bei vielen Desinfektionsanstalten in Deutschland, sind aber meines Erachtens überall nothwendig wo Angehörige Infektionskranke oder infizirte Gebrauchsgegenstände, welche immer in nassen Leinensäcken verpackt sein sollten zum Krankenhause oder zur Desinfektionsanstalt befördern.

Als Muster eines Desinfektionsapparates dürfte die jetzige Einrichtung in dem Institut für Infektionskrankheiten zu nennen sein, welche wie die von Washington und Lion in Nottingham hergestellten Apparate, allen neueren Anforderungen Rechnung trägt. Haupterforderniss bei allen solchen Anlagen, welche durch strömenden Dampf über 100 Grad wirken, bleibt immer, dass todte Ecken vollständig vermieden und der Dampf nicht von unten, sondern von oben in den Apparat eintritt, wie das bei den Henneberg'schen im Koch'schen Institut und den von Washington und Lion konstruirten, in England sehr beliebten Apparaten der Fall ist.

Verkehr mit den Kranken.

Um den Angehörigen einen Verkehr mit den Kranken zu ermöglichen sobald der Zustand derselben es erlaubt, eine Massregel, die wesentlich dazu beiträgt, die Abneigung der Bevölkerung gegen die Unterbringung der Kranken in Absonderungshäusern zu mildern, kann man verschiedene Wege einschlagen: Wenn die Kranken sich bereits im Rekonvaleszentenraum aufhalten, können die Angehörigen sich durch ein Fenster mit ihnen unterhalten: wo ein solcher Verkehr nicht möglich ist oder unzulässig erscheint, wird sich eine telephonische Unterhaltung immer ohne grosse Schwierigkeit durch geeignete Einrichtungen herstellen lassen.

Beförderung der Erkrankten.

Wenn auch nicht zum Bau und zu der Einrichtung von Isolir-Krankenhäusern gehörig, so doch ausserordentlich nothwendig für die richtige Absonderung Kranker, ist die Beförderung derselben von ihrer Wohnung zum Absonderungshause. Dieselbe wird am

schnellsten, sichersten, zweckmässigsten und angenehmsten für die
Erkrankten erfolgen, wenn sie nicht Privatunternehmern überlassen
bleibt, wie es in Berlin der Fall ist, sondern von der Verwaltung der
Absonderungshäuser ausgeführt wird; eine Einrichtung, die meines
Wissens in Amerika, insbesondere in New York, für alle Kranken-
transporte schon besteht.

Die in London seit 1867 geübte Beförderung von an ansteckenden
oder Geisteskrankheiten Leidenden durch das Metropolitan Asylum
Board ist vielleicht die grossartigste aller derartigen Einrichtungen
in der Welt, namentlich seit dem noch eine Beförderung zu Wasser
durch Indienstellung von drei besonders für diesen Zweck gebau-
ten Dampfern hinzugekommen ist, welche Pockenkranke nach dem
15 englische Meilen unterhalb London Bridge gelegenen schwim-
menden Hospital für Pockenkranke überführen. Dieses aus zwei
Schiffen bestehende schwimmende Krankenhaus ist auf 350 Betten
berechnet und mit einem vier englische Meilen weiter unterhalb
gelegenen Schiffsheim für 800 Genesende verbunden.

Grundsätzlich sollten alle derartigen Kranken durch Fahrgelegen-
heiten, welche von der Krankenhaus-Verwaltung geleitet wird,
dorthin befördert werden; wo dies nicht zu ermöglichen ist, dürfte
die Beförderung stets seitens der Gemeinden zu übernehmen, oder
mit den Einrichtungen einer gut geleiteten Feuerwehr zu verbinden
sein. Die Wehrmänner sind durch ihren ganzen Beruf mit derartigen Nothlagen vertraut, haben in Deutschland vielfach, besonders in
Berlin, als Samariter nach Esmarch'schen Grundsätzen ihre Ausbildung erhalten und wissen daher auch mit schwer Erkrankten viel
besser umzugehen, als mancher Krankenfleger oder gar ein gewöhn-
licher Arbeiter bei der von Privatpersonen geleiteten Krankenbe-
förderung. Finanziell aber wird jene Verbindung zwischen Feuerwehr und Krankentransportwesen für die Gemeinden nicht unvor-
theilhaft sein.

Absonderungsräume.

Wenden wir uns nun von der vollkommeneren Einrichtung der
Sonder-Hospitäler zur Unterbringung von an ansteckenden Krankheiten Leidender zu den in kleineren Gemeindewesen erforderlichen
Einrichtungen, so muss auch in Städten unter 5000 Einwohnern
entweder durch *besondere Räume* im allgemeinen Krankenhause
selbst, oder aber in der Nähe desselben durch eine Baracke von
geeigneter Konstruktion, sei es in Holz-, sei es in Steinbau, Eisenbau
und so weiter für die Absonderung solcher Kranken jeder Zeit die
erforderliche Gelegenheit geboten sein. Man kann nicht fordern,

dass in solchen Ortschaften für jede ansteckende Krankheit ein
besonderer Raum zur Verfügung steht, muss sich vielmehr daran
genügen lassen, dass für gewöhnliche Zeiten überhaupt nur ein oder
mehrere Räume für solche Zwecke vorhanden sind.

Absonderungsräume für ansteckende Kranke in oder bei allgemeinen Krankenhäusern müssen von allen übrigen Krankenzimmern
nebst Nebengelass nicht allein getrennt sondern auch abgeschlossen,
das heisst, so belegen sein, dass sie einen eigenen Zugang haben und
weder durch Thüren noch durch Gänge mit den für die übrigen
Kranken bestimmten Räumen und Nebenräumen in Verbindung
stehen. Baulich sind solche Absonderungsräume nach ganz denselben Grundsätzen herzustellen, wie die Räume in den festen Baracken.
Stets wird eine besondere Bade- wie Aborteinrichtung, ein eigenes
Wärterzimmer, gesonderte Heiz- und Lüftungseinrichtung vorhanden
sein, auch dafür gesorgt werden müssen, dass eine Kochvorrichtung
für gefährliche Fäkalien für den Bedarfsfall schnell angelegt werden
kann. Der Desinfektionsapparat des allgemeinen Krankenhauses
kann bei gehöriger Sorgsamkeit stetz mitbenutzt werden. Auch
erscheint es nicht bedenklich, die Wäsche aus den Absonderungs-
räumen, nachdem dieselbe in nasse Beutel von starker Leinewand
gehörig verpackt ist, in das allgemeine Waschhaus der Krankenanstalt zu befördern, unter der Bedingung, dass der gefüllte
Wäschebeutel sofort in einen Kessel mit siedendem Wasser geworfen
und darin mit seinem Inhalt 30 Minuten gekocht wird. Bei *sorg-
samer* Beobachtung solcher Vorsichtsmassregeln ist meines Erachtens jede Uebertragung von Krankheitskeimen aus den Absonde-
rungsräumen fast ausgeschlossen.

In epidemiefreien Zeiten, wie sie in kleineren Gemeindewesen auch
bezüglich Scharlach, Diphtherie, Darm-Typhus oft längere Zeit
eintreten, können jene Sonderräume nach sorgfältiger Reinigung
mit Wasser und Seife, Desinfektion der Gebrauchsgegenstände und,
mindestens 14-tägiger Durchlüftung zur Sommerzeit, anderweit
benutzt werden.

Bewegliche Baracken.

Wo auch solche Sonderräume fehlen, oder bei Verbreitung ansteckender Krankheiten zur Aufnahme der Erkrankten nicht ausreichen, da bleibt als sehr gutes Auskunftsmittel die bewegliche
Baracke, welche ihre vollkommenste Form in der Döcker'schen
Konstruktion erhalten, heizbar ist und sich überall auch in ungün-
stigen klimatischen Zeiten bewährt hat. Ihre Konstruktion als

bekannt voraussetzend, beschränke ich mich hier darauf hinzuweisen, dass in neuester Zeit ähnliche Einrichtungen mehrfach hergestellt worden sind, welche sich im Wesentlichen von der Döcker'schen Baracke wenig unterscheiden, so auch eine von Selberg & Schlüter neuerdings hier aufgestellten Baracke, deren wesentlicher Unterschied von der Döcker'schen in dem zu den Wänden benutzten Material liegt; die Wände bestehen aus zwei Linoleumplatten, zwischen welche Drahtgaze gelegt ist; durch maschinellen Druck sind beide Platten mit dem Drahtnetz unzertrennlich verbunden. Derartig hergestellte Platten werden auf Holzwerk innen und aussen aufgenagelt und auch zur Dachkonstruktion verwendet. Diese Art der Dach- und Wandbekleidung soll sich für Wohnhäuser in den Tropen bewährt haben.

Dass die aus solchen Sonderräumen, Einzelbaracken, kommenden infizirten Gebrauchsgegenstände sofort der Desinfektion sich zu unterwerfen sind, versteht sich von selbst. Es muss daher eine wirksame Desinfektions-Einrichtung für strömenden Wasserdampf, welcher Art sie auch sei zur Verfügung stehen; eine solche ist aber auch leicht zu beschaffen in Gestalt eines gehörig grossen Blechtopfes mit Einsatz, wie solchen Merke in der Berliner klinischen Wochenschrift, Jahrgang 1892, Nro. 37, zuerst zur Desinfektion für Verbandmaterial beschrieben und abgebildet hat. Weitere von dem Genannten angestellte Versuche haben erwiesen, dass derselbe Apparat in erforderlicher Weise vergrössert zur Desinfektion für Matratzen, Betten, Decken und andere Gebrauchsgegenstände ebenfalls brauchbar ist.

Einrichtung der Krankenräume.

Betreffs der Einrichtung der Räume empfiehlt es sich, die Lagerstätten aus Eisen möglichst einfach und so bequem wie möglich für die Kranken herzustellen. Ob man zu dem Zweck Drahtspiralen in Mannesmannröhren mit aufgelegter Decke oder aufgelegtem Betttuch verwendet, ob man auf Spiralfedern, wie vielfach in England, Haferstrohsäcke legt, deren Inhalt dann verbrannt, deren Bekleidung desinfizirt wird, das bleibe dahingestellt. Nur das wird sich empfehlen, Matratzen und Decken nach Möglichkeit von der Benutzung durch ansteckende Kranke auszuschliessen, um eine Desinfektion dieser Stücke zu vermeiden, die immerhin schwieriger ist, als die Reinigung waschbarer Gegenstände oder wollener Decken. Wo indessen derartige Einrichtungen nicht möglich sind, da nimmt man zur einfachen Matratze und zum Bett wieder seine Zuflucht; nur muss auf die Desinfektion durch strömenden Wasserdampf die grösste Sorgfalt verwendet werden.

Beleuchtung.

Man sorge für eine gute Beleuchtung bei Tage durch reichliche Fensterfläche, und sperre blendendes Sonnenlicht durch entsprechende Vorrichtungen, seien es nun leinerne Vorhänge von aussen, seien es Holzvorhänge, oder verschiebbare Läden, endlich Sonnensegel und so weiter, und bei Abend wo es angängig ist, durch gut abgeblendetes elektrisches Glühlicht, oder auch durch entsprechend gemildertes Bogenlampenlicht. Wo elektrische Beleuchtung nicht zu erlangen ist, tritt Gaslicht ein, und wo auch dieses mangelt, wird man sich mit Petroleumlicht begnügen müssen, in beiden letzteren Fällen aber ganz besonders sorgfältig für Regelung der Temperatur und Abzug der Verbrennungsgase Sorge tragen.

Ausstattung der Räume.

Sämmtliche Räume für die Aufnahme ansteckender Kranke sind so einfach wie möglich—in Eisengeräthen mit Glas oder Porzellan, Marmorplatten und so weiter herzurichten; alle überflüssigen Geräthe, Möbel, namentlich staubfangende Dekorationen, wie Vorhänge zu vermeiden; sie werden nur Ablagerungsstätten für Infektionskeime.

Dagegen empfiehlt sich nach englischer Sitte die Ausschmückung der Räume durch blühende Gewächse, welche aber keinen starken Geruch verbreiten dürfen; durch solche Pflanzen werden die Krankenräume behaglich und freundlich gemacht.

Wirthschaftsräume, Wohnungen für Aerzte und Pflege-Personal.

Zum Schluss sei noch ein Wort über Wirthschaftsräume, Aertze, und Pflegepersonal hinzugefügt. Sämmtliche Räume für Speisen und Getränke, wie deren Vorräthe, insbesondere der Speisen, sind isolirt von den Krankenräumen anzuordnen. Auch die Waschküche ist wie in grossen Krankenhäusern von den Krankenräumen abzusondern, kann aber neben der Speiseküche, nur ganz getrennt von derselben, liegen.

Wo nur Sonderräume oder kleine Baracken für derartige Kranke bestehen, wird die Bespeisung derselben besondere Aufmerksamkeit erheischen, um Uebertragung der Krankheitskeime zu verhüten, es wird Sache der Verwaltung sein, bestimmte Personen allein für diesen Dienst zu verwenden. Dieses Pflege- und Dienstpersonal ist anzuweisen und erforderlichen Falles mit Strenge anzuhalten, jeden Verkehr mit dem übrigen Personal, den anderweitigen Kranken und der Aussenwelt bis zum Erlöschen der Epidemie oder zur Ablösung des Dienstes zu vermeiden und vor Aufnahme einer anderweiten Thätigkeit sich durch ein warmes Bad mit Seife, bei welchem die Reinigung des Haupt- und Barthaares sehr gründlich vorzunehmen ist, und Wechsel von Kleidung und Wäsche sorgfältigst zu desinfiziren.

Am meisten empfiehlt es sich, die Speisen, durch die Bedienung nur an die Krankenzimmer zu befördern und einem in der Genesung befindlichen Kranken wenn möglich die Vertheilung zu überweisen.

Das Pflegepersonal für solche Kranke ist unter den geschilderten Umständen streng von dem Pflegepersonal für die übrigen Kranken abzusondern.

Der behandelnde Arzt soll, falls er gleichzeitig alle Insassen des Krankenhauses behandelt, die abgesonderten Kranken stets zuletzt besuchen und sich selbst dann einer gründlichen Reinigung unterwerfen, um die Ansteckungsstoffe nicht zu verschleppen; auf solche Weise ist es möglich, selbst die leicht übertragbaren Krankheiten dieser Art gleichzeitig mit anderen Erkrankungen zu behandeln und zu verpflegen, ohne die Mitmenschen durch Uebertragung des Krankheitsstoffes in Gefahr zu bringen.

Erste Bedingung bleibt für alle solche Verhältnisse, dass Aerzte wie Pfleger und Bedienung sich der peinlichsten Sauberkeit in der Kleidung und am Körper befleissigen. Es wird daher für alles ärztliche, wie für Pflege- und Verwaltungspersonal Pflicht sein, täglich Bäder zu nehmen. Die dazu erforderlichen Vorrichtungen müssen fest oder beweglich überall vorhanden sein oder beschafft werden. Dass für Isolir-Hospitäler, welche ein besonderes Verwaltungsgebäude und besondere Gebäude für das ärztliche und Pflegepersonal haben, stets derartige Vorrichtungen von Haus aus angelegt werden, sei hier noch erwähnt.

Bakteriologisches Laboratorium.

Den Ärzten an Sonder-Krankenhäusern oder bei Absonderungs-Krankenräumen muss die Möglichkeit gewährt werden, den Krankheitszustand der ihnen zur Behandlung überwiesenen Kranken auch mit allen zu Gebote stehenden Mitteln der Wissenschaft zu untersuchen, festzustellen und den Verlauf der Krankheit zu verfolgen. Für Sonder-Hospitälern ist daher die Errichtung eines bakteriologischen Laboratoriums eine unabweisbare Nothwendigkeit.

Schliesslich sei noch erwähnt, dass für grössere Anlagen der Art besondere Gebäude, welche möglichst entfernt von den übrigen derartigen Einrichtungen gelegen sind, für Pocken- und Fleckfieberkranke, zu errichten sind; in England hat man, wie bekannt, für Pocken stets besonders eingerichtete und abseits der übrigen Fieberhospitäler gelegene Pockenhäuser. Wo es die Verhältnisse gestatten, würde, wie bei London, nach dem Muster des dortigen Schiffs-Hospitals für Pockenkranke derartige schwimmende Krankenhäuser sich am meisten empfehlen. Wenn in jenen Ortschaften und Gegenden, wo die obenerwähnten Krankheiten häufiger auftreten, entfernt von den übrigen Gebäuden der Anlage, besondere Pocken- und Fleckfieberhäuser errichtet und eingerichtet werden, so dürfte dem Bedürfniss genügt sein.

Nur in allgemeinen Umrissen war es mir möglich, die mir gestellte Aufgabe zu behandeln; es würde mir eine besondere Freude sein, wenn es mir gelungen sein sollte, in diesen kurzen Sätzen auch nur einen Ueberblick über die Anforderungen zu geben, welche die öffentliche Gesundheitspflege an Isolir-Krankenhäuser und Isolirräume für ansteckende Krankheiten stellen muss.

ISOLATION WARDS AND HOSPITAL FOR CONTAGIOUS DISEASES IN PARIS.

DR. ALAN HERBERT, D. M., AND DR. W. DOUGLAS HOGG, D. M., PARIS.

We propose in this article to describe briefly the means of hospital isolation as adopted by the "Assistance Publique" in Paris, a committee controlling all the hospitals in the capital of France.*

It is not our intention, however, in this article, to attempt any criticism upon the system of the Paris hospitals. Any discussion bearing upon such a point would be out of place here. At the same time, while limiting this article to a mere summary, our final aim will be to submit to the Section conclusions as to the means to be

---

* For a more detailed account of the organization of the committee see our paper entitled "Paris Free and Paying Hospitals," presented to the Congress.

employed in all large centers, with a view to prevent contagion in hospitals during the treatment of patients affected with such diseases.

The question of hospital accommodation for such patients has for some time occupied the serious attention of the governing bodies of the "Assistance Publique" in France.

The interest bestowed of late years on State medicine, and the rapid progress made in that branch of medical science, has induced them, like others, to seek for improved means of treatment in such cases, both for the patients themselves and the surrounding population.

With this end in view the administration of the "Assistance Publique," the "Conseil Municipal" and the French government have considered it a duty to obtain every possible information on the subject.

Without giving a detailed account of the works which have treated of this subject, we may, perhaps, be permitted to recall to memory that in the years 1884 and 1885,* when smallpox and scarlet fever were raging in London and other large English towns, the Minister of the Interior entrusted one of us with a special mission to England, to study the prophylactic measures then in force in that country.

In 1889† the same ministerial department entrusted him with the mission of continuing these investigations, and of completing them by means of documents collected at the time of the Paris Exhibition.

In Paris considerable efforts have been expended in order to diminish the dangers resulting from the treatment, in the same hospital, of ordinary patients and those suffering from infectious diseases. Since 1882 the principle of isolation has been adopted.

In this year a special building was constructed for the treatment of diphtheria. . Since then new difficulties have arisen, and it would be useless to-day to hide the fact that there still remains much to be done to prevent the spread of disease in hospitals. In order to prevent this propagation of infection in any town it is not sufficient to place the affected person in a hospital, but it is also necessary to take measures to prevent that person becoming a source of infection to the hospital itself into which he has been admitted.

The following statistics, for which we are indebted to the kindness

---

*Isolation Hospitals in England. One vol. in 8vo of 250 pages, with 40 engravings and drawings. (Work recompensed by the Institute of France.) Paris, 1886. J. B. Baillière, Editor.

† New Researches on the Isolation of Contagious Diseases. One vol. in 8vo. Paris, 1890. J. B. Baillière, Editor.

of our excellent colleague and friend, Doctor J. Bertillon, chef du bureau de la Statistique de la ville de Paris, shows the number of cases in which contagious diseases have arisen in the interior of the Paris hospitals during the last ten years.

Statistics.

Years.	1884.	1885.	1886.	1887.	1888.	1889.	1890.	1891.	1892.	Total.
Cholera	62	..	..	..	..	..	..	..	19	81
Smallpox	22	25	61	89	..	11	2	7	10	227
Typhoid	38	71	70	188	78	122	318	108	276	1269
Diphtheria	279	175	205	228	331	239	308	221	184	2170
Totals	401	271	336	505	409	372	628	336	489	3747

It will thus be seen that during these ten years 3747 persons have been affected by contagious diseases which they would have escaped had they not entered the hospitals. It is needless for us to remark that this number would have been much greater if the statistics had included the cases of measles and erysipelas.

Before, however, considering the resources which the Paris hospitals possess for the isolation of contagious patients, it will be well to consider what necessity exists for such isolation. We may judge of this by the figures representing the number of patients affected with contagious and infectious diseases which took place during the year 1890.

DISEASES.	PATIENTS DISCHARGED.				FATAL CASES.				Total.
	Adults.		Children.		Adults.		Children.		
	Men.	Women.	Boys.	Girls.	Men.	Women.	Boys.	Girls.	
Typhoid	823	610	113	120	129	125	10	14	1,944
Smallpox	203	183	25	47	10	14	12	4	498
Measles	171	156	309	328	6	6	158	136	1,270
Scarlet fever	128	162	139	118	3	14	26	19	609
Whooping-cough	4	5	123	151	..	..	37	36	356
Diphtheria (croup)	34	36	424	335	8	8	562	540	1,947
Influenza	1,579	691	28	15	22	14	39	51	2,439
Cholera	2	1	..	..	..	1	6	9	19
Various fevers	476	322	12	8	26	13	..	1	858
Ringworm	..	..	9	8	..	..	..	..	17
Consumption	2,664	1,254	41	43	2,570	1,171	37	61	7,841
General Total	....	...	......	......	......	....	......	......	17,798

If from these numbers we take only those which apply to measles, smallpox, scarlet fever, whooping-cough, diphtheria and cholera, we find that in 1890, 4699 infectious cases were treated in the hospitals of Paris.

We will now examine the facilities which the city authorities have at their disposal to meet these cases.

According to a statement with which Doctor Peyron, director of the committee of the " Assistance Publique," has kindly furnished us, it appears that six hospitals are provided with the following means of isolation : *

The *Aubervilliers Hospital* possesses separate buildings for small-pox, measles, scarlet fever, erysipelas, diphtheria, and doubtful cases; in all, 184 beds.

The *Hospital Trousseau.* Isolation wards are established for children with diphtheria, measles, and scarlet fever (181 beds).

Hospital " des Enfants malades " (Enfant Jésus), which is a hospital for children, receives diphtheria and scarlet fever patients, 52 beds.

In addition to these the following hospitals are provided with isolation rooms : *Lariboisière*, 7 beds ; *La Pitié*, 5 beds ; *La Charité*, 3 beds.

All these taken together make a total of 332 beds.

We will now consider each of these establishments separately.

The Aubervilliers Hospital.

At the time of the cholera epidemic in 1884 the administration constructed at Aubervilliers, near the gates of Paris, small wooden buildings for the isolation of cholera patients. These were intended to be only temporary buildings, as the ground does not belong to the city of Paris, but to the State ; being situated on the military zone surrounding the town, on which the construction of buildings is forbidden.

These buildings, however, proved of so much service that they were maintained, and in June, 1887, were employed for the treatment of smallpox patients.

For some months past patients from the various isolation wards of the different hospitals have been transferred to this establishment.

It is composed of small buildings, entirely separate one from the other, and containing altogether 184 beds. Two of these buildings are reserved for the administration and the general service ; the others, for the treatment of the following contagious diseases : smallpox, measles, scarlet fever, erysipelas, diphtheria, and lastly,

* Up to the present time (February 1893) the *Hospital St. Antoine* possessed an isolation ward, which has just been suppressed.

doubtful cases. Two other small buildings, quite separate, contain, one, an amphitheater, the other, a compressed steam disinfecting apparatus and a sulphur-room.

Each building is provided with a bath-room, water-closet, store-room, and attendants' dormitory. The attendants are strictly forbidden to communicate with the other buildings.

All the buildings are in direct telephonic communication with the central administration.

The male attendants wear their beard and hair very short, are expected to wash their hands frequently in a solution of corrosive sublimate, to carefully brush their nails, and take at least one bath a week. They wear a smock-frock, a vest, and an india-rubber covering over their shoes.

Any person before entering the wards must put on a long, closely buttoned frock. When he leaves the ward this garment is deposited in a special room, from which the visitor is conducted to a disinfecting room.

In the case of any outside workman being required for work within the establishment, he must be able to show that he has been recently vaccinated.

On the arrival of a patient his clothes are disinfected by the steam process, his shoes and hat by the sulphur process. Their correspondence is also subjected to the sulphur process before being posted.

No visits are allowed.

Thanks to these precautions, no case of contagion within the establishment has arisen since they were instituted.

The Hospital Trousseau.

This hospital, situated within Paris, 89 rue de Charenton, contains 558 beds. It is for children only, receiving both medical and surgical cases.

The following facts apply only to contagious cases, for which 154 beds are set apart.

The service comprises: 1. Four isolation pavilions, reserved for the treatment of diphtheria, measles, scarlet fever and doubtful cases. 2. A series of wards for cases of whooping-cough.

Each service possesses a staff of nurses, entirely separate from the other attendants of the hospital. They have their own dormitory and dining-room.

As regards the medical service, it is performed alternately, every two months, by the different physicians attached to the hospital.

Details of each Service.

a. Diphtheria. (*Pavillon Bretonneau*), 36 beds.

    Attendants: 1 lady superintendent.

             1 night assistant.

             3 day nurses.

             2 night nurses.

             1 male attendant.

b. Measles. (*Pavillon d'Aligre*), 53 beds.

    Attendants: 1 assistant superintendent.

             1 day under-assistant.

             1 night   "   "

             4 day nurses.

             3 night nurses.

             1 male attendant.

c. Scarlet fever. (*Pavillon Davenne*), 24 beds.

    Attendants: 1 night assistant.

             1 day   "

             2 day nurses.

             2 night nurses.

             1 male attendant.

d. Doubtful cases. (*Patients under observation*), 16 beds. (This service was only opened on the 23d of November, 1892.)

    Attendants: 1 day superintendent.

             1 night assistant.

             2 day nurses.

             2 night   "

             1 male attendant.

e. Whooping-cough. No. beds, boys, 11 } 25.

                  girls, 14 }

    Attendants: 1 day assistant.

             1 night   "

             3 day nurses.

             3 night   "

Number of cases during the year 1892:

	Diphtheria.	Measles.	Scarlet fever.	Doubtful cases.	Whooping-cough.
Admitted,	1089	586	248	51	216
Discharged,	510	422	214	44	156
Fatal cases,	563	153	25	3	46

The Hospital of the "Enfants malades" (L'Enfant Jésus).

This hospital, which contains 629 beds, is situated in Paris (rue de Sevres), in a very populous district. It receives children from one to fifteen years of age, and possesses both a medical and surgical staff.

The isolation accommodation contains 87 beds, for the following complaints: diphtheria, measles and scarlet fever.

An isolation pavilion, constructed in the year 1882, is especially reserved for the treatment of diphtheria.

Two separate wards on the second floor are reserved for measles and scarlet fever patients respectively.

There is, however, under consideration a scheme which will shortly be put into execution, for the construction of entirely separate buildings for scarlet fever, measles and doubtful cases.

At the present moment the diphtheria ward contains 28 beds, the measles ward 25 beds, the scarlet fever ward 24 beds.

The nursing staff is divided as follows:

Diphtheria:
1 day superintendent.
1 night assistant.
4 day nurses.
2 night nurses.

Measles:
1 assistant superintendent.
1 night assistant.
4 day nurses.
1 night nurse.

Scarlet fever:
1 day and 1 night assistant.
3 day nurses.
1 night nurse.

Number of cases during the years 1891, 1892:

		1891.	1892.
Diphtheria.	Admitted,	957	997
	Discharged,	455	522
	Fatal cases,	502	475
Measles.	Admitted,	509	589
	Discharged,	326	422
	Fatal cases,	183	167
Scarlet fever.	Admitted,	188	197
	Discharged,	173	178
	Fatal cases,	15	19

Cases contracted within the hospital:

	Boys.	Girls.
Diphtheria,	58	34
Measles,	149	116
Scarlet fever,	27	19
	234	169

Total, 403 *

Hospital Lariboisière.

Patients affected with contagious diseases are treated at the Hospital Lariboisière in a small isolated building containing seven beds.

Each patient's room opens directly on to a balcony which surrounds the building. These rooms have no direct communication with each other.

Independently of the medical staff there are three persons attached to this building, who are obliged to take all necessary precautions before absenting themselves from it. They are: 1 assistant superintendent, 1 male attendant, 1 female attendant.

Number of cases in 1891 and 1892:

	1891.		1892.	
	Men.	Women.	Men.	Women.
Diphtheria.............	3	11	3	8
Measles	11	12	4	6
Scarlet fever...........	3	5	4	1
Smallpox	..	1	..	..
Erysipelas.............	36	57	36	45
Cholera................	..	..	6	13
Various cases..........	4	23	7	45
Total.............	57	109	60	118
		= 166		= 178
Cases discharged........		153		153
Fatal cases.............		13		25
		166		178

There remains but little to be said with regard to the other general hospitals, viz. " La Pitié " (716 beds) and " La Charité " (520 beds), which possess five and three isolation rooms respectively.

* We must deduct from this number about 20 cases which, on admission, were placed in the general medical wards when the disease was in a state of incubation, but which were afterwards transferred to the isolated wards as soon as their contagious character became apparent.

These rooms are only intended to meet the contingency of contagious cases arising among the patients admitted whom it has been impossible to transfer to one or other of the hospitals previously mentioned. We must mention, however, that during the last outbreak of cholera in Paris these patients occupied at " La Pitié " a medical ward which was evacuated to accommodate them. This ward, which comprised a division for men and another for women, was situated at one end of the hospital, having a separate staircase.

The staff attached to the cholera patients had no communication whatever with the other employés of the building, and the precautionary measures were strictly adhered to.

During the outbreak 69 patients were admitted. There were 31 fatal cases.

Conclusion.

With regard to the foregoing subject we desire to be permitted to submit to the Congress a few proposals relating to hospital prophylactic measures applicable to large towns.

The question under consideration is the isolation of patients affected with contagious diseases in hospitals, and not prophylactic measures in general.

In our opinion the following are the questions which have to be dealt with :

I. In what manner is it best to isolate contagious patients ?

II. Is it sufficient to have special wards in a general hospital, or is a separate building necessary for each disease ?

III. Can several of these buildings be situated in the same grounds?

IV. Do the same rules apply to hospitals destined for the reception of patients affected with acute diseases and to those for convalescents?

To these questions we should give the following replies :

I. In our opinion, the treatment of cholera and smallpox patients requires a special hospital, situated outside the town, at a distance as far as possible from any habitation.

II. Patients affected with other infectious or contagious diseases can be treated in separate buildings, situated in the same grounds, provided there be a distance of at least thirteen yards between them, and that each building has its own distinct and separate staff.

III. Convalescent hospitals for patients recovering from contagious diseases should be established outside the town, in accordance with the preceding rules.

PARIS FREE AND PAYING HOSPITALS.

Dr. Alan Herbert, D. M., and Dr. W. Douglas Hogg, D. M.,
Paris.

According to French law every commune or territorial division is obliged to provide assistance to any of their indigent members requiring aid. A certain number of "communes" have hospitals within their limits. The law of the 7th of August, 1851, obliges such communes to take charge of their sick poor. The hospitals, however, of these communes, when called upon to do so by the Conseil Général of the Department, are obliged to receive patients coming from smaller and neighboring communes who have no hospital within their limits, at a fixed price. These prices are fixed by the Prefect of the Department.

With a view, however, to extend medical help to the poor, belonging to no matter how small a commune, and whether it be provided or not with a hospital (and it must be remembered that out of 36,121 communes only 1200 are so provided), a project of law was recently (5th of June, 1890) laid upon the table of the Chamber of Deputies.

This bill, which did not become law as did that of 1851, recognized the admission of foreigners into these hospitals, but it did not render their admission obligatory on the commune.

It may be argued that a law rendering the admission of foreigners obligatory should exist only in such cases as the nation to which the foreigners belong gave reciprocity.

These principles of rendering aid to the poor and indigent sick were for the first time legally enforced by the convention of 1793, which decreed " that henceforth the property of all charitable bodies and communities should become national property." Before 1789 all charitable institutions were governed by bodies who had little or no connection one with the other; often they were quite independent. All these charitable institutions were managed by the clergy, who distributed the funds.

The king, it is true, had power to interfere on behalf of the indigent population, and this regal power was employed to insure the execution of decisions taken by the different councils (Councils of Tours, Vienna, Trent, etc.).

As early as 793 Charlemagne decreed that certain hospitals should become royal establishments, and instituted rules for the proper treatment of the poor.

In the thirteenth century St. Louis augmented the number of these hospitals, and in subsequent times these institutions continued steadily to increase. But great as these efforts were, it was only in the eighteenth century that assistance to the needy, which had till then been entirely voluntary, was declared to be a matter of right and became a matter of duty.

The convention of 1789 makes strong declarations to this effect in its exposition of principles. It was about this time (1791) that a central and unique administration for the relief of the indigent classes was established in Paris. This central administration, subject to the higher powers of the state, has continued much the same up to the present date.

A law passed on the 10th of January, 1849, is still in force, and by it the "Assistance Publique" has the direction of hospitals and alms-houses, as also of all relief given at the dwellings of the poor, the guardianship of orphans and abandoned children, and of persons of unsound mind. The administration of the "Assistance Publique" is under the control of the Minister of the Interior and the Prefect of the Seine. The direct management is confided to a director who acts with a "Council of Surveillance."

The funds of the "Assistance Publique" are partly derived from property which was, as we have stated, confiscated by the convention in 1791, and also from an annual grant of about the same amount, voted by the Municipal Council of Paris.

In 1890 the sum expended for the maintenance of hospitals, including the establishments for insane patients and abandoned children, amounted to 22,883,163 francs.

In 1889 the published account states that the "Assistance Publique" had under its control 11,989 hospital beds and 12,370 beds in almshouses. There are also 330 beds for confinements, to which 88 midwives are attached.

The medical body attached to these hospitals consists of 88 physicians, 40 surgeons, 9 physicians treating mental cases, 9 accoucheurs. There are also acting under the physicians and surgeons 212 internes or house-surgeons, 22 pharmaciens, with assistants acting under them.

All these officers are appointed after a competitive examination.

The large number of applicants renders this competitive examination very difficult.

We have already stated that every commune is bound by law to give medical relief to its indigent sick. Paris is, of course, bound by the same obligation and admits the indigent sick into its hospitals free of all charge. This gratuitous treatment, however, extends only to the indigent. After admission to the hospital an inquiry is instituted, and if it be found that the patient is in a position to pay, the sum of 3 francs 30 centimes a day is required of him. The charge for a child is 2 francs 6 centimes only.

As a matter of fact this sum is rarely claimed. In 1886 the total sum paid by patients or their families for hospital assistance was only 2501 francs, whereas the total expended was 778,840 francs.

It is therefore fair to consider the hospitals as being practically free.

The following statistics will give an idea of the important work done by the "Assistance Publique":

Number of patients in the hospitals of Paris in 1889:

General Hospitals.	Present on January 1, 1889.	Patients Admitted.	Fatal Cases.
Hotel Dieu,	835	9,575	1,215
Pitié,	729	10,097	1,090
Charité,	577	7,348	705
St. Antoine,	758	11,951	1,371
Necker,	486	7,515	839
Cochin,	348	5,614	454
Beaujon,	445	8,524	912
Lariboisière,	816	13,285	1,466
Cenon,	802	12,620	1,521
Laénnec,	627	4,141	580
Bichat,	192	2,691	370
Andral,	103	1,382	169
Broussais,	258	1,994	235
Temporary hospital,	61	598	55
Total,	7,037	97,335	10,982

Hospitals for special diseases:

	Present on January 1, 1889.	Patients Admitted.	Fatal Cases.
St. Louis,	781	8,825	345
Midi,	265	4,667	12
Lourcine,	173	2,093	25
Accouchement,	188	4,843	189
Clinique,	112	2,341	55
Aubervilliers,	21	706	63
Total,	1,540	23,475	689
General Total,	8,577	120,810	11,671

Children :

Children's Hospital,	484	9.674	1,262
Forges,	194	292	7
Trousseau,	382	5,015	1,028
La Roche Guyon,	88	578	5
Berk-sur-Mer,	573	778	41
Total,	1,721	11,337	2,343
Total of hospitals,	10,298	132,147	14.014
Paying hospitals,	158	2,263	360
	10,456	134,410	14.374

Summary.

	10,456
Patients treated admitted during the year,	134,410
Total,	144,866
Patients discharged,	
Cured or otherwise,	119,079
Fatal cases,	14,374
Total,	133,453

Total of days spent by patients in hospitals, 3,992,548.

The statistics just given will enable one to form an opinion as to the requirements existing in Paris and the various resources that town has at its disposal.

Paying Hospitals.

As we have already stated, the patients received into the hospitals of the "Assistance Publique" are, as a general rule, treated gratuitously, and it is very rare that the small contribution of from two to three francs a day is required of them.

There are, however, some exceptions, and the most important is the "Maison municipale de Santé," in the rue du faubourg St. Denis, 200, which receives none but paying patients. The prices are the following :

Small apartment, 12 francs per day. Small lodgings for medical cases, 7, 8 and 9 francs per day ; for surgical cases, 8 and 9 francs per day. Rooms with 2 beds, medical cases, 7 francs per day ; surgical cases, 8 francs per day. Rooms with 4 beds, medical cases, 5 to 6 francs per day ; surgical cases, 6 francs per day. In these prices are included medical and surgical visits, operations, dressings, medicines, food, firing, linen, baths of all kinds, etc.

The Maison de Santé contains 333 beds, of which 187 are for medical and 146 for surgical cases.

The following are the statistics of the patients treated in 1889:

	Patients admitted during 1889.	Discharged during 1889.	Fatal cases.
Men,	1,492	1,201	230
Women,	871	727	130
Total,	2,363	1,928	360

There are also paying beds at the hospital St. Louis and at the Midi.

At St. Louis (hospital for skin diseases) there are two separate buildings or pavilions where the patients pay from 5 to 6 francs a day, according to the rooms they occupy. There are 42 beds, 29 for men, 13 for women. At the Midi hospital (for syphilitic diseases), where men only are received, there are 21 beds. The price is 6 francs a day.

Private Institutions.

We have only mentioned in this paper those establishments which are of a public nature and are connected with the "Assistance Publique" of the town of Paris.

There are also many private establishments where only paying patients are received.

Such establishments as receive patients of unsound mind are subject to regular inspection by government officials.

HOSPITAL FOR CONTAGIOUS AND INFECTIOUS DISEASES.

By M. L. Davis, M. D., Lancaster, Pa.

The importance of isolating the sick from the well in epidemics of contagious and infectious diseases has been fully appreciated for many years. The red or yellow flag has been nailed to the door, hoisted over the building, or placed at the masthead of the vessel having cases of contagious or infectious diseases within, to warn the well of the danger of approaching. The fact that these emblems of danger do not kill the disease germs or prevent them from working their deadly havoc among the afflicted inmates has been neglected. Many patients with the same disease are congregated in the same room, or in wards constructed in such a manner that no restraint prevents the germs from being carried to any part of the building; the result is that each person appropriates the most malignant germs from the others, and although the disease at first may be of a mild type, the virulence of the contagion will increase until malignancy ensues. In other words, the labors of sanitarians have been directed almost exclusively toward preventing the spread of disease from the sick to the well—no attempt being made to protect those already ill from receiving more of the disease germs and thereby aggravating each individual case. Hence we frequently see the anomaly of building cheap, temporary wooden structures for hospital purposes, so that when they become saturated with poison to such an extent as to render them untenable, they can be burned and rebuilt at less outlay than a permanent building would require. This may be a very effectual method of destroying the germs of disease, but is neither rational nor in keeping with the present state of preventive medical science.

The Municipal Hospital at Philadelphia is too small to accommodate the cases of contagious diseases sent to it, and it is only a few days since we read the suggestion of some of the authorities that temporary wooden buildings be erected, and destroyed when no longer safe to be used; this practice is, therefore, not obsolete. The ideal hospital for contagious and infectious diseases must meet the following requirements:

1. It must completely isolate the sick from the well.

2. It must prevent one patient from receiving and appropriating the malignant germs from others having the same diseases, and thereby preventing aggravation of the disease in both.

3. It must destroy all the disease germs given off from the sick within its rooms.

4. It must prevent the escape of any disease germs to poison earth, air, food and water—the media through which contagious diseases are known to spread.

Description of Hospital.

The ground-floor plan of the hospital building consists of a central building, with wings or wards radiating from it of any desirable number and length. The first floor of this central building is divided into rooms for offices, dining-room, bath-rooms, kitchen, disinfecting chamber, etc. In the corridors is an iron stairway leading to upper stories; back of this stairway are situated the furnaces; one a garbage furnace, the other a reverberatory furnace for cremating the bodies of patients dying of contagious or infectious diseases. The burning gases from these furnaces pass under the boilers and thence into the stack, thus being utilized to produce steam for both heating and disinfecting purposes. The disinfecting chamber is situated at the side of the boiler and the cremating furnace; it is made of boiler plate, and is provided with tight-fitting clamp doors, with rubber packing. This chamber is connected with the boilers and with the retort of the cremating furnace, so that steam, dry hot air, or sulphur fumes can be used at pleasure. Radiating from the central building are the wards for patients. Each ward has a central hallway running lengthwise, with rooms on either side.

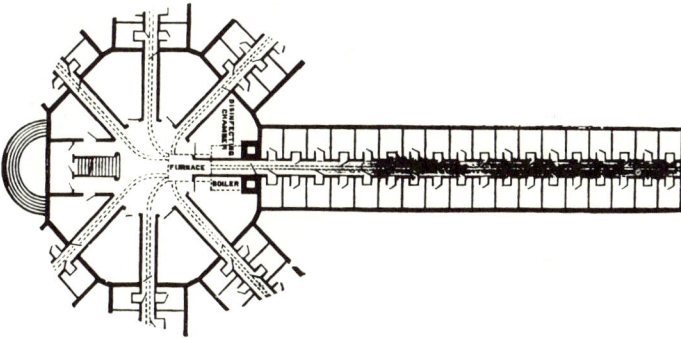

FIG. 1.

Figure 1 shows the central building with one room completed and the other six wards incomplete. These may be added from time to time, as needed, without interfering with the proper working of the plant.

Figure 2 is a cross section through two rooms. Each room is provided with a vestibule having two doors, one opening into the hallway outward, and the other opening inward into the room. These doors are provided with a common spring, so that only one can be opened at a time; they are made air-tight by gum packing. Each vestibule is provided with a vessel containing a disinfectant, and everything taken out of the room is here disinfected before

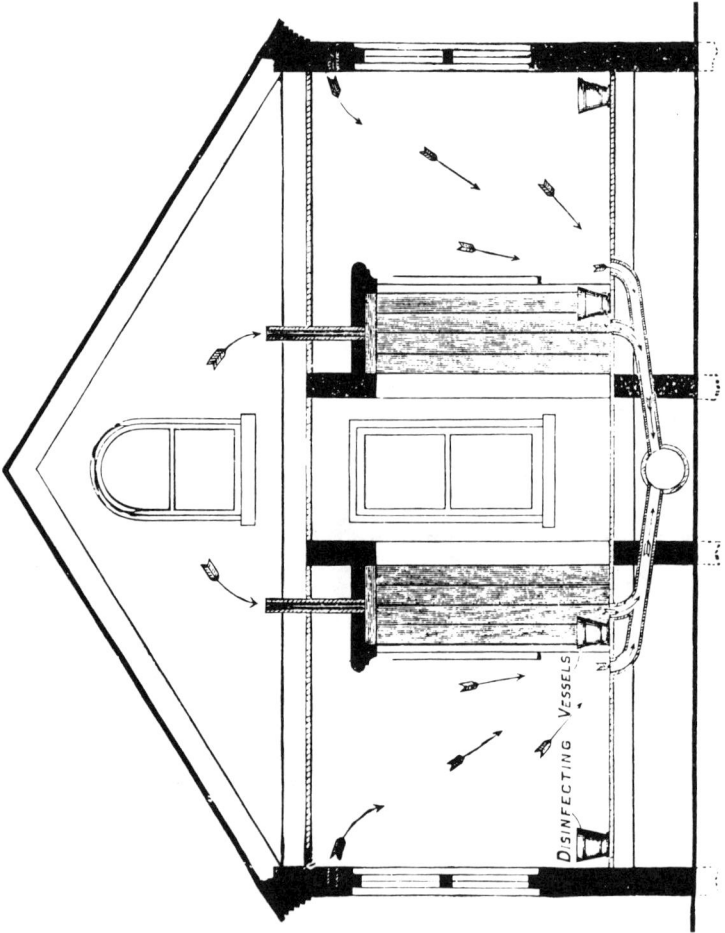

DISINFECTING VESSELS

Fig. 2.

being taken into the hall. The rooms each have one window, which is air-tight; the walls are plastered with cement, to allow disinfection by steam without injury. Under each hall floor is a large air-pipe running the entire length, and indicated by dotted lines in Figures 1 and 2. This is the ventilating pipe, and by its branches to each room and vestibule runs into the central building and ends in the ash-pit of the furnaces. The suction thus produced on this pipe by the furnaces and stack draws the air out of the rooms and vestibules, and with it all the disease germs present, which are consumed in passing through the fire. The heating is by steam pipes from the boilers. Each room is provided with a stop-cock, by opening which the room can be disinfected with steam and rendered pure and clean in a short time. Each room is provided with a metallic waste receptacle with tight lid; all waste is placed therein, disinfected in the vestibule, carried to the garbage furnace and the contents there burned. Each room is provided with electric call-bell and gas-light.

All fresh air admitted to the rooms and vestibules comes through a trapped pipe; it is placed near the ceiling. It is packed with absorbent cotton saturated with any desired antiseptic.

Figure 3 is a vertical section of garbage furnace. As will be seen, it consists of three chambers—the Primary Fire Chamber, Garbage Chamber, and Secondary Fire Chamber. The flame from the primary fire chamber passes through the garbage which has been dumped upon the grate, and dries it thoroughly, the gases driven off passing in the form of smoke to the secondary fire chamber, where they are consumed, and where combustion is so complete that no residual odor can be detected at the outlet from the stack. Liquid waste drips into the evaporating pan, where it is vaporized by means of a pipe running from the bottom of pan to the fire in primary chamber, the steam thus produced passing out of jet at the end of the garbage chamber and assisting combustion at the most needful point in the secondary chamber. When the charge has been thoroughly desiccated the grate is lowered and the dry product is dumped into the fire in primary chamber, where all its organic constituents are finally consumed, being utilized as fuel to dry subsequent charge. This furnace may be built to any scale to meet the wants required, being simple and economical in construction, easy of operation and giving perfectly satisfactory results. Provision is made in the garbage chamber for receiving the vessels containing excrement from the rooms, whereby, after their contents are destroyed, they are easily removed.

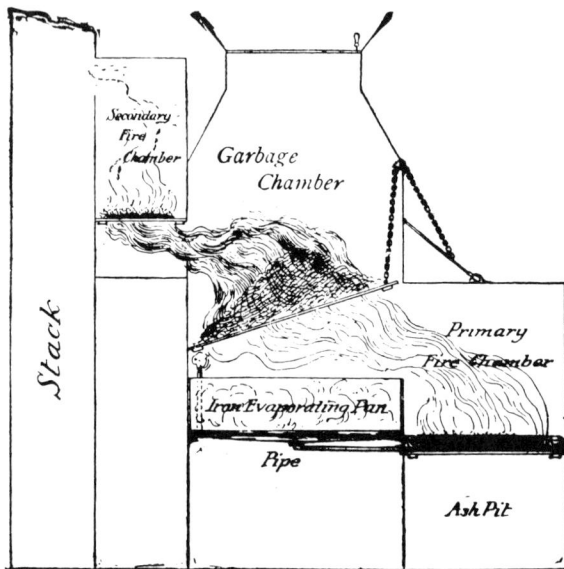

FIG. 3.

Figure 4 gives a cross section and longitudinal section of reverberatory retort furnace for the cremation of the bodies of those who die from pestilential diseases. This furnace is now in use at Swinburne Island Quarantine Station, New York, Municipal Hospital, Philadelphia, and at a majority of the crematoriums in the United States. The body is placed in a tight retort, which is surrounded by flues, through which the fire travels, heating the retort to any degree desired. The heat of the retort distills off the gases from the body ; they are not burned in the retort, but pass through a pipe to the ash-pit, and are there delivered under the grate of the fire chamber, where final combustion is so complete that analysis by Dr. T. B. Baker, of Millersville State Normal School, of what escaped from the chimney gave the following :

	H_2O.	CO_2.	Illuminating Gas.	O.	CO.	N.
Before cremation,	.0011	.00080	.000	.0080	.0000	.016
During cremation,	.0044	.00091	.012	.0065	.0017	.015

The chemist adds that " none of his tests indicated the presence of anything that could pollute the air." The combination of the

CROSS SECTION

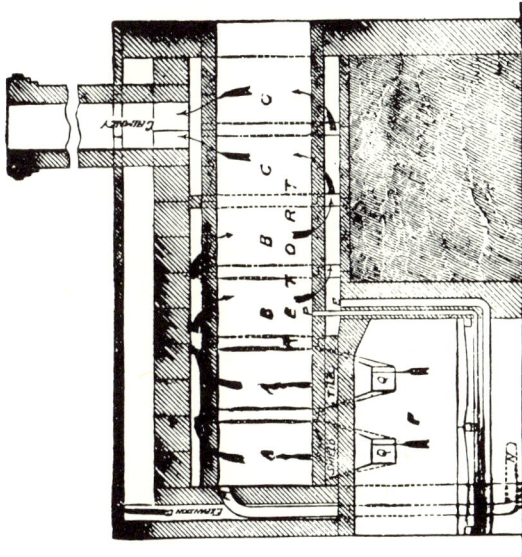

LONGITUDINAL SECTION

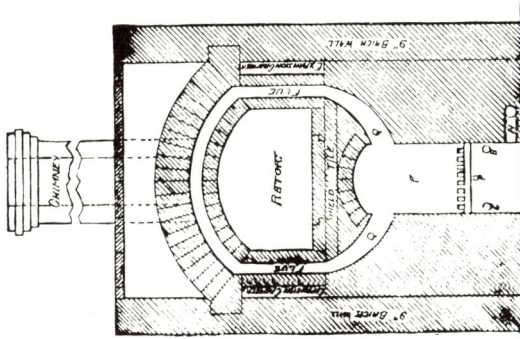

FIG. 4.

garbage and cremation furnaces with the antiseptic hospital, the author believes, covers the whole ground thoroughly and brings the subject abreast of modern science.

DISCUSSION.

THE CHAIRMAN.—The transmission of bacteria through the air in cases of contagious disease is rare, except in the case of measles. The transmission of typhoid fever is always, directly or indirectly, through the discharges, and if those are promptly cared for there is no danger in placing typhoid fever patients in wards with other patients, and in fact it is done every day in almost all hospitals. Scarlet fever is a disease that can be isolated with tolerable ease, if it is taken early. It may be recognized usually within 24 to 36 hours after the outbreak of the initial fever, and physicians usually have no difficulty in isolating scarlet fever cases in private houses where they can place the patients in a separate room on an upper floor, taking special care to remove from the room all things which cannot be treated by boiling or disinfectants.

In diphtheria, if the discharges from the throat and nose be properly taken care of, there is little danger of infection. The special germs of diphtheria and of typhoid fever never rise into the air from moist surfaces, unless carried by insects. If they are allowed to dry and form a crust on the edge of the vessel, or on a handkerchief, towel or sheet, the fragments may pass off in the shape of dust and become very dangerous. The ways in which such diseases as diphtheria may be transmitted are, as you all know, multiple. A patient has diphtheria; the nurse wipes his mouth or his nose with a handkerchief, and leaves the room without washing her hands. She may inoculate the handle of the door, as she goes out, with the bacillus of diphtheria, and the next person who places his hand upon that door-knob may get the germ on his fingers and thence to his mouth. Bacteriology simplifies the construction of hospitals for contagious diseases immensely. With our present knowledge of the causes of wound diseases, it is the business of the surgeon to keep the hospital free from their germs. We do not now expect hospitals to become centers of wound infection; and there is not the same danger in treating surgical cases now that there was fifteen or twenty years ago, when the immediate and special cause of these things was not understood. Dr. Davis proposes to filter all the air that comes into a ward for infectious diseases, through a layer of cotton-wool saturated with a disinfectant. What is the danger of letting fresh air into a ward for infectious diseases? We should rather consider the subject of disinfecting the air as it goes out of the ward or hospital.

It is above all things desirable to get the public to understand that there is very little danger in a hospital for diphtheria, scarlet fever, or measles, separated the width of an ordinary street, even, from the surrounding houses. If there was a hospital of that kind next door to my house, separated by a brick partition wall, I should not have the least fear of anything coming through it or of any contagion coming from it. The details of construction may be made very elaborate, as, for example, in the special isolation ward in the Johns Hopkins Hospital, where each room is separate, with separate air space. The purpose was to have the patient absolutely isolated from all the other patients in that building.

DR. J. L. NOTTER.—I fully agree with you, Mr. Chairman, in the remarks you have made. It is important to recognize that these hospitals are the centers from which disease may spread. Immense numbers of patients are treated in the Hospital Tents in London—smallpox patients—yet not a single case of infection has ever been traced to the proximity of those tents.

Now, on the question of disinfection. The disinfection of the clothing of a patient is one of the most important points in the management of infectious hospitals—not only the clothing which the patient brings in with him and his bedding, etc., but also to see that nothing goes out which can carry any disease germs of any sort. Dry heat is no use whatever. If you use heated air, the temperature is such that it will disintegrate the fiber of any clothing and destroy the material long before it will have any result in destroying the disease germs. The only true method seems to me to be to treat the clothing by atmospheric pressure.

A DELEGATE.—I wish to ask what the effect would be of carrying patients in ambulances through the streets, to hospitals some distance away, in the case of infectious diseases.

THE CHAIRMAN.—If it is done with proper precautions there is little risk. Care must be taken not to scatter anything in the way of infectious dust from such a person; but for all the diseases which are ordinarily sent to contagious disease hospitals no special precautions are required. In the case of cholera, care must be taken, by the use of either rubber sheets or absorbent goods, to prevent any discharges from getting into the street; and the ambulance itself must be thoroughly cleansed with reliable disinfectants.

DIET-KITCHENS IN HOSPITALS.

By Dr. H. B. Stehman,

Superintendent Presbyterian Hospital, Chicago.

Of all the means at the command of the physician in the treatment of disease, none stands higher than a properly selected and carefully prepared diet.

The materia medica furnishes us with various agents which positively modify diseased processes by inhibiting or restraining the force-centers which govern circulation, and thus change physiological or pathological action, or excite nervous and muscular energy, but in doing so one only increases or diminishes the energy which has had its origin in potentialized food properly assimilated.

A drug may call forth or generate action, may rally vital force to bridge a crisis, but any show of strength is but the manifestation and expression of latent force derived from and stored up from food long since appropriated by the organism.

While these facts may be self-evident, nevertheless they are too often forgotten by those who magnify the domain of drugs. Moreover, as physiology and pathology are being better understood, many articles of diet have already assumed a definite place in the treatment of disease.

They not only seem to have a specific action in restraining or increasing tissue change, but in some as yet mysterious manner manifest a selective action in the case of special diseases. They also affect individuals differently ; for example, to some certain vegetables are positively harmful, producing distressing symptoms, while to those of a nervous temperament a juicy beef-steak is almost as stimulating as a glass of wine.

The alert of the profession, recognizing these facts and wishing to utilize them, turn for help to the trained nurse. Her advent is coincident with the modern methods of medicine and surgery.

But for the discovery and practice of asepsis in surgery and allied principles in medicine, her coming into the profession as principal assistant would have been indefinitely postponed. And thus as her services are being more and more appreciated from the view-point of the surgeon, so, as food values become better understood both in the selection and proper administration, her co-operation will be more and more sought after by the physician.

To fit her for this branch of her work is the mission of the diet-kitchen.

As the manual training school is the tangible expression of the dignity with which our modern times recognize manual labor, so the diet-kitchen in its design is the realistic representation of labor once regarded as menial but now genteel. In its relation to the hospital its aim is to supply better food; in its relation to the nurse it is first a laboratory and secondly a dispensary.

The diet-kitchen in the hospital, in our judgment, is not a little kitchen in contrast to the main kitchen.

It is not a place where cooking is done for the mass, or where anything is prepared in gross, but it is a school where a nurse reduces her theory to practice in cooking for the individual as she will be expected to do when she engages in private work, and thus becomes efficient in every branch of her art.

Whether a kitchen such as I have described should form a part of the hospital is a question that is still *sub judice*.

There are many who, having given the subject much thought and study, and appreciating the benefits from having such an important adjunct in caring for the sick, are prevented from adopting it on account of the extra expense; while there are others who prefer to travel the beaten paths of the good old ways and do not take kindly to any innovations.

It thus happens that comparatively very few hospitals in this country have a diet-kitchen proper, and even of these few there is no unanimity as to the relation the kitchen should sustain to the hospital dietary; the one maintains that it should be of and for the hospital, while the other would consider it simply as an experimental laboratory whose products possessed only an incidental value.

We believe that the former is the proper idea for hospitals in general, *i. e.*, that the diet-kitchen should be responsible for a portion of the food supplies; and to make it as practical as possible for the nurse it should furnish only such food as with the preparation of which she ought naturally be familiar. That it should deal directly when possible with the individual, not only that it may stimulate and call forth the best efforts of the nurse, but in having prepared her food she may learn how to present it to the best advantage.

The value of a diet-kitchen to a hospital is estimated entirely by the degree of responsibility it assumes in feeding the inmates.

If it aims to care for such inmates as are upon liquid or special diet it relieves the general kitchen of its most burdensome task, viz., the details. A diet-kitchen in doing this becomes an invaluable help to any hospital; it economizes food, in that it supplies only that which is needed and in such quantities as may be required. If, however, its aim is only to produce so-called dainties and delicacies which have neither sense nor nutrition, and have nothing to recommend them but their ability to foster and feed a fermentative dyspepsia, we had better confine ourselves to simpler methods.

When the kitchen exists only for the nurse, irrespective of the mutual advantage it might be to both hospital and nurse, and as such is an ornament of the former, then it is of little or no benefit. Under such circumstances the hospital is the benefactor of the school to which the nurse belongs and is repaid only indirectly, as the service from experienced nurses is more intelligent, hence more efficient.

The nurse is the one to hail the advent of diet-kitchens; to her it means more than any other part of her training. To know food values, their respective relation to health and disease, is incalculable; but to be able to so prepare the food that by its relish and taste it may not only create its own demand, but become a formidable factor in sustaining life and combating disease, is still a greater advantage. The individual who by her art can devise and suggest means by which the appetite may be coquetted, and distaste be changed to the enjoyment of food, stands in closer relation to the patient than the physician; for the latter may stimulate energies which are latent, while the former gives to the patient the very energy by which convalescence is inaugurated.

To cook efficiently and to furnish proper food is an art which is acquired only by practice. There are general principles which apply to this form of work, the same as to any other accomplishment, and to know these makes the nurse, at least so far, master of her profession; to be ignorant of them renders her liable to failure. As well might one expect a physician to succeed in the treatment of disease by simple book knowledge, as a nurse to cook acceptably for a patient who has had no practical application of the principles which underlie the art of cooking.

Permanency.

To properly manage a kitchen, whether it shall be an adjunct to the hospital or not, requires much tact. To make it what it should be to the nurse requires hearty co-operation on the part of all concerned.

The rule in hospitals varies. In some the nurse goes into the kitchen as a junior and thence becomes a senior, and so on, she in turn teaching those under her; the kitchen in the meanwhile being supervised by some one especially appointed for the purpose.

Didactic lectures are given in classes, while the practical application is made only by twos and threes.

To secure, however, that permanency which is so essential to success in this department, the plan which keeps a permanent tutor in constant attendance, in my judgment, secures the best results.

Diet-kitchens are supported in three ways, by the hospitals with which they are connected, by the training schools, in a measure, whose pupils reap the advantage of the schooling, and also by private individuals.

It is questionable whether any greater charity can be bestowed than to furnish means by which the coming generation could learn how to cook well.

It is a lamentable fact that many of the pupils entering a training school have no more idea of cooking than they have of medicine, and the individual who is generous enough to furnish the means by which they may not only acquire the art of making life enjoyable to the confirmed dyspeptic, but even enter into the secret of saving life, is truly a benefactor of humanity.

It is indeed unfortunate that the introduction of the diet-kitchen has a financial side to it. A department so important, yet so neglected, necessarily comes under this same question, and judgment is deferred until the answer comes, Can it be afforded? No matter how anxious hospital managements may be to turn out efficient nurses (for they after all are their best advertisement), charitable institutions for the greater part have such sickly existences, and funds come in so slowly, that they are obliged to weigh carefully every expense, and in many cases content themselves with what are generally considered actual necessities.

It would take very little argument to introduce a kitchen, well organized and equipped, in most every hospital in this country, provided it could be shown that it would not add to the financial burdens of the respective institutions. And thus it happens that they are found only in such hospitals which feel the necessity of teaching their own nurses whom they agreed to train. Under such circumstances it becomes an expense of the training school, and should be so considered in making a proper charge against the respective departments.

The practical side of this question is, what to do with the food which the kitchen turns out.

It would be hardly right to suggest that in the beginning possibly some of the articles cooked would probably not be considered very wholesome; it is at least fair to presume that in the start some things do not hit.

But this is only in the start, and here is where the great advantage of cooking training comes in. Cooking is a science, true and exact. With proper conditions one can always be sure of positive results, and thus to produce and become familiar with the conditions, to weigh their importance and estimate their relation and value, make cooking an art and a science. As for the use of the kitchen product, I am satisfied that a kitchen, while it may be the laboratory and training school of the pupil nurse, will produce better results if the nurse feels that her effort will be recognized, for there possibly can be no higher incentive for honest, faithful and conscientious work than to know that the product will be of benefit and be appreciated by some invalid. What is a tutor's approbation compared to a patient's appreciation? What is the ability to cook food compared to the pleasure of having an invalid or a friend enjoy it? I am convinced that, as art can be more artistic and that as skill can be more skillful, the consecutive classes of cookery will not only show varying degrees of art and skill, but that the influence of this incentive will be recognized and commented on by the patient. And so I say for the nurse's sake, if not for economy's sake, cook for the patient, and not simply for the sake of practice.

It is not the province of this paper to discuss the general curriculum laid down for nurses in the respective training schools, but it can safely be said that even for the good of the various hospitals the importance of properly selected and prepared foods is too lightly dwelt upon.

Some of the branches now taught have little or no practical value, though they may be necessarily estimated from the standpoint of finish, but with nursing proper they have nothing to do. Not so with practical cooking.

Cooking is not only an art, but proficiency in this respect on the part of the nurse will do more to ingratiate her into the heart of her patient than any other part of her profession.

Nothing so buoys the spirits as good, well cooked food. A dainty meal will dispel the blues, soften the heart, give courage, and bring in a general *bon esprit*.

All this is the privilege of the nurse or the school to which she belongs, and no words can be too strong in urging the schools to provide amply for teaching this branch of nursing. And I am confident that if the person in charge of the kitchen possessed and would cultivate the ingenuity of the French, who construct so great variety from so little, that the kitchen would not only be a good investment for the hospital, but that the trained nurse's work and skill would still further commend itself to the sick public. The diet-kitchen, to be ideal, should be a laboratory. What this is to the druggist in that he combines and makes new formulas, studies reaction, solubility and the various properties of drugs, so the course in the kitchen should embrace the combination of foods in a systematic way, so that in the combination and treatment of exact amounts exact results may obtain.

Previous to entering the kitchen the nurse should receive instructions in food values, its care and preservation.

She should understand the chemical subdivision of food, and what changes occur as it enters the mouth and passes through the alimentary canal, and thus she will more readily arrive at the *rationale* of its administration.

If this preliminary work is carefully done, the field of the diet-kitchen will gradually widen ; and if efficiency in diet-cooking rather than inferior branches shall become among the first requirements for the graduation of a nurse, the public will then more easily be convinced that the trained nurse is a professional whose skill even a new-born will acknowledge.

HOSPITAL DIETARIES.

By Miss M. A. Boland,

The Johns Hopkins Hospital, Baltimore.

It is perhaps not necessary at this late day in the nineteenth century to offer any arguments or apologies for presenting a paper on the subject of food and its preparation, for we have made such strides in the last ten years in what may be called the study of home affairs, that the idea is no longer a new one, and we have already begun to think of system, methods, technique in the cooking of food.

In a short paper of this description, however, it will be quite impossible to do more than touch upon a few salient points, to select what seem to be the greatest defects—for that there are defects one has only to look in order to see—in hospital kitchens and dietaries, and to suggest in a general way remedies therefor.

With this object in view I have visited during the last three months twenty-five hospitals, four Young Women's Christian Associations, one New England Kitchen, and one school in which three hundred persons are furnished each day with dinner at a fair cost. The last six institutions are included because in hospitals the providing of what is known as "ward diet," that is, the greater part of the food consumed, is neither selected nor cooked differently from what it would be if it were designed for those who are in a state of health. These institutions, excluding those not hospitals, located in six of our leading cities—New York, Philadelphia, Boston, Washington, Brooklyn, and Baltimore—represent for the most part types of hospitals. Some are richly endowed, others are poor. Some are marked by the distinctive religious character of the authorities, such for instance as the German Hospital in Philadelphia, in which the entire charge of everything except the medical work, that is, the nursing, buying and cooking of food, and internal management of the institution in general, is in the hands of the order of Deaconesses and most admirably administered. Others are without any special religious motive in their administration. Some are under political control, some are free from it. Some are for the rich alone who pay large prices; others for the poor who pay nothing, and so on. These I have divided into three classes, basing the classification entirely upon the condition of the kitchens, utensils and workers as to *cleanliness*, because it is the very first essential to the attainment of wholesome food. One may have the best of materials in proper variety and entirely fail to secure from them health-giving food without this element.

Class I includes those which are good, that is, with kitchens and appliances, store-rooms, refrigerators, dressers, serving-rooms, dishes, food and food materials, positively clean and well kept.

Class II consists of those institutions in which there is a passable degree of cleanliness, some care, but much indifference; and

Class III those which are positively bad, the neglected kitchens, the "submerged tenth" of kitchens, so to speak. In Class I, those unquestionably good, of which there are six, many excellent features were seen; two have kitchens which were models of neatness, containing modern appliances in excellent order, with corners, insides of dishes, ovens and "out-of-the-way" places as carefully kept as the tops of the tables and more noticeable parts of the rooms, indicating that cleanliness is a reality and not practiced for show. One housekeeper, whose refrigerator I have marked number one of the whole list, told me that twice each week everything was taken out and the woodwork thoroughly washed, scoured and aired. It contained distinct compartments for meats, butter and milk, vegetables, fruits, wines and jellies, and miscellaneous cooked food; the different kinds of vegetables were kept in large sliding drawers on a level with the hand, as were also the fruits. The bread, which was delicious in flavor, was stored in ordinary flour barrels which were immaculately clean both inside and out and stood in a store-room of the same description. All food seen was most wholesome in appearance and appetizing. The tops of working tables were covered with sheets of zinc tacked on at the sides, which can be so easily made clean with hot water and soap, thus saving the necessity of laborious scouring. Granite-ware utensils were in use, and there were several large double boilers, with which only the thorough cooking of cereals can be easily and successfully done. I find on referring to the notes made after each visit that in all of this class of hospitals women are in charge of the kitchen department.

Class II we may pass without comment further than to say that they were simply ordinary—not as bad as possible, but far from being good. Of this class there are also six out of the twenty-five, some of which are in the charge of men, and some in the charge of women.

Of Class III, those which are very bad, three were filthy in the extreme,—drawers, cupboards and corners swarming with vermin, refrigerators and sinks having the appearance of never having been washed, food lying about in the presence of swarms of flies, and many other signs of the entire disregard of all rules of even a decent degree of cleanliness. This of the three classes is unfortunately the largest, thirteen out of the twenty-five composing it. Of these, in five out of the thirteen the buying is done by men, and of the three worst of this class it is noticeable that both the buying and cooking are done by men,—in other words, men have entire charge of the food to the time it is served. It is a surprise to find that of the thirty-one institutions known about, in the three that are pre-eminently good the buying, cooking and entire charge of the cuisine is in the hands of women, while in the three as pre-eminently bad it is in the charge of men. I say it is a surprise, because the question naturally arises whether women in such positions would show the ability to buy to advantage and to provide with the same constancy that characterizes men; but in these days of universal educational advantages, of high-schools in every country town, in the present generation many women are well educated and possessed of discriminating minds, good judgment and that moral balance and tone which guide them to do good work for its own sake; which qualities have been generally lacking in what may be termed the old-fashioned housekeeper, who, with no mental training worth mentioning, lacked the business ability to deal with large quantities and the power to systematize work.

At all events these are interesting facts: the three institutions referred to for excellence are large institutions, two of them hospitals; they have been in existence for some years, have always been in the entire charge of women, and are to-day models of their kind. It would seem that women have the instinct of attention to nicety of detail that men do not possess, and which in cooking is so necessary, as it is largely a work of minutiæ.

If we regard the twenty-five hospitals seen as typical examples of the hospitals of the country, we find that at least one-half of them are far from being what they should be, and of the remaining half, two-fifths are at least capable of being much improved.

The condition of the kitchens as to cleanliness, upon which to base a classification, was selected not because there were not many other factors upon which a classification might be made, but because the condition as to cleanliness is a symptom which indicates in a general way healthful or unhealthful food, and thought and care in cooking it, or the lack of it.

The inspection of these thirty-one institutions has given tangible material upon which to base the conclusions which have been drawn, after much deliberation upon the subject and viewing the food question from many sides.

The conclusions are these : that it is not lack of money, not lack of an abundant and varied food supply in the markets, not lack of necessary help, that gives to the inmates and employes of so many institutions a diet upon which they cannot fail in the long run to degenerate in health, and which for those positively ill is wholly inadequate to tempt the appetite, or, with appetite present, to restore to health. There is, it seems, enough food material, enough money to buy it, and hands enough to cook it. Where then does the difficulty lie? Why then is the subject of food in institutions in which it is not wholly ignored, ever one of constant perplexity and contention? These questions are not capable of being answered simply, of being solved by a single statement; they involve too many factors for that; we may, however, select some of these factors and endeavor to deal with them. I would say that first there is a lack of *affectionate* interest in the subject on the part of many connected with it. The buyer buys, the cooks cook, but no one cares whether the dishes made are acceptable to the eater, or whether they are eaten at all. There is too little loving consideration for the ultimate welfare of the consumer. Few have the motive of preparing "something good" for somebody.

Food is too often bought by contract, by commissioners and others who never even see the people who eat it. The details of selection are frequently left to the sellers, who are often both shrewd and unprincipled enough to send materials that cannot be disposed of to the individual buyer, knowing full well that once in the institution there they will remain, that no one will take the trouble to send them back, or perhaps notice the difference between the good and the bad.

Usually the cook holds much the same relation to the eater that the buyer does, often not knowing anything whatever of those for whom he labors, and therefore having no incentive to please or to take vital interest in the work. The personal element is lacking.

Cooks are human beings who in order to do well need instruction, encouragement and criticism. They should at times be told when a dish is good or when it is bad, and if possible why it is so; otherwise the best of them fall into a state of drudgery, whose round of duties consists in the mechanical turning out of so much bread, meat and vegetables with but little regard to the quality and acceptability of them.

Second, there is an alarming degree of ignorance in regard to the necessity of cleanliness in the care and preparation of food. I have seen a baker smoke day after day as he molded and mixed bread, and in the afternoon when his work was done the same man was in the habit of taking a nap on the molding board, which during his waking moments he occupied instead of a chair. I have seen quarters of beef taken from the bottom of a none too clean cart, thrown upon the filthy floor of a store-room, whence they were carried to a block bearing all the signs upon its surface of the incipient putrefac-

tion of the remains of many previous quarters of beef, chopped up in
the presence of a swarm of flies which had been foraging during the
morning in all sorts of decaying matter, and transported to the kettle
without further care.   I have seen large stationary soup-kettles
washed out with the broom used for the floor.   These are among the
mildest illustrations that I could find in my long list, as the details of
many are too unpleasant to relate.   Many a woman who would be
shocked at a speck upon the snowy whiteness of the table napery
eats bread mixed and molded by hands whose owners know not the
meaning of the word " bath," who are as guileless of soap and water
as the wandering savage ; and many a man who can give to delighted
audiences the fascinating accounts of the life and history of the
infinitely tiny forms of life which his microscope reveals, who can
tell you the number of millions of bacteria that may be found in a
gram of butter, that the dreaded typhoid-fever bacillus finds a comfortable home in milk, that the germ of Asiatic cholera may live in
varying times from one hour to twenty days upon bread, roast meat,
in water, milk, and butter, on the surfaces of fruits, on the bodies of
flies, etc., has not yet thought of taking the kitchen as an experimental field.   This man, if he would enter the average hotel or
hospital kitchen, might find himself in a tropical forest of micro-organisms whose luxurious growth and transforming power might give
the clue to many a case of sickness, degenerated health,—disease.

Esthetically this is not pleasant; hygienically, it is without doubt
one of the serious factors in the food question.   That fermentative
and putrefactive changes take place with great rapidity, under favorable conditions of warmth and moisture, in all kinds of both cooked
and uncooked food, is an established principle.   Of the nature of
these changes and of the products which result from them we are not
yet well informed, but experiments are constantly being made in this
direction, and the day is not far distant when we shall have sufficient
proof to speak with positiveness on more of these subjects.

A recent work—" Lehrbuch der Intoxikationen," by Dr. Rudolph
Kobert, Stuttgart, 1893—contains interesting matter on this point.
According to him, sausage poisoning, which frequently occurs in
Germany and sometimes in this country, depends for the most part
upon a mixture of bases of which ptomatropin is the most important.
Its formation is due to the action of a bacillus.   About 40 per cent
of those attacked die.   The symptoms of the poisoning are fully
described, and then he adds : " Wholly analogous symptoms have

followed the eating of fish no longer fresh, corned beef, tainted ham, old roast fowl (goose and duck), decomposing beef and crabs. It is probable that the same poison, ptomatropin, is the active agent."

The poisoning resulting from the use of canned meats is often bacterial in origin. Poison may also occur, according to the same authority, (1) *in meat from healthy animals which has been improperly prepared or kept too long ;* (2) *in meat from animals which during life have suffered from bacterial infection.*

There are many examples. In man, the eating of such food, *even though it has been boiled or roasted,* gives rise to severe symptoms which Bollinger calls intestinal sepsis. The symptoms are due to the action of the poisons on the intestines and their absorption thence. Dozens and sometimes hundreds of men have been attacked at once from the use of such food.

A sufficient number of similar experiments have been made by Vaughan in this country, and others, to enable us to infer that poisonous substances of deadly character may and often do occur in meats, milk, oysters, lobsters, crabs, and other moist albuminous foods. When these changes have gone so far that we are able to recognize them by bad-smelling gases, changes in color, consistency or reaction, then the danger is not so great, for well-disposed persons know from experience that such foods are unwholesome and cannot be eaten without danger, although it not infrequently happens that they are prepared for the table by the ignorant cook.

The danger lies not only here but in the fact that without extraordinary care, changes begin at once in all of these foods, and that in the hands of the average worker they must often contain poisonous matter in small quantities *which may not be destroyed by any method of cooking,* and that foods of such a nature tend to depress the powers of the body, and if eaten for a length of time may so disturb the economy of the system, either by direct absorption into the circulation or by causing digestive disturbances, as to give rise to actual conditions of sickness, or to put the body in such a state of nonresistance to pathogenic organisms that disease easily gains a foothold. In addition to this, in cases where not actual *poisonous* matter is produced, fermentative changes may take place which destroy desirable nutritive and savory qualities in food. Changes of the last two kinds are the most to be dreaded because of their subtle nature and the difficulty of recognizing them, therefore the ordinary worker should be taught by some one who does understand the means of prevention.

An article recently published by Dr. Cyrus Edson, on " Some Sanitary Aspects of Bread-making," is in the line of this point. He says : " I have not the slightest cause to doubt that diseases have been and will be carried about in bread. I have seen journeymen bakers suffering from cutaneous diseases, working the dough in the bread trough with naked hands and arms. This is an exceedingly objectionable thing, from the standpoint of a physician, for these reasons : while it needs no medical knowledge to cause a person to object to having the bread he eats kneaded by a baker having cutaneous eruptions on his arms or hands, it does need this knowledge to understand that the germs of disease which are in the air, in dust, on stairways, and straps in street-cars, are most often collected on the hands. Any person who has ever kneaded dough understands the way in which the dough cleans the hands. In other words, this means that any germs which may have found a lodging-place on the hands of the baker before he makes up his batch of bread, are sure to be in the dough, where they find all the conditions necessary for subdivision and growth. This is equivalent to saying that we must depend upon heat to kill these germs, since they are sure to be in the bread." He then adds : "I have not the slightest doubt that, could we trace back some of the cases of illness which we meet in our practice, we would find that germs collected by the baker had found their way into yeast-bread, that the heat had not been sufficient to destroy them, and that the under-cooked bread had been eaten with its colonies of germs, the call for the physician rounding off this sequence of events."

Whether this will bear scientific investigation remains to be seen, since bread is generally subjected to a high temperature in cooking ; but whether it will or not, it is a valuable suggestion, as indicating a long line of possibilities in other kinds of food which are not subjected to so high temperature as that usually given to bread.

In addition to this there is always the possibility of getting into the system, through the medium of food, the organisms of the various contagious and infectious diseases, such as tuberculosis,—the organism of which may exist in the air, be blown about with dust and settle upon fruits, food and dishes,—typhoid fever, diphtheria, cholera, etc.

A purveyor, housekeeper, superintendent or other person whose duty it is to look after the affairs of a hospital kitchen should be able to recognize all of these points. Of much importance in hospitals is a supply of unquestionably good milk, which should be stored in absolutely clean vessels, in a clean, well-aired refrigerator. It should be frequently tested for fat reaction and specific gravity, and in cases of epidemics, or when for any reason it is not above suspicion, it should be taken.to a reliable chemist for analysis, or sterilized. A purveyor should be able to intelligently determine the quality of bread made, to prevent the use of alum and alum baking powders in it, as also the use of stale eggs, decaying butter, commonly called rancid, and carbonate of ammonia in cake, and he should be able to do for every other form of food what he does for milk and bread, that is, have an intelligent understanding of the nature of foods, and know the means by which they may be made and kept in the most wholesome condition. The question is here naturally suggested, where can be found a person willing to take such a position who knows enough of chemistry and bacteriology to appreciate these things? My reply is, create the demand and the supply will be forthcoming.

Twenty years ago, when an eastern State decided to have drawing taught in its public schools, the commissioners were obliged to send to England for teachers. Immediately, as soon as the demand was apparent, young men and women in this country began to study the subject, and in five years we had enough teachers of our own. Create the demand and the question of supply is only a matter of time.

I might mention here that which scarcely needs to be said, that is, that the demand must come from the trustees and officers of institutions, otherwise there will be no change, no progress. The servant of himself will not change. We cannot look to him to do so. He never elevates himself, no matter what stress of need or coercion may be brought to bear upon him. He cannot, without opportunity, encouragement, instruction, none of which are at present accorded him. He often struggles to do so, but it is ever a struggle in the dark, and usually ends in perplexity. As for the patient, his voice is never heard in such matters, except in those hospitals fortunate enough to have paying patients whose presence and criticisms are a stimulus to all.

Good quality and proper care of food materials and the most scrupulous neatness of workers, working-rooms and utensils, are the foundations upon which any good system of dietaries must rest.

After this we come to the consideration of system and order in methods of cooking. To illustrate this latter point we may select

any line of dishes,—for instance, soups. A head-cook should have at
hand a list of wholesome and simple soups (it is neither necessary
nor advisable in a hospital to make the more elaborate dishes of any
kind), which will vary somewhat according to the seasons of the
year, but which in the main may be the same for the twelve months.
I would advise dividing them into four groups, and if possible, no
matter how acceptable it may be, that the same soup be served not
oftener than once in two weeks, for the sake of securing sufficient
variety. This is a much more simple matter to formulate than it
seems. It requires only an intelligent head to plan, to direct, to criticise, and the thing is done.

Chicken, Julien, oyster, clam, celery, mock-bisque, asparagus, pea,
bean, lentil, consommé, barley, and bouillon are familiar soups. These
should be made according to some definite and exact rule which has
been proved to be wholesome and savory. For instance, mock-bisque
soup is a compound of tomatoes, milk, flour and butter, with soda,
salt and pepper. Cooked tomatoes are strained and a pint measured.
To this is added a teaspoon of salt, a fourth of a teaspoon of pepper,
and an eighth of a teaspoon of bicarbonate of soda; the latter is used
to partially neutralize the too strong acid of the tomatoes. The process is this : the tablespoon of flour is cooked in the tablespoon of
butter, and a pint of milk added ; the pepper, salt and soda are
mixed with the tomato, the sauce is then poured in, the whole
strained, and the soup is done. This gives a quart of simple but
wholesome soup and one which is usually acceptable to the sick.
These proportions may be regarded as a unit rule by the multiplication of which any quantity may be made. A quart of soup will
furnish enough for five portions. If a hundred persons are to be
supplied, twenty quarts will be required, and by multiplying each
item in the unit rule by twenty and carrying out the process correctly,
exactly the same quality of soup will be obtained. The formula
for twenty quarts will be ten quarts of tomatoes, ten quarts
of milk, twenty tablespoons or two and one-half cups of flour, two
and one-half cups of butter, twenty teaspoons of salt (ten tablespoons)
or one and one-fourth cups, two and a-half teaspoons of pepper, two
and a-half teaspoons of soda.

There are some precautions to be observed in using this rule.

(1) If the flour is not cooked in the butter for a definite time
before the milk is added in making the sauce, the flavor and quality
of the soup are impaired, for the high temperature which the butter

can attain changes the nature of the starch in the flour, rendering it both more palatable and more digestible than it would otherwise be.

(2) The bicarbonate of soda must not be omitted, otherwise the soup will be too acid and will have a curdled appearance.

(3) Any deviation from the proportions will cause a difference in the quality of the soup. It is difficult for the ordinary cook to see this, but it can be demonstrated to him. If the soup be made according to the formula its quality will be constant. It will not be too sour to-day, too salt to-morrow, too thick another time. This point is of great importance, for a vast amount of the waste of food materials is brought about because of this lack of constancy of good quality in the dish made, not to mention the harm wrought by eating such food.

In one of the thirty-one institutions mentioned, I took nearly every meal for a week. We had the same soup for dinner each day. One day it was good, another day it was burned beyond the possibility of eating, and on a third occasion the meat from which it was partly made was tainted. On the two last occasions nearly the whole of the soup must have been a complete loss, and certainly much better lost than eaten. On other days it was indifferently bad, showing that it was made at the discretion of a very poor cook without any desire for the good of the eater whatever.

It is a question whether such conditions are not criminal offenses, and when the eaters of such food fall into a state of fatal disease they should be spoken of not as having died but as having been killed by the sinful indifference of men and women in positions of power whose moral status is wholly insufficient for their responsibilities.

Making soup according to an invariable formula which has been proved to be satisfactory may, to those who have always regarded the kitchen as a place of chaos from which by some mysterious combination of circumstances dishes are evolved three times a day, seem difficult to inculcate, but it is in reality not so, provided there is somewhere in the domain a hand guided by an intelligent head. After a few trials a cook soon learns that it is infinitely easier to make according to rule rather than by guesswork; the element of uncertainty in regard to result is eliminated, the quality of the dish will always be the same, there will be no necessity for tasting, no necessity for hovering over the kettle to see whether it is coming out right; time is saved, and the pleasure which a satisfactory piece of work always gives will be attained. Of course the ultimate and most important thought is the welfare of the eater.

My experience with cooks and other servants is that they are extremely anxious to learn when they find a teacher, and that they are extremely quick in discriminating between the reality and the sham, between those who really know and those who think they do.

I have dwelt upon this single dish because it illustrates the method that should be followed in all cooking. Bread, vegetables, meats, puddings, in fact every kind of food that is made should be made according to a fixed and definite plan as to proportions, process and details of manipulation. Can this be accomplished in institutions? If so, how? I will say that it is not only entirely practicable but that it is already practiced. It is in part carried out in one institution which I visited, which it was my great good fortune by accident to learn about, as it by far and above all others excels in its cuisine.

It is a sort of hotel for women, for working women of the better class, and entirely managed by women. Its various departments are conspicuous for their excellence, but most conspicuous of all for this characteristic is the table. I lived in this establishment for a week, and in no place, either in a private family or at an hotel, have I ever seen a more satisfactory table. The food was of excellent quality, of good flavor, satisfying and inexpensive; the ordinary market food materials, by superior methods of cooking, having been converted into acceptable and health-giving food. The mid-day meal, a luncheon, is served to five hundred persons, so that it will be seen that the food must be cooked in large quantities. From the results seen I became deeply interested to learn the details of the plan of management; for that there were both plan and system in its execution was perfectly evident,—such results could not be accomplished by haphazard. Through the courtesy of the managers I was " let in " to the secret workings of the kitchen and shown all the various details in cooking.

The work is divided into two departments, that of the actual furnishing of food, and that of serving, each with a superintendent. The woman at the head of the food department does the marketing—buying all food materials and caring for their proper storage and preservation—perfects the formulæ and criticizes the food when done. She takes, in a measure, the place of a teacher giving actual instruction in the various divisions of her department—to the pastry-cooks, meat-cooks, etc. Do they resent this? Not at all. The most friendly relations exist between those in authority and the servants. The latter are glad to learn, their work is less worrying, their lives consequently more content and their service of more value.

We had one day a delicious salad. On inquiry, I found that the formula for it had been worked out by the superintendent and cook together until it was perfected, and the proportions thus obtained constituted their working formula, from which no deviation was allowed to be made.

The menus in this institution are interesting. Table d'hôte meals are regularly served, and also one may order à la carte, but the former are so acceptable that it is seldom one cares to order special dishes. The following is one day's menu (Saturday, April 22):

Table d'hôte Breakfast.—Porridge of oatmeal or wheat, beefsteak, soft-cooked eggs, Saratoga potatoes, griddle-cakes.

Lunch.—Vegetable soup, scalloped oysters, potato salad, cold meats.

Dinner.—Royal soup, roast veal, Irish stew, browned potatoes, corn, lettuce, rice-cups with custard, cottage pudding, oranges.

With all the meals corn, Graham and white bread of exceptional quality are served, and tea, coffee or cocoa. This is simple but well constructed and gives some opportunity for choice. A list of this kind is of but little value, however, in conveying ideas, unless one knows the *quality* of the food served; but when we find that the vegetable soup is of excellent quality, savory and satisfactory, that every morsel of it is eaten, that the scalloped oysters are above reproach, and the salad all that one could expect, the lunch becomes ample. Let us compare with this the following dinner menu found in one of the pay-wards of a hospital:

Chicken soup, raw oysters, broiled spring chicken, sweetbread with toast points, roast beef, broiled fish, stewed tomatoes, stewed corn, rice, mashed potatoes, hominy, peach pie, oranges. This is somewhat elaborate. Let us sample some of these dishes. The chicken soup tastes of the iron kettle in which it was made, and is very suggestive of not clean old bones; two or three spoonfuls are enough. The broiled chicken is not well prepared, there are feathers on the outside, and it is raw and red at the joints; portions of the breast are nibbled, and the rest of what should be a most delicious food is thrown away. The sweetbreads savor of rancid butter, and they meet much the same fate as the chicken; the corn, rice, potatoes and hominy all taste alike, and of the peach pie one is afraid to eat, because it has a flavor of tin, which can only be explained by the supposition that the fruit was allowed to remain some time in the can after it had been opened.

Here we have an example of the failure to supply acceptable food to the eater, with every factor present except that of care and understanding in cooking. Varied, wholesome, and valuable food material fails to fulfill its ultimate use. It is evident that money, energy and time in abundance have been put into the menu, and that they, in a measure, have failed to find an adequate value because of ignorance in the methods of cooking. I would suggest that the list be much simplified, and that some of the force here expended be diverted in the direction of perfecting methods, so that there may be sent to the bedside of every sick patient, food that is at least entirely and absolutely wholesome, and prepared according to the very best possible methods known in these matters.

We must take the initiative ; it is more or less our duty to do so. Our charitable institutions, especially hospitals, should be homes in which there is less suggestion of that cold charity which the world practices, and more of the new charity which has already begun to dawn in places,—the charity of the close of the nineteenth century, which as yet is a tiny blossom, but which with hope and joy we look forward to as the only kind which shall characterize the morning of the coming century which is so near ;—that charity which has a living interest in the welfare of its object, which seeks to restore him to perfect physical and mental health and vigor,—to put him upon his feet again, so to speak, that he may have strength and courage to battle with the world and honestly earn his daily bread.

Hospitals should keep high standards of what restoring to health means. Some men, it is true, are wrecked to such an extent that a perfect state of health can never again be possible for them ; but for those who are not wrecks, for how many of them is this done?

In one hospital characterized by the barbarous condition of its cuisine, in which condensed milk is the only milk furnished the sick, and bad bread without butter and boiled cheap tea without milk constitute the evening meal of those able to eat,—I was told on inquiring what food was planned for convalescents, that they never had that class of patients, that as soon as a man could sit up he was sent home, and then my informer naively added, " But it is a bad plan ; they are always coming back to us."

In presenting this subject to you I hope I have not been too radical. Should it seem so, I entreat you to study it for yourselves in every possible light and phase, with the assiduity and methods of a scientist, until point after point are known with exactness; and if this paper arrests the attention of only one among you sufficiently to do this it will not have failed in its object.

DISCUSSION.

CHAIRMAN.—The last two papers are now before the Section for discussion. In regard to Miss Boland's paper, it is a melancholy presentation of the conditions in some kitchens. It is true that bacteria are all about us, but if the bacteria were not there we should be in a very much worse condition. Every person in this room has millions and millions of bacteria in him or her, and if it were not so they would be very sick indeed. The immense majority of micro-organisms are healthful and not harmful. The fluids of the body and the mucous canals all contain them. But it is the dangerous bacteria we have to look to. This does not militate against what Miss Boland said about the necessity of cleanliness throughout the kitchen, but cleanliness is to be maintained without any special reference to bacteria. I don't see the force in Dr. Edson's statement that there are bacteria in the bread. Of course there are bacteria in the bread, and on the outside of it too. There are bacteria in every breath of air you draw. It is housewife cleanliness that you should observe, not bacteriological or chemical cleanliness.

The last part of Miss Boland's paper I think most excellent. The greatest addition we want to our knowledge now is constructive knowledge—to tell how to do things.

MR. BURDETT.—I want to say a word on this question of hospital dietaries. It is a most important one. I think Miss Boland's paper is a most valuable one, because it focuses the present state of things, and will bring home to the minds of people not familiar with the subject the exact facts; and I think further that those of us who have had the pleasure of reading Miss Boland's book and of visiting the Johns Hopkins Hospital and seeing her work there, will recognize that we owe her a debt of gratitude. I would like to say further that I personally feel most grateful that in this section we have had a hospital physician who has gone out of the ordinary path of his work in order that he might emphasize as a medical man the importance which he attaches to this very question of diet-kitchens in hospitals. I think that is a fact which shows development in the right direction.

A DESCRIPTION OF THE PROPOSED NEW LAUNDRY OF THE UNIVERSITY OF PENNSYLVAVIA HOSPITAL,

With Special Remarks and Experiments upon Disinfection in connection with the Work of Hospital Laundries.

By A. C. Abbott, M. D.,

First Assistant in the Laboratory of Hygiene, University of Pennsylvania.

(From the Laboratory of Hygiene, University of Pennsylvania.)

The laundry that is about to be constructed for the University of Pennsylvania Hospital, the floor plan of which accompanies this paper, has not been designed with any special views to architectural effect, but rather as a building arranged for work of a particular character. It is to be supplied with all necessary apparatus of modern pattern that is essential to the saving of labor and the proper performance of the functions of this department, and has been arranged with the special view of putting into practice those methods in the management of hospital laundry work that are essential in preventing the dissemination of disease through this channel.

The building, when complete, will be a one-story structure located upon the lawn of the hospital, within easy reach of the back entry. It is, roughly speaking, to be 90 feet long by 50 feet wide, and at the ridge of the roof has an elevation of 18 feet.

The ceilings throughout are to be 10 feet high. All rooms are to ventilate into the loft between the ceilings and the roof, from which the air is allowed to escape through a slatted cupola. The walls are to be of brick, 13 inches thick, plastered but not furred on the inner surface. The floors are to be of concrete, with a fall towards central openings for drainage. The building is divided into two compartments; the one marked *A* in the accompanying plan, having a floor surface of 48 by 20 feet, not including a drying room of 26 by 8 feet in area, is a private laundry in which the clothing of the resident staff and possibly that of a few private patients will be laundried.

This section of the building is not in communication with the public laundry. It is entirely independent of it, being provided with its own drying room and all apparatus necessary for the performance of the work coming within its scope.

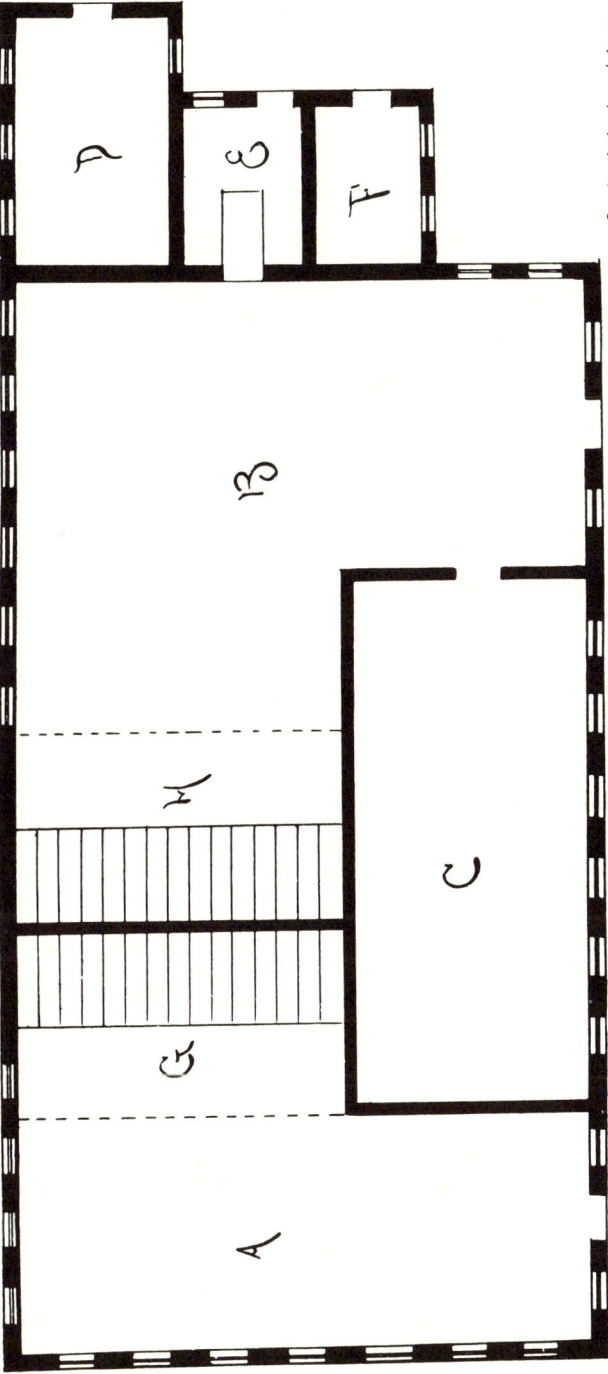

Laundry, University of Pennsylvania Hospital.

Scale $\frac{1}{16}$ inch = 1 foot.

The remaining space *B* and *C* will be devoted to washing and iron-ing the articles from the public wards. The room *B* is the wash-room proper, in which will be located three mechanical washers and a mechanical wringer or centrifugal machine. The room is 48 feet long by 25 feet broad at one end and 46 feet broad at the other, and is in communication with a drying chamber (*H*) that is 26 feet long by 8 feet broad.

Room *C* is the ironing room, in which will be located the mangle and tables for hand work. It has a floor surface of 21 by 44 feet, and is abundantly supplied with light. Each place at the ironing tables in this room is to be provided with a gas heater for the irons, as no stove for the purpose is to be used. The use of gas is prefer-able because the individual can better regulate the temperature of the iron than when it is placed upon the stove. On the stove the iron commonly becomes overheated and is then cooled by dipping it into cold water, much to the detriment of its smooth, polished surface.

The spaces *G* and *H* are the drying-rooms for the private and public laundries respectively. They each have an area of 234 square feet, and will be provided with the ordinary sliding clothes-racks 9 feet in height. Between these racks there will be vertical, direct radiation drying coils, having a radiating surface in proportion to the air capacity of the chamber of about 1 square foot to 5 or 6 cubic feet of air; this, under steam pressure of 55 to 60 pounds, with properly proportioned inlet and outlet openings for ventilation, should insure complete renewal of the air in these rooms about twice per minute.

It should be needless to emphasize the necessity for high tempera-ture and rapid ventilation for drying purposes, for the conditions calling for them are, on physical grounds, too obvious; but it is not uncommon to see such rooms arranged with coils for heating the air but with no provisions at all for permitting its escape when it has become saturated with moisture and no longer effectual as a drying agent. That drying-rooms constructed in this way do serve the purpose for which they were designed is due entirely to the natural exchange of air that occurs by leakage through cracks and crevices, but the amount of work that they are capable of doing in removing moisture under these circumstances is not by any means commensu-rate with what they could do had they the proper arrangements for permitting the free escape of the saturated air with an equivalent ingress of air less rich in moisture. The drying-room of a laundry is no more complete without means for adequate ventilation than would be a drying-kiln for lumber without a fan for forcing air through it.

Room E is the disinfecting chamber provided for the steam disinfecting apparatus. It communicates with the laundry only through the apparatus, the idea being that infected clothing or mattresses, when brought into this room, shall reach the laundry only after having been subjected to the disinfecting action of steam.

Room F is a rinsing room in which chemical disinfection and subsequent rinsing of the disinfected articles can be performed before they are permitted to pass into the laundry proper. It will also contain a metal caldron provided with steam coils for disinfection of small articles by boiling, when it is not desirable to operate the larger apparatus.

Over rooms D, E and F is to be a second story, consisting of a single room in which mattresses and bed-clothing can be stored, aired, etc. It will be reached by a covered stairway located on the outside.

It is not the province of this communication to discuss the various methods of washing clothes, but rather to impress the importance of hospital laundries as factors in preventing the spread of contagion.

Those who are interested in the management of institutions intended for the care of the sick will, I think, agree that there are few departments of a hospital more potent for good in preventing the dissemination of infectious diseases, when well and properly managed, or more liable to do harm when badly conducted, than is the laundry. It is here that are brought underclothing, bed-clothing, mattresses, and in some instances dressings from patients, many of whom are at times afflicted with diseases of a communicable character, and unless the necessity for special precautions intended to render harmless such materials is appreciated, harm may result, and such doubtless often has been the case.

The functions of the laundry are not limited to the space confined within the boundary of its walls, for it is not alone the treatment received by infected clothing when in the laundry that is of importance, but of equal moment are the precautions to be taken in removing it from the patient and conveying it from the ward. In these respects the greatest care is to be exercised by the attendant to whom the duties fall, in order that neither he himself nor others in the vicinity may become infected. A number of plans, having for their object the removal of infected clothing from the wards of hospitals to the laundry, have been suggested, but relatively few of them are put to practical use. The plan to which we give preference, because of its safety and simplicity, is as follows: All bed-clothing and underclothing that are stained with evacuations from the intestinal canal, whether they are of an infectious nature or not, also all articles stained with discharges from wounds, are, upon their removal from the patient, to be placed at once into a covered vessel containing a disinfecting fluid that has been brought to the bedside, and they are to remain in this solution until the time necessary for disinfection has expired before they are permitted to be washed with other clothing.

Objections are occasionally raised to this method of procedure on the grounds that the action of chemical disinfectants is often that of a mordant for white goods stained by blood, fæcal matters and discharges from wounds generally, and for this reason the method has not met with general favor. As opposed to these objections, the advantages possessed by it are obvious, viz. the clothing is not carried through the ward in a dry condition, but is placed, immediately upon its removal from the patient, into a covered vessel containing a reliable disinfectant, and after a very short time is harmless and can be handled without danger of spreading infection. In view of these advantages I have endeavored to determine experimentally how far the objections to this method are based upon fact.

In my experiments which were made upon flannel, canton flannel and muslin, stained both by blood and by intestinal discharges, a number of interesting and instructive results were obtained. The disinfectants with which I have made the experiments were moist heat, in the form of hot water, and steam; carbolic acid in 3 per cent solution; a mixture of 3 per cent carbolic acid and 1.5 per cent ordinary laundry soap in water; and 0.5 per cent solution of chloride of lime in cold water. Throughout, the strengths of the agents employed have been sufficient to ensure disinfection of non-spore-bearing pathogenic organisms within one-half hour.

The results that I have obtained, stated in brief, are these, viz. white goods, including muslin, flannel and canton flannel, when stained with blood or intestinal discharges, and the stains allowed to dry, and subjected to either hot water at a temperature of from 176° F. to the boiling-point, or when immersed for two hours in a solution of corrosive sublimate of the strength of 1 to 1000, have their stains so fixed that it is impossible to remove them subsequently by any of the ordinary methods employed in laundry work. Carbolic acid of the strength of 3 per cent solution in cold water, alone or plus the addition of 1.5 per cent common laundry soap, which renders the acid more soluble, does not have the property of fixing these stains indelibly, even though the goods may be soaked in this solution for as long as 18 hours.

Chloride of lime in the proportion of 0.5 per cent solution in cold water has also no effect in fixing the stains, and has likewise apparently no injurious action upon white fabrics that are exposed to it for a period of one hour. It is to be borne in mind that satisfactory results in disinfecting bed-clothing and underclothing by this method, and at the same time ridding them of all unsightly stains, are only to be obtained when the entire process is carried on at a temperature not exceeding 100° F., for, as I have demonstrated, blood-stains and stains of intestinal evacuations, when partly removed from white goods by soaking them for from one to two hours in cold disinfectant solutions, may still be rendered partly indelible by the subsequent action of hot water.

They should therefore, when the time necessary for disinfection has passed by, be removed from the disinfectant solution and thoroughly rinsed in cold soap and water until all traces of the stains have been removed; they can then be subjected to the usual processes of the laundry. I have found that blood-stains, both recent and old, are, contrary to what I had expected, more easily removed from white goods than are the stains of fæcal matters; the latter, even when recent, but dried, are exceedingly difficult to remove. For the removal from white cotton goods of stains of this character, and at the same time for their complete disinfection, the solution of chloride of lime of the strength of 0.5 per cent acting for one hour has given me the best results, but it is open to two objections—first, the difficulty of obtaining a preparation of this substance in which the proportion of available chlorine is at all constant, and secondly, the objection frequently raised, for which I cannot vouch, that preparations of chlorine, when allowed to act repeatedly on cotton and woolen fabrics, cause them to deteriorate.

For these reasons I have given the preference to the mixture of carbolic acid and soap as recommended by Nocht (Zeitschrift für Hygiene, Bd. VII, 1889). The strength of the mixture is:

Carbolic acid, 3 parts.
Common soft soap, 1½ to 2 parts.
Cold water, 100 parts.

The soap is to be dissolved in the water, after which the acid is to be added and the mixture thoroughly stirred. Experiment has shown that in this strength all non-spore-forming pathogenic organisms are destroyed in one half-hour.

Another mixture that is sometimes recommended, and upon which I have made a few experiments, consists of equal parts of crude carbolic acid and concentrated sulphuric acid dissolved in water to the required strength; this is not to be recommended for laundry purposes, as it not only gives rise to an unsightly, dirty-yellow discoloration of both cottons and woolens, but has also, in my experiments, had some effect in fixing the stains. This preparation of carbolic acid is, moreover, of very doubtful value in the proportion of phenol contained in it, is but a few cents per pound cheaper than commercial carbolic acid, and, as just stated, possesses disadvantages which at once exclude it from use in the laundry. There are three grades of carbolic acid usually on the market, viz. the crude, the commercial and the chemically pure. The first is excluded from use for the reasons just given, while the third mentioned is relatively too expensive; the second, the commercial carbolic acid in the strength given, answers perfectly well for all practical purposes.

Note.—Samples of materials of different character that have been stained with blood and with fæcal matters, and subsequently treated by the chemical methods just referred to, accompanied this paper. Each sample was labeled, and the results of the various methods could be seen.

From these experiments it is manifest that chemical disinfection carried on at a temperature not exceeding 100° F. is to be preferred, and that all efforts at disinfecting these articles by heat, in any form whatever, must necessarily result in permanently fixing the stains. If it is proposed to rinse out the stains prior to subjecting them to the disinfecting action of steam or boiling water, it is evident that the process of rinsing must be carried on at a time when some, at least, of the articles are capable of causing infection. Another advantage in favor of this method is that it does not require the employment of a disinfecting apparatus, an advantage readily appreciated by those having access to such a plant.

For larger objects, such for example as mattresses or outer wearing apparel, the method of chemical disinfection is obviously not applicable, and only steam should be employed. Much has been said in regard to steam disinfection and the requirements of the apparatus designed for this purpose, but unfortunately it has been of such a character as to leave the impression that a steam disinfector is necessarily a complicated and expensive apparatus, and in order for all theoretical requirements to be fulfilled perhaps it is, but a boiler-iron cylinder of the necessary capacity, placed horizontally, with swinging doors at either end, an inlet for steam at the top and a valved outlet for air and water of condensation at the bottom, will be found to answer all practical purposes, providing it is intelligently operated ; and no hospital laundry is complete without such an apparatus.

In size it should be capable of accommodating at least two or three mattresses or their equivalent bulk of clothing. It may be either circular, oval, or rectangular in cross section, and should be located horizontally in a room especially provided as a disinfecting chamber. It should be provided at either end with a door that when closed can be clamped and the joint thus practically hermetically sealed.

It should stand in the disinfecting room in such a way that only one end is accessible from the room, while the other end can only be opened from the laundry, there being no communication between the disinfecting room and the laundry except through the disinfector, which will always be closed, unless for the removal of articles disinfected, or the reception of articles to be disinfected.

It is sometimes undesirable to place an apparatus of this size in operation for the disinfection of a few things from a single patient, and in this event, if heat is insisted upon as the method to be used, a covered metal caldron of 40–60 gallons capacity, provided with steam coils, so that the water contained in it can readily be brought to the boiling point, will be found of great convenience.

There is no doubt that some or perhaps all of these directions will be called into question because of their not taking into account certain theoretical details that are considered necessary in order that disinfection may be complete.

Disinfection as practiced upon such resistant test objects as the spores of the bacillus anthracis might possibly not be complete if attempted by any of the methods that have been recommended in this paper, but it is seldom that objects of this character are to be dealt with in ordinary hospital work. The infectious agents requiring most frequent attention in hospitals, such for example as clothing soiled with the dejections of typhoid patients, the soiled clothing from diphtheria and tuberculosis patients and the articles from surgical cases, will be readily rendered safe by any of the methods here recommended.

DISCUSSION.

DR. J. L. NOTTER, of Netley, England.—There are one or two points I should like to be very clear on, and that is the use of terms. This term "disinfectant"—there is no more misused word than that. What do we mean by disinfectant? We mean some chemical agent which destroys specific poison. Now it is not to be confounded with an antiseptic; and the mere staining of clothing, which I take is the principal object of exhibiting these samples here, which is the result of chemical action itself, whereby albuminous substances which were thrown out in the discharge have been coagulated by the application of heat, is of little importance. The simplest method when you have a discharge to deal with is to receive the sheets or clothing into a solution of mercuric chloride, then subsequently treat the articles in the ordinary way. It is not the chemical action that causes these stains; they are simply produced by heat; it is the fixing of the albuminous compound in the infected clothing due to the discharges.

Now as to the question of disinfectant. Too much reliance has been placed upon them, that is my own personal experience. Disinfectants are good, but cleanliness is better. When I go into a hospital and smell disinfectants I am suspicious. The best destroyer of infected matter is one-half an ounce mercuric chloride, two or three ounces hydrochloric acid, three gallons of water. The addition of hydrochloric acid prevents the mercury from doing any damage.

As to carbolic acid, I have carried on a great number of experiments. It is useful in some cases, but you must have it in not less than five per cent solution.

I used in India, for the destruction of the cholera bacilli, five per cent carbolic acid, and found it a fairly good disinfectant; but we preferred the mercury, in the acid form, for the typhoid.

As regards heat. Now disinfecting chambers are not always available. Wherever they are available they should be used. Not only is it desirable for the clothing, but for the beds and bedsteads, and for everything with which the patient comes in contact, that may require steam or atmospheric pressure, a little above atmospheric pressure, to destroy any germs which it may contain.

These are, I think, the principal points that are dealt with. I most strongly recommend caution about accepting the results of experiments and thinking you have destroyed contagion simply because you have taken out the color. My own experiments do not lead me to place value of any consequence upon chloride of lime.

DR. BILLINGS.—For the disinfection of clothing, bedding, towels and everything that can be boiled without injury, the simplest and most certain method is to boil them. But if clothing soiled with blood and discharges from wounds, or from the intestinal discharges, be allowed to dry, and is then put into boiling water, a permanent stain or discoloration will be produced. The articles to be boiled should go to the laundry without being allowed to dry. If soiled articles are put into cold water for two hours without any chemicals, the pigments will soak out, and then you can put them into hot water, boil them and thoroughly cleanse them without fixing a stain.

In a great hospital receiving cases of typhus and typhoid fever and other infectious diseases, the general laundry receives bedding and clothing from all such cases, and these articles are washed, rubbed and boiled together, yet there has never been a case of infection known to be traceable to the articles treated in the laundry. I believe that there is no danger of infection in a hospital laundry where everything goes in together—the clothing of the doctors, nurses and patients. But there is a feeling of repugnance to such a mixture which I think should be recognized, and in every large laundry it is recommended, as in this paper, to have the articles of the physicians and attendants go to a separate laundry for treatment. Keep the washing of the sick person separate from the washing of the others, but not by reason of any bacteriological necessity, because it cannot be defended on that ground.

NOTES ON NAVAL HOSPITALS, MEDICAL SCHOOLS, AND TRAINING SCHOOL FOR NURSES, WITH A SKETCH OF HOSPITAL HISTORY.

BY J. D. GATEWOOD, M. D., United States Navy.

A Sketch of Hospital History.

Many Christian writers and speakers, both lay and clerical, have claimed and are claiming for Christianity the origin of hospitals. They picture in glowing language this birth as springing from the divine injunction to heal the sick, and from the elevating and softening influence upon the hearts of men of this beautiful religion of our land. One is forced to believe that such statements are made without sufficient investigation, as no teacher can afford to build upon any other foundation than that of truth.

The Jews also have made a like contention, though it would appear, upon a little reflection, that all civilizations and all cultured religions have been associated with the growth of that compassion for suffering which, though at times latent, is an inherent quality in man. It is to this growth that we must look for the origin of hospitals, and indeed for much of the effort of the medical mind in all ages and nations to heal the sick and the suffering.

The pages of history are open to all, and though, in looking through the centuries, formless ashes are almost everywhere, shapes may still be found to more than suggest the beautiful thoughts and deeds of the human mind from almost the very beginning of this never-ending tragedy of life.

The study of this question should begin with that of the physician, for no individual or state would evolve the idea of a hospital without the suggestive existence of minds equipped and available for the performance of hospital duties. Yet, in this short paper, the account of the beginning and rise of that interesting and remarkable personage must be very incomplete.

It is true that in remote antiquity there was, in some parts of the earth, a realization that certain diseases were curable. The people of the far and sunny East had, among other dreams, that of the removal of the hand of suffering and death from certain cases. The sick were exposed on couches in the public places, that they might have the benefit of the experience of the masses. It must have been an interesting spectacle—this approaching of the restored ones to the couches of the sick—to hear their complaints, to listen to the statement of symptoms, that those who had been similarly afflicted might impart the method of their cure. Thus so early in the story of life do we find an extensive attempt to use the guiding hand of experience.

The sight must have impressed the minds of men in many different ways and degrees, and the most educated and observing ones would soon begin to collate methods and results. The empirical led to the question of why, and the question led to the study; and the study of one set of questions by a few always creates a class.

In this case it was a class within a class—the priest-physician. This result is not surprising when one recalls how many centuries were to pass before the mind could be prepared for the separation of medicine from magic, divination and priestcraft.

So it happened that we find the Egyptians writing systematically on medical subjects as early as the 14th century B. C. This medical papyrus in Berlin contains a treatise on inflammation and other subjects, and gives color to the claim of the Egyptians to the invention of medicine. This wonderful people, working out their ideals under the fostering care of their profound religion, soon had a corps of medical men of the sacerdotal order, paid by the state, and as early as the 11th century B. C. there was in that land a college of physicians in receipt of public pay.

The physicians, required by the state to treat the sick poor, practised their healing art in every direction; but it cannot be supposed that they could visit their patients except in particular and grave cases. There were, therefore, establishments set apart by the state, to which the masses could repair at fixed hours. Here we come to the beginning of dispensaries—an interesting fact, as it may be taken as a maxim that the hospital is the development of the dispensary.

The existence of such institutions in that land of high ideals, excites no surprise when one reads on their sarcophagi such remarkable epitaphs as the following : " He succored the afflicted, gave bread to the hungry, drink to the thirsty, clothes to the naked, shelter to the outcast, that he opened his doors to the stranger, and was a father to the afflicted." So this land had long become famous, and a few inquiring minds from the less advanced countries of the North came to seek knowledge.

Thus it is with no surprise that in the early history of Greece we find votive tablets on the walls of the temples. These, while exhibiting the superstition of the age, exhibit also, in some degree, the medical work of the time. They record the history and treatment of individual cases, and are in evidence of the crowds of sufferers who flocked to the temples of Æsculapius at Cos and Tricca, to dream at the foot of the altar and be guided by the advice of their priests.

There is no proof, however, that these particular accounts relate to the poor of that country; on the contrary, they probably express the thanksgivings of the owners of goods and chattels. Yet they were histories of cases, and, one might say, leaves of the medical books of the time.

In the fifth century B. C. the people of Athens were electing and paying physicians and building dispensaries and hospitals. One of these latter, it is stated, was situated at Piræus. Physicians and surgeons had, however, appeared in the history of Greece and Rome much before this date, and accounts of them will be found scattered through the history of that time. Pythagoras had visited the East ; and Hippocrates had appeared, to become the great clinical observer and writer, and to separate Greek medicine from priestcraft.

The Romans were behind the age in refinement and culture, still one is not surprised to find that at the defeat of the Hetrurians (483 B. C.) the wounded Romans were quartered, by the order of the consul Fabius, at the houses of the senators. It was the custom in those days, and had been and was to be for many years, to place the sick and wounded in the houses of the citizens. However, before the time of Hadrian, there probably were government institutions among the Romans for the care of those injured in the defense of the state, though there seems to be no record of such before that period.

But to return to earlier times and a more imaginative and profound people. In India, the history of hospitals many years before the Christian era is most clear and conclusive. The great king Asoka; who died in the third century B. C., established by royal edict these institutions on the routes of travel throughout his dominions. This edict, it appears, is still to be seen bearing the date 220 B. C. It was cut on a rock in Guzerat, probably by his successor. It states that "they shall be well provided with instruments and medicines, consisting of mineral and vegetable drugs, with roots and fruits ; and that skillful physicians are to be appointed to administer them at the expense of the state."* These hospitals were founded at that time (220 B. C.) and continued their good work for more than eight hundred years, when their walls crumbled, after the government under which they existed had passed away.

Here one might mention another civilization which goes back to remote antiquity, and whose origin is shrouded in a mystery that provokes the research of our own time. The land of this people was Mexico. Prescott states, on several authorities, that hospitals were found among that ancient and remarkable race. These hospitals were erected and supported by the government, and, as he expresses it, were "for the care of the sick and the permanent refuge of disabled soldiers." The date when these people constructed their first hospital is a part of the Mexican mystery, but the existence of such

---

*Review of the History of Medicine, by Thomas A. Wise. London, 1867.

institutions in that unknown land is a further proof, if any were needed, that out of all civilizations and all cultured religions comes the growth of that compassion for suffering which is an inherent quality in man.

In the earliest history of the Hebrews the priests were the physicians and surgeons, as has been the case with all races. The Scriptures (Genesis xvii) give the first recorded surgical operation after the Flood, and (Leviticus xiv) show the relation in very remote times of the physician-priest to the people in matters pertaining to the preservation of the public health from the attacks of contagious and infectious diseases. The Bible (Exodus xxx) also mentions the apothecary at an early age, and (2 Kings xx) exhibits the method of treatment in a certain class of cases. It is interesting to observe how early in the history of this ever-memorable people the physician was separated from the priest (Jeremiah viii). These references might be multiplied, but they do nothing towards showing that any provision was made for the treatment of the sick at the public expense. Yet, considering the character of the Hebrews, there must be some record of such provision at some time early in their history.

Returning to less remote ages, it may be observed without surprise, as Rome drew many of her inspirations from Greece, that, 219 B. C., a surgery was provided at the public expense, at the Acilian Crossway, for a certain Greek physician, who came to exhibit the greater advance of his countrymen, and that, as the years rolled by, such places became more common in that land. When Vesuvius threw a pall over the fair city of Pompeii (Aug. 23, A. D. 79) it covered a hospital; and centuries after, when an investigating race uncovered this interesting building, it was found to consist of a large room—the full depth of the house—divided in part into small rooms on each side of a passage. In one of these rooms many surgical instruments, now displayed in Naples, were discovered. These consist of " scalpels, scrapers, elevators, forceps, drills, and a well-made vaginal speculum." Had some benevolent pagan erected this building for the care of the afflicted, or was it a private institution for those able to pay? It was a hospital at any rate, and is worth recording on account of its early appearance in the land of the Cæsars.

As early as the 2d century A. D. there was an organized medical corps in the Roman army, though physicians and surgeons had long accompanied, in a somewhat desultory way, the armed forces of all nations. Xenophon (about 400 B. C.) alludes to them in connection with the Greek armies. As has been said, mention is made of a government hospital for the wounded in war during the reign of Hadrian (117-137 A. D.). In an order of Aurelian (270-274 A. D.) to his soldiers occurs the following: "Let the soldiers be cured gratuitously by the physicians, and let them conduct themselves quietly in the hospitia; and he who would raise strife let him be lashed." In the 2d century mention is made of the valetudinarium in camps, and the proper place for this camp hospital is indicated in plans for winter quarters. In the century preceding, it would seem that the wounded were, as a rule, placed in their tents; as generals are mentioned who excited admiration by visiting from tent to tent the wounded under their command.

Tombstones have been found in England and Rome erected to the memory of members of the medical staff of the Roman army in the 2d century, and in Dresden there appears a tablet "discovered in the Elysian fields near Baiæ, in the vicinity of the famous Pontus Julius, and the station of the imperial Misenian fleet, which is to the memory of M. Satorius Longinus, physician to the Cupid, a three-banked ship." Though this is later, there is reason to believe that at a very early age vessels of war were provided with medical officers, and that the sick and wounded of the navy were received into institutions erected by the government for them, before the time of Hadrian.

There could be no Christianity without effort to help the poor and the suffering. This is a fundamental and essential part of the teachings of Christ. The Christian life began with it, and the care of the poor, the sick and the outcast has been the care of His Church and His people from the beginning. It seems the natural outcome, then, that so soon as the believers in this beautiful religion could acquire property with any reasonable expectation of remaining in possession, the hospital should be made to hold high the flag of the cross. So we learn without surprise that, as the 2d century was about to expire, the Christians seized the idea of hospitals in a practical way, and that their efforts increased as the years rolled by. As early as 300 A. D., several hospitals were founded near Bethlehem under the direction of St. Jerome.

Some of these buildings were retreats for the poorest and meanest, the most diseased and despised—the leper—and were thus a fit exponent of the Christian teaching. Others were used, together with those on the roads to Jerusalem, for the accommodation of pilgrims and the treatment of the sick.

A few years after this, the influence of Jerome had extended to more distant lands, and his friend, the Roman lady Fabiola, expended her wealth in founding in the city of the Cæsars a house for the special care of the sick. In the Council of Nice, early in the 4th century, hospitals were spoken of with the greatest enthusiasm, as representing a glorious part of the church work.

Indeed, so strongly had their influence been felt, that the very intellectual Julian "The Apostate," in his endeavors to re-establish the religion of his ancestors, availed himself of the power of hospitals, by establishing inns for travelers, the indigent and the sick of all creeds and nations.

The famous hospital of Cæsarea was founded 370 A. D., and the Hotel Dieu in Paris, 600 A. D. Many if not most of these buildings, prior to the 11th century, were utilized to encourage pilgrimages, and thus excite religious enthusiasm; but they were also equipped for the treatment of the sick and the sheltering of the poor. They were also, in almost every instance, church institutions, and were employed, among other things, to propagate and extend the teachings of that church.

As cathedrals and monasteries were constructed to hold high the cross all over the European world, hospitals were built close to them and were under the supervision of the bishops and monks. This consideration is an important one, because it has had much to do with the plan and construction of hospitals. The chapel became the most important part of the hospital establishment, and around this all the other buildings clustered. This was also true of many of the convents and monasteries, and furnishes us with the origin of the block plan. This idea of bringing the sick in close contact with the chapel, where they might hear the masses and see the processions, that their hearts, already troubled by sickness, might be touched by religion, culminated at the building of the Grand Hospital in Milan in 1456, when the Church of Rome was at the height of its power.

It is a matter for interesting speculation as to how long hospitals would have been constructed on that plan, if there had not come the separation of hospital and church. But Christendom was in the next century to experience that great religious convulsion known as the Reformation, from which was to come a long period of independence in thought and action. Strangely enough, at the same time, Henry

VIII of England, that fearfully eccentric " defender of the faith," was confiscating church property and converting certain abbeys and monasteries into hospitals ; thus starting in the hospitals of St. Bartholomew and St. Thomas that separation which was to become greater with each succeeding year.

However, much time had to pass before the influence of the old days was far enough removed to allow the scientific mind to grope its way to higher ground. It was not, perhaps, until the eighteenth century, that this air we breathe, and which for centuries the sick had been denied, save in a more or less poisonous state, began to be intelligently considered, and ventilation began to be the cry.

It is thus apparent that it was not until men became free to investigate, and science, born, it may be, under the stimulating hope of a better life, came with religion to bless our race, that improvements in the construction of hospitals took intelligent shapes, and buildings intended for the care of the sick ceased to be grand palatial structures erected for their death.

Let us go back a little, to see how the soldier and the sailor fared during all these years of Christian influence. In the wars under the Cross and against the Crescent, the hospitals of the Church were of course open alike to civilians, soldiers and sailors. These wars stimulated in an unexpected manner the erection of retreats for the sick ; for, as a result of the Crusades, establishments for lepers had to be erected all over Europe, and great numbers of them were built even in England and Scotland.

When Christian nations themselves appealed to the sword, the wounded were in great part distributed in the nearest towns and quartered upon the inhabitants. In this we see a repetition of the practice of pagan peoples. It is true that in some Christian countries, the State insisted that the hospitals of the Church should receive the wounded, but it is fair to say that military and naval hospitals have never originated from a spirit of humanity, but have been born of sheer necessity, and from the spirit of science in war.

It seems that the first record of a separate hospital for the wounded erected by a Christian government bears the date of 1575, when, under the immediate influence of Ambrose Paré, and the general influence of writers on military science at that time, a military hospital was built at the siege of Metz.

In 1666, when Colbert, that wise minister of Louis XIV, founded Rochefort and organized the navy of France, necessity created a naval hospital in the little priory of Saint-Éloy. Thus, amidst the sick and dying in the swampy grounds of the new station, France began the lesson which her many naval hospitals show that she learned so well.

In 1694, the partially erected palace at Greenwich, England, was converted into a residence for worn-out and wounded seamen. In the tax for the maintenance of that hospital can be found the suggestion to the American colonies, which eventuated in the establishment of our own marine hospital service and our own naval hospitals.

It was not until 1756 that the modern ideas of hospital construction found anything like an intelligent expression—when a London architect, named Roverhead, designed a naval hospital which was built at Stonehouse, near Plymouth, England. The design was a compromise between the old block system and the present one of separate buildings. This hospital, with its ten detached buildings, began a new era in hospital construction just seven centuries after the erection of the first general hospital in England.

Since the founding of Rochefort by Louis XIV, since the conversion of the palace of Charles II into a harbor of refuge for the disabled warriors of the sea, naval hospitals have sprung up along the coasts of all civilized nations. Born of no religion, the offspring of sheer necessity, they wait for the tocsin of war. As quiet as the smile of peace on the face of Europe, their polished wards for the most part silent and unused, they stand amid trees and flowers, a ready refuge for the heroic lovers of country and of home, or for the victims of ambition, greed or revenge. They stand on sure foundations, and their walls will never crumble until the day of everlasting peace.

Naval Hospitals.

These institutions are not special hospitals, but general hospitals for the treatment of a special class. They present marked peculiarities, which differentiate them from civil establishments. They are situated, as a rule, near navy-yards, that they may be accessible to the sick of the station and of the various ships, and are surrounded by several acres of ground containing trees, shrubbery, flowers and lawns. The number of patients is liable to very great variations, depending upon the movements of the different squadrons and the varying exigencies of the service. The medical officers are all resident, and have no duty to perform outside of the institution. There are no visiting physicians and surgeons, and consequently no unpaid medical talent.

When a patient is received he has already been under the care of a medical officer, and is accompanied by a hospital ticket stating the diagnosis and history of his case. All the patients are practically under absolute control, and have their movements and dates of discharge determined for them. The sick are of different ranks and grades, thus requiring more or less segregation, and necessitating additional expense to the government, without increased compensation. The sick must be kept until they are fit for service at sea, or for discharge from the navy. This leads to a much lower general intensity of disease than exists in civil hospitals, and to a large number of convalescents and semi-convalescents who may perform light work about the building.

All the naval hospitals of one nation are conducted under the same rules and regulations; and to guard against improper claims for pensions, much work is done on Boards of Survey, and in making out papers and writing journals.

The fact that all the medical officers are permanent members of a corps including different ranks, requiring good records for promotions, and necessitating a life under navy regulations, leads to more caution, and, may be, to less independent action; and while it throws an increased responsibility upon the medical officer in charge, it tends, perhaps, to diminish the originality and ambition of the juniors.

NAVAL HOSPITALS OF ENGLAND.

The English navy has 711 ships, 58,142 men and 13 hospitals. These hospitals contain 3617 beds, and have daily under treatment about 1100 patients. The sick berth-staff on shore numbers 230, and is maintained at an annual expenditure of $65,000. At the head of the medical department is the Medical Director-General at the Admiralty.

The following titles designate the various ranks included in the corps: Deputy Inspector-General of Hospitals and Fleets, ranking as rear-admiral (does not serve at sea in time of peace); Deputy Inspector-General of Hospitals and Fleets, ranking as post-captain (does not serve at sea in time of peace); Fleet Surgeon, ranking as commander; Staff Surgeon, ranking as lieutenant of eight years service; and Surgeon, ranking as lieutenant under eight years service.

Candidates for admission to the Medical Corps enter an open competition before a specially selected board that sits in London. When successful, the candidate is ordered at once to Haslar for special instruction. The hospitals are situated at Haslar, Plymouth, Chatham, Haulbowline, Great Yarmouth (lunatic asylum), Malta, Bermuda, Jamaica, Ascension, Cape of Good Hope, Hong Kong, Yokohama, and Esquimalt.

It is believed that a study of most of these, and of the Medical School and Training School for Nurses, will furnish some desirable information.

The Royal Naval Hospital at Haslar.

At this hospital, which is on the water's side, close to Gosport, in view of Spithead, and about a mile and a half from the town of Portsmouth, is concentrated much of the activity of the Naval Medical Service on shore. This one institution comprises not only a large hospital, but also the Naval Medical School, the Training School for the Nursing Staff of the service afloat and ashore, and a depot of medical supplies for the various ships and stations.

The buildings (52 feet high) are of three stories, made of brick, supplied with many of the modern improvements and conveniences, and arranged around three sides of a square in two rows, one within the other, leaving the rather narrow space between of 35 feet. Around the inner row on the ground floor is a corridor, which thus borders the large enclosed area, and furnishes an outside means of communication. The fourth side of the square, 400 feet long, is partially occupied by the chapel, which faces the middle or executive part of the building (Fig. 1).

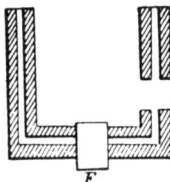

FIG. 1. NAVAL HOSPITAL, HASLAR. *F*. Front.

The wards (60 × 24 feet), which are divided into medical and surgical, are, as a rule, supplied with open fireplaces, and with windows on both opposite sides. They are thus fairly well ventilated, but are rather too wide for their length, and the ceilings (10 and 12 feet) are too low. They contain as a rule about fourteen beds, and give an average of 1100 cubic feet of air space and 103 feet of floor space to each bed. The walls are colored plaster, and the floors ordinary deal, but some of the surgical wards have teak floors laid in cement. The polish of these, under an application of beeswax and turpentine, adds to the appearance of cleanliness visible everywhere.

The plan of this hospital is a singular one, and presents in more than the usual degree all the grave objections inseparable from the block system. This establishment was built in 1762, at a time when ventilation was being considerably discussed. It is fair to presume that economy prevailed, as well as a tendency to cleave to old traditions.

The grounds in which this building stands extend over 60 acres. They are beautified with lawns, trees, shrubbery and flowers. Some of this could very well have been devoted to more ground space in construction, lessening the number of floors, and separating and increasing the number of buildings. However, this hospital has been continuously occupied for more than a century, and the mortality rate is small even now. This is doubtless due in part to the superior administration incident to it as a government institution, and to the number of patients being as a rule much below the capacity. This latter enables the wards to be more frequently renovated, and allows an additional air space.

This immense hospital has accommodation for 1298 patients, including 68 sick officers ; but the average number under treatment is somewhat less than 500. The staff consists of seven medical officers, including an inspector-general, who is in charge. There are several large residences in the grounds near the hospital for most of these, while others are accommodated within the building. The staff seems small when one considers the large amount of work in the hospital and schools. There can be but little time for more than the very closest attention to duties.

An interesting portion of the Haslar hospital is its kitchen, which is situated on the top floor. It is connected with the wards by elevators, which enable the food to be conveniently distributed. But little coal is used in this kitchen. Steam is used to do all the boiling, and broiling is done by gas heat. The crockery upon which the meal is to be served is kept hot on iron tables heated by steam. One can see that this arrangement must be very satisfactory for several reasons, not the least of which is the absence from the wards of the kitchen odor.

The surgical cases in this hospital are about four times the medical. About one-half of them are venereal cases, which cause the largest amount of invaliding. Several hundred wounds are treated annually, with a very small mortality and a reasonable percentage of invaliding.

The medical cases average about 1000 a year; the principal diseases being rheumatism and pneumonic phthisis. The latter is the most frequent cause of death and invaliding. Many cases of remittent fever reach this hospital, chiefly from the Mediterranean Squadron. A large proportion of the sick from that and the home squadron is received, as well as all the sick from the neighboring dockyard.

A short time ago there was no separate building for contagious diseases, and all such cases were treated in one of the end wards. Possibly, this very unsatisfactory arrangement has been changed. The laundry is in a separate building, and is supplied with modern improvements.

The storehouse is also separate, and it is large, as it is here that many medical supplies are kept for distribution to the various ships and stations. In connection with this work there is a permanent board, consisting of the senior medical officer and others from the hospital staff, for examining and inventing improvements in naval medical appliances. The method of packing and transporting medical and surgical outfits in expeditions on shore, appliances for moving the wounded in battle, improvements in operating cases, medicine chests, ventilating apparatus, water filters and the like, receive special attention in the effort to keep the service supplied with all possible improvements. As soon as anything is approved it is sent to one or more ships in actual service for the only true test of merit.

The Naval Medical School.

The Naval Medical School is for the purpose of giving the medical officers recently admitted to the service, instruction in hygiene, military medicine and surgery, pathology, and all subjects necessary for the most efficient performance of those special duties created by naval life. Instruction was formerly given at Netley, but, in 1880, the Naval School was removed to Haslar.

The reasons for this change were many. The young naval surgeon was desirous of learning naval duties, while the army school naturally emphasized those pertaining to its own service. Another consideration, probably more potent, was that nothing stimulates a corps and develops its talents so much as a school taught by itself.

In teaching a class formed of recent graduates in medicine who have built upon a good general education, the older members of the corps are stimulated to greater activity, and a new force is introduced to prevent that stagnation to which there is such a marked tendency. Haslar, with its larger number of cases, many representing diseases incident to naval service, and with its proximity to the great naval station at Portsmouth, furnished a place pre-eminently calculated to facilitate the special instruction desired. Besides, who are so competent to teach the requirements of any service as those who are familiar with them by long experience?

As soon as the graduate has passed the required examination for entrance, and has received his commission, he is ordered to Haslar for this instruction. The course lasts for four months, and though it does not establish precedence in the service, this having been previously determined, it does determine the degree of adaptability and has much to do with the assignment to duty. All the papers and marks of the first examination are sent to this school by the Medical Director-General of the Navy. These must furnish eventually some interesting data bearing upon the competency of any examination to determine that essential quality known as adaptability.

The class, as a rule, consists of about twenty members, more or less. Quarters are provided for them in the hospital, two wards being fitted up for this purpose. They also have a special dining room and a sitting or reception room. A billiard room is also provided, and outdoor sports are encouraged.

The school is well equipped for its special work. The library or lecture room is well provided with the best literature on medical and kindred subjects. The museum, which receives additions from almost all the medical officers in the service, is provided with collections of materia medica, alimentaria, natural history, pathological and geological specimens, and the appliances used in the service. There are also models of ships, and diagrams showing ventilating apparatus in use, and proposed.

The laboratory contains many microscopes and all the apparatus necessary for bacteriological research, and the analysis of urine, water, soil, food, air, and clothing.

In the wards of the hospital much instruction is given in minor surgery and case-taking. Each member of the class is also made thoroughly familiar with the various blank forms used in the service, the system of making sanitary reports, and the method of keeping medical journals.

Autopsies are made as opportunities occur, and written reports are made of all pathological conditions.

The work of the day begins in the wards. This is followed by work in the laboratory, and by a lecture in the library. This lecture is often illustrated by various models and diagrams. In the afternoon perhaps the dry dock may be visited, where ships in ordinary and in various stages of construction are inspected from a sanitary point of view, and a draughtsman explains the plan being followed in the construction.

The final examination is made up of oral and written questions and practical work. All written questions have been submitted to the Medical Director-General of the Navy. The possible total mark is 3,000. To the principles of hygiene and practical hygiene are assigned 1,000 each, while journal-keeping, pathology, and military medicine and surgery absorb the other 1,000.

This school is so practical in its teaching, so praiseworthy in its object, and so far-reaching in its influence that it is well worthy of imitation by all nations.

The Training School for the Nursing Staff.

This school was established at Haslar shortly after the medical school. It was the outcome of a report by a special commission made in 1884. The old system of civilian nurses led to the change, as the material supplied by this method was very often exceedingly poor. Now, nearly all the nurses for the navy afloat and ashore are being obtained primarily from the Greenwich Hospital School.

At that school a fair general education is given, and various mechanical trades are taught. After some service at sea, if the boy, who is about 17 years old, desires to become a nurse in the navy, he makes application, and after a rigid physical examination is received at Haslar. Here he finds himself with others quartered in a large ward in the third story of the administration building.

Nine or ten trained female nurses of the highest respectability have been procured to facilitate the education, and he is taught by lectures and in the wards by seeing the things done that he is to learn to do. A certain amount of minor surgery, such as bandaging, is also taught, and when the student is considered qualified, he is sent to sea. After a cruise he is eligible, if his record be good, for service in the hospitals, and can enlist under special regulations providing promotions and increased pay.

The Royal Naval Hospital at Plymouth,

or rather at Stonehouse, was built in 1764, and is next in importance to that at Haslar. It consists of ten separate buildings, or rather eleven, including the chapel, each constituting a separate hospital. These surround a large square laid out in grass plots and gardens. A colonnade ornamented by one hundred and fifty monoliths connects them, and extends around the sides next the court.

There are 44 wards. Each ward contains fourteen beds, separated by over five feet. They accommodate six hundred and sixteen patients, and give an air space of twelve hundred cubic feet to each. The ventilation is good, the buildings are remarkably clean, and the absence of hospital odor is noticeable. The plan of this hospital permits a free circulation of air within the court, a good general ventilation, and a very desirable segregation of patients. House cleaning and painting can be carried on with little or no inconvenience or annoyance.

Generally there are six wards in each building in use for the sick. Quarters are provided for fifty-one sick officers, and room is given for a smoking room and library. The water supply is good, and there are rooms supplied with hot, cold and vapor baths. The water-closets are excellent.

The plan of this hospital is considered the best of any of England's naval hospitals, and it has frequently served as a model.

The total capacity of this institution is considered to be six hundred and sixty-seven, but in 1780 the remarkable number of fourteen hundred and twenty-three were treated here at one time. Probably many were placed under canvas.

It has an easy approach for boats by way of Plymouth Sound, and receives sick, not only from the fleets, but also from the dockyard and marine barracks.

The total number of admissions each year approaches thirty-five hundred. The surgical wards receive about twice as many as the medical. The average number daily under treatment is about three hundred.

In the medical wards rheumatism and pneumonic phthisis are the principal diseases, the latter being the chief cause of death. In the surgical wards, venereal troubles are in the large majority, these amounting in a year to about one thousand. Syphilitic and gonor-rhœal troubles divide the honors. About two hundred cases of injury are treated annually. The loss by death is small, but the invaliding is not inconsiderable.

There are over fifty in the nursing staff, while the hospital staff consists of an inspector-general in charge, a deputy inspector-general, two staff surgeons, and three surgeons. The wards are visited four times daily or oftener by the surgeon having the day's duty, while those in charge of particular wards make routine visits morning and evening. A very good library is provided for the medical officers, and the seniors have separate residences for themselves and families.

Royal Naval Hospital (Lunatic Asylum) at Great Yarmouth.

Great Britain has made generous provision for the insane of the navy. Probably there is no institution better supplied and more ably managed than the asylum at Great Yarmouth.

So desirous is the Admiralty that the guiding shall be by the most experienced hands, that there is no rotation of officers assigned to this special work, the inspector-general in charge retaining the duty permanently. All recommendations made by this officer, who has absolute local control, meet with more than the usual compliance, and all requisitions for supplies are considered in a spirit more than usually generous.

No government can really afford to do otherwise; for nothing increases the tendency to cheerful work, or acts so constantly to maintain discipline in a service, as the belief on the part of all that they will be well cared for in sickness, misfortune, or death. This consideration has at times been forced upon the attention of authori-ties, and has had much to do with improvements in all services in all governments.

The hospital at Great Yarmouth was built early in this century, but was used for a naval hospital only a few years. In days of peace it passed into the hands of the army for use as a barrack. However, when the century was a little more than threescore years old, it became a naval establishment again, and was devoted to the care of those wrecked in mind as well as in body—patients living in a realm of their own.

This hospital is another illustration of the block plan, but in this case there are four two-story brick pavilions arranged around a square of one and three-quarter acres, with the corners sufficiently open to allow the free circulation of air (Plate I). There is an arched corridor eight feet wide around the lower inner face of each building, and forming their only connection. This plan or arrangement is considered one of the best of any of the older hospitals in the United Kingdom, and though the situation is rather bleak, the selection of this hospital for the present duty is regarded as most wise.

Each pavilion is two hundred and sixty feet long, and, with the exception of the one in front, is divided into two sections by a central structure unoccupied by beds. These sections are subdivided by staircase and nurses' rooms. This results in the formation of eight well separated wards in the pavilion. However, the wards on the lower floor of the rear pavilion have been divided into rooms opening on the corridor, for the use of those too restless to occupy beds near others.

The wards are forty feet long, twenty-three wide, and fourteen and a half high. They have windows on both opposite sides, with beds between. They were originally designed to be occupied by fourteen persons, but the number under treatment is so very much less than the capacity that this overcrowding is made impossible. Indeed, the space unoccupied by beds is so great that it is used for several dining rooms and day wards.

The water-closets are in small towers outside of the line of the wall, and the connections have lattice-work sides, to allow the air to sweep through. The bathing facilities are ample, and include even a Russian bath. This part of the building is not for show, but is used regularly and systematically under the rules of management.

The front pavilion has the second story divided into rooms for the officers under treatment. There is a dining room in connection with these, while a very large parlor on the first floor is set apart for the reception of friends. This lower floor is used, however, chiefly for administration purposes. All the buildings are heated by hot water pipes, and to a certain extent by open fireplaces.

The position of the nurse rooms between wards facilitates their work very much, as, with a suitable division of patients, two wards can often be watched at night by one nurse.

Wherever practicable, a certain amount of ornamentation is used to give as homelike an appearance as possible, and even curtains have not been discarded. This is probably more or less wise as a part of the treatment.

Regulations are strictly enforced in regard to a frequent change of bedding. This change is made immediately when needed in cases confined to bed. Close-stools are cleansed at once, night and day, and frequent visits are made to the restless ones in the separate rooms. There are padded rooms in this institution, but the idea governing the treatment leads to only an occasional use of them.

There is one nurse for eight patients. This does not seem a large allowance. Yet much work is done by the patients themselves. Such occupation is considered a valuable part of the treatment in many cases. It keeps the mind from (as it were) feeding upon itself, and, in the accomplishment of something that can be seen, tends to bring back the interest in life. Trades are encouraged, and places are provided for the pursuit of such pleasant occupations. The nurses are carefully selected, and can be instantly discharged for incompetency or carelessness.

This institution is surrounded by more than nine acres of ground, some of which is divided by walls into exercising courts. Arbors and covered ways have been built for use in bad weather. The outdoor plan of treatment is pursued here whenever advisable, as it often is, and every attempt is made to take away from the mind the idea of prison life.

The kitchen is in a detached building, and is well equipped and managed. The laundry, which is near it, is kept as busy as all such should be. Comfortable houses are in the fore-court of the hospital for the two medical officers comprising the staff. At present there are about one hundred and fifty patients, including forty officers, more or less.

The mortality averages ten per cent, and the recoveries are relatively many. Mania designates more than one-half the cases; and dementia, melancholia, and paralysis of the insane, follow in the order named. The admissions are sufficient to keep the total number under treatment about the same.

Royal Naval Hospital at Malta.

This hospital is situated near the walled city of Valetta, on the north side of the island of Malta, in the Mediterranean Sea. Malta is a sand and limestone formation, eighteen miles long and eight wide, with its long axis approximately northwest and southeast. A range of hills forms its backbone. It is from these that an ancient and leaking aqueduct conveys a limited supply of good water into

Valetta. Cisterns are used for storing this and rain-water; but as these are often polluted by leaks, intestinal disorders and typhoid fever are not uncommon.

The climate is very delightful from October to April, the thermometer ranging from 50° F. to 70°; the atmosphere, under the north winds, fairly dry, and the days almost invariably full of sunshine. This enables invalids and convalescents to live out-of-doors. During this period the rainfall is over twenty inches, but, most conveniently, it falls as a rule during the night, and upon a soil that drains rapidly. Snow is unknown, and the formation of ice is a surprise.

The heat during the summer makes sunstroke not infrequent, while in early autumn the moist sirocco or southeast wind debilitates mind and body, and predisposes to neuralgia and malarial diseases.

Valetta is a terraced city, on the end of a high tongue of land that makes out to the northeast within one of the many indentations of the coast. Its end, however, St. Elmo Point, is so far out as to be on the general coast-line, and forms with Ricasoli Point the entrance to the harbor or bay which is southeast of the city.

Across this bay, half a mile from the city, and on a bold promontory between Forts Ricasoli and St. Angelo, is the largest foreign naval hospital of Great Britain. It has a beautiful site, overlooking the city and harbor, and its Doric two-story stone buildings present an imposing appearance.

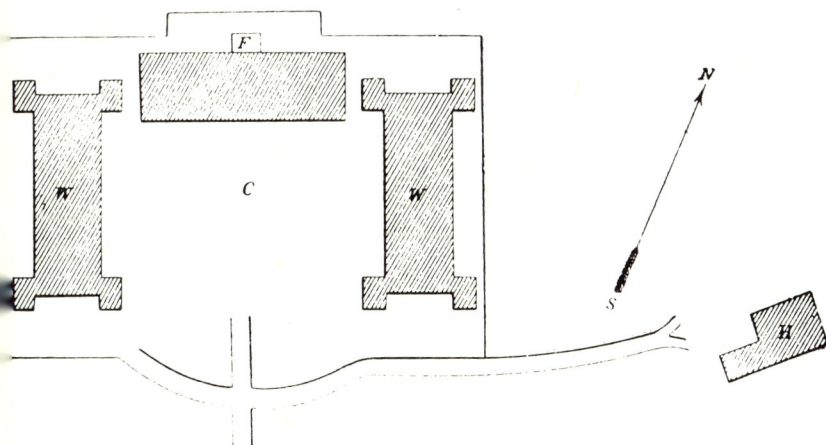

FIG. 2. NAVAL HOSPITAL, MALTA.
F. Front. W. Wings. C. Court. H. Inspector's House.

The building that forms the front looks to the northwest, and the detached building on each side extends back perpendicular to the line of the main structure. There is a corridor around the inner face of each, and the enclosed court, which covers an immense cistern, is paved.

The wards are nearly one hundred feet long, twenty-five wide and twenty-two high. There are, however, smaller wards, and many rooms for sick officers. They furnish nearly 1800 cubic feet air space per bed, and are supplied with a fair number of high windows, open fireplaces, and large openings near the ceilings. The ward furniture is reduced to a minimum. The beds are iron, and the mattresses always look new, as they are frequently re-made. There is a good smoking-room and a library.

The bath-rooms are supplied with modern improvements, and the water-closets, though near the wards, are well supplied with seats and water and are easily flushed. The floors of these, being tiled, are easily kept clean and present a good appearance. A small building about three hundred yards from the main buildings, is used for contagious diseases. There is also a large storehouse, which is kept well filled with medical supplies for the fleet.

The nursing staff consists of ten, and these are fairly well provided with quarters. The kitchen and laundry are on the ground floor. The medical inspector in charge has a large residence east of the buildings. This hospital has accommodations for two hundred and eighty patients, including fifty-eight sick officers.

The wards are divided into medical and surgical, and the average number under treatment is about eighty. The number treated annually approximates one thousand—about equally divided between medical and surgical cases. The number of cases of remittent fever treated annually often approaches one hundred; about fifty per cent of these are eventually sent home to recover from the consequent debility. Typhoid fever is not uncommon, there being, perhaps, fifteen or twenty cases each year, with a mortality, it seems, of about twelve per cent. The general death-rate of this hospital is not very large, but a considerable number of invalids are sent home by the troop-ships to escape the summer and early fall.

The authorities of this port are exceedingly sensitive on the subject of epidemic influences, and as a result the quarantine regulations are very rigid. The large number of troops in the garrison, and the importance of the island as a naval station and base of operations, necessitate, however, the greatest caution. There have been sad experiences with cholera, which is the disease most dreaded, as the island is on the line of travel from the East.

The Royal Naval Hospitals at Bermuda, Jamaica, Ascension, Cape of Good Hope, and Esquimalt.

These hospitals present nothing especially worthy of attention. They are, of course, of inestimable importance to the naval service, and from that point of view demand some notice. It is believed that the following short notes will be considered sufficient:

Bermuda.—The hospital is situated on Ireland Island, the naval station, and occupies rather high ground, overlooking the water to the west. It is three stories high, and contains four wards, two on the second and two on the third floor. These wards are thirteen feet high, twenty-four feet wide, and sixty long. They contain fifteen beds each, and furnish a little more than twelve hundred cubic feet per bed. Considering the climate, this space should be at least doubled. Ordinarily this is the case, as the average daily number under treatment in time of peace is only thirty, including sick officers, who have rooms on the first floor and are provided with a private dining-room and library.

The whole building is entirely surrounded by broad verandas, which are necessarily supplied with Venetian blinds. There are water-closets and bath-rooms on each floor. As the ground furnishes a rather steep slope the drainage is good. Innumerable gutters conduct off the surface water, while the water-closets have a sewer leading out into the bay.

The kitchen and laundry are in a small detached building; but, unless there has been a recent change, meals are served on small tables in the wards for lack of space for a messroom. It is needless to criticise this undesirable condition of things.

There is no separate building for contagious diseases. Suspicious cases are allowed to develop in the hospital, and then, if necessary, are transferred to the common pest-house on the island. The water supply is rain-water collected in cisterns.

The deputy inspector in charge has a separate house. He and two surgeons comprise the staff. The number of nurses allowed is four. The total number of cases treated annually is about two hundred and fifty. The number of surgical cases is double that of the medical. Venereal troubles form about twenty percent of the total.

Remittent and typhoid fevers are rather frequent. The average number of days under treatment per case of all diseases is nearly fifty.

The climate of the Bermudas is exceedingly pleasant and equable in winter, but in spring, summer and fall the heat is frequently oppressive, though much modified by breezes. The average temperature during this period is about 77 degrees F.

Jamaica.—At Port Royal, the naval hospital is an extensive building, but only a part of it is kept in operation or in fair condition. In the early part of this century, events seemed to necessitate a large building for the sick in this part of the world. Its capacity is now considered to be one hundred and twelve, including rooms for twelve sick officers; but the average number of cases daily under treatment is only ten. Five nurses are allowed, as the intensity of disease is liable to sudden changes in this climate. In 1882, forty cases of yellow fever were treated in this hospital.

In the event of any increase of the naval force in these waters, or even of any interference with the cruise to the north in summer, the number of cases and the intensity of the disease would be much increased in this building. As it is, the total number of patients during a year is usually only one hundred and fifty, the medical rather exceeding the surgical cases. About eight percent are invalided, and the loss by death frequently approaches the rather large number of fifty per thousand. This mortality is due in great measure to fevers of various types. Venereal cases number fifteen or twenty annually.

Three medical officers compose the staff. These, in addition to usual duties, have charge of the large amount of medical supplies kept here for the fleet.

Yellow fever receives little attention at the quarantine station across the bay, but smallpox is regarded as the great enemy, demanding constant watchfulness.

Ascension.—This building is in Georgetown, a very small naval settlement on the west coast of Ascension Island. This volcanic island has a diameter of six miles. Its surface consists of many hills and mountains, intersected by innumerable watercourses and deep valleys. The mountains frequently attain an elevation of fifteen hundred feet. Much of the coast is formed of rough lava-rocks, while the hills and mountains present many well-formed craters.

The hospital is at the extreme south of the settlement, high above the water, from which it is distant a fraction of a mile. It has accommodations for sixty-five sick, including fourteen officers. There is only one nurse allowed, but the average number of patients daily is but six. About one hundred cases are treated annually. The medical cases are about double the surgical.

As might be expected, venereal troubles are rare, and malarial fevers are very common. These latter are brought by the ships cruising in the rivers and on the coast of West Africa. Indeed, this island is used as a sanitarium. Vessels are sometimes almost entirely deserted, and the crews placed in the barracks on Green Mountain, near the center of the island. From near this mountain, water of good quality is supplied to Georgetown.

At this hospital the mortality is frequently only about ten per thousand; the invaliding, ten percent; and the average number of days treatment per case, less than twenty-five.

Cape of Good Hope.—The naval hospital here is small. There are accommodations for eighty patients, including rooms for six sick officers. The average number of patients daily under treatment is twenty-five, and the total yearly is three hundred. The surgical cases are three times the medical. This is to be expected, as venereal troubles are common.

Ships cruising in these waters have few places where liberty can be given. Cape Colony is one of these. About one hundred venereal cases find their way to hospital in the course of a year. Of course, this is a small proportion of the total number of cases.

Ships cruising on the West Coast bring, from time to time, large numbers of malarial cases to this hospital. The death-rate is relatively small, but the invaliding is over eighty per thousand. Summer is the most healthy season, as it is then that the southeast winds prevail.

Esquimalt.—This is the smallest of all the royal naval hospitals. It can accommodate but forty patients. The average number daily under treatment is only five, and the total number yearly, less than fifty. Only one or two are invalided during the year, but the average number of days treatment per case is generally over forty. The building is wooden, well-lighted, but poorly ventilated, with two wards. It has ten acres of ground on the west coast and south side of Vancouver Island, and overlooks Constance Cove, a part of Esquimalt harbor.

The surgeon has a house about thirty yards from the main building. In this there are also rooms for four sick officers. There is a structure for contagious diseases.

Across the Cove and distant a small fraction of a mile is the dockyard. This is the British naval station in the Pacific.

Royal Naval Hospital at Hong Kong.

This hospital is situated in the eastern suburb of the city of Victoria, on the island of Hong Kong. This island, which is just within the tropics (latitude 22° north, longitude 114° east), is eight miles long and averages about three miles in width. The long axis is nearly on the parallel. A great part of the surface is formed by barren mountains of volcanic rock which rise in many places over fifteen hundred feet, and are swept during the winter months by the northwest monsoon, and in the summer by the southwest.

The north wind sometimes in January forces the thermometer at Victoria down to 40° F., when snow may appear on the mountain tops. The mean annual temperature of the city is 73° F. The hottest month is July, when with a mean temperature of 86° F. and with a humidity of ten grains per cubic foot, sunstrokes are not uncommon. The coldest month is January, with a mean of 52° F. and a humidity of four grains per cubic foot. The highest barometer is in November and the lowest in July.

The wet months are June and July, and the dry months, January and February. The rainfall averages eighty inches, and the rainy days over one hundred.

Victoria, which is on the north side of the island, and one mile from the mainland, has a population of over two hundred and twenty thousand, including two thousand Europeans and Americans. The English rule is strict, so that in spite of the large number of Chinese, cleanliness is observed and epidemics are rare.

The houses are built upon volcanic rock or its derivative laterite, which retains the water during the wet and hot months, and increases the marked tendency to malarial troubles. Turning up the soil is dangerous on that account, but the English authorities have done much, by paving and other sanitary precautions, to improve the general health. Dysentery and diarrhœa have become less common, but smallpox, on account of inoculations, still clings to the Chinese homes.

In the eastern suburb of the city is situated the Royal Naval Hospital, two hundred feet above high water, and overlooking the city and harbor.   It is a fraction of a mile from the coast-line and dock-yard.

The hospital was a private residence, and was bought by the government for £7000.   It consists of four buildings, each thirty feet square, built of stone, two stories high, and shaded by verandas. The enclosed square, which receives the breeze through the space between the buildings, is paved.   The water-closets and bath-rooms of each building are separated from the wards and placed in offsets.

The upper stories are the four wards, each containing twelve beds, and furnishing thirteen hundred cubic feet to each bed.   These wards have high ceilings, windows on both opposite sides, and are lighted by gas.   In the lower stories are storerooms, dispensary, nurses' and officers' quarters.   The Deputy Inspector in charge has a good residence.   He and two surgeons comprise the staff.

The water supply is derived from mountain streams and reservoirs. Provision is also made for the dry season by storing in tanks.   The English authorities have done much to protect the water from pollution, and have succeeded in increasing its reputation for being the best on the coast.

The hospital has accommodation for fifty-six patients, including eight officers.   During the year, about three hundred patients are treated—the surgical being only slightly greater than the medical. The cases of venereal diseases average about fifty annually.   Dysentery, smallpox, and remittent and typhoid fevers are not uncommon. Occasionally cholera claims a victim.   The number of cases invalided, averaging about eight per cent, is chiefly from the medical wards. The death-rate sometimes does not exceed one per cent of the total number treated.   In the early spring many patients go with the fleet to Yokohama, as the moist summer heat materially delays convalescence.

Royal Naval Sick Quarters at Yokohama.

This hospital, which was formerly a barrack for English troops, is a plaster and tile building of one story, built on three sides of a rectangle (Plate II).   It is situated on a bluff which rises from the sea to the height of one hundred and twenty-five feet.   The trend of the coast here is toward the northwest.   As the building faces the east, and the sea from which the prevailing winds come, the enclosed court is shut off from the breeze.   The length of the front is about one hundred and twenty-five feet, while that of the wings which extend back at right angles is more than two hundred. Around the inner face of the entire building there is a veranda which is much used in warm weather, and furnishes an outside communication.

This main structure can accommodate over eighty patients. The front and north wings are divided into four wards, each about sixty feet long. These wards have windows on both opposite sides, and have additional ventilation through openings near the ceiling, which discharge near the roof into the air. All these wards are for the treatment of seamen and marines. The south wing is divided into rooms for non-commissioned and warrant officers.

The average cubic space per bed is nearly 1500 feet. The building is heated by stoves and open fireplaces, the latter, of course, assisting much in the ventilation.

The grounds comprise about five acres, ornamented by grass slopes, lawns, groves of trees, and flowers. The locality is a desirable one, and it is on this bluff that most of the foreign residents live, and the United States has established its hospital.

The dispensary and stewards' quarters are two buildings outside of the quadrangle, but facing the unoccupied side. To the south of these, and on the other side of the main gate, are the dwellings for the two medical officers comprising the staff. These houses have a detached kitchen and servants' quarters.

South of the main building, and separated from it by about seventy-five feet of lawn, are the quarters for sick officers. These consist of rooms well fitted up, and usually more than one room is assigned to each invalid.

The mortuary is at the extreme north end of the grounds, and is about 50 yards distant from the main building, from which it is hidden by a grove of trees.

At the extreme southwest corner of the grounds are two separated buildings for the treatment of contagious diseases. Near-by is a spring, a storehouse and a disinfecting chamber. This part of the ground is cut off by a grove of trees. A fire-engine house is near the north wing of the hospital.

The nursing staff consists of seven. These are quartered in a building near the general kitchen, storehouse and coal shed, at the northwest border of the grounds, and distant from the main building about thirty feet.

The method of dealing with the water-closets is one common in the East. They can, almost all, be reached from the outside of the building, and natives, under contract, remove every night the large earthen jars.

The water supply is from wells, a spring, and a tank in which rain water is stored. All the drinking water is filtered, and in the summer is also boiled.

The total capacity of this hospital is ninety-five (95), including accommodations for thirteen sick officers. The average number under treatment approaches thirty (30). The surgical cases are nearly double the medical. The death-rate is relatively small, and the invaliding, which is influenced by the patients received from the hospital at Hong Kong, amounts to about five per cent. The total number of patients treated annually is about two hundred. Phthisis is common, and the number of venereal cases possibly reaches fifty —twenty-five percent of the total. Malarial fever and occasional cases of smallpox help to make up the record.

The record of this hospital is influenced by the practice of the fleet to cruise north from Hong Kong in the spring. The ships arrive at Yokohama about April, bringing all patients from the Hong Kong hospital who can be safely moved. They return to the coast of China in the fall and carry back with them all who in the intervening months promise to be ready for duty, or who would be benefited by the change. These transfers, however, are chiefly due to the relaxing and debilitating summer at Victoria.

NAVAL HOSPITALS OF FRANCE.

The French navy has 378 ships, 75,915 men and 5 hospitals.

The following titles designate the various grades in the medical corps : Inspecteur général, directeur du service de santé, inspecteur adjoint, médecin-en-chef, médecin professeur, médecin principal, médecin de première classe, and médecin de seconde classe.

Each member of the medical corps has obtained his professional education at one of the three naval medical schools at Rochefort, Toulon, and Brest.

The hospitals are situated at Rochefort, Cherbourg, Brest, Toulon, and Saint Mandrier, and offer with the medical schools no uninteresting study.

Naval Hospital at Rochefort, France.

At Rochefort, on the Charente river, the French made the beginning of a regular organized navy. Here in 1666 Louis XIV, under the influence of his able minister, Colbert, devoted some of his easily squandered money to the praiseworthy object of founding a naval station. However well chosen the site was from a naval point of view, from that of a sanitarian it was most unfortunate. The work was carried on at the frightful cost of many lives. The swampy ground, when turned up, engendered intense malarial disorders, making a hospital an early necessity. This was established in the old priory of Saint-Éloy at Tonnay (Charente).

Happily there was a village fortunately situated, and abundantly supplied with good water. The old priory was soon insufficient, but it was not until 1683 that the hospital at the new naval station was completed. At that date Tonnay Charente was abandoned and the sick were removed to Rochefort. This new hospital consisted originally of eight wards, each containing fifty beds. These were placed in two buildings, connected by a central structure for administration, two wards on the ground floor of each and two on the floor above. The beds were of wood, and each constructed for two occupants. They were also supplied with green serge curtains. There was additional room in each building for 40 couches—thus making the total capacity 480.

In a short time, however, in spite of the large mortality brought about by the terrible crowding, there was not room for the many demanding admission, and, fortunately, tents had to be used. At one time there were as many as 700 patients. This occurred during the frightful epidemics in the navy during the ten years prior to 1750. It was in this latter year that an addition was made in the form of a new pavilion.

It seems that the large mortality and overcrowding continuing, plans for a new hospital were devised in 1782, and extensive grounds were bought in a more elevated situation outside the ramparts. Here work was begun in 1783 on a hospital to cost 400,000 francs, and to contain 1002 single beds, with 1400 cubic feet of air to each.

In the middle of 1787 the work had progressed so far that these beds were moved in. Iron beds they were, the first used in French hospitals. In 1788 this hospital, the present one (Plate III), was opened with much ceremony, and in three days the old one was abandoned, one may suppose with a sigh of relief; for during the 105 years it had been occupied, 30,000 dead had been carried out of its doors.

Naval Hospital at Toulon.

In writing of the naval hospital at Toulon, one feels that the task is more or less disagreeable. The French Government should have destroyed it long ago. It was never suitable for a hospital, and yet it has been used as such for more than a century.

In much less time, even the best-planned hospital is in danger of suffering from hospitalism ; but an old seminary, wretchedly designed, shut off from sunlight and pure air, when used for the treatment of the sick, soon becomes contaminated, and each patient entering its doors encounters a new danger, in spite of the best directed and most skillful efforts of those having him in charge.

The walls of this institution have been standing since 1686, at which time the Jesuits began the education here of chaplains for the navy. A similar enterprise had been initiated the year before at Rochefort. The government, at such an early date, considered it advisable for priests serving in the navy to have special training.

Twenty-three years after this, by the effort of that memorable medical officer, M. Dupuy, a like conviction was instilled into the mind of the king's minister, in regard to the medical officers of the service, and, in 1725, a school was established at Toulon for a like purpose, six years after a similar one had been founded at Rochefort. At that time, however, there was no regular constituted naval hospital at Toulon. The sick of the navy had been treated for some years in the arsenal.

In 1716, this proving inadequate, the system was inaugurated of paying a civil hospital for this service. This, for several reasons, always proves very unsatisfactory, and, as a result, the project of establishing a naval hospital was constantly being discussed.

Time passed, and Toulon increased in importance as a naval station. Economy still prevailed ; but the need becoming more urgent, the king, in 1774, signed the transfer of the house of the Jesuits to the medical department of the service. The clergy and the municipal authorities naturally objected, and their influence was so great that the change was delayed.

In 1783, just after peace with England was signed, the French fleet broke its rendezvous at Cadiz, and many of the vessels came into the harbor of Toulon, having eleven hundred sick on board. There were not accommodations for such a large number, and tents were used for this purpose.

The necessity for a naval hospital was thus greatly emphasized, and the long-delayed transfer was made in 1785. The school and hospital have worked together in this building ever since.

The building has a front five stories high, facing the south, and occupying the shorter parallel side of a trapezoid; the wings going back on the two adjacent sides, and joining a rear building parallel to the front. This rear building is again connected with the front by two additional perpendicular wings, thus dividing the enclosed ground into three small unequal courts—all the wings, and rear of three stories, and the extreme west wing extending beyond the rear structure its own length. Some idea of this plan is obtained by Plates IV and V.

A massive structure it appears, set down in a densely populated city, and separated by narrow streets from the many neighboring buildings. There is a court in the rear, a continuation of the trapezoid, with continuous one-story buildings around it, containing store-rooms, attendants' quarters, and the like; and projecting into it, a building for a pharmacy, dissecting room, mortuary, laboratory, and other offices. But little air stirs within or without such a hospital, and the sunlight shining on its high front reaches but little else.

There are twelve wards, many of them practically being one, as the only separation is an arch. They are one hundred feet long, thirty wide and fifteen high. They contain, as a rule, twenty-four beds each, between and near six windows on each side. There are no additional means for ventilating the fairly great allowance of nearly nineteen hundred cubic feet per bed. The floors are tiles laid in cement, and the walls are whitewashed. A patient, looking out of a window, sees, as a rule, nothing but walls, though he may catch a view of the sun for a short while.

The water-closets are separated from the wards by a narrow passage. They have a fairly good upward ventilation, though requiring frequent disinfection. The drainage is into open gutters, swept by a rapidly moving stream of water.

The total capacity of this hospital is about three hundred, over two hundred and eighty being in wards, and the remaining accommodations, for the officers mainly, being in rooms in the front. These rooms are supplied with open fireplaces, and, fronting on the south, are more cheerful and comfortable. The greater part of the building is, however, heated by stoves.

It is almost needless to say, that in spite of all the skill practised within its walls, the mortality is great, and patients admitted with slight injuries are liable to develop grave troubles.

The kitchen, though an excellently managed one, is in the basement, directly under a ward. The bath-rooms are also in the basement, but at a considerable distance from the wards, thoroughly equipped, and commanding admiration. The laundry work is done at a distance, in large stone basins supplied with water by a natural stream. There is every attempt made at cleanliness and comfort. The linen is frequently changed, and the beds have each two good mattresses on well-made springs.

The efforts of the staff are worthy, too, of every praise, for they fight a good fight against a constant and ever-present enemy. This staff consists of eight officers, including the médecin-en-chef in charge. In addition to other duties, many of these conduct the school.

The whole work is performed in the most excellent manner. Most of the nursing is done by men, but the Sisters have the general supervision of them, as well as the care of special cases. These superintend also the storerooms, kitchen, linen-room, and the general distribution of material.

The Naval Hospital at Toulon is most ably conducted. It could not be otherwise, under men who hold their high position by great merit only. But France considers herself too impoverished to build another, though she listens to the earnest requests and representations of her well-informed medical officers, and continues to expand her wonderful navy and army.

Naval Hospital (Clermont- Tonnère) at Brest.

Prior to 1666, the sick of the navy were treated in the civil hospital at Brest. At that date, this hospital was destroyed by fire, and an old deserted guard-house was taken for this purpose. The building was small, in a bad situation, and soon overcrowded. As a result of this unfortunate situation, the government was compelled, in 1684, to construct a naval hospital. This hospital contained three hundred beds, but was too small to accommodate the large number requiring treatment, and an addition was built in 1689.

In 1776, this first naval hospital at Brest was destroyed by fire, and it is stated that convicts there under treatment, and still in chains, were burned in their beds. After the fire, there was an immediate necessity to find accommodations for the many sick. An old Jesuit seminary was taken for this purpose—it then being used as quarters for the marine guard. The sick were put in this building, and, in time, certain additions were made to it, so that it was able to contain five hundred beds.

This seminary was used as the Naval Hospital at Brest until 1834, when the present structure was finished. The corner-stone of the present hospital was laid in 1822, by Clermont Tonnère, the Minister of Marine, from whom it received its name. The site is the same as that of the old building burned in 1776. It is an extensive granite structure, on a plateau back of the city of Brest, and on the left bank of the Penfeld river, commanding a fine view of the city and the roads. It has two stories and an attic, and contains 1200 beds.

It is a pity that this large hospital has such a defective plan (Plate VI). Though symmetrically arranged, its wards bear such a relation to one another that but little light and air are admitted to them. All the wards are parallel, and are connected at one end by a corridor, or rather gallery, to which they are all perpendicular. From this gallery, or rather in the continuation of the wards into it, are the stairs connecting the two stories. The wards are joined in the rear, mostly in pairs, by passages in which are the water-closets, and from which are back stairs connecting the two stories, and also steps leading down into the gardens and courts which the various buildings enclose. The whole comprises a series built upon the block plan, and containing its worst features.

Each ward is over 170 feet long, 26 wide and 15 high, containing, usually, 50 beds, and furnishing over 1200 cubic feet of air space per bed. There are sixteen windows on each opposite side, but no other means of ventilation, save the two doors. The next building across the court is distant less than fifty feet. The beds are iron, and have two mattresses on springs. Strange to say, officers are treated in wards just as enlisted men, there being a ward on the second floor reserved for them. The number of rooms is very small. These are well furnished and contain every convenience, but have to be kept for serious cases only.

There is no separate building for contagious diseases, and at a date not very remote, many cases of smallpox were treated in the wards. The venereal ward is at the extreme end of the building, and this connects through a small room with an annex generally used for other contagious disorders. This annex is continued so as to form a court around the chapel, and contains smoking-room, baths, mortuary and post-mortem room. The kitchen is to the left of the second entrance, near the quarters of the junior officers on duty, and to the right of this entrance is the administration. The grounds contain a botanical garden, and a promenade bordered by trees. Between these is the building for the medical school.

The sisters, who have special quarters assigned them near the entrance court, nurse special cases and have the supervision of the male nurses. They also superintend the kitchen, laundry, store-rooms, and the like. There is one nurse for every twelve patients. The number of patients treated here is several thousand a year, and the mortality frequently exceeds four per cent. The hospital is in charge of a médecin-en-chef.

Naval Hospital of St. Mandrier.

The coast in the immediate neighborhood of Toulon forms, as it encloses the two roadsteads, a curve somewhat like a parabola, with the axis nearly east and west. Toulon is on the north side of the curve, and the hospital Saint Mandrier on the south, distant from the city more than two miles, and overlooking the Grand Roads. Here the ground is high, and the extreme point is commanded by a fort, to guard the entrance to the roads. This fort is 900 yards distant from the hospital, which is sheltered by the intervening hills and the bluff formed by the excavation necessary for a site.

Unfortunately, in the desire to protect the hospital from shells in time of war, so much excavating was done that the wind from the south is entirely excluded from it. In doing this a tremendous amount of labor was required, so that, though the work was commenced in 1817, under the design of M. Raucourt, an hydraulic engineer, it was not completed until 1830. Much of this work was done by convicts. The building erected at that time for their occupation still stands (800 feet long), and is used now for venereal cases, the laundry, and quarters for workmen.

The grounds are 675 yards long and 255 wide, and exhibit by the amplitude the great amount of excavation required. The shore here can be approached by small boats, for which there is constructed a small dock; but the main landing extends out 400 yards (Plate VII).

The main buildings consist of three detached pavilions, one fronting the bluff to the south, and the other two placed laterally nearer the water, and perpendicular to the first. They are each three hundred and sixty feet long and twenty-seven wide, but the breadth is doubled by strong covered balconies on the faces next the court.

These immense buildings, with their three stories, and adjoining grounds containing a botanical garden, beautiful walks and trees, and many detached buildings, including a classical chapel with its dome supported by many Ionic and Corinthian columns, present a glorious memorial of the greatness, gratitude and justice of France. And yet, the never-ending questions: should there be any grand hospitals anywhere?—should not all hospitals be cheaply built, and frequently destroyed?—present themselves even here.

There are 1200 beds within these walls and the many detached smaller structures. Most of them, however, are placed in the wards of the lateral buildings. These wards are 120 feet long, 27 wide and 14 high, and contain 36 beds each, with more than 1200 cubic feet per bed. The floors are tiled, the walls plastered, and the ceilings wofully cut up by arches. There are windows on both opposite sides, but no other means of ventilation. The necessary heat is supplied by three open stoves, symmetrically placed in each ward. The climate, however, is remarkably mild, as is demonstrated by the tropical growth in the gardens.

The front building contains, on the first floor, offices for the administration, and quarters for the chaplains, chief medical officers, and sisters. These last superintend the kitchen, storerooms, laundry, and the nurses. On the second floor of this building are quarters for the junior officers, and small wards for the treatment of sick officers. In the basement or ground floor are the laundry, kitchen, linen room, and the like, and also the pharmacy.

Strangely enough, there is not a water-closet in the whole building. The system employed is that of perambulating closed stools, which are kept, for the most part, in the balconies, and emptied into an earth-pit. This, of course, entails many inconveniences, and makes cleanliness exceedingly difficult.

Associated with this hospital are many detached buildings. In the rear of each lateral building is a series of parallel, temporary, detached wards, accommodating many patients. In front of the administration building are three enormous cisterns, remarkable for the capacity of 10 million litres. In regarding these caverns, one is impressed by the great work of those galley-slaves.

Among the objections to this great hospital are the nearness of the bluff, and the obstruction presented by those very wide balconies to the admission of sunlight to the wards. But this large receiving hospital has been of immense value to France in her many wars; notably, in the Greek, Algerian, Crimean, Italian, and German campaigns; and to Toulon in her many epidemics.

In 1850, the botanical garden was transferred here from the hospital at Toulon. Every year, its connection becomes closer with the naval medical school in the south of France, and much work is done here now by the students, especially in surgery and clinical medicine.

Naval Hospital at Cherbourg.

Cherbourg was not designated as a naval station until 1781, from which time until 1793, the sick of the navy were treated in a civil hospital. When the large number of workmen in that locality made it impossible for this hospital to receive all the sick, an ancient abbey was placed at the disposition of the navy, which, after many changes, was converted into a naval hospital. Soon this became insufficient, and a new pavilion was added, containing three wards, holding forty beds each. The capacity was thus increased to three hundred beds. The grounds of this hospital contained a chapel, and many small buildings for mortuary, laundry, and quarters for workmen; and also a botanical garden.

As Cherbourg increased in naval importance, additional quarters for the sick were obtained in a barrack. There were disadvantages in having the sick in two establishments so far apart, and, besides, the total number of beds was not sufficient for emergencies. Thus, after much consideration, large grounds were purchased west of the city, for the erection of a large modern hospital to contain 1000 beds. This hospital was not completed sufficiently for occupation until 1870, and a portion of the plan still remains to be carried out. (Plate VIII.)

It consists now of three detached pavilions, arranged like those at Saint Mandrier, except that the front one extends beyond the others, sufficiently for two additional outside rear-pavilions to be built in accordance with the original plan.

The front looks to the north over the dockyard and Grand Roads, so that the rear pavilions have the great advantage of being north and south, thus receiving much of the sun. All the buildings are three stories high, and contain about six hundred beds, though, usually, there are only two hundred and fifty patients. In front is a large garden and promenade. The enclosed court is also laid out as a garden, and is surrounded by a covered way which connects all the buildings, and which can be closed in bad or cold weather.

The main structure in front is used for the same purposes as the corresponding building in Saint Mandrier, while the long, narrow wards are chiefly in the rear pavilions. The wards have polished oak floors laid in cement, and are warmed by stoves with porcelain sides. Besides numerous windows on both opposite sides, there are ventilators near floors and ceilings. Each ward contains forty-eight beds, which are supplied with two mattresses and good springs. There are water-closets, urinals, and sinks near every ward, but well separated from them. A male nurse looks after twelve patients, but as in all French naval hospitals, the sisters nurse special cases and have the general superintendence.

The rear pavilions, which are over four hundred feet long, are distant from each other more than 200 feet. Occupying a part of the space between their rear ends is a large chapel, while in the corresponding space at the other end are the baths. These are most complete, containing in addition to the usual tubs, a swimming pool, a large variety of douches, and shower, sulphur, vapor, and hot-air baths.

The laundry is in a separate building in the west rear corner of the grounds. It is complete in every respect, and has been recently erected at the cost of 300,000 francs. The mortuary is in the corresponding corner on the other side. There is a small wooden structure, rather too close to the main buildings, for the treatment of contagious diseases.

The Naval Medical Schools of France.

A description of the naval hospitals of France, however short, can scarcely be separated from some account of the Naval Medical Schools so closely connected with them. The French naval hospital dates back to the beginning of the regular organized navy in 1666, but the school did not follow until more than a half a century had elapsed. There were several conditions which finally necessitated their establishment. Soon after the foundation of Rochefort it became necessary to have capable medical officers at the various naval stations where so many officers and workmen were being employed.

Considerable care was exercised in their selection, with the result of obtaining good men. The inducements were sufficient to retain them in these positions for many years, as is shown in the case of Ollivier, who was, "1er médecin du port de Brest" for more than forty years. These in turn were succeeded by others, all remaining for many years, and attaching importance and dignity to the titles

" Médecin du port" and " Chirurgien-major du port." Some of these gentlemen represented the best talent in the whole kingdom, and were doctors of medicine of the best faculties in France.

On the other hand, the medical service afloat was made of different material. For some time, commanding officers of ships selected their own surgeons from such material as presented, and they held their places for short times only, and under other great disadvantages. Then a few surgeons were appointed at each port who were available for sea service, but their assistants continued to be appointed in the same manner. At this time there existed in the navy, as on shore, both the physician and the surgeon. The latter was, as a rule, illiterate, and had obtained his small knowledge as an apprentice in the office of some surgeon in the large cities.

The former, though the better educated, was generally one of little worth, who, in spite of the disadvantages of life at sea, resorted to the navy as a means of livelihood. In their education they had also imbibed à contempt for the surgeon as a class. Out of this condition of things only dissatisfaction could come.

The various medical officers of the ports soon became aware of the great need of improvement. A short time after M. Dupuy was appointed " 1ᵉʳ médecin" of the port of Rochefort (1712), the establishment of a naval medical school became the great object of his life. This gentleman, who was a graduate of the faculty of Toulouse and a member of the Academy of Sciences, repeatedly urged upon the government the necessity for such institutions.

Disheartened by no failure, he finally accomplished his object, and succeeded, in 1722, in having a suitable building erected for the purpose, at which time this school was opened at Rochefort, with much formality. The success of the project was soon assured, and its influence became so apparent that two other schools were soon established, the one at Toulon, in 1725, and the other at Brest, in 1731.

These schools have commanded the admiration of the world ever since ; and in spite of the many successions of kings and of the Reign of Terror itself, they have always been fostered and prized by the French people.

M. Dupuy is marked in naval history by his thorough grasp of a subject so important to the future welfare of his country. In England the purpose of the Naval Medical School is to *complete* the education of their assistant-surgeons acquired at the various medical schools of the country, but in France the object is to *begin* that education, and carry it on to a high grade of perfection. These schools have been so ably described by Medical Director Richard C. Dean, of the United States Navy, that all the remaining remarks upon this subject may be considered as a résumé of his remarkably complete report.

The student is taken as a youth over eighteen years of age, and impressed, from the beginning, with naval methods. He must be a citizen of France, without physical fault, and have arrived at the dignity of an A. B. or a B. S. Dismissal from one school for deficiency in studies, or infractions of discipline, bars him from the other schools and from naval life. There are two divisions in the school, and promotion from one to the other is determined by examination at the end of one year. This is a good arrangement, as two failures (one year interval) to pass from the lower to the higher division, leads to dismissal and rids the school of the trouble of working and spending money upon unsatisfactory material.

The professors are permanently attached to the school. They are assisted by " fellows " who have arrived at that dignity after a special examination. These latter are liable in time to sea service. Every subject is lectured on three times a week, and each course is completed once in two years. Thus, after two years study, the successful candidate becomes an assistant-surgeon; and, after two years more study, if successful, a surgeon of the second class.

An assistant-surgeon is not considered prepared for service at sea, as he has been examined only on the following subjects:

1. Anatomy, performance of dissection (oral).
2. Pharmacology, extemporaneous pharmacy (oral).
3. Minor surgery, application of apparatus and bandages (oral).
4. General pathology and semiology (written).

After this examination he remains under instruction for another two years, with the exception of six months at sea, and is then examined for promotion to the grade of surgeon of the second class. This examination is on the following subjects:

1. Anatomy and physiology (oral).
2. Materia medica and therapeutics (oral).
3. External pathology, operative surgery, obstetrics (oral).
4. Internal pathology, hygiene, legal medicine (written).

Having passed this examination, he is granted six months leave for the purpose of procuring the degree of "doctor of medicine" from one of the faculties of France. The government defrays all the expenses entailed by this leave in the event of success, and in return demands a written contract to remain in the naval service for ten years.

The examination for promotion to the grade of surgeon of the first class is also held at the school, and embraces the following subjects:

1. Physiology (oral).
2. Clinical medicine (oral).
3. Operative surgery, obstetrics, performance of one surgical and one obstetrical operation (oral).
4. Naval hygiene, pathology, a report on medical jurisprudence (written).

The whole curriculum of studies is as follows:

1. Legal and administrative medicine.
2. Clinical medicine, medical pathology.
3. Materia medica and therapeutics, toxicology.
4. General and naval hygiene.
5. Clinical surgery, surgical pathology.
6. Operative surgery.
7. Anatomy and physiology.
8. Obstetrics, diseases of women and children.
9. Chemistry.
10. Pharmacy and medical physics.
11. Natural history (medical), pharmacology.
12. Descriptive anatomy.
13. General pathology and semiology.
14. Minor surgery, apparatus and bandaging.
15. Extemporaneous pharmacy, chemical manipulations.

To teach these various branches there are various amphitheaters, a library, a botanical garden, and a museum of natural history, pathology and anatomy. In addition to all this, the wards of the hospital form the great school, and in them clinical instruction is given in the most thorough manner.

The final examinations for each grade are conducted at each school by professors from all of them. The examination is presided over by the director of the school at which the examination is held. He is assisted by one professor from that school, who has been determined by lot. The other two come, one from each of the other schools, and have been selected in the same manner. All the questions to be asked have been chosen by the medical council in Paris, from the number sent from all the schools. These questions, in a sealed envelope, with each question also sealed, and those for the different grades separated, are sent to the board of examiners after they have met in session.

The candidate to be first examined is determined by lot, as well as the question to be first asked. All other candidates then withdraw, and are placed under guard in a distant room. As soon as the question is answered, the same question is put to each of the others, the order being determined by lot. Thus a separate question is drawn at each day's session. As a candidate answers, each professor places after the name his estimate of the value. When the answer is written, it is placed in a sealed envelope, and is read aloud next day by the candidate in public. After the last question has been answered, there is prepared, in secret session, a list of all the candidates, with the marks of each professor opposite his name. This list is sent to Paris, where a superior commission is appointed, to consider these marks and make the final classification. The minimum for each grade is 200, and 20 is the maximum for each question. No one can serve as a member of the examining board who is, in any degree, a relation or a connection of any student. An alternate, selected by lot, is available for any such emergency. This remarkable method demands no criticism here, but suggests many. At any rate, it precludes all prejudice, favoritism, and mercy.

Before leaving this subject, something must be said about the daily routine. The work begins at eight o'clock, before breakfast, and starts with an hour's clinic in the wards, followed by an hour's lecture. The lecture is generally from manuscript. Attendance is obligatory, and the subjects to be lectured upon, with the day for each, are posted on the bulletin board every week. After the lecture comes the hour for breakfast, followed by another lecture lasting an hour. After this, there are three hours passed in the dissecting-room or laboratory. This routine seems to demand a great deal from young men before breakfast, but is in accordance with the French method of living. There are generally over 100 students at each school, and of these, about 10 per cent come up to the requirements.

NAVAL HOSPITALS OF THE UNITED STATES.

The history of the navy of the United States begins as early as October 13th, 1775; but there was no attempt to establish naval hospitals until February 26th, 1811. However, much before that date, provision had been made for the treatment of the sick and disabled seamen of both the navy and merchant service.

When the partially erected palace of Charles II at Greenwich, England, was, in 1694, converted into a naval hospital, the tax for its maintenance was levied, not only at home, but also in the American Colonies, where each seafarer was required to pay a portion of his earnings to support an institution so far distant. The collectors were educating the American people then, and continued to educate them for many years, in a system which they themselves were to adopt after a century, with its many dark days, had been added to the past. 1776 came, and a new flag was unfurled, which was soon carried at mastheads rapidly increasing in number.

By July 16th, 1798, the number of American seamen had become so great, that Congress passed an act for the relief of the many sick and disabled. By this act, twenty cents per month were deducted from the wage of each seaman in a merchant vessel of the United States, and directors were appointed to control the expenditure of this hospital fund at the various ports. This was the beginning of the Marine Hospital Service, under which the sick of the sea could find refuge in various civil hospitals designated by the directors. On March 2d, 1799, the act of the previous year was extended so as to embrace the naval service ; the Secretary of the Navy being authorized to deduct twenty cents each month from the pay of every officer, seaman, and marine. The benefits and advantages were to be the same as those accorded to the crews of merchant vessels of the United States.

However, as might have been predicated, it was soon apparent that the navy could not, without many disadvantages, depend upon civil hospitals for the treatment of its sick. The men, passed from the control of their own officers, lingered in hospitals for considerable periods, and in many instances finally disappeared. It soon became the opinion that the good of the naval service demanded that it should have its own hospitals. Accordingly on February 26th, 1811, Congress passed a law establishing naval hospitals.

By this law, the Secretaries of Navy, Treasury, and War were appointed, for the time being, "Commissioners of Navy Hospitals," and to them the hospital tax accruing from the navy was to be paid, together with all fines imposed upon officers, seamen, and marines.

This fund was augmented by $50,000 appropriated out of the unexpended balance of the marine hospital fund ; this being considered the amount belonging to the navy from payments made prior to the passage of the act. These commissioners were authorized to procure sites for hospitals, and, where suitable buildings could not be purchased with the sites, to cause such to be erected. They were also required "to provide, at one of the establishments, a permanent asylum for disabled and decrepit navy officers, seamen, and marines."

The act goes on further to say, that when any officer, seaman, or marine shall be admitted into any hospital, that that institution shall be allowed one ration per day during his continuance therein, to be deducted from his account, and that when any one is admitted who was previously entitled to a pension, this, during his continuance therein, shall be paid to the commissioners, and deducted from the account of the pensioner.

Little, however, was done for ten years by these commissioners. The Secretary of the Navy, Mr. Hamilton, had hospital plans prepared by Mr. Latrobe, and was very anxious to execute, as soon as possible, the very desirable and very plain law. The other two commissioners were not in sympathy with the plans of the man knowing best the urgent needs of the service of which he was the head ; the opposition being based upon its permanency and stability. The importance of the subject increased by time; its advocates becoming more earnest each year. The good of the service demanded a better provision for the sick than was made by the inconsiderable establishments at some of the navy-yards. These were, in some cases, cast-off buildings and wretched hovels, destitute of every necessary comfort. The method of caring for the sick was constantly undermining the discipline of the service, and diminishing the spirit of cheerfulness and content.

It was more than ten years after the passage by Congress of the "act establishing navy hospitals," that the commissioners, changed by the various political currents, began to carry out the real intent of the law under which they were created. Then, land was purchased at Boston, New York, Philadelphia, and Norfolk, and appropriations were made for buildings. The difficulty with which the three commissioners worked together, led, shortly after this (10th July, 1832), to Congress investing the Secretary of the Navy with all their powers. After this the work progressed more rapidly, and the navy was soon provided with hospitals in keeping with its promising future. As the history and description of each hospital are found below, it is only necessary here to give some idea of their internal organization and government.

The book of " Instructions for Medical Officers of the United States Navy " gives most of the required information. The medical officer in charge of a naval hospital is responsible for the care and treatment of the sick, and for the discipline, cleanliness, and economy of the institution, which it is his duty to keep always in an efficient condition ; and to this end he shall exact from his subordinates, employés, and patients, a proper obedience to his orders and to the laws and regulations of the navy. Medical officers, and all persons employed in the hospital, shall perform such duties as may be assigned to them by the officer in charge.

No changes, except in cases of emergency, which shall be immediately reported to the bureau, shall be made in the hospital buildings, furniture and grounds—such as destroying or removing trees, or disturbing the soil around them ; and no bills for purchases or repairs shall be contracted without permission of the bureau.

The medical officer in charge shall inspect all medicines, provisions, supplies, etc., that may be received, or shall cause them to be inspected by a subordinate medical officer, who shall report to him their condition, etc. A record of the inspection shall be entered on the daily journal. He shall direct the medical officers in charge of the wards to present their case-papers to him once a week for examination, and will assure himself that they are accurately and carefully kept.

The officer in charge of the hospital shall detail a medical officer who, in addition to such professional duties as may be assigned him, shall perform the duty of "officer of the day" for twenty-four hours, commencing at 10 A. M. The officer of the day shall make a tour of inspection through the wards, kitchens, mess and other rooms occupied by patients and employés, upon going on duty at 10 A. M., and during the afternoon at a different hour daily, and finally at night after the patients are in bed. A list of patients and employés who have received passes shall be furnished him, as early as practicable every morning, and all patients and others will be required to report their return to him.

A journal shall be kept by him, which he shall sign at the end of his term of duty, at 10 A. M. ; in which he shall make a brief record of the following points, which are to be noted at the time of occurrence : the condition of the wards, kitchens, mess, smoking and other rooms, at each inspection ; the condition of the meals served, as to quality and quantity ; the names and diseases of the patients admitted, and the places from which they are received ; the names, number of days subsisted, and disposition of patients discharged, and whether the necessary papers in each case are correct and complete; the names and conditions of patients and employés who have returned, or who have overstayed their leaves; the confinement and discharge of offenders; the reporting and detachment of officers, or their going upon and returning from leave; the record of inspection of all articles received; the object and finding of all boards of survey; and finally such other matters occurring during his term of duty as it may be desirable to record.

Medical officers in charge of wards shall be held responsible for their order and neatness, and for the good condition of all within them. They shall exercise a personal supervision over the comfort and welfare of the sick, visiting them at least twice daily, and oftener in severe cases; and they shall assure themselves that their directions as to medicines, dressings, regimen, etc., are accurately and promptly carried out. They will, personally, take the temperature of patients, and will never allow this duty to be performed by the nurses.

Patients should be accompanied, upon admission, with hospital tickets, but in cases of emergency they may be admitted without this paper, when the medical officer shall report the fact to the commandant of the station, with a statement of the emergency, and cause the necessary hospital ticket to be supplied.

Convalescents may be detailed for light service, but shall not be retained in the hospital for that purpose after they are fit for duty.

No patient in hospital shall be entitled to any service except that of the regular hospital attendants, nor shall any one except medical officers on duty, patients and employés of the hospital, be subsisted or lodged, without permission of the bureau.

In hospitals the following diet table will be followed for patients when practicable, but the allowances to attendants' messes may be varied at the discretion of the medical officer in charge, provided the value of the ration be not exceeded:

BREAKFAST.		DINNER.		SUPPER.	
Sunday.					
Coffee (oz. 1),	pt. 1.	Roast beef,	oz. 12.	Tea (oz. ½),	pt. 1.
Bread,	oz. 6.	Bread,	oz. 4.	Bread,	oz. 6.
Butter,	oz. 1.	Potatoes,	oz. 10.	Butter,	oz. 1.
Stewed mutton,	oz. 4.	Other veg's,	oz. 4.	Sugar,	oz. 1.
Sugar,	oz. 1.	Pickles,	oz. 1.	Milk,	oz. 2.
Milk,	oz. 2.				

Monday.

Coffee (oz. 1),	pt. 1.	Mutton,	oz. 12.	Tea (oz. ¼),	pt. 1.
Bread,	oz. 6.	Bread,	oz. 4.	Bread,	oz. 6.
Butter,	oz. 1.	Potatoes,	oz. 10.	Butter,	oz. 1.
Beef hash,	oz. 4.	Other veg's,	oz. 4.	Sugar,	oz. 1.
Sugar,	oz. 1.	Pickles,	oz. 1.	Milk,	oz. 2.
Milk,	oz. 2.				

Tuesday.

Coffee (oz. 1),	pt. 1.	Boiled beef,	oz. 12.	Tea (oz. ¼),	pt. 1.
Bread,	oz. 6.	Bread,	oz. 4.	Bread,	oz. 6.
Butter,	oz. 1.	Potatoes,	oz. 10.	Butter,	oz. 1.
Mutton hash,	oz. 4.	Other veg's,	oz. 4.	Sugar,	oz. 1.
Sugar,	oz. 1.	Pickles,	oz. 1.	Milk,	oz. 2.
Milk,	oz. 2.				

Wednesday.

Coffee (oz. 1),	pt. 1.	Beef soup,	pt. 1.	Tea (oz. ¼),	pt. 1.
Bread,	oz. 6.	Pork,	oz. 12.	Bread,	oz. 6.
Butter,	oz. 1.	Beans,	oz. 4.	Butter,	oz. 1.
Beef hash,	oz. 4.	Bread,	oz. 4.	Sugar,	oz. 1.
Sugar,	oz. 1.	Potatoes,	oz. 10.	Milk,	oz. 2.
Milk,	oz. 2.	Pickles,	oz. 1.		

Thursday.

Coffee (oz. 1),	pt. 1.	Roast beef,	oz. 12.	Tea (oz. ¼),	pt. 1.
Bread,	oz. 6.	Bread,	oz. 4.	Bread,	oz. 6.
Butter,	oz. 1.	Potatoes,	oz. 10.	Butter,	oz. 1.
Pork and beans		Other veg's,	oz. 4.	Sugar,	oz. 1.
(warmed),	oz. 6.	Pickles,	oz. 1.	Milk,	oz. 2.
Sugar,	oz. 1.				
Milk,	oz. 2.				

Friday.

Coffee (oz. 1),	pt. 1.	Fish,	oz. 12.	Tea (oz. ¼),	pt. 1.
Bread,	oz. 6.	Bread,	oz. 4.	Bread,	oz. 6.
Butter,	oz. 1.	Potatoes,	oz. 10.	Butter,	oz. 1.
Fish chowder,	oz. 4.	Other veg's,	oz. 4.	Sugar,	oz. 1.
Sugar,	oz. 1.	Pickles,	oz. 1.	Milk,	oz. 2.
Milk,	oz. 2.				

Saturday.

Coffee (oz. 1),	pt. 1.	Bean soup,	pt. 1.	Tea (oz. ½),	pt. 1.
Bread,	oz. 6.	Stewed mut'n,	oz. 12.	Bread,	oz. 6.
Butter,	oz. 1.	Bread,	oz. 4.	Butter,	oz. 1.
Beef hash,	oz. 4.	Potatoes,	oz. 10.	Sugar,	oz. 1.
Sugar,	oz. 1.	Other veg's,	oz. 4.	Milk,	oz. 2.
Milk,	oz. 2.	Pickles,	oz. 1.		

A special diet list shall be kept for each ward, which shall be revised and corrected every morning by the medical officer in charge of the ward.

Admission of Patients.

The following forms are to be observed:

(*a*) When the hospital ticket is found correct, endorse and file it, with accompanying papers relating to the case; if defective, return to the medical officer signing, when he is at hand; or otherwise, through the bureau.

(*b*) Enter name, etc., as follows: (1) In the general alphabetical register of patients, which is the permanent hospital record, for future reference. (2) In the abstract of patients.

(*c*) Open case-paper.

(*d*) If seaman from the receiving ship or other vessel, send ration notice to commandant of receiving ship as paymaster's notification; if a marine from the neighboring barracks, send the ration notice to the commanding marine officer through commandant.

Discharge of Patients.

No person shall be discharged from the service for physical disability, without having been previously surveyed by a board of medical officers. A copy of the report of survey and of any other paper relating to the patient, shall be appended to the case-paper, which shall be signed at its conclusion, or on detachment of the officer, by the medical officer in charge of the patient's ward. Case-papers will be verified by the signature of the medical officer in charge of the hospital. When a patient is discharged from hospital, the fact shall be entered upon the register of patients, and also upon the case-paper, which is then to be filed with the hospital ticket attached. The ration notice shall be forwarded through the commandant of the station. On every Monday, a report of the sick for the preceding week shall be made in triplicate, one copy of which shall be sent to the commandant of the station, one to the bureau, and the other retained for the files of the hospital, as a basis for the report of the following week.

Medical Department, United States Navy.

By an act of Congress, 31st August, 1842, reorganizing the Navy Department, the various bureaus were created, and the management of the medical department was vested in a single head, denominated Chief of Bureau of Medicine and Surgery. It was required that this officer should be chosen from the surgeons of the navy. On September 1st, 1842, William P. C. Barton, M. D., was appointed the first chief of that bureau. On March 3d, 1871, the title of Surgeon-General of the Navy was conferred, and with it the relative rank of Commodore.

At the same time the relative ranks of the officers of the medical corps were designated as follows: Medical Directors, with relative rank of Captain; Medical Inspectors, with relative rank of Commander; Surgeons, with relative ranks of Lieutenant-Commander and Lieutenant; Passed-Assistant Surgeons, with the relative ranks of Lieutenant and Lieutenant (Junior Grade); and Assistant Surgeons, with the relative rank of Ensign. With the exception of the Medical Directors, these officers serve both afloat and ashore.

Candidates for admission to the medical corps are examined at the Naval Hospital, Brooklyn, New York, by a specially selected board. Permission to appear before this board is obtained from the Secretary of the Navy.

Attendants on the sick at the various hospitals are male nurses, selected from civil life by the medical officer in charge of the institution. They are paid from $15 to $25 per month, and are subject to instant dismissal for incompetency or misbehavior. The number employed is about one to every eight patients.

The naval hospitals of the United States are situated at Widow's Island, Maine; Portsmouth, New Hampshire; Boston, Massachusetts; Brooklyn, New York; Philadelphia, Pennsylvania; Washington, District of Columbia; Annapolis, Maryland; Norfolk, Virginia; Pensacola, Florida; Mare Island, California, and Yokohama, Japan. The total capacity of these is 823 beds, and the daily average number of patients is about 225. In the navy are 10,500 officers and enlisted men.

Naval Hospital on Widow's Island, Maine.

On Widow's Island, Penobscot Bay, Maine, is a naval hospital, specially constructed for the quarantine and treatment of the sick with yellow fever. It is a novel hospital, in that the permanent building is chiefly for administration, while the wards are portable Ducker hospitals, packed away until necessity shall require their use.

The history of this institution is rather peculiar. In 1885, the Isthmus of Panama was the scene of considerable naval activity, as the United States was under the necessity of having a force on shore and a squadron in that locality. The presence of so many ships in a part of the world so often the home of yellow fever, induced the idea that it would be wise to provide a suitable refuge for infected vessels. This situation was the exciting cause of the construction on Widow's Island, but a strong predisposing cause is found in the proximity of the old quarantine station near Portsmouth, New Hampshire, to sections frequented by summer visitors.

The island had been purchased by the government for lighthouse purposes, but, as it was not required for that use, it was offered to the Navy Department to meet the supposed necessities of the time. It contains 15 acres, has a height of 100 feet above sea-level, is bounded by East Rockland Bay and Fox's Island Thoroughfare, and is 12 miles from Rockland and 2 miles from North Haven. The place could scarcely be more segregated, but, in time of need, special transportation of supplies from Rockland could be easily provided for.

At the time of its selection it was almost barren, being destitute of trees and shrubs, and even water. However, the deep water near at hand, where the largest ships could swing at anchor, and the situation so far north in a summer climate opposed to the spread of the yellow scourge, made it a desirable place for the purpose. A well, furnishing potable water, was soon made by boring, and a temporary wooden building was constructed in 1885, under the design and direct guidance of Surgeon A. C. Heffenger of the navy. There was fortunately no occasion for its use, but as the idea still prevailed that some future time might develop a pressing need for such an establishment, Congress appropriated $50,000 for a permanent structure.

This was begun June 4th, 1887, and completed, together with the pump-house and mortuary, on the following February. A wharf was also constructed on the southwest side of the island, where the land slopes gently to the water. All the rest of the coast is precipitous. By the approval of the Surgeon-General, Surgeon Heffenger furnished the design, and the work was also carried on under his supervision.

The following description was written by him in 1888:

" The plan of the present hospital embraces a finished basement of eight feet, and two stories of twelve feet each. Its dimensions are ninety-six by fifty feet. The basement is built of granite, with granite water-table; and the walls are built of brick, with a thickness of sixteen inches. It is placed on the highest point of the island, founded upon solid ledges, and facing the southeast. A wide verandah extends across the entire front and for some distance on either side of the hospital. The roof is of slate, and is surmounted by a cupola and flagstaff.

In the basement are the laundry, ironing room, drying room, disinfecting room, and numerous storerooms. On the first floor are the dispensary, reception-room, officers' dining-room, patients' dining-room, attendants' dining-room, kitchen and pantry. On the second floor are three officers' wards, three wards for men, a linen room and two attendants' rooms. A dumb-waiter extends from the basement to the second floor. In the north corner in the basement, and upon both floors, is a room fitted with lavatory, water-closets and bath-tub; thus there is but one soil-pipe in the building, and that runs direct from the basement through the roof, where it is properly covered with a ventilating cowl. All the plumbing and plumbing fixtures are exposed, and have been thoroughly tested.

Two water-tanks, with combined capacity of three thousand gallons, are placed in the attic, and water is pumped into them from the artesian well by a Rider caloric engine of six-inch cylinder, and deep well pump. To ensure a sufficient volume of water for using this pump, a reservoir six feet in diameter and twenty feet deep was blasted from the upper end of the well tube, the capacity of which more than equals that of the combined tanks. A two-inch distributing pipe runs from the tanks down to the basement, and a fire-plug with hose attachment is provided on each floor and in the basement. The tell-tale and overflow lead into the laundry tubs.

The drainage is excellent; the main sewer pipe running down the southwest slope from the rear of the hospital into Fox Island Thoroughfare, where it terminates below the level of ebb-tide. A manhole and trap are provided just outside the building, and again immediately above high-water mark."

"The barren and altogether unprepossessing aspect of the island rendered it advisable to make such improvements upon the grounds as the limited amount of the appropriation would permit. A number of walks were laid out and graveled. About two hundred and fifty spruce, fir, and hardwood trees were planted on the borders of these walks, and upon other parts of the island, and a lot for a cemetery was ploughed up, leveled and planted in grass seed. The ground immediately around the hospital was graded, terraced, covered with sea gravel for some distance, and sown in grass seed outside the margin of gravel.

The hospital furniture was received and put in place during June, 1888. It is plain in design, of excellent quality, and ample for the probable requirements of the station. The iron bedsteads with woven wire mattresses manufactured in Hartford, Conn., merit special notice. The pneumatic tubes and bells which connect all parts of the hospital are also worthy of special mention.

The provision of Ducker Portable Field Hospitals is of great value to this station, as it makes it possible, under any ordinary demands, to treat all contagious cases outside of the main hospital, which can thus be reserved for treatment of non-contagious cases, and administrative purposes.

A small dead-house, with a cast-iron revolving autopsy table and concrete floor, is placed some distance from the other buildings, and affords excellent facilities for post-mortem examinations.

The station as now equipped, including main hospital building and Ducker pavilions, accommodates fifty patients, and this number could be doubled or quadrupled by simply adding more Ducker pavilions."

U. S. Naval Hospital at Portsmouth, New Hampshire.

There are two islands close to the Maine coast-line and the city of Portsmouth, New Hampshire, that are used by the United States for naval purposes. They are called the Puddington Islands, and are connected by bridges with each other and the Maine mainland, to which State they once belonged. They were a part of the discovery of Martin Pring in 1603, charted by John Smith in 1614, and included in the grant to Sir Fernando Gorges in 1639.

In 1800 the government purchased from William Dennett the one nearer the mainland, for $5500. The other to the south, known as Seavey's Island, did not become the property of the government until 1866, when the 26 owners parted with it for $105,000.

The navy-yard was established on the one first bought, soon after the purchase. There was, however, no local provision for the care of the sick until 1834, when a small vacant frame building, constructed in 1802, was repaired and furnished for that purpose. It could accommodate but ten patients with any comfort, though occasionally 15 were treated there at one time. In 1865, certain alterations were made, increasing its capacity to 25. It was then, however, more than 60 years old, and soon the necessity for a new building became apparent. This subject was agitated from year to year, until in 1888, the Surgeon-General reported the old hospital beyond repair, and in every respect unfitted for the treatment of the sick.

Congress, on March 2, 1889, and on June 30 of the next year, appropriated $43,000 for the construction and furnishing of a new building. Work was commenced in September, 1890, and the building, with its various outhouses, was finished in a year, and commissioned on December 21, 1891, when the old hospital was abandoned. The old frame structure still stands in its dilapidated condition—one of the few wooden relics of the early days on the island.

The new site is on the west shore of Seavey's Island. This island was selected because it was important to have the hospital outside of the yard, and yet easily accessible. Next the Piscataqua river, and between it and the road connecting the bridges in the north with Fort Sullivan in the south, 3½ acres were set apart for hospital purposes.

The building, which is about 83 feet long and 54 wide, is constructed of brick, and fronts the south, with its length north and south. It consists of a cellar, 3 stories and an attic, under a pyramidal roof, surmounted by a ventilating cupola. The front projects for two stories, forming a small tower, on each side of which are short enclosed piazzas.

The hospital, though new, is built on the corridor plan, there being a single central hall 10 feet wide on each floor, connecting the back and front. On each side of this are placed the wards and rooms. Little more need be said about the arrangement, as a reference to the plan submitted will be sufficient. The three wards are on the second floor. Sick officers and the resident medical officer have quarters on the third floor. The first floor is given up to administration, the dining-room and kitchen. (Plate IX.)

The pitch of the first floor is 10 feet ; of the second, 12 feet 3 inches, and of the third, 11 feet. There are beds for 26 patients, with 1060 cubic feet of air space to each. In the officers' wards the air space is 2970 cubic feet for each.

The floors of all the wards are of Georgia pine, on an under-flooring. The windows have double sashes, this being necessitated by the severe winters. They are provided with hinged lights. There are also 3 brick air-shafts extending the whole height of the building and connecting with the ventilating stack, while registers are near ceilings and floors, and cold air ducts from the exterior lead to the bases of the radiators. The radiators, which are placed at convenient points throughout the building, are supplied with steam from the boiler-house in the rear. Gas for lighting purposes is made on the premises.

The water-closets are at the back of the building, as well separated from the wards as the ground plan permits. They are supplied with overhead tanks and all modern improvements. The bath-rooms near by are well furnished. The traps to all fixtures have ventilating ducts, which finally discharge above the roof. The sewer system is an independent one, and empties into the adjacent waters.

The source of the water supply is the ponds formed by damming the overflow from the springs near the center of the island. The boiler and laundry house is about 30 feet in the rear. The laundry has a concrete floor and wood ceilings, and is supplied with the modern machinery of the Troy Laundry Company. The dead-house is at the northwest boundary of the grounds, near the water.

The staff consists of a surgeon and a passed-assistant surgeon. The former is also the surgeon of the navy-yard, where he is provided with a residence. The total number of patients treated last year was 86.

Seavey's Island contains 105 acres of uneven and hilly ground, well suited for farming purposes. The surface soil is, however, generally shallow and covers granite. The views from the island are extensive and attractive. The winters are long and severe, while the summers are short and mild. Storms are not uncommon, and fogs are not rare in summer. July and August are the warmest months, the thermometer perhaps reaching 85° F. February is the coldest month, as then the mercury may be 10° or 15° below zero F. The mean annual temperature is 44° F. The location is free from malarial influences, but rheumatism, neuralgia and bronchial disorders are common. However, the climate seems conducive to a long life, though typhoid fever is not uncommon in the city, and cases of phthisis last, as a rule, but a short time.

Naval Hospital at Chelsea, Massachusetts.

As the policy of the government during recent years has been toward the concentration of the work of construction and repair of ships at two yards only, the navy-yard at Boston has, for the time being, diminished somewhat in importance, and, with it, the naval hospital, where the average daily number under treatment last year was only 17.

This hospital is beautifully situated at Chelsea, a suburb northeast of the city of Boston, and separated from it by the Mystic river, spanned at this point by a substantial bridge, across which street cars closely connect the thickly populated suburb with the city proper. It is near the Boston end of this bridge that the navy-yard lies, less than a mile from the hospital. The hospital grounds are on the left bank, and occupy the angle formed just above the bridge by the Mystic and Mill rivers.

On September 22, 1823, this tract, consisting then of 115 acres, was purchased for $18,000 from Dr. Aaron Dexter, of Boston, by the Secretary of the Navy, Secretary of the Treasury and Secretary of War, representing the government as " Commissioners of Navy Hospitals." This tract has been reduced to nearly 75 acres by several encroachments, but this has been since the hospital was commissioned on January 7, 1836.

The hospital then was much smaller than it is now, as on July 14, 1862, $71,500 were appropriated by Congress for its extension and repair. Adams and Jenkins were the contractors, who, completing the new portion by March 2, 1864, and thus furnishing room for the sick, were able to remodel and repair the old portion by June 1, 1865. While this work was going on, Morris Tasker & Co., of Philadelphia, completed for $18,000 the arrangement for heating the new portion, and for the laundry and culinary work, placing the boiler and laundry in a detached building in the rear.

Considerably prior to these changes, the surgeon's house was built. This is a large residence, 250 feet south of the hospital. It was erected at a cost of $11,500, this amount appearing in the appropriation bill for the year ending 1857.

The hospital is a large granite house, devoid of any special hospital plan, 148 feet long and 70 wide, with pyramidal roof, attic, three stories and cellar. It is on a slight elevation, and faces the river to the southwest, from which it is distant about 100 feet. The first floor is only slightly above the ground level, so that there are only one or two short steps at the main entrance under the projecting portico. The portico is 27 feet long and 13 wide, extends to the level of the second floor, and has four columns of the Doric order placed in front. The first story is divided by a central hall, 23½ feet wide, connecting the front and rear entrances. On the north side of this hall are the dining-room (21½ by 66 feet), well lighted by seven large windows, the dispensary, the kitchen, and two storerooms. On the south side are dining-room for the junior medical officers on duty, the administration office, reception room, storeroom, and linen closet.

From the rear of the main hall a stairway ascends to the second story. The pitch of all the stories is 14 feet, and the arrangement of the 2d and 3d stories is the same. There is a hall ward, 23½ by 26½ feet, supplied with one window and containing eight beds, all against dead walls. To the north are two wards of nearly the same size and arrangement as the preceding one, and a large ward running crosswise and corresponding with the dining-room below. This ward, 21½ by 66 feet, with a window at each end and five on one side, contains 20 beds—ten against the dead wall and ten between the windows opposite.

The nurse rooms, bath-rooms, and water-closets are between the long and smaller wards. The bowls in the water-closets are porcelain, and well flushed from overhead tanks. The closets containing no windows are lighted by gas, and ventilated by an air-duct leading to the roof. Their very objectionable situation is inseparable perhaps from the general plan.

To the south of the main hall, on the two upper floors, are large well furnished rooms for sick officers and resident medical officers. The bath-room and water-closets are between the end rooms. Of course, all these various rooms and wards are arranged along intersecting halls or corridors. The accompanying plate (No. X) shows the arrangement on the second floor, and more than suggests the obstruction to the free circulation of air throughout the building.

It is useless to make any comment on the many beds against dead walls, and the many intersecting corridors. Every hospital should, of course, be considered with all the beds full, as this is the situation which best tests its plan. Here there are 100 beds with from 985 to 1090 cubic feet air space and from 71 to 78 feet floor space to each ; but, as the number under treatment at one time rarely exceeds 30, these figures mean ordinarily but little. The beds in the wards are iron, and supplied with a hair and a wire woven mattress.

The floors are painted soft pine, and the walls are calcimined. However, in the third story hard pine floors have been laid, and the walls are painted plaster.

In addition to the windows and doors, ventilation in some of the rooms and wards is assisted by shafts leading to the roof. There is, however, no complete system of ventilation.

Electric call-bells are placed throughout the building, and electric lights are now being introduced—the work to be completed by July 1st, 1893. Gas is supplied by the city, as is the case with water, which comes from the reservoir of the Mystic Water Company. The water is abundant and of excellent quality. The sewer system is complete and independent; it discharges into the adjacent waters.

The Walworth system is used in heating the hospital, the surgeon's house, and certain other rooms, such as the smoking-room in the wooden annex. The steam heat is, however, difficult to control, and this in the variable climate leads to too great variations in temperature.

The naval hospital grounds surround those of the marine hospital, which are off to the east and comprise ten acres. These ten acres were inadvertently given by Congress to that service. When it was discovered that they, a part of the original purchase of 115 acres, had been paid for by money held in trust, $50,000 were added to the hospital fund in lieu of them.

The original purchase was further reduced by several acres taken at the beginning of the Civil War for ordnance purposes. It is not clear how the Bureau of Ordnance acquired this ground, nor how many acres are claimed.

The acreage left to the hospital is, however, most ample; it, indeed, represents quite a farm. Much of it contains many fruit trees, while about the building and in other sections are ornamental trees, shrubbery and flowers.

Off to the west, a quarter of a mile from the hospital, and in the low and moist ground near the point where the two rivers join, is the smallpox hospital, completed on 25th April, 1869, by Geo. W. Clark, of Chelsea, at a cost of $8000. To the north, and at the same distance, is the cemetery. This is separated from the hospital by a line of hills 100 feet high. These hills, on whose slope the hospital is really built, shelter the building from the strong northeast winds which often prevail.

Nearer the hospital, about 40 feet from the north end, is the brick mortuary completed in 1865. There are also near-by many coal sheds, a new barn, stable, carpenter shop, conservatory, hotbeds, paint-shops, and other outbuildings. The grounds are enclosed by water and by brick walls.

The staff consists of a medical inspector and two assistants. During the last twenty years the total number of patients treated has been nearly 3000.

Until recently this was the only naval hospital on the Atlantic coast of the United States entirely free from malarial influences. This renders it a desirable place for the treatment of the many malarial troubles originating during the southern cruise of the home squadron.

U. S. Naval Hospital, Brooklyn, New York.

This establishment increases daily in importance as the navy gathers strength, and the navy-yard near-by becomes more and more the center of great activity in construction and repair. It is situated in the city of Brooklyn, in the State of New York, and, facing the west, overlooks the navy-yard, half a mile distant, and separated from it by a narrow intervening strip of the city. The grounds, now enclosed by high brick walls, comprised, originally, 33 acres, but, on July 2, 1890, the United States Government sold to the city a little more than two acres.

These 33 acres were the hill portion of the Schenck farm, purchased on May 1, 1824, together with the mansion and farm buildings, for $7650. In this purchase the government was, of course, represented by the " Commissioners of Navy Hospitals," while the parties of the first part were Sarah and Jane Schenck, widows, and Jacob and Ida Harris and Isaac and Mary Ann Harris. On April 19, 1833, the State of New York ceded to the United States its jurisdiction over this property. However, at the time of the purchase, the mansion and farm buildings were made ready for the reception of the sick of the navy, then treated in a house rented by the government, and were so employed until 1838, when the front or main portion of the present hospital was first commissioned. In 1840 the wings were added and the original plan completed. At the same time was constructed the building to the east of the north wing, which is now designated as the laboratory, but was originally used as a pest-house.

The hospital is on an elevation 56 feet above high water, and the wall in front, separating the grounds from the city, is distant 200 feet, while that to the south, where the main gate is, is 360 feet away. The building, fronting 197 feet, and consisting of full basement, two stories and attic, is constructed of marble from the Sing Sing quarries, originally white, but now a decided gray. The ground plan is like a modified H, the wings perpendicular to the front, and 49 feet wide, extending *back* 73 feet, but to the *front* only 11 feet. These forward extensions are really a part of the front or main building, the intervening space being occupied by an imposing portico 11 feet wide and 100 feet long, which, with its 8 square columns, supports a frieze and cornice suggesting remotely the Doric order.

Though the columns extend from the ground, the floor of the portico is on a level with the first floor. As the ground immediately in front of the building is higher than that in the rear, the basement is partly covered in front; and the broad stone steps leading up to the portico spring from a terrace. This terrace is paved with stone flagging, and extends along the whole front, and for more than thirty feet on each side, where from each end steps ascend to a side entrance on the first floor.

The paved court, which is open to the east, is 100 feet from wing to wing, and 60 feet deep; this being also the depth of the main building, which has, at the back and thus toward the court, 8 square columns similar to those in front, but supporting piazzas 100 feet long and 10 wide for each floor. As the court is on a level with the ground floor, it is in the rear that the hospital presents its full height.

A corridor nearly 10 feet wide extends the whole length of the mid-line of the front on every floor, and is joined by similar ones from the wings. On each side of these are the rooms and wards. Thus it is seen that this is a corridor hospital on the block plan. The different stories are reached by very broad staircases within the front where each wing joins. The staircase wells allow with the corridors a free communication of air throughout the building.

All the sick, except commissioned officers, are on the second floor. Here are found 15 wards of varying sizes for the treatment of enlisted men, and rooms for laboratory employés and sick warrant-officers. The wards, which are divided into many classes in accordance with the character of the cases, are in the south wing and the front. The rooms are in the north wing, though there are rooms for nurses in both wings, and there is an operating room in the south wing. This latter is on the south side of the corridor. Its floor, 15×11 feet, is of hard pine shellaced, and its height is 17 feet, this being the pitch of both stories. It contains one large window, and is bountifully supplied with instruments and all things necessary for successful work ; but, opening upon the corridor, its atmosphere is that common to the whole hospital (Plate XI).

The largest wards are, of course, the four in the front extensions. These are 27 × 21 feet, and two are supplied with four windows each, and the inner two with three each. These windows are necessarily on adjacent sides ; thus, as is the case throughout the building, leaving dead walls ; and like all the windows, though large, not extending nearer the ceiling than 3 feet. All the other wards are about 15 × 21 or 22 feet, and have two windows in each on the same side. The floors are, for the most part, painted soft pine, but recently a few hard pine floors have been put in. The walls are painted plaster.

The beds are iron, and supplied with a hair and also a wire-woven mattress. Near each bed is a locker, a chair, and a small carpet-rug. The number of beds in a ward varies with the size of the ward, but as a rule, the allowance of floor space per bed is 65 feet, and the cubic space 1100 feet. As this hospital, with accommodations for 125 patients, has most of the time less than 50, the floor space and air space given each patient are ordinarily most ample. However, occasionally the number of patients reaches 100, and probably hereafter this will occur more frequently. The rooms on the second floor of the north wing are chiefly for sick warrant-officers. These are fairly well furnished, and have associated with them a dining-room and reception-room.

On the first floor there are in the south wing, quarters for the three junior medical officers on duty ; in the north wing, a counting-room, quarters for the apothecary, and 5 rooms for sick commissioned officers, with reception and dining-room attached ; in the front are administration offices, board rooms, a mess-room for resident medical officers, 3 rooms for sick commissioned officers, a chapel and library, and a dispensary. The rooms for sick officers are well furnished, and have a homelike appearance.

In the basement, which has a height of about 10 feet, and where the corridors are paved with stone flagging, are smoking and mess rooms for the men, kitchens, carpenter shop, storerooms, and quarters for laborers. The mess-rooms are two, one being for those on full diet.

There are water-closets and bath-rooms on each floor, off the corridors at the ends of the wings ; those on different floors being imme-

diately above one another. The bath-rooms are 8 × 16 feet, while
the rooms for water-closets are about half the size. Some of the bath
tubs are porcelain and others are copper. There are also appliances
for various special and medicated baths. The water-closets are supplied with seats, porcelain bowls, flushed from overhead tanks, and
urinals. The floors are concrete, and there is a large window in
each room. The doors of these rooms open directly on the corridors, but the water supply for flushing is unlimited, and the sewer
connections are well guarded by traps.

There are in the building a dark room, and electrical appliances
for surgical and medical treatment. Fireplaces are in almost all the
wards and rooms, but the hospital is heated by steam and hot air
supplied from the engine and boiler house in the rear. The same
machinery that drives heated air into the building in winter, supplies
cool air in summer. The means of ventilation are, besides doors,
windows, and chimneys, air shafts in the walls, and roof ventilators
over the staircase wells.

The system of sewers is extensive and complete, not only for this
building but for all others in the grounds. The manholes and vents
are open, and the highest point of the system is connected by a ventilating duct with the chimney of the steam building. The pipes
connect finally with the sewers of the city.

The water supply is the same as that of the city, connection being
made with the city mains. This allows many fire-plugs about the
grounds. From the city is also obtained the gas which lights the
whole building. However, the work of introducing electric lights
has been begun and will soon be completed.

Walking about the grounds, one notices the laundry close against
the engine and boiler house, 50 feet in the rear of the hospital. This
laundry is relatively new and is supplied with every necessary apparatus. There is also the long stone building like the wings, and
built on the same line as the north wing, though 60 feet in the rear.
It is 100 feet long and 50 wide, was constructed in 1840 at the same
time the wings were built, and was known then as the pest-house.
It is now called the Naval Laboratory, though it is simply a large
reception and storehouse, with basement and two stories, from which
medical supplies are distributed to the various ships and stations. It
is in charge of a medical director, who has a commodious house in
the north division of the grounds. This division is made by a high
brick wall, extending approximately east and west, about 80 yards

north of the hospital. Between the wall and the hospital are the mortuary, chapel, and a two-story building for contagious diseases. This latter building, called the smallpox hospital, is 200 feet from the main building to the northeast. Near it is a disinfecting chamber.

The medical director in charge has a large residence in front of the north end of the main building. It faces the south, is forty-five feet square, with a large back building and has two stories.

120 yards in rear of the hospital is the cemetery, whose register now numbers over 1250.

The staff of the hospital consists of a medical director, a surgeon and two assistant-surgeons. The number of patients is, of course, liable to great variations. The mortality ratio has also been very variable, at times comparatively small, and at others relatively large.

U. S. Naval Hospital at Philadelphia, Pennsylvania, and Naval Home of the United States.

Immediately after the passage of the law of 1811, entitled "An Act establishing Navy Hospitals," it became necessary for the navy to take charge of its sick on shore. It was, however, very poorly equipped for such work, as there was not under its control a suitable building anywhere for such an undertaking. Necessity demanded something in the way of sick quarters at all the navy-yards. At the old navy-yard on the Delaware, in the city of Philadelphia, a very small building was appropriated to this use. It was represented in 1813 as a wretched hovel, destitute of every necessary comfort for sick persons, and calculated to hold eight patients. At that time it was holding twenty-four, and the thought of each was simply to gather strength enough to desert. This state of affairs demanded immediate correction, and a frame building was accordingly erected by order of the department issued the same year. This was regarded at the time as only a temporary structure, but it was not until the 26th of May, 1826, that the commissioners created by the act of 1811 made a move to carry out in this locality the real intent of that law. Then the purchase was made of the "Abbot lot," the site of both the Naval Hospital and the Naval Home of to-day.

This lot of 23 acres is situated on the left bank of the Schuylkill river, in the western section of the city of Philadelphia. It cost the government $17,000, and, as a part of the Pemberton estate of 150 acres, has a long and interesting history. It is sufficient here to state that the Pembertons bought their "plantation" from the Penns in 1735, built a large square brick house and several brick outhouses on it, beautified it, and lived outside the city in good old colonial style. The British officers, attracted by the beauty of the place and its natural advantages, occupied it frequently during the war of the Revolution. Surgeon Thomas Harris, of the United States Navy, many years afterwards, influenced by the same qualities, impressed upon the "Commissioners of Navy Hospitals" the desirability of acquiring possession of the lot of 23 acres, then the property of the Abbot family and containing the buildings.

By the act of 1811 the commissioners were required to provide at one of the hospitals a permanent asylum for disabled and decrepit navy officers, seamen and marines. It was decided to carry out here in Philadelphia this provision of the act. Accordingly, immediately after the purchase in 1826, the buildings were made ready to receive the sick and also a few beneficiaries, and the hospital at the navy-yard was abandoned. Then, under Mr. Strickland as architect, and Surgeon Harris as superintendent, the work of constructing the asylum was begun. It was called "Asylum," as it had been so designated in the act establishing it, but soon there were many who regarded the selection of that term as unfortunate. The difficulty of making asylum and home synonymous was insuperable, but it was not until July 1, 1889, that the official designation became "Naval Home."

In 1832 the building was under roof, but the Hospital Fund was so nearly exhausted that Congress, in July of that year, had to come to its relief by appropriating $33,900. So the work progressed, and toward the close of 1833 certain parts of the building were occupied. The old buildings were then deserted and the sick and the beneficiaries were transferred to the new home. A short time after this the other buildings were demolished and the bricks utilized to improve the walks. Work continued on the asylum, and it may be said that the building was not really finished until 1848. Over $195,000 were expended in construction, and Congress appropriated $93,000 of this sum, the remainder having been supplied out of the Hospital Fund. It remains now to give a short description of the building and grounds before passing on to the Naval Hospital, which is of much more recent construction.

The grounds, in a great part surrounded by high brick walls, approximate the trapezoidal shape. The longer (1226 feet) of the nearly parallel sides is formed by the Gray's Ferry road, and the shorter (583 feet), to the west and near the river, by Southerland avenue. The side (947 feet) nearly perpendicular to these is at the south, and the long (1364 feet) side at the north. The home fronts the southeast and the long parallel, from which it is 223 feet distant. It is a building 380 feet long, composed of a central structure, with a pavilion on each side, entering into the formation of the front and ending in a transverse building. A basement, two stories and an attic, broad verandas on the two floors of the wings, broad stone steps with a marble colonnade for the central structure, fine marble stairways in the interior, and vaulted masonry ceilings, and a domed chapel, give a general idea of the building.

The beneficiaries number over 100, and each has a small room, three good meals a day, and a pound and a half of tobacco and a dollar each month. All the laundry work is done without any expense to him, and every reasonable convenience is supplied. Twenty years service, or serious disability in the line of duty, allows admission. On entering, all pensions must be allotted to the hospital fund. Before the building of the present hospital, the home was, of course, as much a hospital as an asylum. For hospital purposes the second floor of the south pavilion, the rooms in the transverse building and the attic were employed.

It was in this Home that the germ of the Naval Academy originated, as it was under its first "Governor," Commodore Biddle, that a class of midshipmen was formed, and professors were employed to teach them. The students were those preparing for examination, and the class was renewed year after year, until the founding of the Naval Academy in 1845.

The Naval Hospital is in the same enclosure, 350 feet in the rear of the Naval Home, and 225 feet from the shorter parallel side of the grounds near the river. It is, with the exception of the stone basement, a brick building. It is 320 feet long, faces the southeast, and consists of a basement, two stories, and attic with mansard roof. It was designed by John McArthur, an architect, in 1865, when the appropriation for its erection was made. The work was begun in 1866, with Dobbins Bros., Philadelphia, as contractors. After an expenditure of $172,500, the hospital was commissioned in July, 1868.

It consists of a central structure and two wings, all entering their full length into the formation of the front. The wings are pavilions, over 100 feet long, ending in transverse buildings, and containing the wards,—the central structure being the administration portion. The wings, denominated northeast and southwest respectively, were originally alike, but in 1886 the former was divided into rooms for beneficiaries from the "Home"; but these rooms have never been occupied by them. Indeed, no one lives in that part of the building but the chaplain of the Home, who has his quarters in the second story.

The southwest wing remains as it was originally designed—on each floor is a long ward, 81 by 24 feet, and in the transverse portion a smaller ward, 21 by 20 feet, with nurse rooms, and in the rear and across a short corridor, water-closets. The floors are all soft pine painted, and the walls are painted plaster. The full height of the ceilings is 15 feet. There are 14 windows in the large ward, placed symmetrically on the opposite sides, while in the small ward there are seven. Twenty beds are in one ward, and five in the other. These are of the usual pattern, and are supplied each with a hair mattress on a wire-woven base. There are the usual lockers and chairs and electric call-bells. As the other wing is not used, the total number of beds is just fifty—twenty-five on each floor. The air space for each bed is 1400 cubic feet. The hospital was, of course, designed for fifty additional beds in the other wing.

This total of 100 can be increased 50 by using the wards under the mansard roof. This space is not used for the sick, as the ceiling of the long ward is low. However, in the transverse portion of the mansard are two rooms, 20 by 21 feet, with fairly high ceilings. These at present are used, one for a bag and hammock room, and the other for microscopic and photographic work. In the basement of the pavilion are a smoking-room corresponding to the long ward and two storerooms.

The central structure occupies 118 feet of the front, and has a depth of 74 feet. This does not include its further extension of 52 feet in an addition consisting of a basement and one story, containing in the former the kitchen, and in the latter the dining-room and several pantries. In the basement of the main or central portion, there are, besides this kitchen, many storerooms, and quarters for employés. On the first and second floors are the administration offices, quarters for resident medical officers and for sick officers, reception-rooms, dining-room, dispensary, diet-rooms, bath-rooms and water-closets. Under the mansard roof are an autopsy room, and a ward 28 by 45 feet, now used as a lumber-room. In the rear of these, and separated by the corridors, are quarters for the servants. (Plate XII.)

The entire building is lighted by gas and abundantly supplied with good water from the city. As the water pressure is insufficient, tanks have been placed under the roof, which are kept filled by a steam pump. Steam for heating purposes is supplied from the boiler house in the rear, where also is the laundry, well supplied with all necessary appliances. There is good natural ventilation, and consequently it is seldom necessary to use the artificial means provided. These consist of openings near the floors, through which hot air comes, heated in its passage by the steam pipes contained in brick casings, and openings near the ceilings, through which the air is drawn into the chimney of the boiler-house by a fan. The sewer system is not altogether satisfactory, as it is too closely connected with that of the city, as there is a large sewer running through the hospital grounds which has an objectionable manhole not far from the building.

To the north of the Home is the residence of the governor of that institution, and to the south is the residence for the senior medical officer of the Hospital. There is a garden south of the hospital, and various outbuildings, but no separate place for contagious diseases. The dead were once buried in the grounds, but the government now owns a place in one of the city cemeteries.

The staff consists of a medical director and two junior officers. The beneficiaries from the Home furnish most of the patients. These are placed on the lower floor; the paralytics and other helpless cases in the small ward. These old men, already near their end, furnish, of course, a large mortality, though they have the advantages of an almost model hospital. From July 1st, 1868, to December 31, 1892, there were 5346 persons treated in this institution. Of these, 648 were discharged from the service or transferred to the Government Hospital for the Insane, and 392 died. As 303 of these were beneficiaries, the ratio of 73.32 deaths per thousand should excite no surprise. The largest number of patients under treatment at one time was 54 in 1872. The average number now is 25.

U. S. Naval Hospital, Washington, D. C.

The first naval hospital at Washington was established in a building near the navy-yard, rented for that purpose. The price paid was $200 a year. This was succeeded by the one established at the navy-yard, and which was discontinued in 1843, when the sick were transferred to the Marine Headquarters. Afterwards, the Civil War caused these accommodations to be insufficient, and on June 8, 1861, a temporary naval hospital was established in the "Government Hospital for the Insane" near Washington; certain wards having been "appropriated by the Secretary of the Interior for naval purposes." These wards continued to be used until October 1, 1866, and 1488 patients were treated, with a recorded death-rate of 31.6 per thousand.

The increasing importance of the navy-yard, the number of naval vessels in the Potomac, the uncertainty attending the condition of war, and the disadvantages of having a naval hospital under the same roof with insane patients, induced Congress to appropriate $25,000, on March 14, 1864, for the construction of a new building. The cost of work and material being then very great, additional appropriations had to be made, until the total aggregated $115,000. The building was completed in July, 1866, and commissioned October 1st of the same year.

The grounds comprise three-fourths of an acre, and are situated near the navy-yard. About one-half was purchased June 4, 1821, and the remainder, March 30, 1865; the total cost being $7819.50. They form a trapezium, bounded by the streets of the city, and enclosed by a handsome iron railing, and present with the building, walks, grass and trees, an attractive appearance.

The hospital is back from the street, fronts the south, and is 90 feet long and 60 deep. A part of the depth is made by small extensions back and front, so that the ground plan resembles a cross with short arms. It is built of brick, and includes a basement, two stories, and an attic under a mansard roof. The pitch of the basement is 9 feet, and of the two stories 14 feet. The rooms and wards open on corridors. A central hall, 10 feet wide, connecting back and front, is crossed perpendicularly by a narrower one extending the length of the mid-line. The corridors thus form a cross, and divide each floor into four sections (Plate XIII).

In the basement, the floor of which is somewhat below the ground level, are the apothecary's quarters, the kitchen, laundry, boiler room, coal-bunker, storerooms, bath-room and water-closets. On the first floor are offices, mess-room for the men, and quarters for all the medical officers on duty. On the second floor are dispensary, officers' ward, nurses' room, and four wards for enlisted men. The two rear wards are 18½ × 35 feet, and the other two, one at each end of the front, are 24 × 22 feet. They contain many windows, and have pine floors and painted plaster walls. The bath-rooms and water-closets on each floor are in the rear extension, which is 9 feet deep and 43 long. They contain good tubs, and well trapped bowls with overhead tanks. The sewer pipes connect with those of the city.

In spite of the plan of this building, the ventilation is remarkably good. The large number of windows, the walled duct under the hospital communicating at each end with the outside air, and dis-charging into stacks containing the steam pipes, and the ventilators throughout the building near floors and ceilings, accomplish an excel-lent result.

The water is from the city, but, as the pressure is insufficient, a steam pump is provided in the basement, to force the supply into two iron tanks placed in the attic. All the water is passed through a Loomis filter, to free it from the large amount of matter held in suspension. The building is heated by steam supplied from the boiler in the basement, and is lighted by gas from the city, but elec-tric lights are now being introduced.

The present number of beds is 26, with an air space of 1392 cubic feet to each; but the average number of patients daily under treat-ment allows over 3000 cubic feet to each. The hospital was designed for 50 beds, with 1155 cubic feet of air to each. In 1871 there were 63 patients under treatment at one time. The staff consists of a Medical Director and a Passed Assistant Surgeon, both of whom reside in the building.

"*Sick Quarters,*" *U. S. Naval Academy, Annapolis, Maryland.*

The United States Naval Academy, situated at Annapolis, Mary-land, on the right bank of the Severn river, is separated from the city by a high brick wall, which, with the river, encloses more than 60 acres of ground. These are beautified with walks, lawns and orna-mental trees, and contain the many buildings necessary for the school.

This school was established in 1845, on 9 acres of ground trans-ferred to the Navy Department from the War Department, which had here a small fort. Additions have been made by purchase from time to time, until the present ample dimensions have been attained.

The hospital is near the south end of the main building, or "cadet quarters," and was built in 1853, to take the place of a small two-story frame structure near the fort. It is a brick building, 42 feet wide and 67 deep, fronts the east, and consists of a half-cellar, three stories and attic. Originally much smaller, it was enlarged and altered in 1876, and again in 1886. The cellar has a depth of 7 feet, is well ventilated, and its floor is of concrete. The storerooms situated here are therefore dry and ample. On each story there is a wide central hall connecting back and front, and having rooms or wards on either side. Broad iron stairways connect the different floors.

The hall on the 1st floor is tiled, and ends in a rear vestibule, from which the back stairway ascends. This stairway well is connected with the water-closets and bath-rooms on each floor, and is shut off from the rest of the building by doors. Contagious disorders can thus be treated on the 3d floor without any communication with the other parts of the hospital.

It is true that a detached pavilion would be preferable, but the writer has known scarlet fever, mumps, diphtheria, and other communicable diseases, to be repeatedly treated here without any extension, thus apparently demonstrating the tendency of infection to confine itself to the horizontal plane.

The water-closets and bath-rooms are separated from the wards by doors and the staircase well. They have concrete floors and slate walls, two or more windows each, good tubs, and bowls well flushed from overhead tanks. All the fixtures are well trapped, and the sewer pipes connect with those from the "cadet quarters," and empty into the river near by. The first story has a pitch of 8½ feet, the second 12 feet, and the third 14 feet. On the first floor, on one side of the hall, is a large dispensary, communicating in the rear with a convenient laboratory, the dining-room, and nurses' room ; on the other side is the officer-of-the-day's room, communicating in the rear with a waiting room, the kitchen, and dentist's room. The kitchen is only used to keep the meals hot before serving. All the cooking is done in the kitchen of the "cadet quarters." The laundry work is also done outside of the building in the main laundry. On the second story, the hall room is the operating room. This is lighted by three large windows occupying most of the walls, and contains the necessary appliances. On one side of the hall is the medical inspector's office and library, and two wards; on the other, two wards and the apothecary's room.

The third floor has a dark room and six wards, one of which is called the board room, as the physical examinations of all the candidates for admission to the school and of all cadets are conducted there. The wards are all well supplied with windows extending nearly to the ceilings, and with ventilators near floors and ceilings, connecting with ventilating shafts. The attic is surmounted by a large ventilating cupola.

Electric call-bells are distributed throughout the building. Large steam radiators are in suitable places, and connection is made with the boiler-house, from which most of the houses in the grounds are heated. Gas is obtained from the Naval Academy tanks, and water from the city reservoir, five miles distant. The source of this water is a small stream fed by springs. It contains 4 grains of solids to the gallon, of which 2.5 are non-volatile.

The patients having accommodations in the hospital are chiefly cadets, of whom there are generally about 250 in the school. Officers connected with the academy have, as a rule, quarters within the grounds provided for them and their families.

There are, however, many enlisted men in the marine barracks and on the ships located here. Serious cases among these are admitted into the hospital, and indeed from this source is almost all the mortality—there not having been a death among the cadets at the academy for several years.

The medical officers on duty look out for the sick of over 1000 people, including many women and children. The official returns include, of course, only such cases as occur among the persons in the naval service. During the last 3 years there were 3059 cases treated; of these, 14 were invalided and 5 died; the causes of death being phthisis, suicide and tetanus. In 1890, out of 240 cadets, 172 were attacked with epidemic catarrh, but none of these cases ended fatally.

The staff consists of a medical inspector, a surgeon and two passed assistant surgeons. The hospital can accommodate 50 patients and furnish 3500 cubic feet of air space to each bed. The number in sick quarters is, however, as a rule much below this, and each one probably has not less than 5000 cubic feet of air.

In the spring and summer the broad verandas on each floor furnish to convalescents opportunities that are not neglected of remaining out-of-doors in good weather.

The mean annual temperature is 55° F., while that of summer is 76°, and winter 35°. The rainfall is about 45 inches. The atmosphere in summer occasionally furnishes a high degree of humidity, but the climate is remarkably good most of the year for a place situated on the Atlantic coast. There is a mild malarial influence in summer and early autumn, but it is only occasionally noticeable, as the grounds are kept in beautiful order and are well drained. Indeed, it may be said that few places urnish such grass and trees and opportunities for outdoor life.

U. S. Naval Hospital, Norfolk, Virginia.

After 1811 the sick on this station were treated in a temporary hospital established at the navy-yard. It was a very poor structure, and in a few years after its occupation was unfit for use, by reason of decay and other causes. It was not, however, until 1826 that the commissioners caused the various sites near Norfolk to be examined with a view to the erection of a permanent building. Craney Island was first selected, and its transfer from the War Department was secured in November of that year.

This site was not very satisfactory, and the conditions attached to the transfer not altogether agreeable. Therefore on January 8, 1827, a request was made to the Secretary of War, himself a member of the Board of Commissioners, to transfer Fort Nelson, near Norfolk, and the public land attached to it, to the Navy Department for hospital purposes. The transfer was made, and 25 acres or more of adjoining land were purchased for $5000 from Col. Thomas Newton, then a member of Congress. The conveyance of the latter was not completed until November 29, 1827.

In December, 1826, a plan for the hospital had been accepted from John Haviland, an architect in Philadelphia, and the work was commenced early in 1827, under his personal supervision. He also made all the contracts for material and labor and was responsible for the payments. On July 17, 1830, the sick, together with all furniture and appliances, were moved from the temporary hospital at the yard to the one wing of the new building sufficiently completed. This transfer was effected by Surgeon Thomas Williamson, U. S. Navy, the first medical officer in charge of the present naval hospital at Norfolk. In 1832, after an expenditure of $270,000, the building was still more or less incomplete, and indeed the work continued from time to time for several years.

The hospital is well located on the left bank of the Elizabeth river, opposite the city of Norfolk, and separated from the navy-yard by the city of Portsmouth. The grounds comprise 80 acres, of which 50 in the rear of the building are covered by a pine forest, cleared of undergrowth and traversed by roads. The land in front is a broad stretch of lawn, ornamented by walks and trees, and surrounded by a sea wall terminating in a point projecting into the river 1000 feet away.

This hospital, constructed of granite, presents an imposing appearance; its basement and 3 stories being adorned by a portico 110 feet long and 17 feet wide, approached by broad stone steps, and containing 10 lofty Doric columns supporting a handsome entablature and pediment. The block plan was chosen, with a front of 195 feet facing the northeast, and two perpendicular wings extending 170 feet. The width of each is 44 feet, except for 123 feet of the wings adjacent to the front. Here the deficiency is supplied by an outside balcony on each floor. The fourth side of the square is occupied in part by a two-story annex, 60 feet long and 20 wide. This is joined to the wings by balconies that extend on every floor around the entire court.

All the wards are in the wings; each wing has eight on a floor, five being 26 × 15 feet, and three 35 × 10 feet. They all connect by arched openings forming alcoves on each side, and except on the third floor have vaulted ceilings with a maximum height of 11½ feet. Each has two opposite windows, painted wood floors and plaster walls. Each contains 4 beds and furnishes 1087 cubic feet of air and 98 feet floor space to a bed. (Plate XIV.)

A hall 12½ feet wide traverses the length of the floors of the main building, having the rooms in front. Stairs from these halls connect the various floors. On the 1st floor are offices, reception-room, and officers' dining-room. On the 2d floor are quarters for resident officers and for sick officers. On the 3d floor are storerooms, apothecary's room and quarters for employés. The nurses' rooms are in the wings, one at each end of the row of wards in the narrower portions, with water-closets opposite, and stairs connecting the different stories. These closets are used only by special cases, as the main water-closets are in the annex, where also are the smoking-rooms, wash-rooms, and barber-shop. In the general basement are kitchen, laundry, mess-room, storerooms and quarters for employés.

The court covers large cisterns, into which water is pumped from a deep well extending into a natural underground current supplying 30,000 gallons daily. There are also large iron tanks on top of the annex for storing this water. The pump and boiler-house are in the rear. Steam is supplied for heating the building, for the pumps in storing water, and in connection with a perfect fire system. Ventilation is accomplished by doors and windows; the long summers and mild winters allowing a free circulation of air most of the time.

The sewer system is complete and independent. All fixtures are trapped and the abundant supply of water allows frequent flushing. The pipes discharge into the river north of the building.

A number of electric lamps supply light; though, of course, the gas fixtures are retained, and connection with the gas-works of the city of Portsmouth.

Well situated in the midst of pine trees is a frame building used for contagious diseases. There are also, of course, the usual outhouses, such as woodsheds, stables, greenhouse, and boathouse.

To the south is a good residence for the medical director in charge. His assistants, a passed assistant surgeon and two assistant surgeons, reside in the main building. The south wing of the hospital is not used, as the average number daily under treatment is 30. This hospital was, however, designed for 200 beds.

During the last 3 years 593 patients have been treated.

The climate is rather debilitating in summer, on account of the high temperature; though at night during this period there is generally a pleasant breeze, allowing refreshing sleep. The spring and autumn are delightful, and the winters, as a rule, mild ; though snow and ice are common in January and February.

In the early autumn, cases of malarial fever are not infrequently admitted from the navy-yard, and typhoid fever is not rare in the cities. Pulmonary troubles do better than in any of the other naval establishments, and patients are occasionally transferred here for that reason.

The increasing importance of the Norfolk navy-yard, and the large number of naval vessels seeking these waters, make it very desirable to have a hospital so delightfully situated, and so entirely free from epidemic influences.

U. S. Naval Hospital, Pensacola, Florida.

This hospital is a light frame structure, situated three-quarters of a mile to the west of the navy-yard. The hospital and the navy-yard, with the little village of Wooster at its north, and the larger straggling village of Warrington at its west, are on the naval reservation, 5 miles by water southwest of the city of Pensacola. This reservation is part of the ungranted Spanish royal domain, which became the property of the United States by the treaty of 1819, ratified by Spain in 1821. Florida ceded its jurisdiction over this tract to the United States in 1845. The coast here forms an angle that includes the reservation, the south and east sides of which are both on the Bay of Pensacola, while the Grand Bayou, formed by an arm of the bay extending west, forms the north boundary of the "reserve." The apex of the angle is called Tartar Point, and it is here that the navy-yard is situated. The soil is white sand, sparsely covered with grass. The trees are pine, and water and live oak.

In seeking a site for the hospital, the higher ground at the west of the naval reserve was selected, and 15 acres were set apart by high brick walls. The building is 566 yards from the bay, and 42 feet above sea-level. It is a simple pavilion of five wards arranged in a row. Each ward has five beds, with 1047 cubic feet of air to a bed. This simple structure is 126 feet long and 30 wide, is surrounded by a balcony, and faces the south. The surgeon's house, near by, and to the west, has much the same appearance, and is but little smaller. In addition to his quarters it contains two rooms for sick officers. These rooms have each 2260 cubic feet of air space.

The two buildings, with their kitchen in common, were completed in October, 1875, by R. E. Anson, contractor, at a cost of $18,872, and were immediately occupied. They occupy the site of the old hospital destroyed by fire during the Civil War. Reminders of the old structure can be found in the remains of such outhouses as the mortuary, bakery, laundry and engine-house. Since the building of the hospital, nothing has been done to improve the grounds by repairing or taking away these old relics. This is probably due to the relatively small importance of the institution. The sick of the fleet seek the northern hospitals, and the navy-yard is now one chiefly in name. Money, however, is expended in the way of preservation, and the hospital is kept clean and ready for emergencies.

The ventilation is very good, as, in addition to windows and fireplaces, there are doors provided with transoms, and in the ceiling of each ward are two movable blind ventilators. These latter open into the attic, which is ventilated by stationary blinds. The water supply is provided for by a cistern in which is collected the rain water from the shingle roof of the surgeon's quarters. The annual rainfall is 90 inches.

A portion of the grounds in front of the buildings is low, and here collect the drainage waters from the slope to the west around Fort Barrancas, and the opposed slope of the hospita grounds. The result is a sluggish pond, 210 feet long. The warm climate and the decaying vegetable growth so near the hospital furnish, in the early fall, conditions not favorable to the health of the locality. The winters are very mild, giving but little frost, and the summers are long and exceedingly hot. July and August are the warmest months, but September is probably the most debilitating. The mean annual temperature is nearly 70 degrees F., and the range in 1880, an exceptional year, was between 118 degrees and 7 degrees.

The prevailing diseases are intestinal and malarial. Yellow fever is an occasional visitor—the years 1863, 1867, and 1875 and 1883 marking some of its visits. This disease is not indigenous, but sometimes passes from the quarantine station to the southeast on the long island of Santa Rosa. The hospital has no separate building for such cases, and in 1883, eight were treated in the wards.

The staff consists of one surgeon, who, in addition to hospital duties, does much work among the poor of the two villages. The navy has supplied only 271 cases since the hospital was commissioned in 1875. Of these, 12 died (6 from yellow fever), 209 were discharged to duty, and 50 were invalided. During a part of 1888 there was not an unoccupied bed, as 24 patients were under treatment at one time. But during the last four years there have been only 14 sick, as the naval force at the yard has been reduced to a minimum.

U. S. Naval Hospital, Mare Island, California.

The naval station of the United States on the Pacific is Mare Island, a tract of land acquired by the government on January 4, 1853, at a cost of $83,000. It is situated 25 miles from the city of San Francisco, on San Pablo Bay, the northern extension of San Francisco Bay, and was originally a grant to Señor Castro, who parted with it for money, as several others did before its final purchase.

This island is very extensive if all the marsh land be considered, but only 930 acres are at all suitable for naval purposes. These include the rolling land, forming approximately an ellipse, comprising the southern portion. The long axis of this is 2¾ miles, extending northwest and southeast, while the short axis is ⅝ of a mile.

Between the island and the town of Vallejo on the mainland is the Mare Island Strait. At the southern extremity (the Carquinez Strait) the waters of the Sacramento and San Joaquin rivers empty into the bay. The formation of this part of the island is sandstone, covered by 2½ feet of black loam. The climate and soil have been so favorable to the cultivation of trees and flowers that the island has become celebrated even on that coast.

Soon after the purchase, the navy-yard was established on the side opposite Vallejo, the intervening waters furnishing a quiet anchorage for ships of any size. A building was set apart for "sick quarters," and for storing medical supplies for the squadron and station. This is employed now as the dispensary and surgeon's office of the yard ; the large number of officers and workmen requiring medical and surgical assistance near at hand. It ceased to be used as "sick quarters" when the present hospital was completed in 1870.

This hospital has an isolated position outside and to the south-east of the yard, being one mile from the workshops, and on a slope facing Mare Island Strait, and ending in an intervening marsh. It is 66 feet above low water, and consists of a central structure, and two pavilions terminating in small transverse buildings. It fronts the east and is 250 feet long. It is built of brick, and has a basement, two stories, and an attic under a mansard roof. The spaces in front between the projecting central structure and the transverse portions of the pavilions are occupied by broad verandas on each floor. Each floor of a pavilion is a ward ; the transverse projection containing bath-room and water-closet.

Each ward is 68 feet long, 24 wide, and 15 high, and contains twenty beds between windows, and furnishes over 1200 feet air space and 81 feet floor space to each. There is an open fireplace near each end, 10 windows on both opposite sides, and an end window. The windows are 9½ feet high, and extend within 3 feet of the ceiling. The floors are painted Oregon pine, and the walls painted plaster. Fresh air is admitted by openings near the floor, connecting with ducts. A current is induced by ventilators near the ceiling communicating with large Emerson ventilators opening above the roof and provided with steam coils. The water-closets and bath-rooms are in the transverse projections on opposite sides of the wards. They are included in the ventilating system, have concrete floors, windows and all modern improvements.

The basement has 5½ feet of its pitch below the ground level. It contains mess-room, reading-room, kitchen, storerooms, and quarters for employés. The floors of the central building contain offices, resident medical officers' quarters, rooms for sick officers and for special cases, operating rooms, and apothecary's room. (Plate XV.)

The whole building is heated by steam and lighted by electricity. The sewer system is independent. All fixtures are well trapped, and the pipes join the 10-inch sewer in the rear, which connects with a well ventilated brick sewer nearly 500 feet long, emptying at an inclination of one foot in forty into the adjacent waters.

The steam laundry, drying-room and boiler are in a building 140 feet south of the hospital. In an annex to this is the mortuary. The boiler supplies steam for heating the building, and for forcing water into the iron tanks under the hospital roof. Water is obtained from the water-works of Vallejo and from the reservoir on the island. The latter holds 13,000,000 gallons of rain-water, but this supply is regarded as a reserve: the large number of people living on the island making it unadvisable to trust entirely to the connection with Vallejo.

The staff consists of a medical director, who is provided with a delightful residence, a surgeon and a passed assistant surgeon. Patients are received from the Pacific and Asiatic squadrons, from the station, and the Yokohama hospital. The 80 beds are, however, rarely filled, as the average number of patients daily under treatment is about 40. During the last three years 581 cases have been treated.

The climate is regarded as salubrious. During six months of the year there is almost no rain. The rainy season begins in May and lasts until October, though during this period there are usually considerable periods of fine weather. The mean annual temperature is 57° F. The thermometer occasionally falls to 28° in January, the coldest month. In summer there is a period of northwest winds, fogs and dust, that produces influenza and various respiratory troubles. Malarial influences are rarely noticeable, and epidemics unknown.

U. S. Naval Hospital at Yokohama, Japan.

This beautiful little establishment, constructed in 1872, and commissioned on May 16 of that year, accommodates 34 patients, including 8 officers. It is delightfully situated amid the residences of the foreign population, and near the English and German naval hospitals, on the bluff southeast of the main or lower section of the city of Yokohama.

It consists of a main quadrangular building of two stories and two detached buildings of one story. One of these, called the wing, is situated to the east and rear, so that its front is nearly on a line with the rear of the main building, with which it is connected by an outside passage. The other building, containing the dining-room, kitchen, pantry, cooks' room and store-rooms, is nearly 30 feet in rear of the main portion, and is connected with the wing by a passageway. The whole hospital is constructed of tile and plaster, fronts the south, and is nearly surrounded by verandas on all stories.

A smallpox hospital, with a disinfecting chamber near by, is 110 feet from the main building, and near the northwest limit of the grounds. It is a one-story building, containing a ward 25 × 54 feet, and two rooms 14 × 15 feet. The ward has 8 windows and a door, and contains 18 beds, with only 644 cubic feet of air space to each. Each room has 3 windows, a door and two beds, with 987 cubic feet to each bed. All these doors are 87 × 41 inches, and the windows are 58 × 85 inches.

The main building is 85 feet long and 35 feet deep. On the first floor are quarters for the resident medical officer, offices, dispensary, bath-room and water-closets. On the second floor is a ward containing 8 beds, with 902 cubic feet to each; 4 rooms, having 2 beds each, for sick officers, with 1200 cubic feet to each bed, and 2 rooms for nurses. The ward has 4 windows and 3 doors, and each room 3 windows and a door. The windows are 87½ × 45½ inches, and the doors 88 × 38 inches.

In the wing are the main ward, 54 × 24 feet, and nurses' rooms and water-closets. The ward contains 18 beds with 1717 cubic feet to each. It is lighted by 8 windows, each 76½ × 43 inches, and has 4 doors 83½ × 47 inches each. The water-closets all have earthen jars under the seats, which are removed from the outside of the building every night.

The grounds contain 1¾ acres, and are shaped somewhat like an arrowhead with blunted barbs. They are beautified with grass plots, trees, walks, and a pretty shaded mound 20 feet high. East of the wing is the residence of the medical officer in charge.

The ventilation of this hospital is good, as the many windows and doors are assisted by the badly fitted woodwork. All the buildings and grounds are lighted by electricity. Water is obtained from a well, and by storing rain-water in large iron tanks. The well is 67 feet deep, and furnishes an ample supply of water containing 13½ grains of solid matter to a gallon—silicic acid, chloride of sodium, carb. magnesium, sesquioxide of iron, and sulphate of calcium (trace). All drinking water is filtered, and in the summer months boiled. The rooms and wards of the main building have open fireplaces, but these being inadequate, stoves are employed.

The staff consists of a surgeon and a passed assistant surgeon. The employés are the apothecary, watchman, two cooks, a gardener, and four coolies. Two of the coolies do the cleaning and act as nurses; the other two are laborers. They have detached quarters. The watchman acts also as night nurse, and the cooks also set the tables. The gardener is also a carpenter and gatekeeper. The apothecary, in addition to usual duties, superintends nurses and issues stores.

The daily average of patients last year was 10. The patients come entirely from the fleet, and many of the diseases originate on the coast of China. Venereal troubles, of course, play their part, diarrhœal and malarial disorders are not uncommon, and smallpox is an occasional visitor.

Yokohama itself furnishes a certain number of cases, as the vessels of the navy pass much of the year there, to escape the debilitating summer of the south. This city, frequently spoken of as a desirable sanitarium, has a delightful climate, though July and August have a mean temperature of 80 degrees F. with a minimum of 70 degrees F. January, the coldest month, has a mean of 38 degrees and a minimum of 30 degrees. The dew-point in January is 30, and in July and August is 70. The annual rainfall is 50 inches. The prevailing winds in May, June and July are southeast, and during the rest of the year northeast. The main portion of the city is intersected by numerous canals, and has northwest of it many rice fields which are frequently flooded. Malarial disorders are therefore common, but on the bluff this influence is not noticeable.

Variola is present all the time, and occasionally becomes epidemic, beginning among the native population. Rubeola, frequently attacking adults, is also occasionally epidemic. There is also a disease among the natives known as kakke, and considered identical with beri-beri.

Closing Remarks.

The subject is far from a conclusion. England, France and the United States are only *three* of the many nations who send their sons upon the sea as warriors. Austria, Brazil, China, Germany, Italy, Russia, Spain, Turkey and others, represented by 2000 ships of war with 200,000 men, have established naval hospitals well worthy of study. These institutions furnish a part of the histories of these countries and offer to him who seeks, much of interest and profit. Yet they cannot be considered here, as an apology is due for the many pages already written. This apology is found in the little attention *these* important hospitals have received from the various writers on that subject.

DISCUSSION.

THE CHAIRMAN.—The Section is very greatly obliged to Dr. Gatewood for this paper, which is valuable from an historical point of view, and for permanent consultation when published. The paper is accompanied with plans of a number of French, English, and American naval hospitals; and it would be very desirable if this could be completed for other nations, as Dr. Gatewood suggests, because, so far as I know, there is no treatise or article upon naval hospitals which is complete.

UEBER MILITÄRLAZARETHE.

VON DR. GROSSHEIM,

Königlich Preussischer Generalarzt, Berlin.

Für die Erbauung und Einrichtung der Militärlazarethe müssen die grossen Grundsätze massgebend bleiben, welche sich für den Bau von Krankenhäusern überhaupt durch die Anforderungen der in stetem Fortschritte befindlichen hygienischen Wissenschaft herausgebildet haben. Diese Anforderungen haben sich im Laufe der Jahre wesentlich gesteigert und einen erheblichen Aufschwung erfahren durch die für alle Zeiten denkwürdigen Lazarethbauten während des nordamerikanischen Secessionskrieges, deren Beschreibung in dem überaus werthvollen Circular No. 6 des Generalstabsarztes der Vereinigten Staaten-Armee vom 20. Juli, 1864, niedergelegt ist.

Eine praktische Verwerthung und ausgezeichnete Weiterentwickelung jener Erfahrungen fällt bei allen seit jenen Tagen in Nordamerika entstandenen Krankenhausbauten dem fremden Besucher in ange-

GROUND PLAN OF NAVAL HOSPITAL, YARMOUTH–310 BEDS,

exclusive of Sick Officers Accommodation

PLATE I.

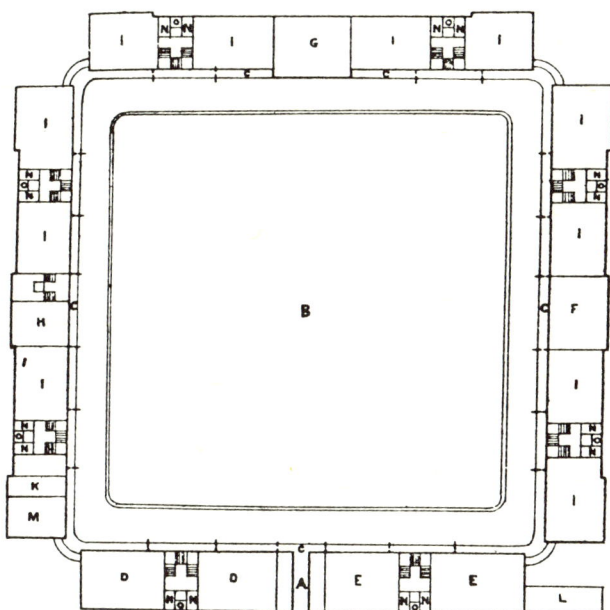

A Entrance archway.
B Garden.
C Open arched corridor, one story high, surrounding the garden.
D Rooms for sick officers.
E Steward's stores.
F Chapel
G First floor; operating theatre; ground floor, billiard room

H Committee room, surgery, &c
III, &c: Wards, 14 beds each.
K Padded room.
L Bath rooms, washhouse, &c.
MM Sculleries.
NN Nurses' rooms.
OO Waterclosets.

Royal Naval Hospital, Yokohama.

PLATE II.

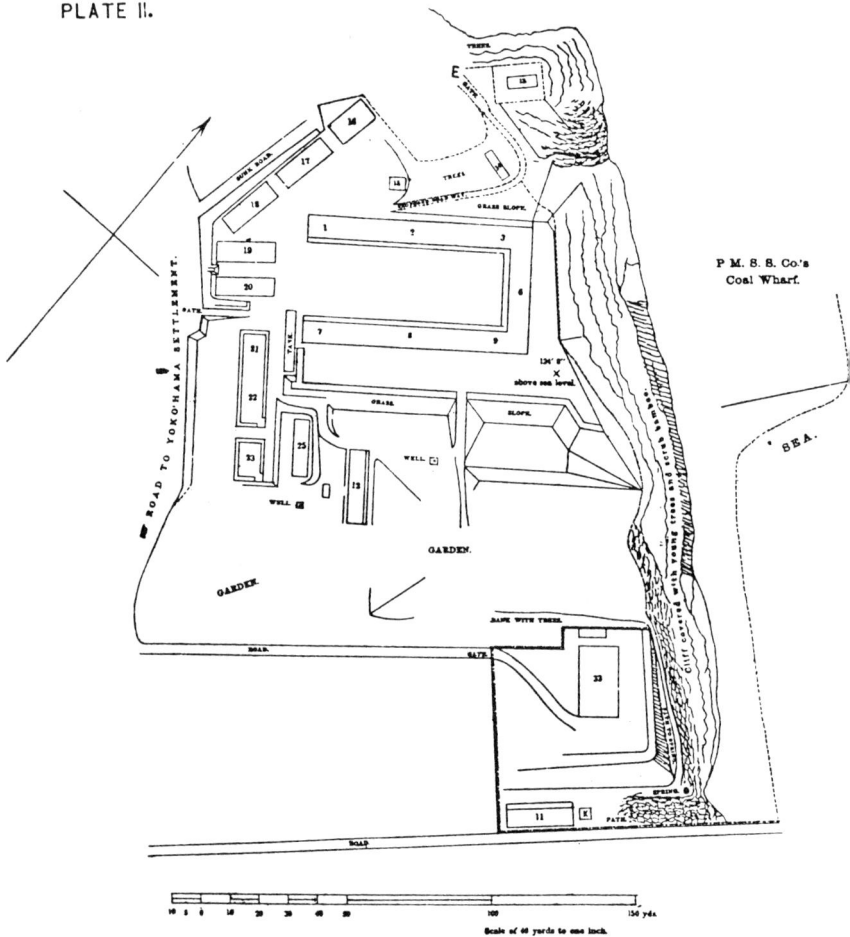

KEY TO PLATE II.

1, 2, 3, 6. General Wards.
7. Gun-room and Engineer's Ward (rooms).
8. Warrant Officers' Ward (rooms).
9. Non-commissioned Officers' Ward (rooms).
11. Contagious Ward.
12. Ward-room Officers' Ward (rooms).
13. Mortuary.
14. Latrine.
15. Fire-engine House.
16. Quarters for Natives.

17. General Cook and Bath House.
18. Nurses' Quarters, Clothing Store, Coal Store and Larder.
19. Steward's Quarters and Bedding Store.
20. Dispensary, Survey Room, and Provision Store.
21, 22. Senior Medical Officer's House.
23. Second Medical Officer's House.
25. Servants' Quarters, Kitchen, Stores, etc., for Medical Officers.
33. Contagious Ward.
K. Kitchen, Disinfecting Rooms, etc.

PLATE III.

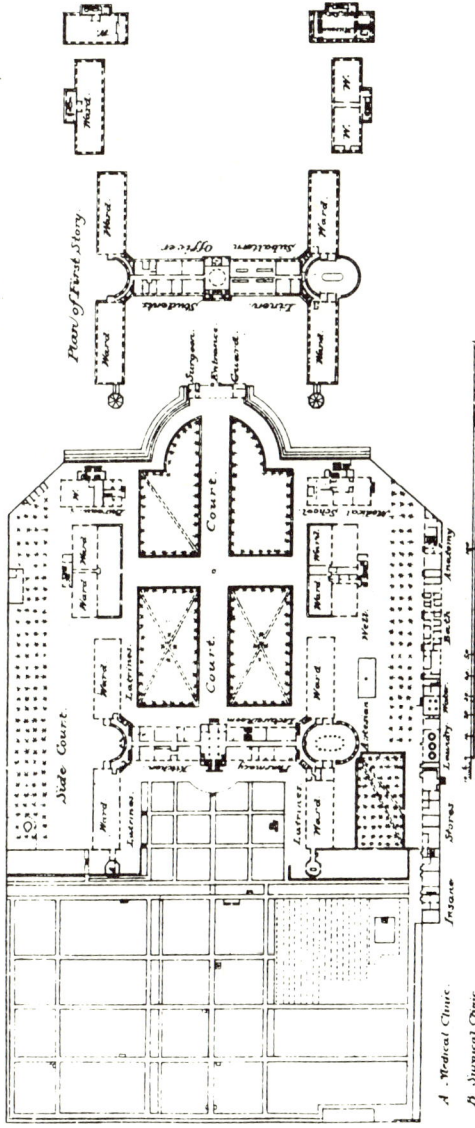

Naval Hospital at Rochefort.

Centre 1st Story.

Chapel   Officers

Plan of First Story.

Ward   Ward   Subaltern Officer   Ward   Ward

Students   Linen

Surgeon   Infirmary   Guard

Plan of Basement

Side Court   Court   Court

Latrines   Latrines

Ward   Ward   Ward   Ward   Ward

Insane   Stores   Laundry   Bath   Academy

A. Medical Clinic.
B. Surgical Clinic.

PLATE IV.

Naval Hospital, Toulon.

—— BASEMENT. ——

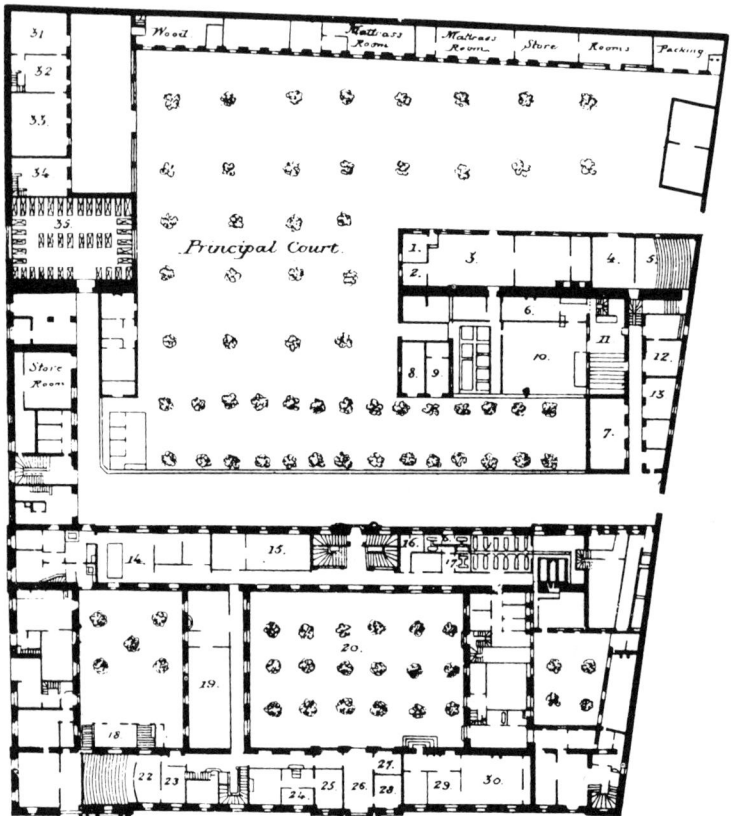

KEY TO PLATE IV.

1. Bureau of Pharmacy.
2. Office of Apothecary-in-Chief.
3. Laboratory.
4. Mortuary Chapel.
5. Anatomical Lecture Room.
6. Chemical Room.
7. Dissecting Room.
8. Mineralogical Room.
9. Botanical Room.
10. Garden.
11. Chemical Lecture Room.
12. Dead Room.
13. Professor of Anatomy.
14. Cuisine.
15. Linen Room.
16. Surgeon on Duty.
17. Baths.
18. Laboratory.
19. Grand Pharmacy.
20. Court.
21. Court of Sisters of Charity.
22. Lecture Room on Practice of Medicine.
23. Professors' Cabinet.
24. Control.
25. Office of Entries.
26. Entrance
27. Guard Room.
28. Sentries' Room.
29. Office of Director.
30. Council Room.
31, 32, 33, 34. Rooms for arranging Linen.
35. Sleeping Room of Attendants.

PLATE V.

Naval Hospital, Toulon

2ND Story.

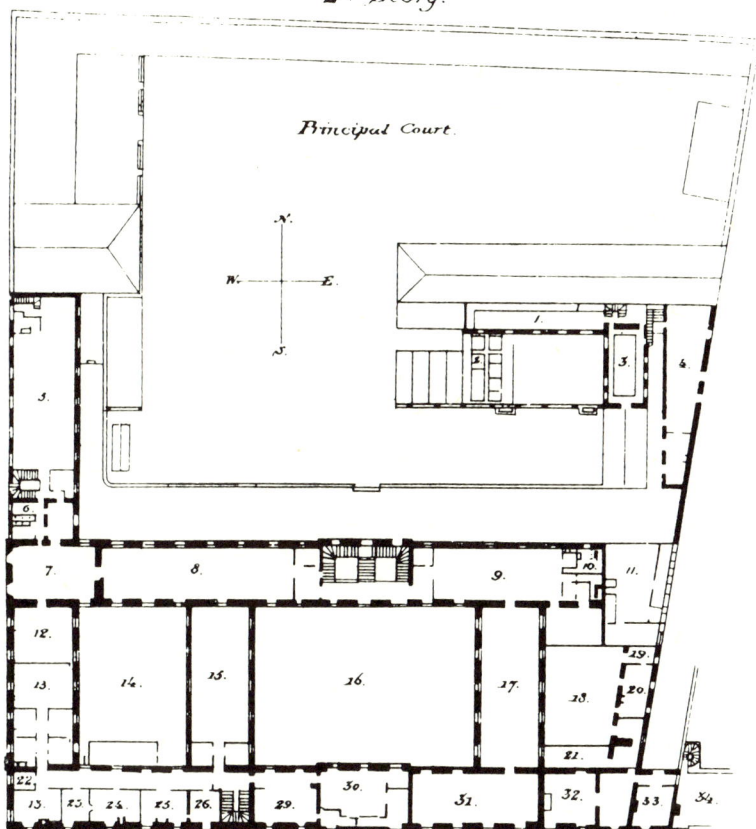

KEY TO PLATE V.

1. Museum.
2. Basins for Leachers.
3. Lecture Room for Chemistry.
4. Anatomical Collections.
5. Ward.
6. Water-closets.
7. Ward.
8. Ward.
9. Ward.
10. Water-closets.
11. Storeroom Pharmaceutical Utensils.
12. Room for Confinement of Patients.
13. Officers' Room.
14. Court.
15. Ward, Medical Clinic.
16. Large Court.
17. Ward.
18. Court for Sisters of Mercy.
19. Pharmacy for the Sisters.
20. Chamber for the Sisters.
21. Gallery.
22. Office.
23. Salle-a-Manger.
24. Room for Pupils.
25, 26. Superior Officer's Room
27, 28. Cabinet.
29. Cabinet of Natural History.
30. Library.
31. Ward.
32. Chapel of the Sisters.
33. Room for the Sisters.
34. Superintendence.

PLATE VI

PLATE VI.

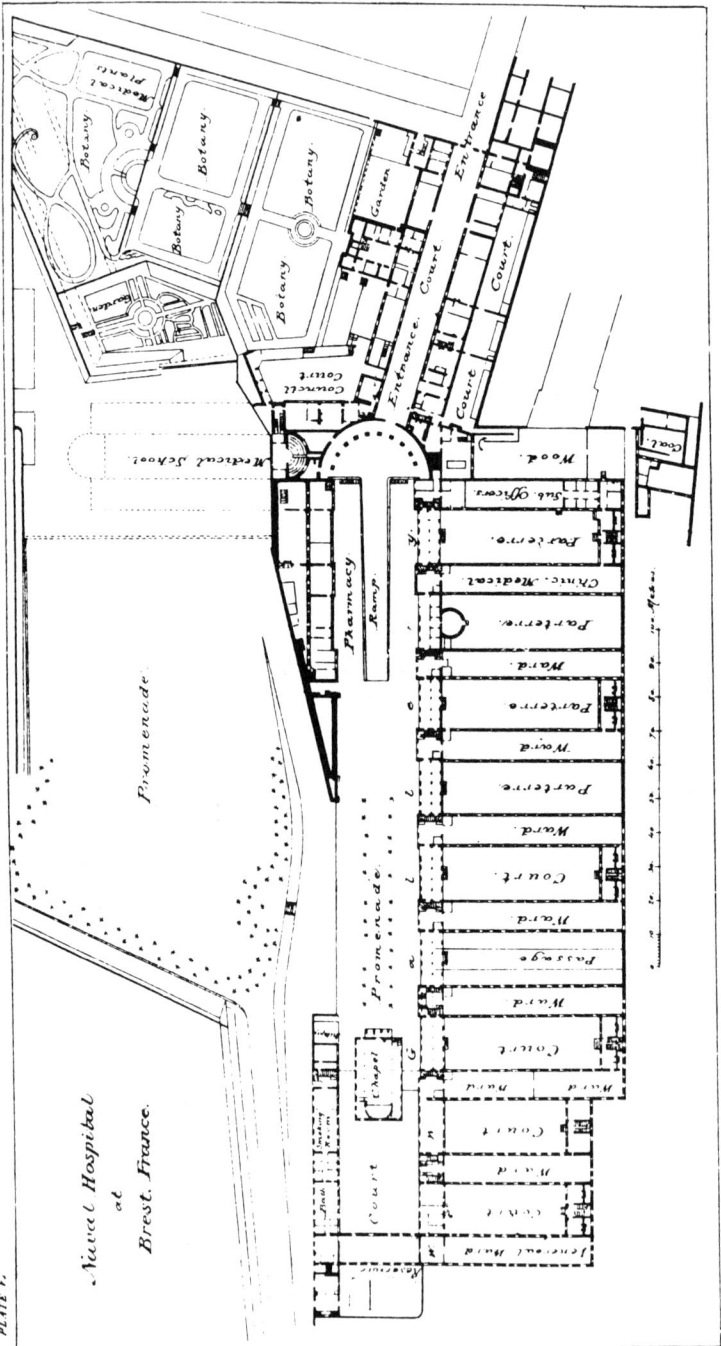

Naval Hospital
at
Brest, France.

Hôpital maritime de St Mandrier.

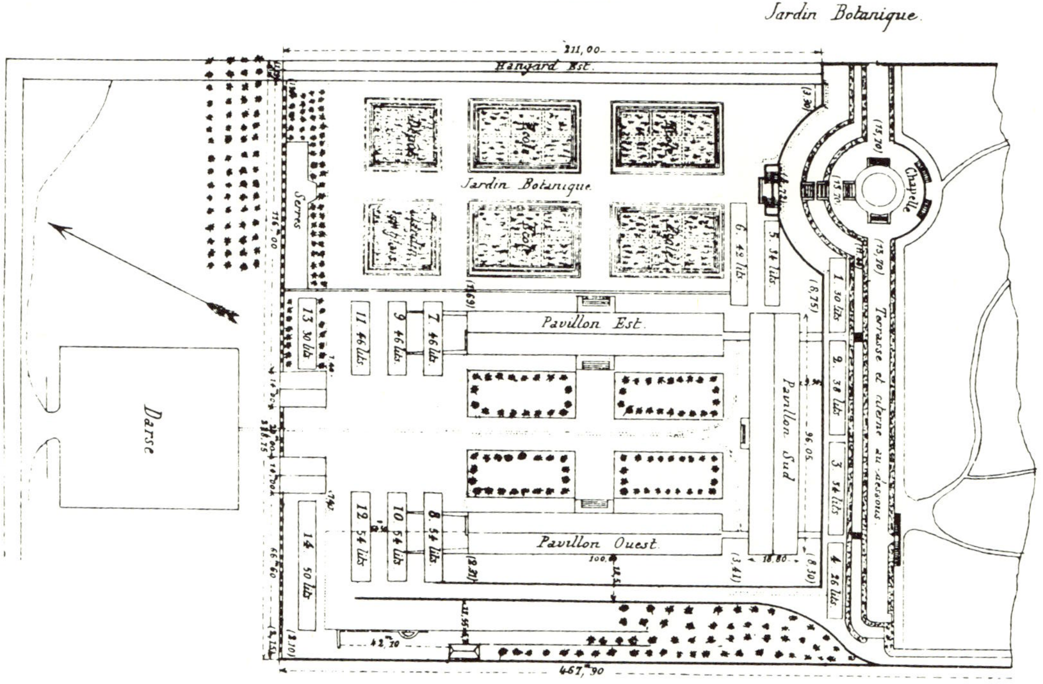

PLATE VII.

Jardin Botanique.

Chapelle

(13,70)   (13,70)   Terrasse et citerne au dessous

(13,70)

(3,70)   1. 30 lits   2. 38 lits   3. 34 lits   4. 26 lits

(8,75)   96,05   (8,30)

(4,22)   Pavillon Sud

5. 34 lits

6. 42 lits   (3,41)

École   École

Hangard Est   311,00   457,90

École   École   Pavillon Est   Pavillon Ouest

Dépôt   Jardin Botanique

(1,69)   7. 46 lits   8. 54 lits   (2,31)

9. 46 lits   10. 54 lits

11. 46 lits   12. 54 lits

Serres   13. 30 lits   14. 50 lits   (3,10)

116.00   288.75   66.60

Darse

PLATE VIII.

Cherbourg.
Nouvel hôpital maritime.

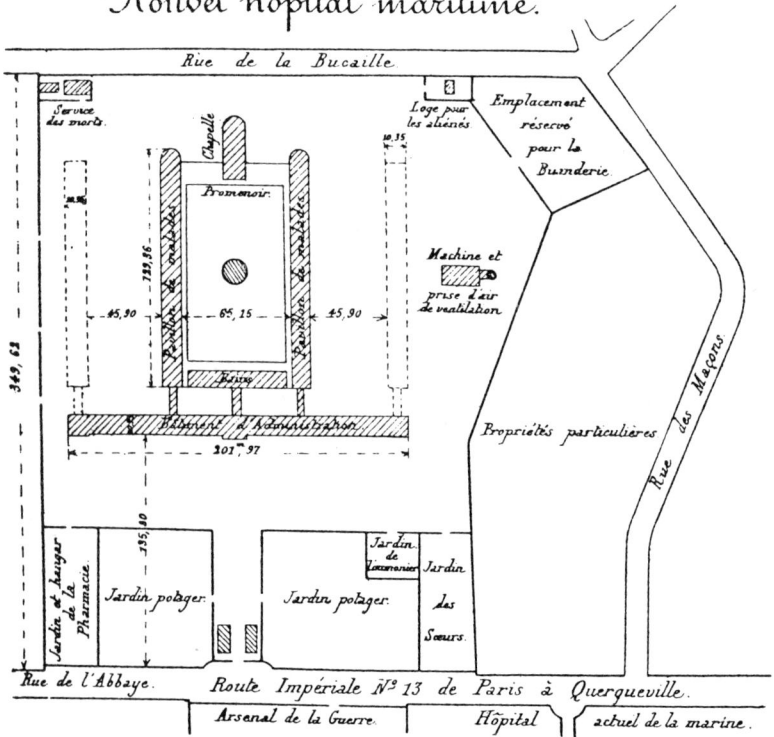

Rue de la Bucaille

Service des morts.

Loge pour les aliénés

Emplacement réservé pour la Buanderie

Chapelle

Promenoir

10.35

Machine et prise d'air de ventilation

135,36

Pavillon de malades

Pavillon de malades

45,90

65,15

45,90

Bains

Propriétés particulières

Pavillon d'administration

101,97

135,10

Rue des Maçons

Jardin et bûcher de la Pharmacie

Jardin potager.

Jardin potager.

Jardin de l'aumonier

Jardin des Sœurs

349,63

Rue de l'Abbaye.

Route Impériale N° 13 de Paris à Querqueville.

Arsenal de la Guerre.

Hôpital

actuel de la marine.

U.S.N.HOSPITAL
AT
Portsmouth N.H.

PLATE IX.

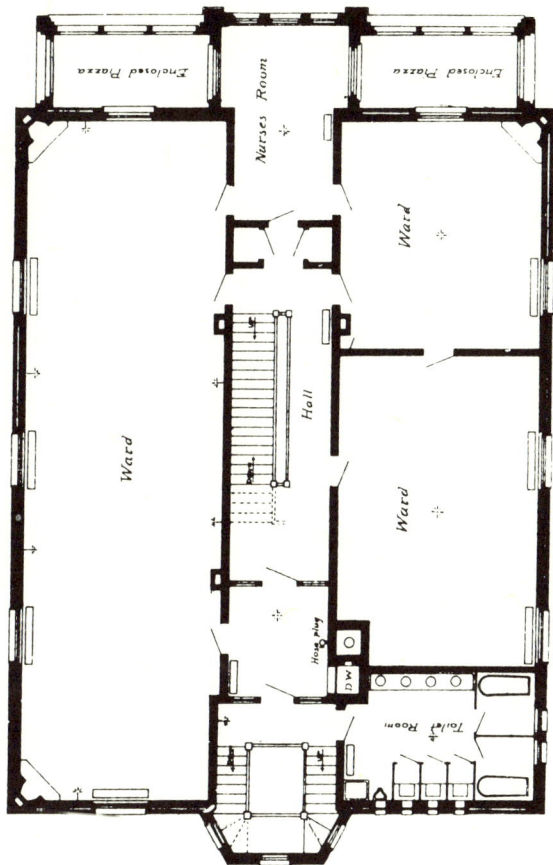

Enclosed Plaza

Enclosed Plaza

Nurses Room

Ward

Ward

Hall

Ward

Housekeeping

D.W.

Toilet Room

— 2ᴰ FLOOR —

PLATE X.

U.S. HOSPITAL. CHELSEA.

2ᴰ FLOOR.

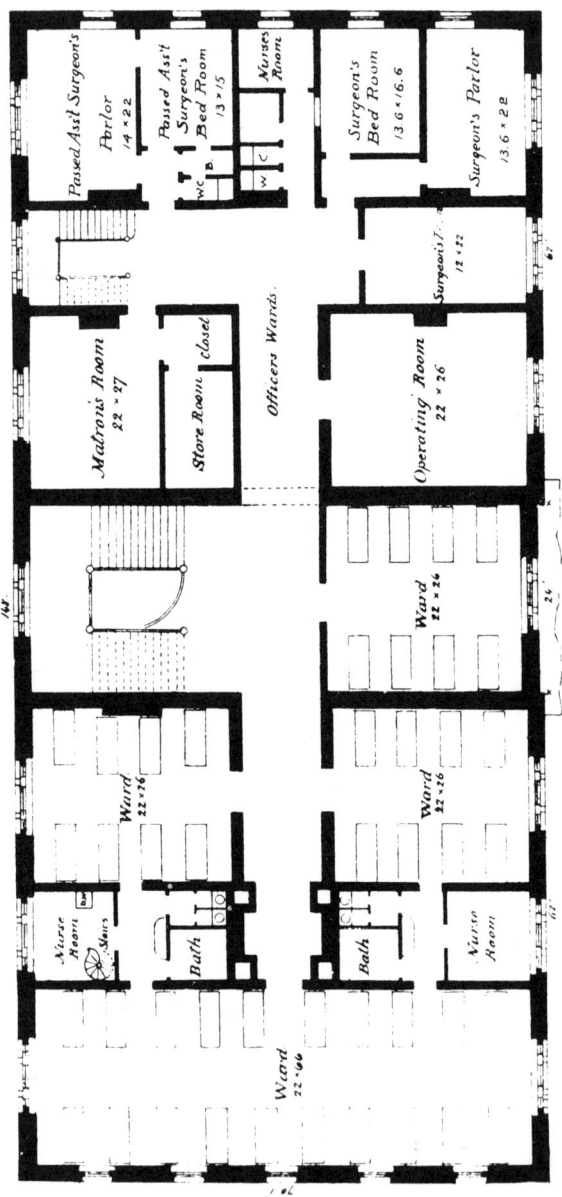

Scale 7⁄8 = 10 Ft.

PLATE XI.

U.S.N. HOSPITAL. — BROOKLYN.

—— 2D FLOOR. ——

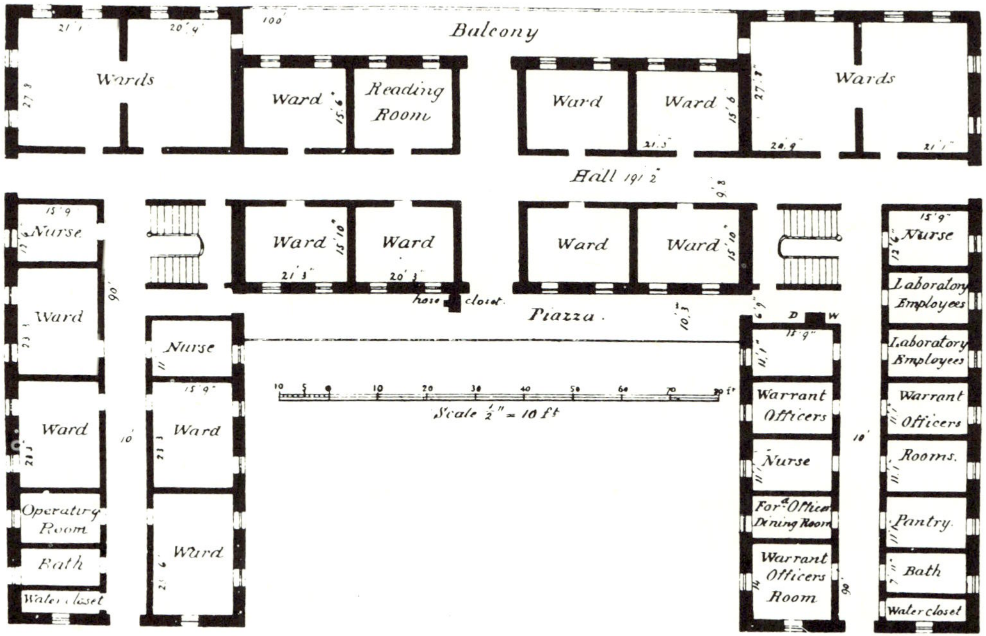

Wards

Ward

Ward

Balcony

Reading Room

Ward

Ward

Hall 19·2

Ward

Ward

Ward

Ward

hair closet

Wards

Piazza

Scale 1/8" = 10 ft

Nurse

Laboratory Employees

Laboratory Employees

Warrant Officers

Rooms

Pantry

Bath

Water closet

Warrant Officers

Nurse

For Officers Dining Room

Warrant Officers Room

Nurse

Ward

Ward

Nurse

Ward

Ward

Operating Room

Bath

Water closet

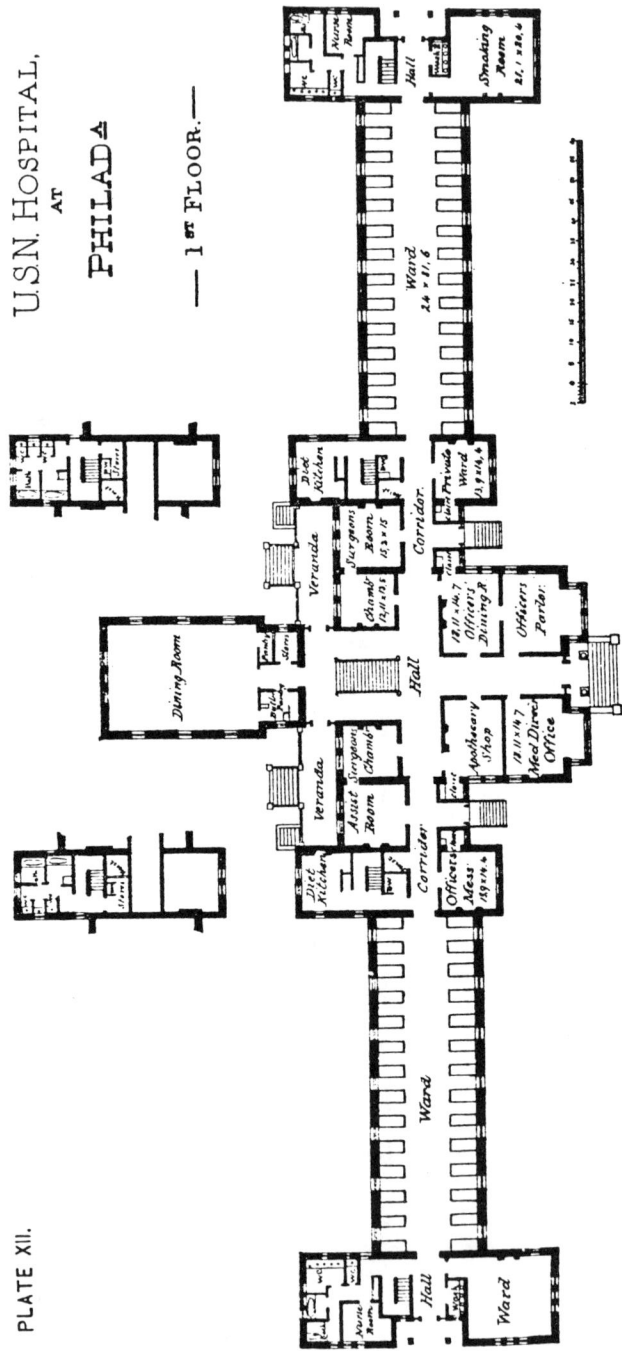

PLATE XII.

U.S.N. HOSPITAL,
AT
PHILAD.ª

— 1ˢᵀ FLOOR. —

U.S. Naval Hospital, Washington.

—2d Floor.—

PLATE XIII.

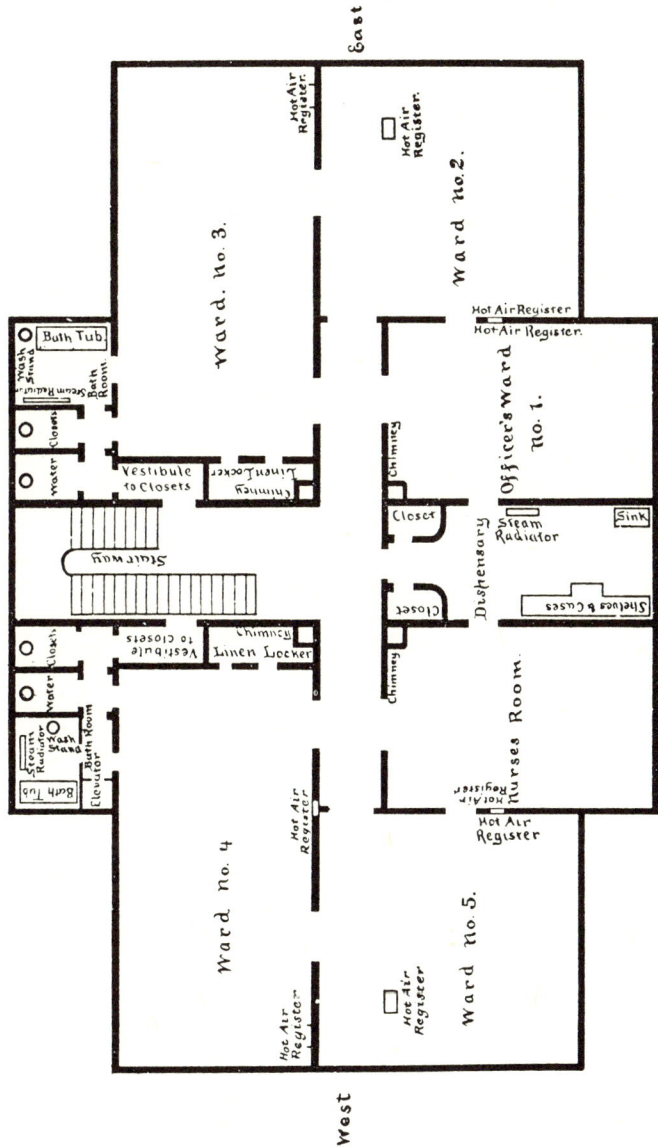

North

East

South

West

Ward. No. 3.

Ward No. 2.

Bath Tub

Wash Stand

Steam Radiator

Bath Room

Water Closet

Vestibule to Closets

Chimney

Linen Locker

Stairway

Vestibule to Closets

Water Closet

Linen Locker

Chimney

Steam Radiator

Wash Stand

Bath Room

Elevator

Bath Tub

Hot Air Register

Hot Air Register

Hot Air Register

Hot Air Register

Hot Air Register

Hot Air Register

Hot Air Register

Hot Air Register

Hot Air Register

Ward No. 4

Ward No. 5.

Nurses Room.

Dispensary

Chimney

Closet

Closet

Chimney

Officer's Ward No. 1.

Steam Radiator

Shelves & Cases

Sink

PLATE XIV.

U.S.N. HOSPITAL.

NORFOLK.

— 2D FLOOR —

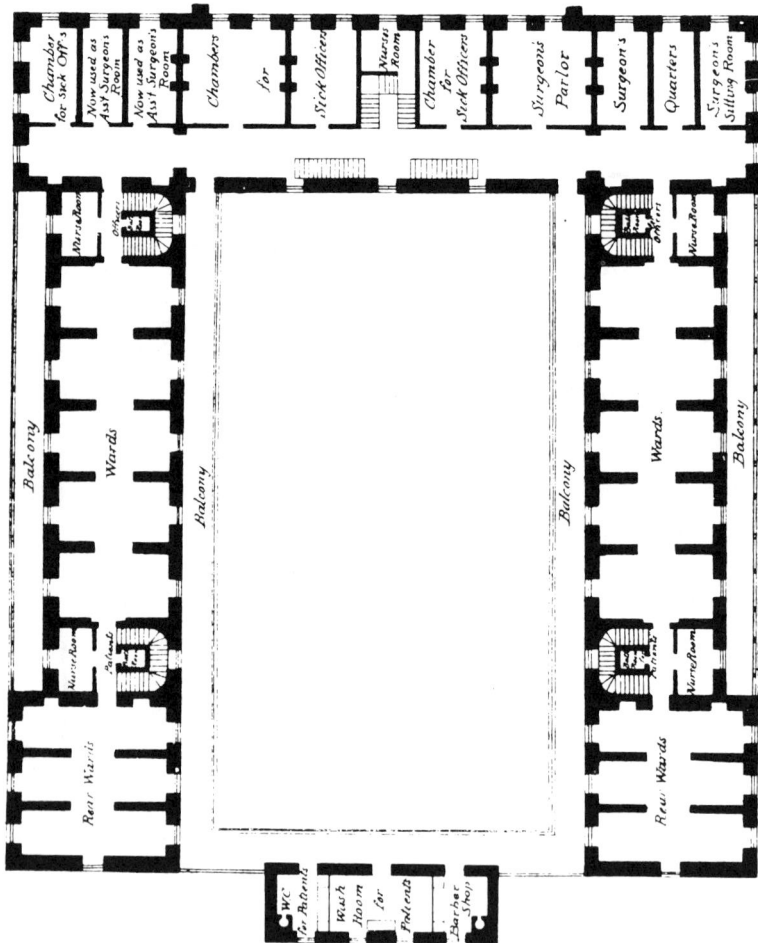

Scale ½ = 10 Feet.

Chamber for Sick Off's

Now used as Ass't Surgeon's Room

Now used as Ass't Surgeon's Room

Chambers

for

Sick Officers

Nurse's Room

Chamber for Sick Officers

Surgeon's Parlor

Surgeon's

Quarters

Surgeon's Sitting Room

Nurse Room

Offices

Balcony

Balcony

Wards

Balcony

Balcony

Wards

Nurse Room

Offices

Nurse Room

Patient

Rear Wards

Rear Wards

Patient

Nurse Room

W.C. for Patients

Wash Room for Patients

Barber Shop

PLATE XV.

U.S.N. HOSPITAL
AT
Mare Island Cal.

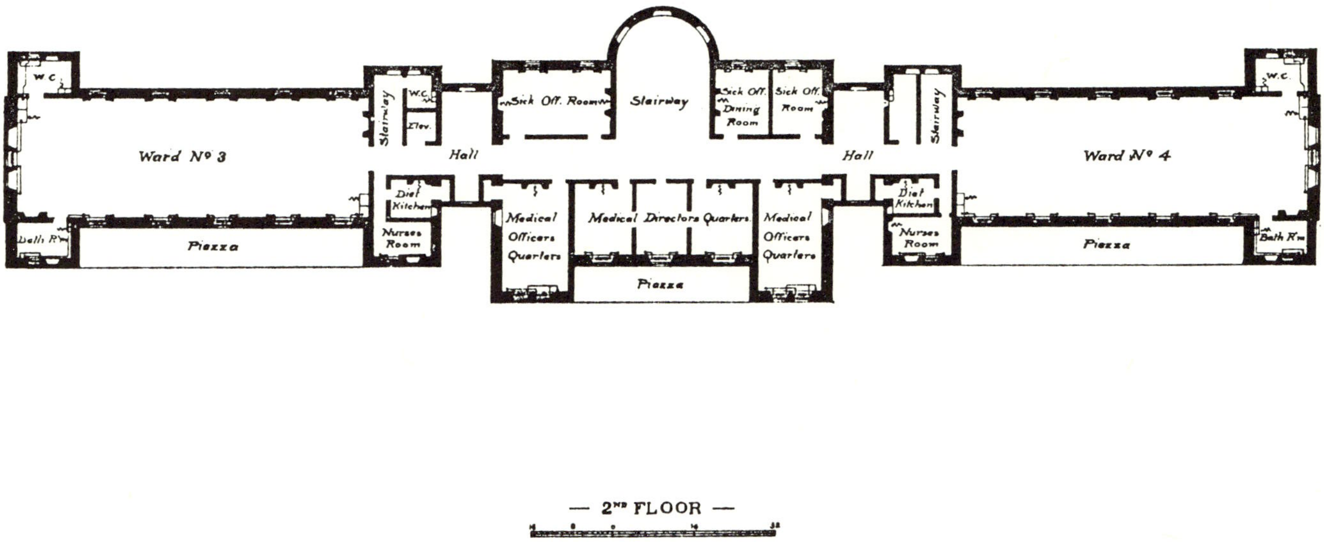
W.C.
Bath R'm
Ward No 3
Piazza
Stairway
W.C.
Elev.
Diet Kitchen
Nurses Room
Hall
Sick Off. Room
Stairway
Sick Off. Dining Room
Sick Off. Room
Medical Officers Quarters
Medical Directors Quarters
Piazza
Medical Officers Quarters
Hall
Stairway
Diet Kitchen
Nurses Room
Ward No 4
Piazza
W.C.
Bath R'm

— 2ND FLOOR —

PLAN OF THE U. S. NAVAL HOSPITAL AND GROUNDS, YOKOHAMA, JAPAN.

PLATE XVI.

Fig. 1. Mound 20 ft. high, covered with trees, and former site of a Japanese temple and tombs.

2. Flagstaff.   3. Vault.   4. Tennis Court.
5. Carpenter.   6. Laborer.   7. Watchman.
8. Cooks.   9. Officers.   10. Store Room.
11. Carpenter Shop.   12. Coolies' Quarters.
13. Assistant Surgeon's Dining-room.
14. Parlor.   15. Ass't Surgeon's Bedroom.
16. Pantry.   17. Light Room.
18. Surgeon's Office.   19. Officers' Room.
20. Dispensary.   21, 22 Apothecary's Quarters.
23. Cell.   24. Men's Smoking Room.
25. Men's Diningroom.   26. Lavatory.
28. Ward.   29. Porter's Lodge.
27, 27. Servants.   30. Main entrance to Hospital.

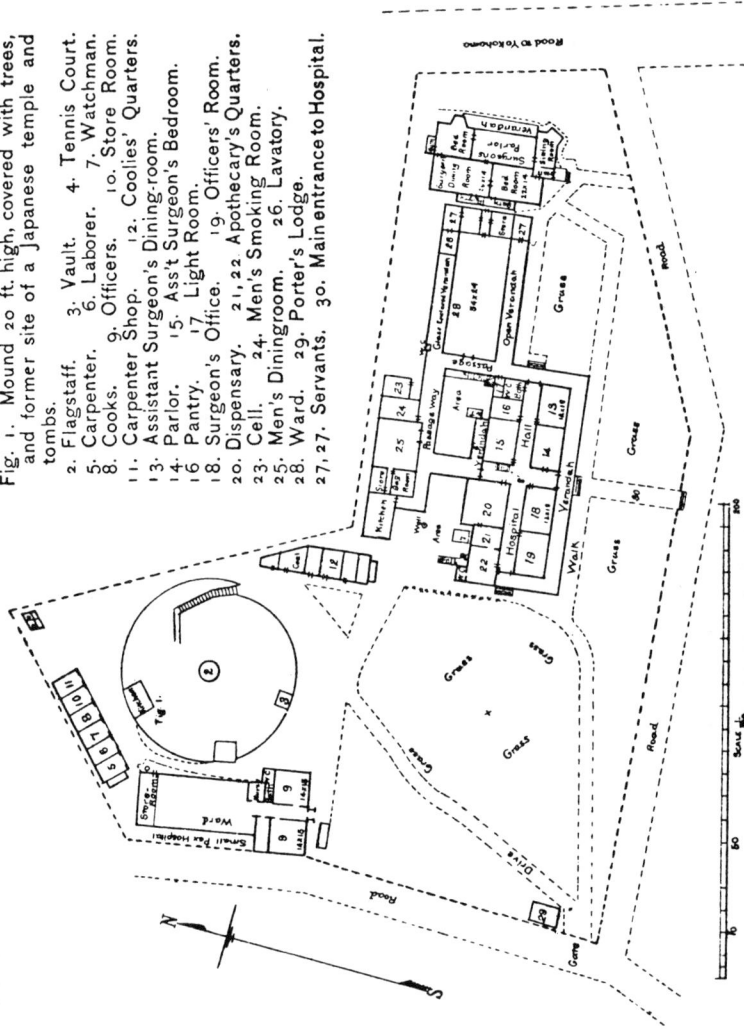

nehmster Weise ins Auge und allen denjenigen Männern, welche
thätig und erfolgreich an jener Entwickelung Theil genommen haben,
gebührt daher innigster Dank. Insbesondere auch unserm Herrn
Vorsitzenden, dem Surgeon John S. Billings, welcher mit einem
seltenen technischen und ärztlichen Scharfblick die Bedürfnisse für
Krankenanstalten nicht nur in klassischer Weise formulirt, sondern
auch die Erbauung solcher Musteranstalten energisch gefördert hat.

Seiner geehrten Aufforderung entspreche ich heute, wenn ich
einige Bemerkungen über Militärlazarethe vorzutragen mir erlaube,
wobei ich mich schon aus Rücksicht auf die zu Gebote stehende
Zeit im Allgemeinen nur auf die Verhältnisse in der Deutschen
Armee beziehen möchte.

Zwei wichtige Zahlen können als hygienischer Markstein aus der
Entwickelung des Deutschen bz. Preussischen Lazarethbauwesens
an die Spitze gestellt werden. Erstens die Zahl, welche den für den
einzelnen Kranken erforderlichen Luftraum bezeichnet und zweitens
die Zahl, welche als Massstab für die Grösse des Lazareths einer
Garnison zu Grunde gelegt werden soll,—die Normalkrankenzahl.

Im Jahre 1852 schrieb das Reglement für die Friedenslazarethe der
Preussischen Armee vor, dass jedem Kranken ein *Luftraum* von
450–540 Kubikfuss zu gewähren sei. Wer könnte heute noch eine
solche Zahl als Norm für ein Krankenhaus festsetzen? Das 3 und
4-fache derselben wird nicht nur verlangt, sondern gilt überall für
unerlässlich. So ist denn auch schon seit dem Jahre 1868 in der Preussischen Armee der Luftraum von 1200 Kubikfuss=37 Kubikmeter
für jeden Kranken Vorschrift. Die seit diesem Jahr in den mannig-
fachsten Lazarethen gemachten Beobachtungen haben die Ansicht
gereift, dass dieser Luftraum als ausreichend erachtet werden kann,
wenngleich zum Beispiel in den Isoiirpavillons, welche vorzugsweise
zur Unterbringung für ansteckende Kranke dienen sollen, nicht
selten über jenes Mass hinausgegangen wird. Die im Jahre 1891
herausgegebene Deutsche Friedens-Sanitäts-Ordnung enthält dem-
zufolge auch die Bestimmung, dass der normalmässige Luftraum für
jeden Kranken durchschnittlich 37 Kubikmeter betragen soll. Und
zwar sollen die mit horizontalen Decken versehene Krankenstuben
in der Regel eine Höhe von 4 bis 4.20 Meter erhalten. Für jedes
Bett ergiebt sich dann eine Grundfläche von 9 bis 9.5 Meter.

Was die Grösse der Stuben anbelangt, so sollen dieselben im
Krankenblock nicht mehr als zwölf, in Pavillons nicht mehr als 18
Betten erhalten. Neben diesen grossen Stuben sind in jedem Krank-

engebäude einige kleinere für 1 bis 3 Kranke eingerichtet. Der
Abstand der Betten von der Wand wird auf 0.5 bis 0.7 Meter, die
Zwischenweite auf 1 Meter, der Gang zwischen den Fussenden
zweier sich gegenüberstehenden Reihen Betten auf 2 bis 2.5 Meter
angenommen. Bei dieser Aufstellung ist vollkommen Platz zwischen
den Betten vorhanden, um den zu jedem Bett gehörigen Kranken-
tisch zu placiren und dem ärztlichen Personal und den Pflegern freie
Bewegung zu gestatten.

Es ist ja bekannt, dass die angegebenen Masse betreffs der Höhe
und der für jedes Bett zu gewährenden Bodenfläche in einer Reihe
von Krankenhäusern überschritten werden, aber es muss gerade für
Militärlazarethe daran festgehalten werden, nicht über das Noth-
wendige und Bewährte hinauszugehen. Ein Mass wie das in Preussen
übliche ist um so mehr ausreichend, als peinlich darauf gehalten wird,
dass alle unnöthigen Möbel wie Utensilienstücke und so weiter aus
den Krankenzimmern fern gehalten werden und die Betten niemals
mit Vorhängen versehen sind.

Der Fussboden der Krankenräume besteht in der Regel aus
einer Dielung von Kiefernholz, welche mit Oelfarbe gestrichen wird.
Doch findet sich der Holzfussboden oft und namentlich in den nicht
unterkellerten einstöckigen Pavillons durch einen Belag von hart-
gebrannten, glatten Thonplatten ersetzt, wobei zur Abhaltung der
Bodenfeuchtigkeit und Verminderung der Abkühlung eine Asphal-
tirung auf flachseitigem Ziegelpflaster oder eine Betonbettung erfolgt.
Auch Riemenfussboden in Asphalt verlegt findet vielfach Anwendung.

Dabei bleibt der Raum unter den Dielen hohl und wird einerseits
durch Schlitze in den Fussleisten mit der Stubenluft, andererseits
durch ein Thon- oder Metallrohr mit der Heizanlage in Verbindung
gesetzt.

Die Wände und Decken in den Krankenzimmern sind mit Oel-
oder Lackfarbe gestrichen und zwar die Wandflächen gewöhnlich
in graugrünlichem, die Decken in mattweissem Tone.

Die Fenster müssen möglichst hoch bis nahe an die Decke hinauf-
geführt werden, während die Höhe der Fensterbrüstung etwa 0.75
Meter beträgt. Sie sind meistens 1.2 Meter breit. Dabei gilt als
Vorschrift, dass die Mindestfläche für jedes Bett in den Krankenblocks 1.2 bis 1.5 Quadratmeter, in den Pavillons auf 1.8 bis 2.3
Quadratmeter ausmacht. Die Flügelthüren sollen eine Abmes-
sung von nicht weniger als 1.5 Meter in der Breite und 2.5 Meter

in der Höhe haben. Die Heizung der Krankenzimmer erfolgt fast durchweg durch Kachel- oder eiserne Oefen. Zentralheizung ist nur ausnahmsweise bei neuren Anlagen vorhanden. Ob es vorzuziehen sei, alle Krankenzimmer mit Zentralheizung zu erwärmen oder bei der Einzelheizung durch Oefen zu bleiben, ist oft Gegenstand eingehender Erwägungen gewesen. Bis jetzt hat man sich für die Einzeloefen entschieden, einerseits weil dieselben nach den jahrelangen Erfahrungen den Ansprüchen durchaus genügt haben, andererseits die laufenden Kosten für Kohlen und sonstiges Heizmaterial erheblich geringer sind. Die Oefen sind derartig eingerichtet, dass sie neben dem Heizzweck gleichzeitig der Ventilation dienen und sowohl zur Zuführung frischer Luft als zur Abführung verdorbener Luft ausgenutzt werden.

Ein besonderer Werth wird auf die Ventilationseinrichtungen gelegt, jedoch gleichzeitig grösste Einfachheit dabei beobachtet. Ein Luftwechsel von 60 Kubikmeter pro Bett und Stunde wird als angemessen erachtet und grundsätzlich angestrebt. Die Lüftungsanlagen zur Erreichung dieses Zieles sind verschieden je nachdem es sich um Krankensäle in einstöckigen Pavillons oder um Krankenstuben in Blocks handelt. Die Krankensäle der Pavillons erhalten eine Firstlüftung entweder durch eine Anzahl von Luftschlotten, welche an der untern Mündung eine stellbare Verschlussklappe und über Dach einen Saugkopf erhalten, oder auch durch einen Dachreiter, welcher seitlich durch bewegliche stellbare Klappen verschliessbar ist. Wenn neben dieser Vorrichtung die Fenster geöffnet und die in der untern Thürfüllung angebrachten durch Schieber verschliessbaren Schlitze benutzt werden, so kann man im Sommer einen ganz entsprechenden Luftaustausch bemerken. Für den Winter wird die frische Luft den Kranken durch einen Kanal zugeführt, welcher unter dem Fussboden verläuft und einerseits durch die Frontmauer hindurch nach aussen mündet, andererseits mit dem Raum zwischen Heizkörper und Ofenmantel in Verbindung steht. In der Regel sind zwei Oefen vorhanden, von denen der eine der Aspiration der andere der Circulation der Luft dient. Den Abzug der verdorbenen Luft bewirken Lüftungsrohre, welche von dem Fussboden der Stube beginnend neben den Rauchrohren befindlich und über Dach mit einem Saugkopf versehen sind.

In den Krankenstuben der Blocks sind Lüftungsrohre angebracht, welche zwei mit stellbarem Verschluss versehene Oeffnungen haben. Von diesen wird die obere, unter der Zimmerdecke befindliche für den Gebrauch im Sommer, die untere, dicht über den Fussboden befindliche für den Gebrauch im Winter, offen gehalten. Der Ofen saugt auch hier im Winter durch einen Kanal frische Luft an.

Einen wesentlichen Fortschritt gegen früher hat die Beleuchtung gemacht, insofern in einer grösseren Anzahl von Lazarethen elektrische Beleuchtung eingeführt ist. Bei allen Neubauten wird dieser Beleuchtungsart mit Recht den Vorzug gegeben. In den Krankenstuben sind Glühlichtflammen von 12–20 Kerzenstärke, auf den Höfen Bogenlicht in Gebrauch.

Ich habe diesen kurzen Ueberblick über die Haupteinrichtungen, welche für einen Krankenraum eines Militärlazareths in Betracht kommen, zusammengefasst, ohne bisher auf das eigentliche System, in welchem ein solches Lazareth zu erbauen ist, eingegangen zu sein.

Die Frage nach dem System hängt innig zusammen mit der zweiten oben als Markstein in der Entwickelung der Militärkrankenhäuser bezeichneten Zahl, mit der *Normalkrankenzahl* zusammen. Der Umfang eines Garnisonlazareths wird nach der Garnison-Kopfstärke und der zu erwartenden Krankenzahl derselben bemessen. In dem alten Lazareth-Reglement von 1852 wurden 6⅔ Prozent dieser Kopfstärke—also 15 von 100—als krank und der Lazarethpflege bedürftig angenommen und demgemäss zum Beispiel die Grösse eines Lazareths für eine Garnison von 4500 Mann auf 300 festgestellt.

Inzwischen haben sich die Mortalitätsverhältnisse ausserordentlich gebessert. Der Generalstabsarzt der Preussischen Armee, Seine Exzellenz von Cöler, dessen hohe Verdienste um das Armeesanitätswesen Ihnen bekannt sind, konnte in einer am Stiftungstage des medizinisch-chirurgischen Friedrich Wilhelms-Instituts in Berlin gehaltenen Rede als einen glänzenden Erfolg der auf die Verbesserung der Gesundheitsverhältnisse im Heere gerichteten, unermüdlichen und sachverständigen Bestrebungen hervorheben, dass „in dem 20-jährigen Zeitraum von 1868–1887 die Zahl der jährlichen Gesammterkrankungen in der Armee um 46 Prozent herabgesunken und die jährliche Sterbeziffer von 6.9 Prozent auf 3.2 Prozent sank, was eine Verminderung um 54 Prozent bedeutet. An Typhus hatte das Heer im Jahre 1868 einen Zugang von 10.9 auf 1000 der Kopfstärke, im Jahre 1887 nur 4.4, also um mehr als die Hälfte weniger, und der Verlust des Heeres durch Tod in Folge dieser Krankheit verringerte sich während dieses Zeitraumes in stetiger Abnahme von 2.1 Prozent auf 0.32 Prozent, also auf nahezu ⅐ der früheren Höhe.

Durch den geringen Krankenzugang sind im Jahre 1887 verglichen mit den entsprechenden Verhältnissen des Jahres 1868 allein 2,000,-000 Behandlungstage weniger erforderlich gewesen und, was vielmehr ins Gewicht fällt, die allmählich erzielte Verminderung der Sterbeziffer in der Armee bedeutet allein für das Jahr 1887 einen Gewinn von 1539 Mann, die in diesem Jahre dem Heere, dem Staate und ihrer Familie erhalten sind."

Diesen Ausführungen entspricht die höchst bemerkenswerthe Thatsache, dass die Normalkrankenzahl, das heisst, wie oben bemerkt, die Zahl der für den Bau eines Lazareths in Aussicht zu nehmenden Krankenzahl, von 6⅔ Prozent der Kopfstärke allmählich herabgesetzt werden konnte, so dass sie jetzt nur 4 Prozent der etatsmässigen Garnisonkopfstärke beträgt und in günstig gelegenen Garnisonen sogar auf 3½ Prozent sinkt. Um bei dem obigen Beispiel zu bleiben, werden also bei einer Kopfstärke von 4500 Mann—nicht mehr wie ehedem, für 300 Kranke, sondern nur für 180 Kranke Lazaretheinrichtungen zu treffen sein. Welche unendlichen Vortheile sich aus diesem Zahlenverhältniss ergeben, liegt auf der Hand. Es bedeutet—abgesehen von dem daraus für die Gesundheit der Truppen hervorleuchtenden günstigen Zeugniss—nicht nur eine ausserordentlich wichtige Ersparniss an Anlage- und Unterhaltungskapital, sondern auch eine erhebliche Entlastung des ärztlichen und Verwaltungs-Personals.

Es sei übrigens ausdrücklich bemerkt, dass diese Normalkrankenzahl bei der thatsächlichen Belegung der Lazarethe durchaus nicht immer erreicht wird, sondern dass ausreichend Räume zur Verfügung stehen, um einen steten Wechsel in der Belegung der einzelnen Krankenräume vorzunehmen. Ein solcher Wechsel ist ausdrücklich vorgeschrieben und muss auf einer in jedem Krankenzimmer hängenden Tafel durch Notirung über die Belegungszeiten ersichtlich gemacht werden. Auch ist eine vollständige Isolirung ansteckender Kranken bei der nach obigem Massstab festgesetzten Lazarethgrösse durchführbar.

Von der Grösse des zu erbauenden Lazareths hängt das System ab, nach welchem es errichtet werden soll. Wir unterscheiden Blocksystem und das Pavillonsystem.

Unter *Krankenblocks* verstehen wir, wie bekannt, Gebäude von einem oder mehreren Geschossen, in denen die miteinander nicht verbundenen Krankenstuben an einem gemeinschaftlichen Längsflur liegen, während wir als *Pavillons* Gebäude von einem Geschoss oder von zwei Geschossen mit grösseren die ganze Tiefe des Gebäudes einnehmenden, von einem Vorraum oder Mittelbau zugänglichen Krankensälen bezeichnen. Bei kleineren Lazarethen wird noch gelegentlich *ein* Krankenblock gebaut, in dessen unterem Geschoss die Verwaltungsräume liegen, doch wird auch für diese schon vielfach das System der eintstöckigen Pavillonbauten für die Krankenunterkunft gewählt und für die Verwaltung ein besonderes kleines Gebäude errichtet.

Für grössere Anlagen wird je nach dem klimatischen und sonstigen lokalen Verhältnissen entweder der Bau von zwei- und einstöckigen Pavillons in Verbindung mit Verwaltungsgebäuden oder das gemischte System, das heisst, theils Blocks theils Pavillons für die Krankenunterbringung gewählt. Als Beispiele für solche Bauten gemischten Systems darf ich aus neuester Zeit die Lazarethe in Mainz, Potsdam, Stettin nennen, während Ihnen ja aus früheren Jahren das Garnisonlazareth Tempelhof bei Berlin, welches immer noch als mustergültig dasteht, bekannt ist. Als Lazarethbau, welcher nur aus einstöckigen Pavillons besteht, sei das in neuester Zeit vollendete Lazareth in Strassburg angeführt.

Auf eine nähere Beschreibung der Anordnung und sonstigen Einrichtung der Gebäude, hier einzugehen, würde zu weit führen. Erwähnt sei aber, dass abgesehen von modernsten Wasch- und Kücheneinrichtungen, insbesondere die Einrichtung von Operationszimmern, sowie die Beschaffung von Desinfektionsapparaten und transportablen Lazarethbaracken eine grosse Berücksichtigung erfahren hat.

Für die Operationszimmer wird selbstredend verlangt, dass sie allen Ansprüchen, welche die anti- bz. aseptische Wundbehandlung erfordern, in vollstem Umfange entsprechen. In Folge dessen werden Fussboden und Wände aus glattem, undurchlässigen, leicht zu reinigenden Material hergestellt, alle zur Ablagerung von Keimen geeigneten Ecken und Vorsprünge vermieden und alles der peinlichsten Reinigung zugänglich gemacht. Die Ausstattung mit Operationstisch, Instrumentenschränken und so weiter erfolgt in demselben Sinne.

Die Desinfektionsapparate arbeiten mit strömendem gesättigten Wasserdampf von mindestens 100° C. und sind entweder mit einer für sonstige Zwecke schon im Lazareth vorhandenen Dampfmaschine in Verbindung gesetzt oder haben ihre eigenen Dampfentwickler. Es sind mit der Zeit eine ganze Anzahl von Fabriken mit der Anfertigung solcher Apparate hervorgetreten, die bekanntesten sind Rietschel und Henneberg in Berlin, Schimmel und Co., in Chemnitz, Budenberg in Dortmund, Schmidt in Weimar, Rohrbeck in Berlin und Andere. Die Apparate müssen so geräumig sein, dass Matratzen und grosse Packete von Kleidern, Wäsche und so weiter leicht darin Platz finden, und dass sie namentlich auch für die schnelle Desinfektion grösserer Mengen von Uniformstücken der Truppen brauchbar sind.

Transportable Lazarethbaracken, denen eine unschätzbare Wichtigkeit für die Militärkrankenpflege im Frieden und im Kriege beizulegen ist, sind in grossem Umfange für die Preussische Armee beschafft und haben sich ganz vortrefflich bewährt. Sie gewähren im Sommer und Winter den Kranken einen sehr angenehmen Aufenthalt und eignen sich in jeder Beziehung ausgezeichnet zur Krankenunterkunft. Sind sie schon bei stehenden Lazarethanlagen für gewöhnliche Verhältnisse zur Isolirung der Kranken von grossen Nutzen, so gewinnen sie zu Zeiten von Epidemien und zu Kriegszeiten eine ganz ausserordentliche Bedeutung. Sie sind überall hin schnell versendbar und leicht auch von ungeübten Händen aufstellbar, dabei sowohl für Krankenunterbringungs- als für Lazareth-Wirthschaftszwecke trefflich verwendbar. Beim Garnisonlazareth Tempelhof (Berlin) war vom Juli bis Ende Dezember 1891 eine vollständige Lazarethanlage aus transportablen Militärlazarethbaracken eingerichtet, mit Kranken belegt und dauernd in Betrieb gesetzt. Die dabei gewonnenen Erfahrungen waren glänzende und sprachen in jeder Beziehung für die Brauchbarkeit der Baracken. Eine kurze Beschreibung derselben ist in der Deutschen Friedens-Sanitäts-Ordnung von 1891 enthalten; ausführlicher und ausgehender finden sie sich in dem weltbekannten Werke „die transportable Lazarethbaracke von von Langenbeck, von Cöler und Werner" geschildert. Vielleicht trägt dieser Hinweis auch dazu bei, die Verbreitung und Verwendung transportabler Baracken in der Krankenpflege, namentlich auch seitens kleiner, pekuniär nicht sehr leistungsfähiger Gemeinden zu fördern. Ich möchte Ihre Geduld aber nicht länger in Anspruch nehmen. Wenngleich ich mir bewusst bin, wichtige Punkte für den Bau und die Einrichtung von Militärlazarethen nur ganz oberflächlich gestreift und viele ganz übergangen zu haben, darf ich doch der Besprechung eine weitere Ausdehnung nicht geben und nur noch zum Schlusse hervorheben, dass die Militärlazarethe in Deutschland unter dem Befehle und der Verwaltung

von Chefärzten stehen und sich unter diesem Befehle in erfreulich-
stem Zustande befinden. Nur der Arzt ist im Stande die Bedürfnisse
eines Krankenhauses voll zu würdigen und den ganzen Kranken-
hausdienst, der kein anderes Ziel kennt, als den Verwundeten und
Kranken die bestmöglichste Pflege zu sichern und ihrer baldigen
Genesung zuzuführen, fachgemäss zu leiten.

THE UNITED STATES MARINE HOSPITAL SERVICE.

BY GEORGE W. STONER, M. D., Surgeon, U. S. M. H. S.,

Baltimore, Maryland.

The Marine Hospital Service is not quite as old as the Declaration
of Independence, the adoption of the Constitution, or the establishment of the government of the United States, but it has already
reached a very respectable age and is fast approaching its cen-
tennial.

England had a marine hospital at an earlier date, the celebrated
Greenwich Hospital, but this was essentially a military institution,
established for the benefit of seamen of the Royal Navy. The marine
hospital service of the United States was established, or rather provision for its establishment was made by act of Congress approved
July 16, 1798. By this act Congress imposed a tax of twenty cents a
month on every seaman employed on foreign or coasting vessels of
the United States, and out of the moneys collected by authority of
this act, the President of the United States was authorized to furnish
temporary relief to sick and disabled seamen, the moneys to be
expended in the districts wherein collected. This, however, was
amended the following year, March 2, 1799, by an act authorizing
the expenditure of hospital money within any part of the State where
collected, or in the State next adjoining. An amendment was also
passed at this time extending the operations of the law so as to
include the officers and seamen of the navy.* The sentiment that
led up to the passage of the act establishing the marine hospital
service was forcibly expressed by the Boston Marine Society in a
petition as early as 1791; and in the House of Representatives,

---

* In the year 1811 separate hospitals were established for the navy.

November 19, 1792, in his speech on the improvement of commerce, the Hon. Mr. Williamson said:

"Wherever it is probable that sailors may be sick, there I would make provision for their support and comfort. Hospitals should be erected or lodgings hired, as the case may be, at every port of entry in the United States, for sick and infirm seamen, where they may be properly attended during their indispositions. The money to be collected at the several ports as hospital money should be expended at such port and no other place, under the care of such person as may be designated for that purpose. Let a small deduction be made from the wages of every seaman, to be paid at the several ports of entry for their use. I have mentioned a deduction from their wages, because this mode of raising money would probably be more acceptable, and because it is the most equitable tax that can be levied." *

Hospital treatment or its equivalent was given to sick and disabled seamen by the marine hospital service in Boston as early as 1799, the year following the establishment of the Service. The first marine hospital owned by the government, and established under the act of 1798, was located at Washington Point, Norfolk County, Virginia. It was purchased by the United States in 1800. Three years later, in 1803, a marine hospital was completed for the port of Boston. It was located at Charlestown on the Mystic river, an appropriation of fifteen thousand dollars having been made for the purpose by act of Congress approved May 3, 1802. By this act the money collected for the benefit of sick and disabled seamen was constituted a general fund; and provision was also made for the establishment of the marine hospital service at New Orleans (not then belonging to the United States). The following is the text:

"That the moneys heretofore collected in pursuance of the several acts for the relief of sick and disabled seamen, and at present unexpended, together with the moneys hereafter to be collected by authority of the before-mentioned acts, shall constitute a general fund, which the President of the United States shall use and employ as circumstances shall require, for the benefit and convenience of sick and disabled American seamen: *provided*, that the sum of fifteen thousand dollars be, and the same is hereby appropriated for the erection of an hospital in the district of Massachusetts."

Section 2. The President is authorized to cause such measures to be taken as, in his opinion, may be deemed expedient for providing

* Hamilton, *Appleton's Cyclopædia*, 1879.

convenient accommodations, medical assistance, necessary attendance and supplies for the relief of sick and disabled seamen of the United States who may be at or near the port of New Orleans, in case the same can be done with the assent of the government having jurisdiction over the port.

Section 3 required masters of boats, rafts, etc., going to New Orleans down the Mississippi to render true accounts of the number of persons employed on board, and imposed a tax of twenty cents a month for every person so employed, which sum the master was authorized to retain out of the wages of such person.

Section 4 authorized the President to appoint a director of the marine hospital at New Orleans.

Section 5 authorized the admission of sick foreign seamen into marine hospitals of the United States upon certain conditions, and fixed the rate of charge at seventy-five cents a day.

The following letters from American state papers quoted by Supervising Surgeon-General Hamilton, in a paper read at the annual meeting of the National Board of Steam Navigation, held at Cairo, Illinois, several years ago, also in his article in Appleton's Annual Cyclopædia, show, as he says, "the state of affairs which rendered action on the part of Congress necessary":

"NEW ORLEANS, *August* 10, 1801.

A great number of American citizens, especially seamen and boatmen from the Ohio, die here yearly for want of a hospital into which they might be put and taken care of; not that they are refused admittance into the Spanish Poor Hospital, but that building is by much too small for the purpose.

No public house of any reputation will take them in, and consequently they lie in their ships or boats or get into wretched cabins, in which they die miserably, after frequently subjecting the humane among their countrymen to much trouble and expense. Will not this be an object, sir, worthy the attention of the government of the United States? And might not a fund be easily established for the preservation of these poor people, by imposing a light tax upon every vessel and boat that comes in as well as upon every seaman and boatman? About two hundred vessels have entered here from sea during the twelve months past, and allowing eight men only to each, it makes 1600. Perhaps from 350 to 400 boats have come down from the Ohio, etc., during the same time, and allowing four men to each, it would make about an equal number of men. A small sum from each, added to something from every vessel and boat, would probably produce a capital equal to the exigency.

(Signed)   EVAN JONES."

E. M. Day, Esq., in a letter addressed to the Secretary of State, dated November 8, 1802, said: "It will readily occur to you, sir, that thousands of our fellow-citizens must soon be employed in navigating the ships and boats which must ever be used as the means of transporting these commodities (those of the western country) from one place to another. Now, sir, when we take into consideration the climate and the season of the year when this commerce must be carried on, the risk to our citizens must be multiplied in a high degree. It is well known that the western rivers cannot be conveniently navigated into the Mississippi until the breaking up of the frost in the spring of the year. It is then that the great river begins to rise, and it generally remains up until July. The great distance and unavoidable impediments naturally in the way always carry over these commercial transactions to so late a period as to leave the great bulk of those employed in them at or about New Orleans in the sickly season of the year, which in that low, flat, unhealthy southern climate is fatal in the extreme to the strong, robust constitutions of our western brethren; hence many of them fall victims to climate and disease, leaving families and friends at a great distance from them. The want of proper accommodations for sick and infirm seamen and boatmen at New Orleans is another very serious inconvenience our poorer class of fellow-citizens are much subjected to in that place. It is really pitiable to see such numbers of distressed objects as sometimes present themselves to view in the sickly months, who have been left to shift for themselves, after their employers have made their markets. Something like an hospital establishment, to be superintended by American physicians, would go a great way to alleviate the distresses of those useful men. I mentioned American physicians because our people are strongly prejudiced against those of the Spanish faculty; and generally not understanding the language, they derive little or no benefit from them."

The first U. S. marine hospital at New Orleans was not erected until a number of years later, but provision was made for the care of sick and disabled seamen in the local hospitals as early as 1804, and a physician appointed to look after their welfare, the same as had been done originally in Boston, and which is now (since the reorganization of the Service) the custom at the smaller ports of the country, that is to say where the Service is not large enough to warrant the assignment of a regular medical officer or the establishment of a station of the first class.

For a number of years after the establishment of the Service the expense had to be met out of the fund created by the tax upon seamen, and as the amount collected was not sufficient to meet the demands, restrictions were from time to time necessary to keep the expenditures within the available fund. Chronic and incurable cases were excluded from the benefits of the Service, and in no case was relief allowed for a longer period than four months.

Patients in some ports were cared for in local hospitals and were farmed out to the lowest bidders, and in places where there were no hospitals medical charges were restricted to twenty cents a day, with boarding, lodgings, nursing and washing at two dollars and fifty cents a week. For districts south of the Potomac an addition of twenty per cent was allowed. The hardships attending the life of seamen and the administration of the fund for the relief from this period were set forth by the late Supervising Surgeon-General Woodworth in the following language (Annual Report, 1872):

"It was claimed that the fund was to be considered as auxiliary to the provision made by the municipal authorities, rather than as a full compensation for the relief which was due to the wants of sick and disabled seamen. In view of the inadequacy of the fund, a more liberal ruling was impracticable. The administration of the fund on this principle worked the greatest hardships in the new cities and towns which sprang up on the banks of the western lakes and rivers, where few accommodations were to be had for the care of sick strangers left helpless upon their shores. Those who engaged in the commerce of the western rivers were subjected to climatic changes that were to them very pernicious. The numbers who perished in the long descending voyages of the flat-bottomed boats which left the upper waters of the Mississippi and its tributaries, in summer and early autumn, to find a market for the fruits of their toil, at New Orleans were very great. Nothing was more common than for two out of five hands who generally managed those boats to die, and it sometimes happened that the whole crew perished from disease and that the boat with its cargo was left deserted. The steamboats ascending the Mississippi and its tributaries brought up every year a great number of deck passengers, chiefly the sons of farmers returning from their flatboat voyages, many of whom died on board, while others were left on shore at the river towns helpless and among strangers. The cholera epidemic of 1832 and 1834 added greatly to the catalogue of their ills. Moved by a feeling of common humanity for the large class of our young men who had surrendered the endearments of a life spent at home, and united their fortunes with strangers by embarking in the more daring, precarious and toilsome interests of commerce—a pursuit, more than most others, beset with temptations to risk of health and life, to recklessness of character and insensibility to future wants,—sensible also of the sufferings attendant upon such an improvident life, whole communities, both on the seaboard and in the interior districts, petitioned Congress for additional appropriations and the enactment of laws providing increased facilities for the relief of this unfortunate class. From one port it was reported that no better place could be offered to sick seamen than the warehouses and the deserted tenements along the wharf; from another, that they had to be sent to the city almshouse, which was also connected with the penitentiary for common vagrants and petty convicts; and from another the sad story was told that seamen, sick with various diseases, cholera, smallpox, etc., were often forced promiscuously into the same chamber, where the dying and the dead were alike neglected."

Beginning in Boston in 1799, the Service was soon extended to the principal ports along the Atlantic coast, and gradually, as Congress made special appropriations for the same, marine hospital buildings were erected at other ports than those already named. The expenses attending the erection of the original hospitals at Norfolk and Boston were defrayed from the marine hospital fund (the tax collected from seamen for their relief when sick and disabled) in accordance with the law of 1798, which also provided "that when there should be a sufficient surplus after defraying the expenses of temporary relief to seamen, it should be used in erecting marine hospitals." This provision was made probably in view of another provision of the same act, which authorized the President to receive donations of personal property or real estate and which contemplated a surplus. During the earlier years of the Service there was occasionally a small surplus, more frequently a shortage; and as years went on the expenses were greatly increased, and entirely out of proportion to the increase of the collections, and Congress was called upon to make necessary appropriations to meet the difference. These appropriations varied in amounts from one thousand dollars to two hundred and seventy-five thousand dollars a year, and up to 1873, when the last appropriation was made, amounted to the sum of $4,830,994.34. The collections during the same period footed up the amount of $7,096,968.89, making a grand total of $11,927,963.23, while the expenditures were $11,639,-934.66, leaving at the close of the fiscal year 1873 a balance in favor of the fund amounting to $288,028.57.

In the year 1837 (act approved March 3, 1837) Congress appropriated seventy-five thousand dollars for the erection of a marine hospital in the city of New Orleans, and for the purchase of lands on which to erect said marine hospital.

The President was also authorized to select and cause to be purchased for the use and benefit of sick seamen, boatmen, and all other navigators on the western rivers and lakes, suitable sites for marine hospitals, *provided* that the number thereof shall not exceed for the Mississippi river three, for the Ohio three, and for Lake Erie one. By this same act the collection of hospital tax was suspended for one year, and instead of said tax the sum of one hundred and fifty thousand dollars was appropriated. A later act (August 29, 1842) confirmed the act of 1837 and authorized the purchase of sites for marine hospitals at Natchez, Miss., Napoleon, Ark., St. Louis, Mo., Paducah, Ky., Louisville, Ky., Pittsburg, Pa., Cleveland, Ohio. An appropriation for the erection of the first marine hospital in Chicago was made by act of Congress approved August 3, 1848, and was located on land adjacent to old Fort Dearborn. The second, the present hospital in Chicago, was erected under authority of act of Congress dated June 20, 1864, and located on the lake shore, about five miles north of the harbor. The land was not purchased, however, until 1867. The building was completed and ready for the reception of patients in 1873, and was pronounced "the finest structure of its kind in the country, far superior to the marine hospitals hitherto constructed." Before this building was completed, however, the Supervising Surgeon-General (the late Dr. Woodworth) "believed that one-fourth of the amount required to complete the building and fit it for occupation would have been sufficient to construct a hospital which would meet the wants of the Service equally well." He then evidently had in mind the pavilion which was subsequently adopted, and has been continued up to this time as the style of marine hospital construction. He was in "favor of constructing all the hospitals of wood, and destroying them after ten or fifteen years, both as a sanitary and an economical measure, and building new ones in their stead." Fire is no doubt the best and surest antiseptic, but in these days of medical progress less heroic measures answer every purpose, and if buildings are properly constructed, drained and ventilated, the torch need never be applied. The erection of the marine hospital at Detroit, Michigan, was authorized by an act of Congress dated August 4, 1854. This same act also made appropriations for the construction of marine hospitals at Burlington, Iowa, Pensacola, Fla., and for the second hospital at New Orleans. The marine hospital at Detroit is a three-story and basement solid brick building, constructed somewhat after the Mills style of architecture, except that the ground plan is in the shape of the letter T instead of H, and differs in this respect from all or nearly all other marine hospitals the plans of which were drawn by Robert Mills, architect, in the year 1837, and followed by the government, without material change, for a period of about thirty years, or until the construction of the imposing structure previously referred to designed by the late A. B. Mullet and located in this city (Chicago).

The marine hospital service on the Pacific coast was first established at San Francisco in 1851 (the contract system), and a U. S. marine hospital was in use at that port in 1854. It was large and well built, but was injured by an earthquake in 1868. The contract system was then resumed, and continued until the completion of the present pavilion hospital. Besides the places already named, hospitals were located before the reorganization of the Service at Mobile, Ala., Charleston, S. C., Portland, Me., Ocracoke, N. C., Evansville, Ind., Vicksburg, Miss., St. Marks, Fla., Burlington, Vt., Wilmington, N. C., Galena, Ill., and Port Angelas, Washington Territory. Most of these buildings were large, substantial structures, erected at great expense, and some of them were sold afterward at a great reduction, especially those built at places where they were not needed at all, as for example at Paducah, Ky., Burlington, Iowa, Galena, Illinois, and Burlington, Vermont. During the war of the Rebellion many of the marine hospitals north and south were used as military hospitals, and the hospitals at Norfolk and Boston were in similar use during the war of 1812.

The marine hospital service was reorganized in pursuance of an act of Congress approved June 29, 1870: "An Act to reorganize the Marine Hospital Service, and to provide for the relief of sick and disabled seamen. Be it enacted, etc.

" That from and after the first day of August, eighteen hundred and seventy, there shall be assessed and collected by the Collector of Customs at the ports of the United States, from masters or owners of every vessel of the United States arriving from a foreign port, or of registered vessels employed in the coasting trade, the sum of forty cents per month for each and every seaman who shall have been employed on said vessel since she was last entered at any port of the United States, which sum the said master or owner is hereby authorized to collect and retain from the wages of said employees." Section 4 of this act required that all moneys received or collected by virtue of this act shall be paid into the treasury like other public moneys, without abatement or reduction, and appropriated all moneys so received for the expense of the marine hospital service and to the credit of the marine hospital fund. Section 5.—That the fund thus obtained shall be employed under the direction of the Secretary of the Treasury, for the care and relief of sick and disabled seamen employed in registered, enrolled and licensed vessels of the United States. Section 6.—"And be it further enacted, that the Secretary of the Treasury is hereby authorized to appoint a surgeon to act as Supervising Surgeon of Marine Hospital Service, whose duty it shall be, under the direction of the Secretary, to supervise all matters connected with the marine hospital service, and with the disbursement of the fund provided by this act, at a salary not exceeding the rate of two thousand dollars per annum and his necessary traveling expenses, who shall be required to make monthly reports to the Secretary of the Treasury."

The office of Supervising Surgeon was first filled in April, 1871, by the appointment of Dr. John M. Woodworth, of Illinois. The work of reorganization was commenced at once, and had so far progressed by the end of the fiscal year 1872 that the Supervising Surgeon (Dr. Woodworth) in his annual report for that year was enabled to show a " marked increase in the facilities for affording relief, a considerable decrease in the per diem cost for the care of each patient," and an actual saving to the government of $56,819.31 as compared with the preceding year. In the original work of reorganization, or rather in anticipation of the law reorganizing the Service and before a supervising surgeon was appointed, the Secretary of the Treasury received valuable aid from Surgeon John S. Billings of the army (the distinguished chairman of this Section). Twelve thousand three hundred and two sick and disabled seamen were furnished hospital relief during the year 1872, and by a system of outdoor or dispensary relief inaugurated this year, eight hundred and fifty-four seamen were furnished medicine, making a total number of thirteen thousand one hundred and fifty-six. It need hardly be added that the Service soon became self-sustaining and that no appropriation was received or required after the year 1873, except for the erection of new hospital buildings. The work of reorganization had now fairly begun. Surgeons and assistant surgeons, after passing a satisfactory examination before a board of surgeons, were appointed by the Secretary of the Treasury on the recommendation of the supervising surgeon. Hospitals were divided into two classes, viz: Class 1. United States Marine Hospitals. Class 2. Local Hospitals, where seamen were received at rates authorized by the Department.

Provision was also made for the care of sick and disabled seamen at ports where there were no hospitals. One medical officer was assigned to duty at each hospital (Class 1) as surgeon in charge, and when an assistant surgeon was also assigned at the same station, one of the two was required to be on duty at the custom-house during business hours, to examine applicants for admission to hospital, to issue a permit if necessary, to prescribe for cases not requiring treatment in hospital, and at the same time to guard the Service against the irregularities and abuses which had formerly crept in and made the reorganization necessary. At the hospitals of Class 2 where the Service was large enough to warrant the assignment of a medical officer, his duties were essentially the same as if on duty at the custom-house office or dispensary of a station of Class 1; and he was also required to inspect the hospitals where seamen were admitted and to supervise all matters relating to the Service at the port. At the smaller ports the customs officer was authorized to provide for the care of sick seamen by arrangement with a local physician, or to furnish transportation to the nearest hospital where provision was made for relief. The surgeon in charge of a marine hospital was given authority over all officers and employes of the hospital, and he was empowered to enforce regulations for the management of the hospital, subject to the approval of the supervising surgeon. He was held responsible for the proper and economical administration of the hospital under his charge, and for the care and preservation of the building, furniture and stores, but he was not entitled to any stores (subsistence supplies) for himself. He was required (as he is now) to supply subsistence for himself and family, and household help. The steward and other employes were (as they are now) subsisted by the hospital. The compensation of all officers and employes of the Service (except the supervising surgeon, whose salary was fixed by act of Congress) was fixed by the Department.

Regulations covering the foregoing and all other requirements of the Service and duties of medical officers were issued in book form during the latter part of the year 1873, and these regulations have served as the basis and model upon which all subsequent regulations, made necessary by later acts of Congress or Department decisions, have been framed. Within three years after its reorganization the work of the Service began to attract attention from abroad. The London medical journals were profuse in their praise of this peculiarly American institution. The *Lancet* recommended that a "leaf be taken out of the book of the Marine Hospital Service of the United States," and remarked that "our transatlantic neighbors, ahead of us in many things, are most decidedly in advance of the old country in providing for the care of their sick sailors."

In the year 1875, just four years after the reorganization of the Service, Congress enacted (act approved March 3, 1875) that hereafter the salary of the Supervising Surgeon General of the United States Marine Hospital Service shall be paid out of the Marine Hospital Fund, at the rate of four thousand dollars a year, and the Supervising Surgeon-General shall be appointed by the President, by and with the advice and consent of the Senate. In another act approved the same day, provision was made for the care of seamen of foreign vessels at such rates and under such regulations as the Secretary of the Treasury may prescribe.

This act also provided for the increase of compensation before mentioned for the Supervising Surgeon-General. It was during this fiscal year, too, that the department issued the first circular letter to United States officers defining their duties with reference to quarantine and public health. The medical officers of the marine hospital service were especially directed to inform themselves fully as to the local health laws, and regulations based thereon, and in force at their respective ports and stations; and strict compliance with such laws, and prompt assistance in the enforcement of the same, when requested by competent authority, were enjoined. The quarantine law under which these instructions were issued was passed as far back as 1799 (R. S. 4792). It was during the year 1875 also that the first marine hospital of the pavilion style of architecture was opened. This hospital is located in San Francisco and is now in active operation. Similar hospitals have since been built and are in use at New Orleans, La., Memphis, Tenn., Cincinnati, Ohio, St. Louis, Mo., Cairo, Ill., Baltimore, Md., and Evansville, Ind.

Hospitals of the older or block style are still in use at Boston, Mass., Portland, Me., Louisville, Ky., Wilmington, N. C., Mobile, Ala., Cleveland, Ohio, and Detroit, Mich. The present hospital at New York (leased from the Marine Society) is also an old-style building. Some of the old block hospitals have bad histories, but they are now, thanks to improved plumbing and better administration, in good sanitary condition, and the results of treatment, medical and surgical, compare very favorably with the best results in the pavilion hospitals.

The sanitary condition of the old hospital at Detroit, for example, was so bad only a few years ago that the medical officer then in charge recommended that permission be granted to admit and treat all surgical cases in one of the local hospitals or in rented rooms, so as to avoid the invariable complication of erysipelas. Suffice it to say that for the last four years not a single case of contagious or infectious disease or wound infection of any kind originated in this hospital, while more surgical operations have been done than ever before. And this is practically the report of improvement at all the older hospitals where modern methods prevail and "the next thing to godliness" is the rule.

It is not the purpose of this paper to discuss the general question of hospital construction, nor by any means to discourage the erection of pavilion marine hospitals. The pavilion plan is probably the best, all things considered, that has yet been devised. But if the older style hospitals were as bad to-day as they were reported to be when the pavilion was introduced, they should be destroyed forthwith. As a matter of fact they are not so bad, and, as before intimated, results considered, they must now be pronounced good.

Differences of opinion as regards the relative merits of different style hospitals are to be expected. Surgeon John Vansant, who has had extensive experience in hospital work, expressed his views a number of years ago as follows : *

"I have to say that I was once a strong advocate of the pavilion plan for all hospitals, but I have now modified my views, though I have not positively decided what other plan I would substitute for the pavilion. In time of war the pavilion plan is undoubtedly the best, for then there are as many nurses and other attendants, as well as officers, money and supplies of all sorts, as can be wished for; but in times of peace, and for a civil hospital, I think the pavilion plan

*Annual Report M. H. S. 1883.

is more expensive and more difficult to administer. It would also be less comfortable in a cold climate or in winter, and on the score of healthfulness or ventilation, etc. I doubt if it has any advantages over a two- or three-story hospital. I think as a general thing the wards of our hospitals are too large; I prefer a greater number of smaller rooms."

A few days ago I addressed a letter to Surgeon Henry W. Sawtelle, of the United States marine hospital service, requesting his opinion on the merits of pavilion hospitals as compared with the block style of marine hospitals. The following is a copy of his remarks sent to me by return mail:

"As hospitals are for the care and treatment of the sick and wounded, the merits of the various hospitals should be decided upon the results of treatment as shown by their records, assuming, of course, that the administration and care of the hospitals have been careful and efficient. Unfortunately I have no such data at hand, and I shall therefore content myself by giving my views based upon experience at the different hospitals, without reference to statistics. I have served at one pavilion hospital, the one at San Francisco, and at several of the older or block style, namely, St. Louis, New York, Detroit, Portland, Me., and Boston. Ventilation for these hospitals is obtained mainly through the windows and doors, and the appointments generally are below the standard of requirements of hospital buildings according to modern ideas. From these remarks it will be seen that both styles are open for improvement. In regard to the old hospitals of the Service, their bad histories are matters of record —outbreaks of erysipelas, gangrene and pyæmia were frequent prior to the reorganization of the Service in 1871, and for some time thereafter. Such a record was undoubtedly due very largely to the fact that for many years the marine hospital service had been under the control of politicians, and political doctors, who happened to be friends of the collectors of customs, or political allies of sufficient importance to attract the attention of the appointing power, were the medical heads of the hospitals, who paid but little attention, comparatively, to their duties, while the collectors of customs were the custodians of the hospital buildings, and all matters pertaining to the service passed through their hands for approval or disapproval. It is not wonderful then, considering such a history, that at the date of reorganization in 1871 the marine hospitals throughout the country which were of the block plan were found to be in such an infected condition that the result of treatment was unsatisfactory and the percentage of deaths large. Cleaning up old hospitals means prevention of disease in the same sense that proper environment and personal cleanliness mean prevention of cholera. Hence it will be understood that after a general cleaning and repairing of the old hospitals, it was observed by the medical officers that the success attending their treatment of patients increased correspondingly. After about twenty years service in these hospitals, including three and one-half years at the San Francisco hospital, which, as before stated, is of the pavilion plan, my experience in relation to the success of treatment of patients in the old-style hospitals as compared with the pavilion hospital is about the same. For example, at the Boston hospital, which was built in 1859 and which has a bad history, not a case of erysipelas has developed in the wards during the past two years, and no complications have succeeded surgical operations. Primary union after operations is a common occurrence, and I may say that the same is true at other hospitals of similar design where I have served. No greater success was observed at the pavilion hospital. In conclusion I may say that for economical reasons and convenience of management I am in favor of pavilion hospitals for the Service, though I am free to admit that, in case expense is no object, hospitals constructed on the block plan and provided with proper ventilation and all modern appointments, would meet all the requirements for the successful treatment of the sick and injured in as large a measure as upon any other plan."

Supervising Surgeon-General John M. Woodworth, who had been chief officer of the Service from its reorganization, died in the month of March, 1878, and Surgeon John B. Hamilton, who had been ordered to Washington for temporary duty in charge of the bureau during the illness of the chief officer, was soon thereafter appointed by President Hayes to the office made vacant by the death of Dr. Woodworth.

In 1879 the regulations governing the Service were revised. Several of the provisions contained in the original regulations of Oct. 1, 1873, had since the latter date been repealed or modified by circular, etc., and new paragraphs were added in conformity with the law passed in 1875.

During the year 1878 a law was passed establishing a national quarantine, and the Supervising Surgeon-General of the marine hospital service, under the Secretary of the Treasury, was empowered to frame regulations governing quarantine, but no appropriation was made to carry the act into effect. During the same year the terrible epidemic of yellow fever occurred in the Mississipi Valley, and in February following, Congress passed another law (act approved Feb. 3, 1879) establishing a National Board of Health. The latter act embodied all the essential provisions of the former, but changed the executive authority by substituting a board (national board) composed of seven members, and carried with it a large appropriation. The act of 1879 was limited to a period of four years, and upon its expiration the law of 1878 was revived, and became operative by means of the contingent fund appropriated by Congress to be expended by the President of the United States, in his discretion, in preventing the spread of epidemic disease and in maintaining quarantines at points of danger. This discretion was used by the President as above indicated, and the work contemplated by the appropriation act was performed through the agency of the marine hospital service, in aid of State and local boards of health, and in accordance with the act of April 29, 1878.

It is hardly necessary to add that the precedent thus established has been followed up to this time, or until the passage of the recent act (approved February 15, 1893) granting additional quarantine powers, and imposing additional duties upon the marine hospital service.

In thus briefly reviewing the history of the national quarantine service, and the provisions contained in the several acts, the remarks of the late Supervising Surgeon-General Woodworth must not be forgotten. After reading a paper before the International Medical Congress in Philadelphia in 1876 (two years before the enactment of the law of 1878), he said : " From what has preceded, the following conclusions seem to be justified : 1. The supervision of ocean travel ought to be directed to securing good sanitary conditions for vessels at all times, out of as well as in port. 2. A system of port sanitation should be adopted and administered for each country or place separately, and should be modified in particular cases by taking into account the liability of the port to infection, the period of incubation of the disease, the length of time consumed in the voyage, and the measures enforced by the vessel *en route*. 3. In some countries the detention of passengers and crews of ships hailing from infected ports is warranted, but for such time only as is necessary to complete the period of incubation of cholera or of yellow fever, counting from the date of departure from an infected port or of landing from an infected vessel; in no instance should passengers or sailors be held for observation on board an infected vessel, and such vessel should not be detained beyond the period required for inspection and for thorough disinfection and cleansing. 4. Recognizing the fact that the morbific causes of infectious diseases may sometimes elude the most vigilant sanitary supervision of shipping, the importance of wisely directed internal sanitary measures can scarcely be overestimated. 5. As far as America is concerned, it is desirable that prompt and authoritative information should be had of the shipment of passengers or goods from districts infected with cholera or yellow fever, thereby insuring the thorough disinfection of infected articles. 6. The endemic homes of cholera and yellow fever are the fields which give the greatest promise of satisfactory results to well directed and energetic sanitary measures, and to this end an international sentiment should be awakened, so strong as to compel the careless and offending people to employ rational means of prevention."

These views of Dr. Woodworth were recognized in the act of 1878. In fact the said act is sometimes called the Woodworth law. But as before indicated, the law of 1879 changed the executive authority from the Supervising Surgeon-General to the National Board. Under these laws national quarantine stations were established at several points on the Atlantic coast, and inspection stations at various times, when necessary, were maintained at points of danger on the frontier. Sanitary inspectors were also stationed at Havana and Vera Cruz to give prompt notification relative to the sailing of vessels bound for the United States, so as to aid in the prevention of the introduction of yellow fever.

At London and Liverpool inspectors were appointed to give timely information of the shipment of Egyptian rags or any other articles sent through those ports from infected localities. Inspectors were also appointed at the principal European ports to inspect vessels and emigrants bound for the United States.

In 1885 the regulations of the marine hospital service were again revised. A section for the government of national quarantine was added, and the whole was approved by the Secretary of the Treasury and by the President of the United States. In January, 1886, Supervising Surgeon-General Hamilton resumed the publication of the Weekly Abstract of Sanitary Reports, as required by the act of 1878. During the same year or the year preceding, he recommended that the national quarantine stations "be made permanent, and that they be equipped with all the necessary appliances known to modern sanitary science for the treatment of infected vessels and their cargoes, so that not only may immunity from the importation of contagious diseases be secured at those stations, but such security be had with the least possible obstruction to commerce." In 1887 he recommended the establishment of a station on the Pacific coast. In 1888 a law was passed (approved August 1) making the national quarantines on the Atlantic and Gulf coasts permanent institutions, and providing for the establishment of three stations on the Pacific coast.* An appropriation of five hundred thousand dollars was made to carry out the purpose of this act. In 1890 an act was passed to prevent the introduction of contagious diseases from one State to another and for the punishment of certain offenses.

In June, 1891, Supervising Surgeon-General John B. Hamilton, under whose administration of the marine hospital service all the national quarantine work up to date had been performed (except during the active period of the national board of health) resigned his commission as Supervising Surgeon-General, and Surgeon Walter Wyman, then on duty in the bureau as chief of purveying and quarantine division, was appointed by President Harrison to be Supervising Surgeon-General in place of John B. Hamilton, resigned. Dr. Hamilton was at the same time and by his own request reappointed by the President to be a surgeon in the marine hospital service, and assigned to duty at Chicago, Ill.

The latest and most comprehensive legislation affecting the marine hospital service, and of course through it the national quarantine service and the country at large, is contained in the act (approved February 15, 1893) granting additional quarantine powers and imposing additional duties upon the marine hospital service. Under the provisions of sections 2, 3 and 4 of this act, medical officers of the marine hospital service have been detailed to serve, and are now on duty, in association with the consuls at various foreign ports, and from them all necessary information is received relative to the sanitary condition of vessels, cargo, crew and passengers about to depart for the United States. By this means the

---

* National Maritime Quarantines are located at North Chandeleur Island, La.; Tortugas Islands, Fla.; Blackbeard's Island, Ga.; Cape Charles, Va.; Delaware Breakwater, Del.; Reedy Island, Delaware River ; Port Townsend, Washington ; San Francisco and San Diego, California.

ordinary consular bill of health is made to be a certificate of actual observation by a responsible officer whose sole duty is to aid in the prevention of the introduction of contagious disease into the United States.

New quarantine regulations have been framed by a board of surgeons under the direction of Supervising Surgeon-General Wyman, who convened the board for the purpose, and the said regulations have been promulgated by the Secretary of the Treasury. A very large appropriation is now available, and the Supervising Surgeon-General, under the direction of the Secretary of the Treasury, is making extensive improvements at all stations and in various ways increasing the efficiency of the Service. At New York, Boston and New Orleans the maritime quarantines are owned and operated by the state or municipality, but the law requires the Supervising Surgeon-General, under the direction of the Secretary of the Treasury, to co-operate with and aid state and municipal boards of health in the execution and enforcement of the rules and regulations of such boards, and in the execution and enforcement of the rules and regulations made by the Secretary of the Treasury to prevent the introduction of contagious or infectious disease into the United States; . . . . and also requires that all rules and regulations made by the Secretary shall operate uniformly and in no manner discriminate against any port or place; . . . . and at such ports and places within the United States where quarantine regulations exist under the authority of the state or municipality which in the opinion of the Secretary of the Treasury are not sufficient to prevent the introduction of such diseases into the United States, the Secretary shall, if in his judgment it is necessary and proper, make such additional rules and regulations as are necessary, ... but if the State or municipal authorities shall fail or refuse to enforce said rules and regulations, the President shall execute and enforce the same, ... and may detail or appoint officers for that purpose."

It is to be hoped that the relations between the national and the State quarantine will always remain within the bounds of co-operation and aid, and that both may strive how best to work and agree, until such time as the combined efforts may result in better understanding, and above all, in the accomplishment of the objects sought to be accomplished by modern quarantine. An observance of the minimum requirements of the regulations will be a sufficient guard against any conflict of authority.

Medical officers of the marine hospital service are also under the laws of March 3, 1891 and March 3, 1893, required to serve as medical inspectors in the immigration service. The proper performance of this duty must also of necessity result in valuable aid to public health.

From the foregoing compilations and remarks it will be observed that the marine hospital service covers a large field. The Service proper is a peculiarly American institution. It was originally established and is at present maintained for the benefit of the sailors of the mercantile marine. From its beginning in 1798 until 1884 every seaman employed on a vessel of the United States contributed to its support by the payment of a small tax, at first at the rate of twenty cents a month, and later forty cents a month while actually employed. In 1884 by an act of Congress the hospital tax was abolished, and in its stead the tonnage tax received from foreign vessels was made available for the ordinary expense of the Service (for the care and treatment of sick and disabled American seamen). In addition to the treatment in hospital a system of outdoor or dispensary relief was inaugurated when the Service was reorganized, and this has gradually increased year after year until there are now about forty thousand cases furnished outdoor relief annually, while the hospital cases number about sixteen thousand. During the year 1892 there were 37,588 of the former and 16,022 of the latter.

The physical examination of candidates for appointment in the revenue cutter service, and of officers for promotion in that service, is made by medical officers of the marine hospital service. Applicants for employment as keeper or surfman in the United States life saving service are also examined as to their physical condition and, if appointed, instructed in methods for the resuscitation of the apparently drowned. Pilots must also pass an examination before a medical officer of the marine hospital service as to their ability to distinguish the colored lights used at sea.

The regular corps of the United States Marine Hospital Service consists of the Supervising Surgeon-General, surgeons, passed assistant surgeons, acting assistant surgeons, hospital stewards and hospital attendants. The Supervising Surgeon was made a commissioned officer in 1875 and the title of his office was changed to Supervising Surgeon-General. In 1889 statutory provision was made for the appointment of all subordinate medical officers, the requirements being essentially the same as had previously governed by regulation and under which an average of about eighty percent of the applicants had been rejected. The following is the text:

"Medical officers of the Marine Hospital Service of the United States shall hereafter be appointed by the President by and with the advice and consent of the Senate; and no person shall be so appointed until after passing a satisfactory examination in the several branches of medicine, surgery and hygiene, before a board of medical officers of the said Service. Said examination shall be conducted according to rules prepared by the Supervising Surgeon-General and approved by the Secretary of the Treasury and the President. Section 2.— That original appointments in the service shall be made to the rank of assistant surgeon; and no officer shall be promoted to the rank of passed assistant surgeon until after four years service and a second examination as aforesaid, and no passed assistant surgeon shall be promoted to be surgeon until after due examination: provided that nothing in this act shall be so construed as to affect the rank or promotion of any officer originally appointed before the adoption of the regulations of 1879; and the President is authorized to nominate for confirmation the officers in the Service on the date of the passage of this act."

Medical officers are subject to change of station as the exigencies of the Service may require, and are not allowed to remain at any one station for a longer period than four years, unless specially authorized by the Department.

Acting assistant surgeons are appointed by the Secretary of the Treasury upon the recommendation of the Supervising Surgeon-General. They are are not usually subject to change of station. Hospital stewards are appointed to the general service by the Secretary of the Treasury, after passing a satisfactory examination before a medical officer of the Service. Hospital attendants are employed by the medical officer in charge of a station subject to approval of the Department. The different details for attendants are engineer, fireman, cooks, nurses, watchmen, night nurse, ambulance driver, gardener, launderer or laundress, and general service men in dining-room and about buildings and grounds, and dispensary attendant. The marine hospital office or dispensary is usually located in or near the custom-house. Medical officers are required to visit patients in hospital at least once a day, and oftener if necessary, to make a general inspection at least once a week, and to supervise all matters pertaining to the service of the station of which they are in command.

At the larger stations two or more medical officers are usually on duty; at the smaller hospital stations only one. And at stations where there are no hospitals belonging to the government, but where the service is large enough to warrant it, one medical officer is assigned to duty and placed in charge of all Service matters at the port. At the still smaller stations acting assistant surgeons are appointed; they are also sometimes designated sanitary inspectors, if required for duty of that kind, and occasionally when additional medical services are needed and eligible candidates are not available for appointment as assistant surgeons, acting assistants are appointed temporarily to assist the medical officer at a station. Internes are appointed by the medical officer subject to approval of the Department. The latest regulations governing the marine hospital service proper were issued in 1889. New regulations for the government of national quarantine stations have been issued since the passage of the law and are now in active operation.

The Supervising Surgeon-General's office is a bureau of the Treasury Department. It is located in Washington, D. C., at present in the Butler Building on Capitol Hill. The officers and employees now on duty in the bureau are the Supervising Surgeon-General, two surgeons (one detailed as chief of the purveying division, and one chief of the quarantine division), two passed-assistant surgeons (one in charge of the bacteriological laboratory, and one as executive officer or acting chief clerk), one assistant surgeon, assigned to duty on the Weekly Abstract of Sanitary Reports, one chemist, and the necessary clerks, messengers and laborers. The medical officers in the bureau are detailed from the corps by the Supervising Surgeon-General, and are subject to orders the same as if on duty at any other station.

The writer served as chief of the purveying and quarantine division from January 1885 to November 26, 1888.

DISCUSSION.

THE CHAIRMAN.—We are very much obliged to Dr. Stoner for his paper. I am somewhat familiar with the history of the Marine Hospital Service in recent days, because I once had occasion, as Dr. Stoner states, to look into the subject, having reported for special duty to the Secretary of the Treasury in 1869 or 1870, and inspected almost every marine hospital in the United States. I recommended the appointment of a special supervising medical officer and the giving him full power. The condition of affairs at that time was very bad; there was dishonesty in a number of the hospitals, and there were only one or two that were in good condition. The result was that a new law was passed and a medical officer, Dr. Woodworth, appointed, a very excellent appointment. The regulations that have been made (Dr. Woodworth on his death being succeeded by Dr. Hamilton, and he on his resignation by Dr. Wyman) have, I believe, resulted in bringing the Service into a very excellent condition; the hospitals that they manage themselves being in good order, and a very careful scrutiny of the hospitals in which the patients are treated by contract being maintained. As Dr. Stoner remarks, it is purely an American institution; there is nothing like it precisely in any European country, and our foreign friends find it hard to understand, because they are always getting it mixed up with the naval service. I am very glad that we shall have this paper published in the proceedings of this congress, as it will give many persons a more definite notion of the scope and purpose of this Service than they at present have.

HOSPITAL CONSTRUCTION ILLUSTRATED BY STEREOPTICON VIEWS.

BY L. S. PILCHER, M. D.,

Brooklyn, N. Y.

DR. PILCHER.—"I would like to say at the outset that the object of the present demonstration has been in connection with essays and discussions upon ideal hospitals, to present views of existing institutions, with their defects and limitations, with their advantages and lessons.

Slides for this purpose have been solicited by the committee from various sources, but the failure of many hospital superintendents to co-operate limits the views which we shall present this afternoon to the Johns Hopkins Hospital, Baltimore, the Boston City Hospital, and to the institutions of New York and Brooklyn.

Thanks are due to Dr. Hurd, to Dr. Rowe, and Mr. A. R. Pardington, and especially to Dr. H. P. DeForest, of Brooklyn, to whose skill and interest are due a great many of the slides that are to be exhibited.

It is safe to say that an appreciation of the requirements of adequate hygiene in the construction of a hospital is a thing of the last half of the present century. I propose to first present a series of institutions illustrative in some measure of the progressive development of hygienic hospital construction."

The speaker then presented several views of Bellevue Hospital, New York, the eastern façade, the floor plan of the hospital, exterior and interior views of the Sturges ward, Townsend ward, various pavilions and tents, and the morgue; showing the gradual growth of the hospital since it was first constructed, and illustrating the many defects in its construction. Kings County Hospital was then illustrated, the interior and exterior, also views of the various wards and pavilions. The Brooklyn Hospital was next shown, illustrating the old style of ward, with windows on one side only. The other hospitals of New York and Brooklyn illustrated were Long Island College Hospital, St. Vincent's Hospital, St. Peter's Hospital, St. Luke's Hospital, The Norwegian Deaconesses' Hospital, Mt. Sinai Hospital, the New York Hospital, New York Cancer Hospital, Roosevelt Hospital (this hospital being very fully illustrated and being referred to by the speaker as the first hospital in New York City answering the full requirements for isolated pavilion wards), and the Presbyterian Hospital, the most recently planned and built hospital in New York City.

The speaker also presented several views of the Johns Hopkins Hospital, Baltimore, a series of views of the Methodist Episcopal Hospital, Brooklyn, and of the Boston City Hospital.

DETENTION HOSPITALS FOR THE INSANE.

By Matthew D. Field, M. D., New York,

Examiner in Lunacy.

It was my privilege, in the summer of 1892, to read a paper before the American Social Science Association, on the "Examination and Commitment of the Public Insane in New York City." The discussion and comment called forth by this paper showed the almost total absence in this country of reception hospitals for the insane while under observation and examination to determine their mental condition and the propriety of commitment to some institution for treatment. It was related by members from various sections of the union how the unfortunate individuals of both sexes, who were apprehended by the authorities as insane, were sent to prisons and county jails, there to remain in contact with vagrants, tramps and criminals, to await the appointment of physicians to make examinations regarding their sanity. During this detention they received little or no medical treatment for the relief of their condition, but on the contrary, their surroundings and companions were about the worst possible for persons in their state, omitting to say anything of the moral effect on very many, and the great wrong perpetrated upon sick persons, by associating them with criminals and allowing them only the same quarters, food and care that the liberality of county officials bestows on tramps and vagabonds.

The evolution of the reception pavilion for the insane at Bellevue Hospital, and the present system of care and the examination and commitment of the public insane, are of some interest; they grew out of the lunacy legislation of 1874.*

* *Acts of* 1874, *Chapter* 446.

Section 1. No person shall be committed to or confined as a patient in any asylum, public or private, or in any institution, home or retreat for the care and treatment of the insane, except upon the certificate of two physicians, under oath, setting forth the insanity of such person. But no person shall be held in confinement in any such asylum for more than five days, unless within that time such certificate be approved by a judge or justice of a court of record of the county or district in which the alleged lunatic resides; and said judge or justice may institute inquiry and take proofs as to any alleged lunacy before approving or disapproving of such certificate, and said judge or justice may, in his discretion, call a jury in each case to determine the question of lunacy.

Section 2. It shall not be lawful for any physician to certify to the insanity of any person for the purpose of securing his commitment to an asylum, unless said physician be of reputable character, a graduate of some incorporated medical college, a permanent resident of the State, and shall have been in the actual practice of his profession for at least three years. And such qualifications shall be certified to by a judge of any court of record. No certificate of insanity shall be made except after a personal examination of the party alleged to be insane, and according to forms prescribed by the State Commissioner in Lunacy (with the State Commission in Lunacy); and every such certificate shall bear date of not more than ten days prior to such commitment.

Section 3. It shall not be lawful for any physician to certify to the insanity of any person for the purpose of committing him to an asylum of which the said physician is either the superintendent, proprietor, an officer, or a regular professional attendant therein.

The Commissioners of Public Charities and Correction of New York City, under this law, appointed special examiners in lunacy, whose duty it should be to examine all cases that should come under the care of the department, and in proper cases to make certificates of lunacy and present the same for approval before a judge of a court of record, as required by the law ; after which the adjudged lunatic was sent with such certificate to the insane asylum of the department. Such method has continued till the present day, except that formerly the chief examiner held the position of city physician, and had charge, likewise, of the city prison. Such was the condition of affairs when I was appointed examiner in lunacy for the Department of Public Charities and Correction in November, 1882, my senior being Dr. William I. Hardy, the prison physician. Within the year Dr. Hardy was relieved of all duties in the department save those of examiner in lunacy, and our joint functions became and have continued independent. Upon the death of Dr. Hardy in April, 1886, my present associate, Dr. Allen Fitch, was appointed.

In the earlier days there was no special place for the reception of the alleged lunatic, and he was examined where he might be, in prison or hospital. Then all the suspected insane were sent to Bellevue Hospital and placed in the "cells." These were two wards in the basement of the building, one for males and the other for females. In these wards were received not only the supposed lunatics, but all alcoholic, violently delirious and refractory patients of the hospital ; and frequently criminal patients were sent there, too, for safe-keeping. I remember well visiting the "cells" as an interne of the hospital when all these classes were received. I was called as a surgeon to see a wretched woman, who had received a fracture of the arm in a drunken brawl, and who had been committed there as an alcoholic. It was at night, and the light was dim, and a little child, scarcely more than three years of age, was clinging to the skirts of her mother, who was sodden with liquor. As I examined the arm of the drunken mother, the beautiful, innocent, pleading face looked up to me for mercy for her mother ; and I could not but be gentle with her for the child's sake. I thought if the mother would only look upon the child with but a tenth part of that humanity and sympathy with which the child looked up to me, what a different aspect the case would assume. While this was taking place I could hear the shrieks of fear on all sides from those in delirium of alcohol, by which the disturbed lunatic was continually excited.

The Commissioners of Public Charities and Correction had recognized the necessity of separating the insane from the alcoholic; and their persistent application had obtained an appropriation for the erection of a separate pavilion for the reception of the supposed insane. The year 1879 saw the completion of the present reception pavilion for the insane at Bellevue Hospital. It was erected in the grounds of the hospital, and is a one-story brick building, divided by iron doors into two wards, one for males and one for females. Each side has a corridor, lighted and ventilated from above, containing eight rooms for patients, besides an examination room (which contains record and history books, and a medicine and instrument chest), a kitchen, where not only food is received for the ward from the general kitchen of the hospital, but special diet is prepared as the resident physician may direct, the carving is also done, and all dangerous knives are kept. One room is set apart as a linen closet, where the bedding and necessary clothing are kept for patients. There is also a lavatory, bath-room, and closets, removed from the ward by a passage ventilated and lighted by windows on either side, as well as by windows on either side of the closets. The cells were and still are under the care of the house staff, the medical staff dividing the service in looking after the cells. When the pavilion was first established it was placed under the same care; the house physician, having the supervision of the cells also had the care of the insane admitted to the pavilion. The examiners then only passed on the mental condition and the propriety of commitment or discharge; the treatment of the patient while in the pavilion rested with the house physician, who had no special training in the care of the insane, and who had already sufficient work to care for his patients in his regular service, where his interest and heart really were. The oversight of the alcoholic and insane patients was an extra and entirely secondary duty of a busy physician. Soon after my appointment in November, 1882, Dr. Henry V. Wildman, who had had several years' experience as assistant physician at the asylum on Ward's Island, was appointed resident physician at Bellevue Hospital, in charge of the pavilion for the insane. He resigned in October, 1887, and was succeeded by Dr. Stuart Douglas, who had been assistant physician at the City Asylum for over six years, and who is still resident physician. In 1885 the general oversight of the pavilion was placed under Dr. A. E. MacDonald, the General Superintendent of the New York City Asylums.

We may now ask, Whence come the patients? The majority received at the pavilion are committed by the police justices to the care of the Commissioners of Public Charities and Correction for examination as to sanity. The usual term of commitment is five days. Why *five days* nobody seems to know, except that such has been the custom, and that length of time is usually sufficient for the purpose. The police justices commit for examination regarding sanity such persons as manifest evidence of insanity in these classes:

1st. Those persons who are arrested for petty offenses, the nature and manner of the occurrence indicating an unbalanced mind.

2d. Those who interrupt public meetings or divine service, who preach or orate in public places, their conduct appearing to be irrational.

3d. Persons making complaint before police justices, at police stations, in other courts, to the district attorney, or other public officials, of wrongs and persecutions, or presenting claims that appear to be imaginary.

4th. Where complaint is made by citizens of persons who annoy them upon pretense that seems irrational.

5th. Persons who may be found by the police wandering about the streets in an aimless or purposeless manner, or acting in a strange manner, or who are unable to give a rational account of themselves.

6th. Those who have attempted to commit suicide.

7th. Those who are brought before a public magistrate, where the charge or testimony would warrant the suggestion that the individual might be insane and irresponsible.

It is not infrequent for police justices to commit persons for examination, and to endorse across such commitment, " To be returned to court if found not insane." In fact, police justices endeavor to be just, and to commit no person for lesser crimes, when evidence is produced to indicate insanity and irresponsibility, until the question of sanity has been passed upon by the city examiners. In cases of grave crime, they commit for trial, leaving the court of higher jurisdiction to determine the question of sanity and responsibility.

The superintendent of the poor, acting for the Commissioners in cases that are made public charges, where evidence is furnished that such person is insane and requires care and treatment as an insane person, gives permits for admission to the pavilion for examination.

The examining physician for the department, where admission is sought to some hospital and his examination leads him to suspect insanity, gives permits for admission to the pavilion for special examination regarding the applicant's sanity and fitness for admission to the city asylums or other institutions of the department.

A certain number of patients are brought by ambulance from residences, where the statement of friends or the conduct of the patient leads the ambulance surgeon to conclude that the patient is insane. Some are sent directly from police stations, without a commitment from a police justice. These are usually excited, violent, or sick cases, in which the police feel they are not justified in retaining the individual at the police station for the time required to obtain the formal commitment. A few cases are admitted by the resident physician, where patients are brought by friends, with letters from a family physician, or come voluntarily, or consent to temporary restraint. Where the patient is violent, dangerous, or very sick, the resident physician feels justified in admitting to the pavilion without the formality of a commitment by a magistrate. In other cases it is his. habit to recommend an application to some police justice for formal commitment.

Patients are transferred from the regular wards of Bellevue Hospital and from the alcoholic ward, but only after the examination and approval of the resident physician of the pavilion (he indorsing the card with his signature) before the transfer is made. Patients are received from other hospitals and institutions when brought to Bellevue by ambulance. (I have thus far gone into this subject of admission to show the precautions that are taken to prevent the temporary detention even of any improper case in the examining pavilion.)

Where cases of insanity develop at other hospitals or institutions in the care of the department of Charities and Correction, by order of the general superintendent it is the duty of the resident physician of such institution or hospital to report to the examiners in lunacy, in writing, the existence of such patient and a history of the case, and to state that, in his opinion, the patient is in such physical condition as to justify his transfer to the asylum. The examiners are directed to visit such patients at the various institutions where they may be, and pass judgment on the question of sanity and propriety of commitment to some of the city asylums. The examiners prefer to make their visits separately and to arrive at independent conclusions, though they have subsequently to unite in a dual certificate.

Under the present dual certificate required by law, we are in the habit of dividing the work; and, while one examiner makes out the certificates for the males, the other does so for the females. We alternate each month. The first examiner, after the completion of his examination (if he considers the patient insane), makes out a certificate, and makes oath to it before a notary public, leaving the certificate in the notary's charge. The second examiner, if of the same opinion, signs the certificate prepared by the first examiner, with such additions as his examination may lead him to make; then makes oath, as did the first examiner, before the same notary who acknowledged the certificate, and in this form it is presented to the judge for approval. Should the two examiners disagree in any case, as sometimes occurs, the case is referred to the resident physician, whose opinion decides the disposition of the case.

Discretion is exercised by the examiners and by the resident physician in regard to the discharge of patients to the care of friends and relatives. If the friends show a disposition and ability to care for the patients, they are usually discharged to their care, if they sign a contract agreeing properly to provide for them. If the patient be decidedly dangerous to himself and others, we usually insist that arrangements be made with some institution for proper care and treatment. All that is required is a reasonable assurance that both the patient and the community are properly guarded. When once a patient is lodged in some institution, the examiners consider their responsibility ended. Of course, improper commitment or discharge would be still chargeable to them. Beyond that they could hardly be held responsible. The examiners stand between the patient and the community. They must guard the welfare of the patient, consider his right to enjoy liberty and the pursuit of happiness; and at the same time they must guard and protect the community.

The following table will show the number of patients received during the past four years and their disposition:

	Sex.	Admissions.	Transfer'd to City Asylum.	Transfer'd to other Asylums.	Transfer'd to other Institutions.	Dischar'd.	Died.
1888	Male,	997	650	87	135	109	8
	Female,	854	616	36	104	87	11
1889	Male,	1,075	641	139	87	198	16
	Female,	843	625	46	63	93	12
1890	Male,	1,066	658	71	193	135	12
	Female,	830	601	37	70	103	14
1891	Male,	1,138	724	56	187	144	16
	Female,	866	671	23	54	100	17
Total,		7,669	5,186	495	893	969	106

Total commitments............. ....74.09 per cent.
  "   "   to city asylums...................67.62   "
  "   "   to other asylums.................. 6.47   "
  "   "   transferred to other institutions...11.64   "
  "   "   discharged ....12.63   "
  "   "   died........................... 1.38   "

The percentage of discharges when I was first made examiner was over thirty-three per cent. The percentage has gradually diminished, from the great care exercised in the exclusion of admission of improper cases to the pavilion. The number of admissions has decreased but slightly, but the number of improper admissions has lessened very much. This is due very largely to the oversight of a competent resident physician with increased power.

The reception pavilion is in every respect a hospital, with a resident physician and competent and trained attendants. Unnecessary detention at police stations and prisons and the mingling of the insane with the criminal class, are avoided. All patients transferred from the pavilion to the asylum are accompanied by attendants of their own sex, who remain with them until they are turned over to the care of the asylum authorities. Opportunity is afforded in very many cases to obtain a history of the patient, and to consult with friends and allow them the privilege of providing for the patients in other institutions, if they have the means and disposition to do so.

I have brought this subject, with the description of the workings of the reception pavilion at Bellevue, to your attention in the hope that your interest might be secured in the starting of a movement for the establishing of similar institutions in every large city in the United States. This plain and inexpensive building, with but sixteen sleeping rooms, has received at least twenty-five thousand suspects since its opening in 1879. It has served its purpose well, though at times hasty examinations have been required to prevent overcrowding.

An ideal institution for this purpose would be an hospital constructed upon the pavilion plan, for the reception of the insane, inebriate and neurotic, with a small amphitheater, and sufficient wards for proper classification and detention for a reasonable time.

A competent visiting, examining, and resident staff of medical officers should be chosen and clinical instruction regularly given.

I would insist on full records being kept of all cases admitted, and would make the past history of each patient an important matter, to be patiently and persistently sought after and carefully recorded.

Such a hospital would secure prompt, humane and scientific treatment. The opportunity afforded for longer observation, securing histories and examinations, would result in more complete and accurate certification.

There being no need for hasty transfer to other institutions, the feeble, sick, and certain selected cases could be detained for treatment, and clinical instruction would be easily accessible to the entire medical profession.

THE CONSTRUCTION OF MATERNITY HOSPITALS.

By Barton Cooke Hirst, M. D., of Philadelphia,

Professor of Obstetrics, University of Pennsylvania.

The writer must disclaim at the outset any special knowledge of hospital construction. The only claim he has to write on the subject at all is the fact that he has made the plans for and superintended the erection of a maternity hospital under conditions and limitations that must prevail in many similar undertakings in this country. It may, therefore, be helpful to others who are charged with such a task in the future, to know how certain problems that will beset them have been met by us.

Some five years ago it was determined to erect a maternity hospital in connection with the medical school of the University of Pennsylvania. There were no funds at hand for the purpose. All that the University authorities could do was to grant the land upon which the building was to stand. Everything else—the collection of the money for building, and all the details of the building itself—were left to the newly elected professor of obstetrics. The questions to be faced were the following:

1. The plan of a building of ample capacity for a large number of patients during confinement, and yet of small cost.

2. The best architectural plan to secure to each patient privacy, isolation, ample air space during and after delivery; to allow the use of each patient for clinical instruction for one or two members of the graduating class, without undue exposure; but not to give so much space to each individual patient that the size of the building would be excessive and its cost too great.

The manner in which these requirements were met is best told by a description of the building we have begun and will soon finish. It was decided upon after much thought, and after an inspection of many of the best known maternities in this country and in Europe. The latter, however, did not help us much, as it was necessary to adopt a plan that differs materially from any other the writer knows of.

By a glance at the illustration it may be seen that the building consists of a main structure, with a basement, two stories and a mansard roof, the ground dimensions being about 50×40 feet. From each side of the rear runs a long narrow pavilion, one-story high, with a ridge ventilator. In the interior of this pavilion is a glass-enclosed porch, extending the whole length, an inner corridor, and five separate bedrooms, each about 10 feet square. The bath-room and water-closet are entered from the glass porch, and are walled off from the rest of the pavilion.

The main building (not yet erected) will contain on each main floor two wards with a combined capacity of 14 to 16 beds to the floor. The mansard roof provides extra space for at least 12 more beds. The basement is to be used for dining-room, ward kitchen, storage-room and heating apparatus.

In the main building pregnant women will be received, not longer, if possible, than two weeks before their expected confinement. When a woman falls in labor she is transferred to a room in one of the pavilions, where she is delivered and will remain for about ten days. She is then returned to finish the remaining few days of her convalescence in a ward of the main building. By this plan the bed-rooms of the pavilions may be filled and vacated three times a month, giving us a capacity of 30 confinements in that time; or this number may be increased by moving patients back to the main building on the 5th, 6th or 7th day.

Thus during pregnancy, and late in puerperal convalescence, when it is not necessary that each patient should have more air space than any healthy individual requires, we can economize room; while during confinement, and in the puerperium, each patient has an amount of space to herself, a degree of isolation and seclusion in her own room, that is rarely, if ever, afforded in the most lavishly equipped and expensively erected hospital.

The writer expected from this plan the following advantages, and his expectations have been realized:

Design for Maternity Hospital for The University of Pa.

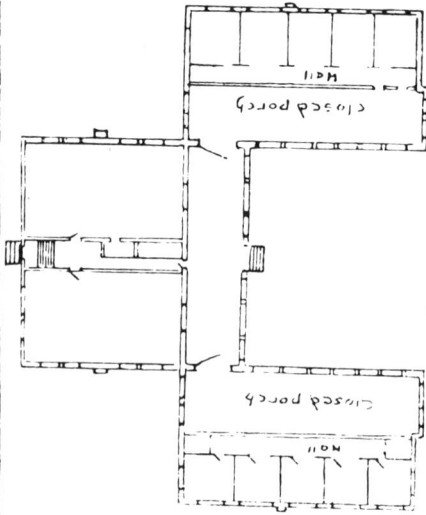

Diagram of Buildings

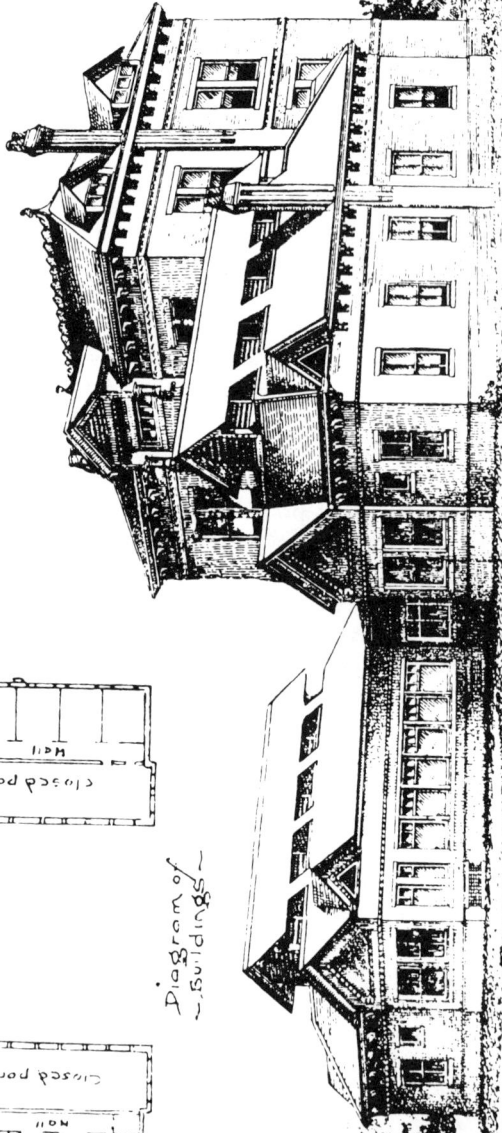

closed porch

No. 1

closed porch

No. 11

1. It is cheap. Each pavilion presenting a handsome appearance, built of pressed brick, with brown-stone sills, and handsomely constructed in the interior, costing $5000. The main building will cost $15,000.

2. It gives the best possible hygienic arrangement of the confinement rooms, separated from one another, each with its own window, a separate ventilator and heating flue, and entered only from the inner corridor, which opens directly upon the well-lighted and ventilated glass-enclosed porch. I have never anywhere seen a maternity hospital so well planned in this respect.

3. It gives the women a privacy during confinement that is rarely enjoyed in a hospital, and enables us to assign an advanced student to the room of the parturient, under an instructor, without exposing her to other patients or to other practitioners engaged in the same work in a common ward.

4. It gives a large capacity at small cost. For $25,000 we have a hospital constructed on the very best hygienic principles, of a handsome appearance, and with a capacity of upwards of 360 confinements a year.

This capacity can be greatly increased at any time by the addition of a story or two to the main building, and by running a third pavilion between the ends of the other two.

The writer would recommend most strongly this system of separate rooms for women in confinement, to any one contemplating the erection of a maternity hospital. The alternatives to this plan are delivery of a number of women in one room, where they remain during convalescence, or a special delivery room in which the child is born, and from which the patient is transported afterward to a ward in which she will lie until she leaves her bed. The disadvantages of the former are obvious. The danger of infection must be increased ; the sight of others in pain, possibly undergoing operation, has a demoralizing influence upon the parturient and puerperal woman; and if the cases are used for instruction of young practitioners, as they always should be, there may be quite a number of students present at one time. The writer will not soon forget an experience while interne in a German hospital; returning one night from the opera, he found in one *gebärsaal* five women in active labor, attended by ten students   Aside from the bad hygiene of such an arrangement, imagine the feelings of any one of these unfortunate women, were she other than a phlegmatic, not to say stupid German peasant ! The second alternative, while better, is still not the best. A special delivery room has the great disadvantage, that, used for a large number of births in rapid succession, it is exceedingly difficult to keep clean. And, moreover, the transportation of the woman to another ward directly after delivery is attended with not a little risk.

It seems indisputable that, from a hygienic as well as a humanitarian standpoint, the plan of single rooms for parturient patients is the best. This admitted, the best and least costly plan of a building will be found to be a combination of a main storage-house for patients and attached pavilions with single rooms.

COTTAGE HOSPITALS.

By Francis Vacher,

Medical Officer of Health for the County of Chester, England.

The First Cottage Hospital.

To Mr. Albert Napper, surgeon, the honor is due of establishing the first "Village Hospital," as he called it. About the year 1855, the desirability of making some provision locally for the treatment of severe medical and surgical cases was forced on his attention, and he made inquiries and interested friends in the subject. Eventually a cottage at Cranleigh was given by the Rector, rent free, and fitted so as to adapt it for use as a hospital at a little over £50. This hospital was opened in 1859, six beds being provided for patients. The general management was placed in the hands of a committee, but an acting manager was appointed, who with the medical officer should be responsible for details and report to the committee. An efficient nurse was placed in charge of the nursing, and subsequently this branch of the hospital work was supervised by a ladies' committee. It was part of Mr. Napper's plan that when the nurse or assistant nurse had spare time she might visit the sick at their own homes as nurse or dresser. The idea has not been put in practice at Cranleigh, but it has elsewhere, and is found to work well.

Mr. Napper remained associated with his hospital till 1880, when he retired, and his work there has since been carried on by his son. The Cranleigh Hospital is yet in excellent working order, treating about 30 patients annually, many of them very severe cases. It shows what can be accomplished with the help of skill, care, and personal attention to detail, for the initial expenditure was most trifling, and the annual income from subscriptions and donations often does not exceed £120. The patients or their friends pay from 3s. 6d. to 5s. per week for maintenance.

Other Early Cottage Hospitals.

The second cottage hospital was opened in 1860 at Fowey, a small town in Cornwall, having a present population of about 2000. A cottage was erected at a cost of £450 (the only annual charge in respect of it being 10s. ground-rent) and partly furnished, eight beds being provided for patients; but the nurse was required to furnish her own apartments, and was only to be paid "when her services were required to attend any sick person or persons in the hospital." When not required, the nurse was allowed to "attend poor women at their own homes during their confinement." An arrangement such as this is so peculiar, one is not surprised to hear that no yearly report is issued, or that some of the patients "are daily supplied with dinner and perhaps with breakfast" by the persons who got them admitted. There is certainly much need of a hospital at Fowey, as it is 25 miles from Truro, where the nearest general hospital is situated; but it should be differently organized, so as to bring it into accord with modern views. The Fowey Hospital is still open and receives upwards of 20 patients annually.

Only two cottage hospitals, so far as I have been able to ascertain, were established in 1861; the first at Bourton-on-the-Water (Gloucestershire) and the second at Woodbridge (Suffolk). The Bourton hospital owes its existence mainly to the exertions of Mr. John Moore, surgeon. An old three-story building was obtained, added to and adapted, and an army pensioner and his wife were put in charge, the latter acting as nurse. It was situated in the outskirts of the village and had a good garden. This building was in use till the middle of the year 1879, when through the efforts of the committee of management an entirely new compact hospital was completed and placed at the service of the district. The new building was erected of brick and tiles at a cost of £1,100, on a suitable site given by a resident. It was designed to accommodate 10 patients, but only 8 beds are provided. The men's ward and women's ward are on the first floor, and there is a ward for convalescents on the ground floor, all being well proportioned, light and airy, but the sanitary arrangements were soon found to be unsatisfactory and had to be put in order. The furnishing of the building cost £180.

The Sekforde Hospital at Woodbridge resembles the Bourton Hospital in having an out-patients' department, but only 6 beds are provided. The annual expenditure at Bourton is a little over £200, and at Woodbridge it is a little over £300.

In 1862 there was a small hospital and dispensary opened at Pembroke, South Wales. Eight beds were provided and about 40 patients received annually, but the number of beds was afterwards reduced to four. The amount of dispensary work done by this institution is trifling and not increasing.

The fifth cottage hospital I find any record of was founded in 1863 at Iver, in Buckinghamshire. A suitable cottage was rented at £20 a year, furnished and provided with 6 or 7 beds and placed in charge of a nurse. It was somewhat enlarged in 1875 and the name changed to the Iver, Langley and Denham Cottage Hospital. There are now nine beds and the income is increased from about £100 to £240 a year. There are no out-patients.

In the same year the first cottage hospital for surgical cases only was founded at Walsall in Staffordshire. A house was obtained and fitted with 20 beds, and patients were treated free. In a few years the number of beds was increased, and in 1880 a new building was erected, the money being obtained by public subscriptions. The institution is now probably the largest cottage hospital in the kingdom. It has 42 beds, the average number occupied being 30, and a large out-patients' department. The number of in-patients treated last year was 494, and the number of out-patients 4,473. The ordinary income and expenditure are about £1,300. The nursing is done by a sister and staff of six nurses.

A third cottage hospital was opened in 1863. It is situated at Redruth, and is called the West Kent Miners Hospital, being originally intended for the treatment of convalescents. It was found to be so successful that in 1871 an accident ward was added. The hospital now makes up 30 beds, the average number daily occupied being 27. Last year there were 198 convalescents and 59 cases of accident treated. There is no out-patients' department, neither is there any medical staff. Each patient selects his own medical man. The special peculiarity of this institution is that it is worked entirely by Lord Robartes, the committee paying him 13s. 6d. per week for each accident case, and 11s. per week for each convalescent case admitted by them. The expenditure last year was £1231. Lord Robartes expends yearly on the hospital more than the amount paid him.

During 1864 was established a cottage hospital at Ditchingham, Norfolk. It secured so much local interest that in the course of a few years a subscription for building was commenced, and by July, 1873, a new hospital was completed at a cost of £3000. This is called All Hallows Hospital, and appears to be the first cottage hospital built on the pavilion principle. It provides 20 beds for patients; the income is about £500 a year. Patients are charged 5s. to 10s. for maintenance.

In either 1864 or 1865 a second cottage hospital in Gloucestershire was opened—the Tewkesbury Rural Hospital. The erection of this building cost only about £1000, yet 20 beds are provided, and there is an out-patients' department. The income is derived almost entirely from subscriptions; last year it amounted to £740.

The next two cottage hospitals opened appear to be those at Wallasey, Cheshire, and at St. Andrews in the county of Fife. The Cheshire hospital originally provided 10 beds, and now has 18; the other originally provided 7 beds, and now has 10. Both were established in 1865.

The Cheshire hospital has an out-patients' department, and an income and expenditure of about £380 a year. At St. Andrews hospital there is no out-patients' department, and the income and expenditure are about £280.

The Cranleigh Hospital and the other eleven cottage hospitals already referred to are all at present active working hospitals. In 1861 a small cottage hospital was opened at Dinorwic in Carnarvonshire; it contained 8 beds, and was kept open for about seven years, when, owing probably to want of funds, it was closed. In 1863, at East Grinstead, Sussex, two cottages were given for the purpose of establishing a cottage hospital. They were altered at a cost of £150, and furnished by subscription, 7 beds being provided. In 1874, on the completion of its eleventh year of work, and after having received and treated 300 patients, it was closed, owing to the difficulty the founder experienced in raising sufficient funds for current expenses. Many years afterwards, i. e., in 1888, the East Grinstead Hospital was resuscitated, 5 beds being provided, and it seems likely to do well. Last year the income was £434.

In 1863 also, a cottage hospital providing 8 beds for surgical cases was opened at Stockton, Durham, a cottage being rented for the purpose at £15. It was successful for many years, but in 1875 a larger hospital was provided in the same town, and this (which now has 60 beds) is prospering well.

The Progress of the Cottage Hospital Movement.

It has been shown that during the first seven years of cottage hospitals, 15 were established, 12 of which now survive. Of the three which failed after many years of active service, one has been re-established, and one superseded by a larger hospital. The spread of the cottage hospital movement after the first seven years was very much more rapid. This will be indicated by the list of cottage hospitals which I have been at some pains to compile, and now submit (*vide* the Appendix). From the list I drew up the following statement, giving the date of the establishment of the whole number of cottage hospitals extant in the United Kingdom at the end of 1892:

1859	1	1871.........	18	1883.........	6
1860.........	1	1872.........	13	1884	10
1861	2	1873.........	13	1885...... ..	4
1862	1	1874.........	8	1886..	7
1863.........	3	1875.........	8	1887........	8
1864.........	2	1876.........	8	1888........	12
1865.........	2	1877.........	4	1889	5
1866.... ...	8	1878.........	7	1890.........	9
1867	15	1879.........	8	1891...... ...	5
1868.........	7	1880........	7	1892	7
1869	14	1881.........	5		
1870.........	15	1882........	4		

Thus, while in the seven years 1859–65 the number of cottage hospitals opened was about two a year, in the seven years 1866–72 the number was about 13 a year; in the seven years 1873–79 the number was about 8 a year; in the seven years 1880–86 the number was just over 6 a year; and in the six years 1887–92 the number was just over 7½ a year.

The fact that the 7 years 1866–72 saw so many cottage hospitals established is exceptionally interesting. It has been explained as follows:

In 1866 a little work on cottage hospital management was published by Mr. Harris and another by Dr. Waring; a third edition of Mr. Napper's pamphlet was issued, and Dr. Swete brought the subject before the British Medical Association, at Bristol.

In 1869 or 1870 Dr. Swete's "Handy Book of Cottage Hospitals" was published, and the extension of the movement was assisted by favorable notices in many influential papers.

More recently a distinct stimulus was given to the movement by the Queen's Jubilee. In 1887 there were established 5 cottage hospitals; in 1888, 6 cottage hospitals, and in 1889 there was established 1 cottage hospital by means of funds collected locally to celebrate the Queen's Jubilee.

It is worthy of note also how wide-spread has been the cottage hospital movement. There are now cottage hospitals in active work in all but three of the English counties (the counties of Huntingdon, Monmouth, and Rutland), in all but two of the counties of Wales (Brecon and Cardigan), in ten counties of Scotland and in three counties of Ireland.

Subjoined is a statement of the number of cottage hospitals existing at the close of the year 1892, and the aggregate number of beds provided in each county:

COUNTIES. England :	Number of Cottage Hospitals provided.	Number of Patients' beds therein.
Bedford	1	18
Berks	8	84
Bucks	5	42
Cambridge	3	58
Chester	5	85
Cornwall	5	69
Cumberland	2	30
Derby	2	18
Devon	14	158
Dorset	7	90
Durham	5	84
Essex	7	53
Gloucester	9	82
Hants	8	76
Hereford	3	20
Herts	6	56
Kent	19	234
Lancashire	7	99
Leicester	2	11
Lincoln	6	107
Middlesex	10	97
Norfolk	3	38
Northampton	1	6
Northumberland	1	16
Nottingham	2	27
Oxford	3	32
Shropshire	4	40
Somerset	8	96
Stafford	9	192
Suffolk	4	31
Surrey	12	167

Sussex..	7	70
Warwick..	1	20
Westmoreland..............	1	25
Wilts...	6	78
Worcester..	3	33
York	16	241
Total in England........................215		2,683

Wales:

Anglesey...	1	5
Carmarthen.......................................	1	20
Carnarvon..	1	14
Denbigh..	1	8
Flint...	1	7
Glamorgan..	3	47
Merioneth..	2	21
Montgomery......................................	1	9
Pembroke..	2	11
Radnor	1	20
Total in Wales...................... 14		162

Scotland:

Aberdeen	4	45
Ayr..	1	14
Banff....	2	23
Edinburgh..	1	12
Elgin...	2	24
Fife..	2	20
Lanark...	1	16
Ross...	1	16
Roxburgh...	1	12
Total in Scotland...................... 15		182

Ireland:

Antrim...	1	22
Down...	1	5
Londonderry......................	1	10
Total in Ireland...................... 3		37
Total in the United Kingdom............247		3,064

Thus is shown at a glance the spread of the cottage hospital movement. It has indeed extended to one of the Channel Islands, for in
May, 1888, the Victoria Cottage Hospital was founded in Guernsey,
providing 10 beds for patients, and the income last year was £755.

Some Cottage Hospitals which have been Closed.

Before remarking on some of the 247 cottage hospitals which have
succeeded, it may be expedient to refer briefly to the cottage hospi-

tals founded during the same period which have not survived. I have not been able to obtain a complete list of these, but the following it is believed is proximately accurate:

Year when founded.	Name of Hospital.	County.	No. of beds provided.
1861	Dinorwic Hospital	Carnarvon	8
1863	East Grinstead Cottage Hospital	Sussex	7
"	Stockton Surgical Hospital	Durham	8
1864	Wrington Hospital	Somerset	5
1866	Crimond Cottage Hospital	Aberdeen	
"	Great Bookham Hospital	York	
"	King's Sutton Hospital	Northampton	6
1867	Charmouth Hospital	Dorset	3
"	Richmond Hospital	York	4
"	Stratton Hospital	Cornwall	6
1868	Alloa Cottage Hospital	Stirling	15
"	Alton Cottage Hospital	Hants	7
"	Knole Cottage Hospital	Kent	
"	Litcham Hospital	Norfolk	8
"	Petworth Hospital	Sussex	8
"	St. Andrew's Home, Weybread	Suffolk	12
1870	Charlton Children's Home	Wilts	10
"	Chipping Norton Cottage Hospital	Oxford	
"	Clearwell Hospital	Gloucester	6
"	Stapleford Hospital	Nottingham	
"	Trowbridge Hospital	Wilts.	6
"	Worksop Hospital	Nottingham	5
"	Yate Cottage Hospital	Gloucester	4
1871	Bovey Tracey Hospital	Devon	6
"	Copland Sodbury Hospital	Middlesex	6
"	Oxlinch Hospital	Gloucester	8
1872	East Rudham Hospital	Norfolk	4
"	Harrow-on-the-Hill Hospital	Middlesex	8
1873	Moreton Hampstead Convalescent Hospital	Devon	14
"	Foston Cottage Hospital	Stafford	3
"	Hilston Hospital	Hereford	5
1876	Llangollen Hospital	Denbigh	6
"	Margate Cottage Hospital	Kent	5
1877	Purton Cottage Hospital	Wilts	5

Thus during 33 years, 34 cottage hospitals have been closed or no longer used as cottage hospitals. I have not been able to ascertain the number of beds provided by five of these hospitals; the aggregate number of the beds provided by the remaining 29 was 198.

The reasons which led to the closing of these hospitals are various. For instance, at Wrington the surgeon was a churchman and the secretary a dissenter, and a discussion arose as to whether the patients when able should attend church or chapel, and this grew into a quarrel, ultimately leading to the closure of the hospital after about five years' work.

At Great Bookham there seems to have been an animus against the hospital, for though only opened in 1866, it was closed as a hospital in 1868 and converted into an institution for providing nurses and sick comforts for the poor.

Richmond Hospital was continued for 11 years in a cottage, the use of which was obtained for a nominal rent, when a large hospital was built by a lady and presented to the town, so that the cottage hospital was no longer required.

Knole Cottage Hospital also appears to have done good work from its opening in 1868 till superseded by the hospital which was erected at Holmesdale in 1873.

Stapleford is reported to have been discontinued owing to the advanced age of the founder and his disappointment in not securing the assistance of his nephew as surgeon to the hospital.

Yate Hospital was closed after about 7 years of useful work, but its closing is reported to be through " no cause suggestive of failure of similar schemes."

The Oxlinch Hospital, which was a farm-house adapted for use as a hospital, and furnished by a lady, was supported solely by the lady except that she charged the patients 6s. a week. It never appears to have been much used, being but four miles from Stroud, where there is a general hospital.

The little hospital at East Rudham is reported to have been closed "because the poor thought that the medical man, whose services were gratuitous, derived some unknown benefit from the hospital."

Hilston Hospital after some years' work closed and kept open the establishment as a dispensary for the treatment of out-patients.

In the case of some of these hospitals the cause of their being closed could not be ascertained, and in many doubtless it was the difficulty in raising the required amount of funds. Some are stated to have been closed only temporarily.

A Few Types of Existing Cottage Hospitals.

I propose now to select out of my list of existing cottage hospitals a few types, not necessarily for imitation, but as fair samples of the whole.

Grantham Hospital in Lincolnshire was erected in 1876 at a cost of £5344, the furniture costing £812, and £1500 being given as an endowment fund. It is built of stone, occupying an excellent site on a hillside and commanding a good view. The two wards for male and female patients are placed as wings on either side of the administrative block, and are large enough for 7 or 8 beds each. Remote from the main building is a small fever hospital, containing 4 beds arranged in two wards. A matron and 3 nurses form the nursing staff for the main building. The drains are all outside and efficiently disconnected and ventilated. On the whole it is perhaps the best and most satisfactory cottage hospital in the country. There is a separate laundry and mortuary. In-patients only are treated, and admission is free by letter of recommendation. Last year the number of patients treated was 180. The income last year was £1355 and the expenditure £1210. The cottage hospital is 22 miles from the nearest general hospital, the Lincoln County Infirmary.

Beccles Hospital in Suffolk was erected in 1874 at a cost of £1500, the furnishing costing £300. The site, valued at £100, was given. There is no endowment. It is a classic building, having a dispensary, waiting-room, accident ward, surgeon's room, matron's room, kitchen, etc., on the ground floor. On the floor above are two wards, 30 feet × 16 feet, two wards 14 feet × 14 feet, and an operating room. The wards were originally fitted with 10 beds in all; 13 are now provided. A matron and 2 nurses form the nursing staff. There appears to be no bath-room, laundry or mortuary. The closets are entered from passages without the intervention of cross-ventilated lobbies. Last year the number of in-patients treated was 75, the number of out-patients 261. The income was £662 and the expenditure £496.

Petersfield Cottage Hospital in Hampshire was erected in 1871 at a cost of £1400, the furnishing costing £234. It has a very small endowment. This little hospital is prettily designed in red brick; the situation being exceptionally well chosen, there is a pleasant country view from the windows. The sanitary arrangements are not well planned, and for many years after the opening of the hospital there was actually no bath-room. The accommodation for patients consists of two wards each 17½ feet × 12½ feet, and two wards each 12½ feet × 10 feet. Originally 6 beds were provided for patients; there are now 8 beds. The wards are placed as wings on either side of the administrative block. There is an excellent, well lighted operating room. A mortuary is provided externally, but no laundry of any kind. Patients are ordinarily charged for maintenance at the rate of from 2s. 6d. to 8s. per week, but many are admitted free. Accidents are received without question at all hours. From 40 to

60 in-patients are treated annually. In the last returns published the income is entered at £363 and the expenditure at £433. At Ryde is a convalescent home in connection with this hospital. The cottage hospital is 17 miles from the nearest large general hospital at Portsmouth.

Berkhampstead Fever Hospital, Hertfordshire, was erected in 1879 at a cost of £2162, including the cost of building a boundary wall, making road and paths through the grounds and sinking a well. The site cost £425 extra; it consists of about 3 acres and has a frontage of about 144 feet on the highway. The expense of erection, etc., was borne by the Berkhampstead Rural Sanitary Authority; the current expenses are also paid by the authority. The buildings as designed consist of two detached ward pavilions, communicating with an administrative block by means of a corrugated iron covered way standing on wooden supports, and also two detached buildings, one containing a wash-house, an ironing room, an ambulance shed, disinfecting room, and a storeroom for dry earth, the other being a mortuary. Only one of the detached pavilions has been built; it contains two wards 24 feet × 24 feet, a nurse's room, store-closet and moveable bath. Each ward has an earth-closet and sink cut off from the ward by a ventilating lobby. The buildings are of white and red brick and stand on a bed of concrete. They are roofed in red tile. Each ward is well lighted with 6 windows, and each ward has an opening from the ceiling to the roof fitted with Boyle's ventilators. The warming is by means of Galton's stoves. The administrative block is a two-storied building; on the ground floor are sitting-room, surgery, kitchen, scullery, store, etc., and on the floor above two bedrooms. The water is derived from a well sunk into the chalk, raised by force-pump into a tank from which constant service can be provided. The sewerage is into a cesspit 350 feet to the north of the well, the flow of the spring in the chalk being from north to south.

I might give particulars of many other cottage hospitals, but these will suffice as examples. Existing cottage hospitals indeed include many varieties. Some, like the hospital at Gorleston (Suffolk) and Winchcombe (Gloucester), provide but 4 beds; others, e. g. Longton Cottage Hospital and Walsall Cottage Hospital, have 42 beds, about double the number first provided.

Most cottage hospitals follow the lead of Cranleigh, being for severe medical and surgical cases; but four hospitals provide for infectious cases as well, and six are wholly for infectious cases, while three or four are for surgical cases only. One hospital receives all but phthisical cases, one is solely for children under 10 years old, one is for patients having ulcerated legs or eczema, one is for hip disease and spinal disease, some are wholly or in part for convalescents, one sets apart half the beds provided for lying-in cases, several provide two or more cots for the treatment of little children.

Many cottage hospitals have been commenced in old buildings altered and adapted for the purpose, and afterwards continued in new buildings. Many have been grafted, as it were, on previously existing dispensaries. Some have prospered from first to last and been able to gather an endowment fund from surplus income, some have had to appeal to the guardians of the poor to augment their subscription list.

Finances.

As regards income, many cottage hospitals are almost entirely dependent on voluntary contributions; a few are wholly supported by their founders and publish no report, while a few are wholly or in part supported from rates levied by the local authority; one is supported entirely by railway workmen. Nearly all cottage hospitals charge for the maintenance of such patients as are considered able to pay. The charge ranges from 1s. to 21s. a week, usually it is from 2s. 6d. to 10s.

Generally it may be said the income of cottage hospitals (with the exception of those provided for the treatment of infectious cases) is commonly derived from subscriptions and donations, church collections, interest on money saved, or given or bequeathed as capital, and payments by patients or their friends.

It is reckoned that, to keep up an interest in the hospital, at least half the income should be derived from local subscriptions. Thus a well managed cottage hospital usually derives about two-thirds of its income from subscriptions and donations. With the help derived in recent years from the yearly " Hospital Sunday," church collections may be counted on to provide a third of the remaining third; there is therefore about two months to be made up by interest on capital and patients' payments. Of course, when a hospital is first opened, and for some years after, there is no capital, and the rule is to require a small payment for maintenance, from patients or their friends. The amount can be adjusted to the means and circumstances of the payer, and in special cases altogether remitted. In course of years a small capital from legacies, etc., is slowly accumulated, and many cottage hospitals have thus been placed in so good a financial position that they have been able to do without maintenance charges from patients. Indeed, in some instances it is difficult to know what to do with capital. After the freehold of land and buildings has been purchased, and there is enough in hand to meet a year's expenses, probably the best use for interest from capital is to make the hospital free. This is certainly better than investing surplus income derived from interest, and so increasing the endowment fund.

It has been found that cottage hospitals, either large or small, taking one with another, can be supported at an annual cost of a little over £46 per bed provided, or £66 per bed occupied. This is certainly less than the cost of ordinary hospitals.

Cottage hospitals for the treatment of infectious diseases are ordinarily provided by the local sanitary authority, and should be maintained by the authority. They are thus more likely to be well managed than if provided and maintained by voluntary subscriptions, etc. Though it is usual to charge the patients or their friends maintenance fees of from 10s. 6d. to 14s. a week, it is not a wise practice. It is for the good of the community that every infectious patient who cannot be properly isolated should be sent to hospital, and every inducement should be held out to patients to get them to consent to their removal to hospital.

Conclusion.

As one who has founded a cottage hospital, and taken an active part in its management for 16 years, I may fairly claim to have some knowledge of the subject I am discussing. My experience in my own hospital, and a study of what has been attempted and done in respect of cottage hospital provision during the last third of a century in the United Kingdom, has naturally led me to some conclusions, and these I shall now state as briefly as possible.

1. The term "cottage hospital" as used in this country means either: (a) A cottage or villa residence adapted and fitted for the reception and treatment of patients; or, (b) a small hospital designed and built as such.

The adapted building, though in some districts all that it is possible to obtain, is never wholly satisfactory; the specially constructed building, with the information at present available, may be arranged to fulfil all the requirements of a rural population as regards hospital accommodation.

2. Cottage hospitals have been found well suited for the treat-

ment of: (*a*) Severe medical and surgical cases, and (*b*) patients suffering from dangerous infectious disease.

They have been also used, but not to any great extent, for the treatment of: (*c*) Obstetric cases; (*d*) convalescents; (*e*) patients suffering from some named disease, skin disease, spinal disease, hip disease, etc.; and (*f*) children.

There is no reason to believe that there is any demand for special cottage hospitals such as these. Obstetric cases are better treated at home. A cottage hospital is no place for convalescents. Children should be admitted in all cottage hospitals.

3. Cottage hospitals receiving severe medical and surgical cases are for villages and rural districts. If the nearest general hospital is 8 or 10 miles away, and the population of the village and rural district within a radius of about 4 miles is 4,000 or 5,000, it may be assumed there is work for a cottage hospital providing from 4 to 6 beds.

4. The smallest cottage hospital should have at least 2 wards for patients, a matron's sitting-room, a medical officer's room or operating room, 2 bedrooms, a kitchen, scullery and wash-house, larder, store-room, bath-room, two water-closets, fuel-house and mortuary external to the house. The drains should be laid outside the house, disconnected and ventilated, and each water-closet in the house should be cut off by means of a lobby having cross-ventilation. In rural districts where there are no sewers earth-closets may be provided in place of water-closets.

5. Every cottage hospital not having a resident medical officer should be within a very short distance of one of the medical practitioners connected with it.

6. Every cottage hospital should be well warmed and lighted and have a good water supply. It should be a detached building, and the site selected should be at least dry and clean, fairly open and reasonably accessible.

7. If the hospital be for the treatment of infectious cases there should be space enough around it for the erection of temporary structures, such as occasion may require. The administrative offices should also be somewhat in excess of the permanent wards.

8. The amount of air space per patient should not be less in ordinary cases than 800 cubic feet, and should not be less in infectious cases than 1,600 cubic feet. If practicable, each ordinary patient should have 1,000 cubic feet, and each infectious patient 2,000 cubic feet.

APPENDIX.

List of Cottage Hospitals extant in the United Kingdom at the end of the year 1892, showing the year when established, the County in which situated, the Number of Beds for Patients provided, and the Average Number occupied.

Year when Hospital was opened	Name of Hospital	County	Number of Beds	Average Number occupied	Remarks.
1859	Cranleigh Village Hospital	Surrey	6	4	For severe medical and surgical cases.
1860	Fowey Cottage Hospital	Cornwall	6	4	Originally 4 beds.
1861	Bourton-on-the-water Cottage Hospital	Gloucester	8		
"	Sekforde Hospital and Dispensary, Woodbridge	Suffolk	6		
1862	Pembroke Infirmary and Dispensary	Pembroke	4		Originally 6 beds, afterwards 8 beds.
1863	Iver Cottage Hospital	Buckingham	9		Originally 7 beds, afterwards 3 beds.
"	Walsall Cottage Hospital	Staffordshire	42	30	For surgical cases only. Originally 24 beds.
1864	West Cornwall Miners' Hospital, Redruth	Cornwall	30		Originally 26 beds.
"	All Hallows Hospital, Ditchingham	Norfolk	20		New building opened 1873. Originally 10 beds.
1865	Tewkesbury Rural Hospital	Gloucester	20	10	Orig nally 7 beds.
"	Wallasey Cottage Hospital	Cheshire	18		Originally 4 beds.
"	Memorial Cottage Hospital, St. Andrews	Fife	10		Originally 7 beds.
1866	Capel Village Hospital	Surrey	10		
"	Congleton Cottage Hospital	Cheshire	8	4	
"	Crewkerne Hospital	Somerset	17	10	Originally 13 beds.
"	Cromer Cottage Hospital	Norfolk	12	8	Originally 7 beds.
"	Oswestry and Ellesmere Cottage Hospital	Shropshire	12 and 1 cot		
"	Reigate and Redhill Cottage Hospital	Surrey	16 and 4 cots	14	Originally 12 beds. Originally 10 beds.
"	Savernake Cottage Hospital	Wiltshire	20	17	New building opened 1872. Originally 20 beds.
"	Yeatman Hospital, Sherborne	Dorsetshire	24		
1867	Bridport Dispensary and Cottage Hospital	Dorsetshire	8	6	Originally 6 beds.
"	Burford Cottage Hospital	Oxfordshire	8		Originally 5 beds.
"	Driffield Cottage Hospital	York	8		
"	Dunster and Minehead Village Hospital	Somerset	7		
"	Mansfield-Woolhouse District Hospital	Nottingham	22	16	Originally 7 beds.
"	Montgomeryshire Infirmary, Newtown	Montgomeryshire	9		Originally 15 beds.
"	Fairford Cottage Hospital	Gloucester	8		Phthisis not admitted.
"	Hambrook Cottage Hospital	Gloucester	6		
"	Hatfield (Broad Oak) Cottage Hospital	Essex	8		

Year	Hospital	County	No.	No.	Remarks
1867	Llanelly Hospital	Caermarthen	20	16	Originally 12 beds. Chiefly for accident cases.
"	Longton Cottage Hospital	Staffordshire	42		
"	Malvern Rural Hospital	Worcester	12		
"	Shedfield Cottage Hospital	Hampshire	7	5	Originally 20 beds.
"	St. Leonard's Hospital, Sudbury	Suffolk	14		
"	Wirksworth Cottage Hospital	Derbyshire	8		
1868	Buckhurst Hill Village Hospital	Essex	6		
"	Hillingdon Cottage Hospital	Middlesex	8	5	Originally 4 beds.
"	Mildenhall Cottage Hospital	Suffolk	6		
"	Melksham Cottage Hospital	Wiltshire	5		
"	Monmouth Hospital and Dispensary	Monmouthshire	9	6¾	Dispensary opened in 1810. Originally 8 beds.
"	Sir Titus Salt's Hospital, Shipley	York	9 and 1 cot.		Originally 6 beds.
"	Tetbury Cottage Hospital	Gloucester	8		
1869	Lloyd Cottage Hospital and Dispensary, Bridlington	York	12	10	Originally 6 beds. Originally 8 beds. New building opened 1875.
"	Bromyard Cottage Hospital	Hereford	18 and 2 cots.		
"	Chesham Cottage Hospital	Buckingham	5		{ Small iron pavilion for infectious cases added in 1871.
"	Darlington Cottage Hospital for Sick Children	Durham	7		{ Miss Peased founded Hospital and supports it entirely. No report.
"	Dowlais Fever Hospital	Glamorgan	25	3	Originally 32 beds.
"	Guisboro' Miners' Accident Hospital	York	13		
"	Market Rasen Cottage Hospital and Dispensary	Lincolnshire	5	10	Dispensary opened in 1856.
"	Newick Cottage Hospital	Sussex	6		
"	Shepton-Mallet District Hospital	Somerset	20	5	Originally 12 beds.
"	Spen Cottage Hospital	Berkshire	6		
"	St. Mary's Cottage Hospital, Tenbury	Worcester	8		
"	Wimbledon Cottage Hospital and Dispensary	Surrey	11		
"	Bangor Cottage Hospital and Home	Down	5		
1870	Ashford Cottage Hospital	Kent	10	6	New building opened 1878.
"	Dowlais Surgical Hospital	Glamorgan	10		Founded and supported by Mrs. Clarke.
"	Devizes Cottage Hospital and Dispensary	Wiltshire	16	8	Originally 6 beds.
"	Erith, Crayford, Belvedere and Abbey Wood Cottage Hospital and Provident Dispensary	Kent	10		
"	Harrogate Hospital and Dispensary	York	25	7	Originally 7 beds.
"	Tyrrell Cottage Hospital, Ilfracombe	Devonshire	26	15	Originally 6 beds.
"	Kendal Memorial Hospital	Westmoreland	25	16	Originally 16 beds.
"	Oakeley Hospital, Blaenau-Festiniog	Merionethshire	12		
"	Charlton Cottage Hospital, Malmesbury	Wiltshire	11	11	Originally 15 beds. { Originally 10 beds and under. For weakly children of 10 years and under.
"	Paxford House Cottage Hospital, Otery-St. Mary	Devonshire	9		{ Founder supports hospital entirely. No report.
"	Royston Cottage Hospital	Hertfordshire	8		Originally 7 beds.
"	Ruabon Accident and Cottage Hospital	Denbighshire	8	6	Originally 6 beds.
"	St. Alban's Hospital and Dispensary	Hertfordshire	14	6	Originally 6 beds.
"	Surbiton Cottage Hospital	Surrey	15 and 2 cots.		Originally 8 beds.
"	Walker Hospital, Walker-on-Tyne	Northumberland	16		Dispensary opened in 1843.

Year when Hospital was opened	Name of Hospital	County	Number of Beds.	Average Number occupied.	Remarks.
1871	Boston Hospital	Lincolnshire	30	4	Originally 12 beds.
"	Braintree and Bocking Cottage Hospital	Essex	5	8	Closed for some years, re-opened 1886.
"	Chumleigh Cottage Hospital	Devonshire	6	8	Originally 6 beds.
"	Dawlish Cottage Hospital	Devonshire	10		For fever patients and convalescents.
"	Dover Cottage Hospital	Kent	20		Originally 15 beds.
"	Dorking Cottage Hospital	Surrey	14 and 3 cots.		Originally 11 beds.
"	Jarrow-on-Tyne Memorial Hospital	Durham	20		Dispensary opened in 1862. Originally 6 beds.
"	Launceston Infirmary and Rowe Dispensary	Cornwall	8		Originally 4 beds.
"	Ledbury Cottage Hospital	Hereford	9 and 1 cot.		Originally 10 beds.
"	Lytham Cottage Hospital and Convalescent Home	Lancashire	20	3	Supported entirely by workmen's subscriptions with the exception of £20 a year from the Great Western Railway Co. Originally 7 beds.
"	New Swindon (G. W. R.) Accident Hospital	Wiltshire	12		
"	Petersfield Cottage Hospital	Hampshire	8		Originally 6 beds.
"	Rugeley District Hospital and Provident Dispensary	Staffordshire	15		Originally 12 beds. Dispensary opened in 1866.
"	Seacombe Cottage Hospital	Cheshire	22	14	Originally 8 beds.
"	Westminster Memorial Cottage Hospital, Shaftesbury	Dorsetshire	13		Originally 7 beds.
"	Stratford-on-Avon Nursing Home and Children's Hospital	Warwickshire	20		
"	Tenby Cottage Hospital	Pembroke	7		
1872	Sunderland Fever Hospital	Durham	20		Originally 30 beds.
"	Beckenham Cottage Hospital	Kent	20		Originally 10 beds.
"	Chalfont St. Peter Cottage Hospital	Buckingham	6		
"	Dinorben Cottage Hospital, Almwch	Anglesey	5		Originally 4 beds.
"	Ealing Cottage Hospital and Provident Dispensary	Middlesex	16	12	Originally 10 beds. New building opened in 1889.
"	Epsom and Ewell Cottage Hospital	Surrey	14	8	Originally 10 beds.
"	Litton Cottage Hospital	Bedfordshire	18	13	Originally 11 beds.
"	Milton Abbas Cottage Hospital	Dorsetshire	6		
"	Moreton-in-Marsh Cottage Hospital	Gloucester	11	9	Originally 7 beds.
"	St. Mary's Cottage Hospital, Northam, Southampton	Hampshire	5		For treatment of patients having ulcerated legs and eczema.
"	Memorial Cottage Hospital, Paulton	Somerset	10		New building opened in 1886.
"	Sevenoaks Hospital for Children with hip disease	Kent	17		
"	Egham Cottage Hospital	Surrey	14		
"	Stony Stratford Cottage Hospital	Buckingham	6		Originally 6 beds.

	Hospital	County	{ 4 and 2 for convales- cents. }		
1873	Charlwood Cottage Hospital	Surrey			Originally 4 beds.
,,	Holmesdale Cottage Hospital	Kent	9		
,,	Lyme Regis Cottage Hospital	Dorsetshire	8		Originally 4 beds.
,,	Monkswearmouth and Southwick Hospital	Durham	14	4	
,,	Newton Cottage Hospital and Dispensary, Newton Abbot	Devonshire	14		Originally 10 beds. Dispensary opened in 1858.
,,	St. Helen's Cottage Hospital	Lancashire	About 20		
,,	Ingham Infirmary and South Shields and Westoe Dispensary	Durham	23		Dispensary opened in 1821.
,,	Ulverston and District Cottage Hospital	Lancashire	14		Originally 12 beds.
,,	Watlington Cottage Hospital	Oxfordshire	8		
,,	North Cambridgeshire Cottage Hospital, Wisbeach	Cambridgeshire	26		Originally 16 beds.
,,	Yoxall Cottage Hospital	Staffordshire	5		
,,	Ross Memorial Hospital, Dingwall	Ross	16	8	{ Originally 8 beds. Half hospital for surgical cases and accidents, half for infectious cases.
1874	Lockhart Hospital, Lanark	Lanark	16		Originally 10 beds.
,,	Beccles Hospital	Suffolk	13		
,,	Cleveland Cottage Hospital, Brotton	York	22		
,,	Hayes Cottage Hospital	Middlesex	5		
,,	Hounslow Cottage Hospital	Middlesex	10		
,,	Lynton District Cottage Hospital	Devonshire	5		Originally 4 beds.
,,	Todmorden Fever Hospital	Lancashire	16		
,,	West Cornwall Infirmary and Dispensary, Penzance	Cornwall	18		Dispensary opened in 1809. Originally 9 beds.
,,	Wells Cottage Hospital	Somerset	8	5	Originally 6 beds.
1875	Cirencester Cottage Hospital	Gloucester	9		
,,	Clevedon Cottage Hospital	Somerset	11		Originally 8 beds.
,,	Enfield Cottage Hospital	Middlesex	9		Originally 7 beds.
,,	Frome Cottage Hospital	Somerset	13	5	Originally 11 beds.
,,	High Wycombe Cottage Hospital	Buckingham	12 and 2 cots	14	Originally 8 beds.
,,	{ Teddington and Hampton Wick Cottage Hospital and Provident Dispensary	Middlesex	9		
,,	Forgue Cottage Hospital	Aberdeen	8		Originally 6 beds.
,,	Wisbeach Fever Hospital	Cambridgeshire	12		Originally 10 beds.
1876	Andover Cottage Hospital	Hampshire	12		Originally 8 beds.
,,	Ashburton and Buckfastleigh Cottage Hospital	Devonshire	10	6	Originally 8 beds.
,,	Birkenhead Fever Hospital	Cheshire	22	5	Originally 16 beds.
,,	Boscombe Hospital and Provident Dispensary, Bournemouth	Hampshire	14	7	
,,	Brackley Cottage Hospital	Northampton	6	4	Originally 4 beds.
,,	Grantham Hospital	Lincolnshire	20		4 beds are for infectious cases.
,,	Keighley Cottage Hospital	York	9		
1877	Berkeley Hospital	Gloucester	9	6	Originally 12 beds.
,,	Lewes Fever Hospital	Sussex	12		
,,	Mold Cottage Hospital	Flintshire	7	3	
,,	Northallerton Cottage Hospital	York	12 and 4 fever beds		
1878	Wimbleton Fever Hospital	Surrey	30		Originally 12 beds.
,,	Batley and District Cottage Hospital	York	21		Originally 20 beds.

Year when Hospital was opened.	Name of Hospital.	County.	Number of Beds.	Average Number occupied.	Remarks.
1878	Beverley Dispensary and Cottage Hospital	York	16	17	Dispensary opened in 1823. Originally 6 beds. New building opened in 1891.
"	Bromgrove Cottage Hospital	Worcester	13		
"	Folkestone Sanatorium	Kent	14	6	For infectious cases.
"	Home for Sick Children, Southsea	Hampshire	19		
"	Morrell Memorial Cottage Hospital, Wallingford	Berkshire	8		
"	Leyton and Walthamstow Hospital, Home for Children	Essex	8		
1879	Barton under Needwood Cottage Hospital	Staffordshire	6 and 1 cot.		
"	Bettes-hanger Cottage Hospital	Kent	7		Originally 8 beds.
"	Maidenhead Cottage Hospital	Berkshire	12		Originally 3 beds.
"	Mount Sorrel Cottage Hospital	Leicester	6		Originally 10 beds.
"	St. John's Hospital, Twickenham	Middlesex	12		
"	Tunbridge Fever Hospital	Kent	12		
"	Fyvie Cottage Hospital	Aberdeen	12	6	Originally 8 beds.
"	Berkhampsted Fever Hospital	Hertfordshire	18		Additions opened in 1884.
1880	Blackheath and Charlton Cottage Hospital	Kent	8	12	New building opened in 1889.
"	Eltham Cottage Hospital	Kent	8		
"	Llandrindod-Wells Cottage Hospital and Convalescent Home	Radnorshire	20	13	Originally 8 beds.
"	Sarah Nicol Memorial Cottage Hospital, Llandudno	Carnarvon	14	7	
"	Tamworth Cottage Hospital	Staffordshire	30	16	
"	Gainsboro Reynard Cottage Hospital, Willingham by Stow	Lincolnshire	17		Originally 12 beds.
"	Turner Memorial Hospital, Keith	Banff	12		
1881	Aberdare Cottage Hospital	Glamorgan	12		Entirely supported by Lady Bute. Originally 7 beds.
"	Rous Memorial Hospital, Newmarket	Cambridgeshire	20		
"	Buchanan Cottage Hospital, St. Leonards	Sussex	19		Originally 7 beds.
"	Johnson Hospital, Spalding	Lincolnshire	20		Established under provisions of will of Messrs. E. H. and M. A. Johnson.
1882	Ballymena Cottage Hospital	Antrim	22	11	
"	Norwood Cottage Hospital	Surrey	16		
"	Garston Accident Hospital	Lancashire	5	4	
"	Hammerwich and District Cottage Hospital, near Lichfield	Staffordshire	13	10	
"	Sidcup Cottage Hospital	Kent	10 and 2 cots.		
1883	Lady Gomm's Memorial Accident Hospital, Rotherhithe	Surrey	6	7	Chiefly for and free to dock laborers. Opened in connection with St. John's Ambulance Association.
"	Falmouth Cottage Hospital	Cornwall	7		

Year	Hospital	County	Beds		Remarks
1883	Sir George Bowles Hospital, Butleigh	Somerset	10		This appears to be chiefly for surgical cases.
"	King's Cliff Hospital, Scarboro'	York	12		Built by Lord Bute. Originally 10 beds.
"	Cumnock Cottage Hospital	Ayrshire	14		
"	Haddo House Cottage Hospital, Tarves	Aberdeen	7		
1884	Bexley Cottage Hospital	Kent	8 and 1 cot.	7	Originally 6 beds and 1 cot.
"	Chislehurst, Sidcup and Cray Valley Cottage Hospital	Kent	14		
"	Halstead Cottage Hospital	Essex	8 and 1 cot.		
"	Eccles, and Patricroft Hospital and Dispensary	Lancashire	12		Dispensary opened in 1877.
"	Potter's Bar Cottage Hospital and Dispensary	Middlesex	9 and 1 cot.		
"	Shirley Children's Hospital and Dispensary for Women	Hampshire	6		
"	Sidmouth Cottage Hospital	Devonshire	5		
"	Victoria Cottage Hospital and Provident Dispensary, Eastbourne	Sussex	6		
"	Ian Charles Cottage Hospital, Grantown	Elgin	10		
1885	Hawick Cottage Hospital and Dispensary	Roxburgh	12	5	
"	Maud Hospital, Exmouth	Devonshire	17 and 4 cots.	8	Chiefly for accidents.
"	Ilkeston Cottage Hospital	Derbyshire	10	5	Originally 8 beds.
"	Newbury District Hospital	Berkshire	12	8	
"	Workington Infirmary	Cumberland	16 and 4 cots.	16	Chiefly for accidents.
1886	Abingdon Cottage Hospital	Berkshire	10		
"	Axminster Cottage Hospital	Devonshire	14	6	
"	Children's Cottage Hospital, Cold Ash, Newbury	Berkshire	20		For children between the ages of 3 and 13 suffering from hip and spine disease and other slow forms of disease.
"	Ludlow Cottage Hospital	Shropshire	9		
"	Wantage Cottage Hospital	Berkshire	8	6	Originally 8 beds.
"	Watford District Cottage Hospital	Hertford	10	7	Originally 9 beds.
"	Whitchurch Cottage Hospital and Dispensary	Shropshire	8 and 2 cots.		Originally 9 beds.
1887	Queen's Jubilee Hospital, South Kensington	Middlesex	12	10	Originally 6 beds.
"	Budleigh-Salterton Cottage Hospital	Devonshire	12	5	Charity established in 1881.
"	Haywood Hospital, Burslem	Staffordshire	31	24	Hospital enlarged in 1891.
"	Dartmouth Cottage Hospital	Devonshire	6		Founded to celebrate the Queen's Jubilee.
"	East Retford General Dispensary and Cottage Hospital	Nottingham	4 and 1 cot.		Dispensary opened in 1865.
"	Emsworth and District Jubilee Cottage Hospital	Hampshire	5		Originally 4 beds.
"	Victoria Cottage Hospital, Kington	Hereford	5		
"	Victoria Infirmary, Northwich	Cheshire	15	3	
1888	Victoria Cottage Hospital, Barnet	Hertford	8		
"	Blandford Cottage Hospital	Dorsetshire	14		Originally 6 beds.
"	East Grinstead Cottage Hospital	Sussex	5		
"	Feversham Cottage Hospital	Kent	10	3½	
"	Gorleston Cottage Hospital	Suffolk	4		
"	Victoria Cottage Hospital, Romford	Essex	9 and 2 cots.	5¾	
"	Victoria Hospital, Southend	Essex	6	4	
"	Victoria Jubilee Hospital, Swaffham	Norfolk	6		
"	Victoria Hospital, Swindon	Wiltshire	12 and 2 cots.		
"	Tavistock Cottage Hospital and Public Dispensary	Devonshire	9		Dispensary opened in 1832.

Year when Hospital was opened.	Name of Hospital.	County.	Number of Beds.	Average Number occupied.	Remarks.
1888	Winchcombe Cottage Hospital.	Gloucester	4		
"	Victoria Cottage Hospital.	Isle of Guernsey	10	6	
"	Stephen Cottage Hospital, Duffown	Banff	10 and 1 cot.	15	
1889	Cornelia Hospital, Poole.	Dorsetshire	17		
"	Chapel Ash Hospital for Women, Wolverhampton	Staffordshire	7		
"	Montague Cottage Hospital, Mexboro	York	14		
"	Woolwich and Plumstead Cottage Hospital, Shooters Hill	Kent	12		
1890	Huntly Jubilee Cottage Hospital	Aberdeen	18		
"	Bingley Cottage Hospital	York	12		
"	Gorebridge Fever Ho-pital	Edinburgh	12	3	
"	Cheshunt Cottage Hospital	Hertford	6 and 2 cots.		
"	Stanmore Cottage Hospital	Middlesex	8		
"	Runworth Fever Hospital, Thirsk	Lancashire	12		
"	Lambert Memorial Hospital, Thirsk	York	6		Hospital built and endowed by Mrs. Lambert. Treatment chiefly by bromo-iodine water.
"	Alexandra Hospital, Woodhall Spa	Lincolnshire	15		
"	Kirkcaldy Cottage Hospital	Fife	10		
"	Kendray Hospital, Barnsley	York	25		
1891	St. Mary's Cottage Hospital, Plaistow	Kent	4 lying-in and 4 general.		
"	Goole Cottage Hospital	York	10	4	
"	Paignton Cottage Hospital and Provident Dispensary	Devonshire	9 and 2 cots.		
"	Coleraine Cottage Hospital	Londonderry	10		
"	Hinckley Cottage Hospital	Leicestershire	5		
1892	Faringdon Cottage Hospital	Berkshire	8		
"	Mary Hewetson's Cottage Hospital, Keswick	Cumberland	10		
"	Herne Bay Cottage Hospital	Kent	4		
"	Smith Hospital, Henley	Oxfordshire	16		
"	Market Drayton Cottage Hospital	Shropshire	8		
"	Horsham Cottage Hospital	Sussex	8		
"	Leanchoil Hospital, Forres	Morayshire	12 and 2 cots.	4	

UEBER DEN BAU VON KINDERKRANKENHAUSERN, ISOLIRUNG UND VERHÜTUNG DER UEBERTRA-GUNG VON INFECTIONSKRANKHEITEN, VER-PFLEGUNG DER KRANKEN.

Von Dr. Adolf Baginsky,

Professor der Kinderheilkunde a. d. Universität Berlin.

Die fortschreitende Kenntniss der Krankheitsvorgänge, gefördert auf der einen Seite durch die theoretischen Hilfswissenschaften, insbesondere durch die Bacteriologie, physiologische Chemie und durch die verfeinerte mikroskopische Technik, auf der anderen Seite durch die eingehendste klinische Beobachtung, kommt nicht allein dem heilenden ärztlichen Wirken in dem Einzelfalle zu Gute, sondern sie führt auch zur Feststellung hygienischer Thatsachen, aus welchen praktische Nutzanwendungen im Grossen für ganze Bevölkerungsschichten hervorgehen. In den hygienischen Einrichtungen der Neuzeit spiegelt sich so gleichsam der jeweilig errungene Standpunkt medicinischen Wissens, und es ist unschwer zu erkennen, wie die ersteren von dem letzteren dauernd beeinflusst und umgestaltet werden.

Ist diese Beobachtung schon an den den Culturmenschen zunächst umgebenden Dingen, an Haus- und Wohnungseinrichtungen, an der Art der Zuführung der wichtigsten Lebensbedürfnisse, wie Nahrung und Wasser, an den Einrichtungen zur Entfernung der Abfallstoffe u. dgl. mehr zu machen, so kennzeichnet sich doch die tief eingreifende Wirkung des Fortschrittes medicinischer Erkenntniss und ärztlichen Wissens nirgends mehr, als dort, wo es sich direct um Einrichtungen handelt, welche dazu geschaffen werden, hereingebrochene Krankheit zu beseitigen, dieselbe von dem einzelnen Erkrankten zu heben und für die Gesammtheit unschädlich zu machen.—Im Krankenhausbau in erster Reihe krystallisirt sich gleichsam das in dem Augenblicke errungene gesammte medicinische Wissen und so ist jedes neu errichtete Krankenhaus, in der Voraussetzung, dass es die höchsten Ziele verfolgt, und dass die fachwissenschaftliche Leistung nicht durch andere, heterogene Einflüsse beengt oder gar verdrängt wird, ein Markstein dieses Gesammtwissens. So kommt es denn—und es ist dies das Geschick auch des besten Krankenhauses—dass dasselbe, während es in dem Augenblicke, wo es errichtet ist, das Ideal zu verkörpern scheint, gerade um deswillen, weil es, gegenüber der fortschreitenden Entwickelung der medicinischen Wissenschaft ein Stabiles, mehr oder weniger Unveränderliches repräsentirt, nach einer Reihe von Jahren veraltet, überflügelt wird, nicht mehr auf der Höhe der Zeit steht. — So ist es ausserordentlich schwierig, ja unmöglich, das wirklich Ideale im Krankenhausbau zu erreichen und man wird sich stets damit zufrieden geben müssen, dasjenige erreicht zu haben, was nach der Gesammtlage der erreichten Kenntniss als das ideal Beste erscheint.

Wenn demnach in den folgenden kurzen Thesen gewisse Punkte für den Bau von Kinderkrankenhäusern als Norm fixirt werden, so kann damit nur ausgedrückt werden, dass dieselben dasjenige zusammenfassen, was nach dem augenblicklichen Standpunkte unseres Wissens gefordert werden muss; von Hause aus aber wird zugestanden werden müssen, dass zukünftige grosse, bahnbrechende Errungenschaften in der Medicin nicht ohne Einfluss auf derartige Normen bleiben können.

In diesem Sinne mögen also die folgenden Thesen aufgefasst werden.

I. *Bau und Einrichtung.*

1. Das Bedürfniss für specielle Kinderkrankenhäuser ist gegeben durch die besonderen physiologischen und pathologischen Verhältnisse des kindlichen Alters, welchen in allgemeinen Krankenhäusern gerecht zu werden kaum möglich, zum mindesten sehr schwierig ist. Die Altersstufen, für welche diese Thatsache Gültigkeit hat, sind diejenigen von 0—12 Jahren, ausnahmsweise bis 14 Jahren. Innerhalb dieser Altersstufen sind die Kinder von 0—7 Jahren diejenigen, welche vorzugsweise die ärztliche Hilfe beanspruchen, während nach der 2. Dentition eine Zeit relativer Widerstandsfähigkeit gegen Erkrankungen eintritt.

2. Säuglinge (Alter von 0—1 Jahren) gedeihen in einer Krankenanstalt erfahrungsgemäss am besten bei Darreichung der Mutterbrust (resp. Ammenbrust). Ein Kinderkrankenhaus, welches Säuglinge aufnimmt, soll daher so eingerichtet sein, dass auch den Säugenden Aufnahme gewährt werden kann. Diese fast unabweisliche Bedingung würde dazu führen, die Säuglingsstation abnorm gross zu gestalten, und mit der Grösse der Abtheilung würden wegen der Schwierigkeit der Gestaltung normaler hygienischer Verhältnisse die Gefahren für die jüngste Altersstufe in gleichem Masse wachsen. Hier kann als wesentliche Aushilfe die ambulatorische Krankenbe-

handlung eintreten.—Die Einrichtung einer *Poliklinik* ergibt sich also, abgesehen von anderweitigen Gesichtspunkten der Zweckmässigkeit, mit Rücksicht auf das Säuglingsalter als eine Nothwendigkeit für ein Kinderkrankenhaus.

3. Eine besondere Stellung nehmen die an ausgesprochen contagiösen Krankheiten leidenden Kinder ein. Es muss Fürsorge getragen werden, dass die Uebertragung ansteckender Krankheiten verhindert wird. Dies geschieht durch möglichst vollkommene Isolirung sowohl der Kranken wie des Pflegepersonals.

4. Für diejenigen Fälle, welche einer contagiösen Krankheit bei der Aufnahme verdächtig sind, ohne dass noch eine präcise Diagnose gestellt werden kann, bedarf es der Einrichtung einer Beobachtungsstation (Quarantaine).—Im Anschluss an die Quarantaine erscheint auch die Einrichtung einer Abtheilung für Kranke mit Mischinfectionen geboten.

5. Demnach zerfallen die Einrichtungen für ärztliche Behandlung im Allgemeinen, wie für Aufnahme und Verpflegung von kranken Kindern im Kinderkrankenhause in folgende Gruppen :

a) Die Poliklinik (Einrichtung für ambulatorische Krankenbehandlung) mit hinreichender Zahl von Isolirzimmern für ansteckende Krankheitsformen.

b) Einrichtungen für Säuglinge mit nicht contagiösen Krankheiten (Säuglingsstation), mit Einrichtungen zur Aufnahme der Säugenden.

c) Einrichtungen für nicht contagiöse Kranke in Altersstufen von 1-12, ausnahmsweise bis 14 Jahren. (Indifferente Station in 2 Abtheilungen zerfallend, *medicinische* (*innere*) und *chirurgische* (*äussere*).

d) Einrichtungen für contagiöse Kranke aller Altersstufen von 0 bis 12 Jahren (Contagien-Stationen). Aufnahme der Säuglinge, wenn irgend möglich, mit den Säugenden.

e) Einrichtungen für noch nicht bestimmbare, aber der Ansteckungsfähigkeit verdächtige Kranke (Quarantaine-Station).

f) Einrichtungen für solche Kranke, welche an Mischinfectionen leiden. Die Abtheilung für Mischinfectionen kann mit der Quarantaineabtheilung im Zusammenhang sein; vielleicht wird es, weil die Quarantaineabtheilung das ärztliche und Wartepersonal voraussichtlich nicht hinlänglich in Thätigkeit erhalten wird, aus Gründen der Verwaltung stets geboten sein, beide Abtheilungen (*e* und *f*) an einander zu fügen.

6. Im Einzelnen knüpfen sich daran folgende Postulate:

a) Die Poliklinik. In dem Ambulatorium treffen contagiöse und nicht contagiöse Krankheitsformen zusammen. Die Gefahr der Uebertragung der Infectionskrankheiten von Kind auf Kind im Ambulatorium ist gross, ebenso gross die Gefahr der Einschleppung von Infectionskrankheiten in die stationären Abtheilungen des Krankenhauses. Daher ist geboten, dass die Poliklinik von den stationären Abtheilungen vollständig getrennt ist, ferner dass in der Poliklinik hinlänglich getrennte Räume vorhanden sind, um die eingebrachten infectiös kranken Kinder vom Augenblicke des Eintrittes von einander getrennt zu halten.—In der Poliklinik begegnet man begreiflicherweise am ehesten denjenigen Krankheitsbildern, welche eine sichere Diagnose nicht zulassen. Daher ist die Verbindung der Poliklinik mit der Quarantainestation sehr naheliegend und die Unterbringung beider in einem Gebäude nicht unzweckmässig. Selbst die Leitung der gesammten Krankenaufnahme, auch für die stationären Abtheilungen, durch die Poliklinik kann bei sorgfältiger Trennung der Krankheitsformen als zweckmässig erscheinen.

b) Die Säuglingsstation wird aus den entwickelten Gründen nicht zu gross zu gestalten sein.

c) Die Einrichtungen für die *medicinische* (*innere*) und die *chirurgische* (*äussere*) Abtheilung (indifferente Kranke) können ohne Weiteres nach denjenigen Erfahrungen gestaltet werden, welche auch sonst auf dem Gebiete des Krankenhauswesens vorliegen.—Im Einzelnen werden an den für chirurgisch kranke Kinder bestimmten Betten Vorrichtungen zu treffen sein, welche eine Verunreinigung der Verbände durch Harn und Stuhlgang möglichst verhindern.—Im Anschluss an die chirurgische Abtheilung wird auf Einrichtung einer orthopädischen Turnanstalt Bedacht zu nehmen sein, während die innere Abtheilung ausreichend mit Tagräumen für reconvalescente Kinder bedacht werden muss.

d) Die Contagienstationen. Der leitende Grundgedanke bei Einrichtung der Contagienstationen muss die vollkommenste Isolirung der einzelnen Abtheilungen von den indifferenten und auch von einander sein. Jedes Contagium hat sich als mehr oder weniger leicht übertragbar auch auf solche Kranke erwiesen, welche von einem anderen Contagium heimgesucht sind. Die für das Kindesalter wichtigsten Krankheitsformen, welche hier in Frage kommen, sind Diphtherie, Scharlach, Masern, Keuchhusten, und in Ländern mit mangelhaft durchgeführter Vaccination auch Variola. Jede dieser Krankheitsformen beansprucht sonach ein eigenes, von den übrigen Gebäuden getrennt stehendes Haus, mit Wohnungseinrichtung für Wärterpersonal und Arzt, und Desinfectionseinrichtung für den eintretenden resp. austretenden Besucher.

e) Die Quarantainestation. Dieselbe erheischt die Einrichtung einer gewissen Anzahl von Einzelzimmern, womöglich mit getrenntem Pflegepersonal für jedes Zimmer.

Dasselbe gilt für (*f*) die Kranken mit Mischinfectionen.

7. Bezüglich Anlage der Wohnungen für den ärztlichen Leiter, den Verwaltungsvorstand, für die Assistenten der indifferenten Stationen, die Apotheke, Bureaux, Waschküche, Küche, Wärterinnenwohnungen (mit Ausnahme derjenigen von den Contagienstationen) können im Wesentlichen die bisherigen, aus allgemeinen Krankenhäusern gewonnenen Erfahrungen zur Anwendung kommen. Nur muss bezüglich der Waschvorrichtungen die Sorge getroffen sein, dass die Wäsche aus den Infectionspavillons (Contagienstationen) noch bevor sie in den allgemeinen Waschraum und in die allgemeinen Waschgefässe eingebracht wird, einem gründlichen, durchaus sicheren Desinfectionsverfahren unterworfen wird. Zu diesem Zwecke kann die Wäsche entweder in desinficirende Lösungen ½—1 % Sublimat eingebracht werden und daselbst einige Stunden verweilen, bevor sie in das Waschhaus kommt, oder sie muss vorher im Desinfectionsapparat (am besten mit strömendem Wasserdampf arbeitend) desinficirt werden.[1] Für die Art der Einbringung der Wäsche in den Apparat aus den Infectionsabtheilungen sind die allgemeinen jetzt geltenden, die Unmöglichkeit einer Verschleppung der Contagien sichernden Grundsätze der Hygiene geltend zu machen. In erster Reihe ist darauf Bedacht zu nehmen, dass die Wäsche einen gewissen Grad von Feuchtigkeit hat, damit nicht Contagien durch Verstäubung verbreitet werden.

Besondere Sorgfalt erheischt die Anlage der Heiz- und Ventilationsvorrichtungen. Bei der Empfindlichkeit der kindlichen Respirationsorgane ist von der schwierig zu regulirenden Luftheizung völlig Abstand zu nehmen. Die Wasserheizung, allenfalls in Combination mit der Niederdruckdampfheizung ist als das vorzüglichste Heizsystem zu empfehlen.

---

[1] Hierbei macht man leicht die Beobachtung, dass die Wäsche durch unvertilgbare Flecken verunziert wird.

Die Ventilation muss von der Heizung unabhängig sein. Am besten ist bei dem starken Luftbedürfniss welches in einem mit Contagien belegten Krankenhause vorhanden ist, und welches einen 3maligen Luftwechsel pro Stunde voraussetzt, die Combination von Pulsionsventilation mit Aspiration, und wo dies zu kostspielig erscheint, zum mindesten die einfache Pulsion.

8. Die bisher entwickelten Anforderungen lassen die normale Gestaltung und die Leitung eines Kinderkrankenhauses nicht leicht erscheinen. Aus diesem Grunde darf ein Kinderkrankenhaus nicht zu gross angelegt werden. 250—300 Betten dürfte die äusserste Zahl der Betten sein, welche für ein einzelnes Kinderkrankenhaus einzurichten wäre.

9. Die Bemessung der Grösse der einzelnen Abtheilungen, insbesondere die Feststellung der Verhältnisse zwischen indifferenten und Contagienstationen ist schwierig zu treffen und wird in jedem Orte nach den langjährigen statistischen Erfahrungen zu machen sein.

10. Die einzelnen Krankenzimmer müssen in Kinderkrankenhäusern nicht für eine grosse Anzahl Betten eingerichtet werden. Die Einrichtung kleiner Krankenzimmer erschwert unzweifelhaft die Pflege und Ueberwachung, sie ist indess gar nicht zu entbehren, weil bei Ansammlung einer grösseren Kinderzahl in einem Saale die Unruhe einzelner Kinder sehr störend wirkt, überdies aber ist, insbesondere bei den contagiösen Krankheitsformen, eine Isolirung von Kindern durch die Art des Auftretens der Krankheiten sehr oft und weitaus häufiger geboten, als bei Erwachsenen. Zimmer für 2—4—6 in den Contagienstationen, bis 10—12 in den indifferenten Stationen sind entsprechend. Der Cubikraum pro Bett auf ca. 32 cbm, die quadratische Fläche auf 8 Quadratmeter (also bei 4 m Höhe) ist bei geeigneter Ventilation völlig ausreichend.

11. Nach diesen Anforderungen ist der Baracken- oder Pavillonbau das für ein Kinderkrankenhaus einzig geeignete System, mit der Einschränkung, dass für die Contagienhäuser der langgestreckte, einstöckige Pavillon, für die indifferenten Stationen und Poliklinik auch der zweistöckige Pavillon annehmbar erscheint, und das generelle Programm gestaltet sich sonach folgendermassen:

a) Verwaltung; Apotheke, eventuell auch Säuglingsstation als selbständiger Bau, beliebig mehrstöckig.

b) Je ein 1- oder 2stöckiger Pavillon für die medicinische (innere) und chirurgische (äussere) Abtheilung mit Operationssaal, Turnsaal (orthopädischem) und Tagräumen.

c) Poliklinik mit reichlichen Isolirzimmern und Quarantaine (zwei-stöckiger Pavillon).

d) 5 Isolirhäuser—je ein für sich stehender lang gestreckter ein-stöckiger Pavillon.

e) Haus für Centralheizanlage mit Desinfectionsapparat, Wasch-küche, Kochküche und so weiter.

f) Leichenhaus mit Sectionsräumen, Studienräumen mit allen Einrichtungen, welche die Wissenschaft erfordert, insbesondere mit Einrichtungen für mikroskopisch-anatomische, bacteriologische und chemische Forschung.

Ueberdies Gartenanlagen in reichlicher Ausdehnung.

II. *Verhütung der Uebertragung von Infectionskrankheiten.*

Es gibt vorzugsweise 3 Quellen der Uebertragung von Infections-krankheiten.—Die Mängel der Diagnostik und die so geschaffene Möglichkeit, infectiöse Kranke direct mit anderen in Berührung zu bringen.—Sodann die Uebertragung durch Mittelspersonen (Aerzte, Pflegerinnen, Beamte, Besucher der stationären Abtheilungen).— Endlich die Uebertragung durch Gegenstände.

Die erste Quelle kann möglichst verstopft werden durch sorgfäl-tige Untersuchung und ausgiebige Anwendung der Quarantaine. Absolut sichere Verhütung der Uebertragung auf directem Wege wird aber nach dem augenblicklichen Stande unseres Wissens kaum möglich sein.

Die Uebertragung durch Mittelspersonen kann verhütet werden durch absolute Trennung des ärztlichen Personals und der Pfleger in den einzelnen Abtheilungen. Ersteres wird nur sehr schwierig durch-zuführen sein, weil es ein sehr umfangreiches ärztliches Personal vor-aussetzt, welches meist nicht zur Verfügung steht. Verständniss für die einschlägigen Fragen und Gewissenhaftigkeit der Aerzte in der Desinfection wird indess diese Uebertragung auf ein Minimum redu-ciren.—Trennung des Pflegepersonals ist leichter durchführbar und deshalb geboten.

Besuch fremder Personen auf den Infectionsabtheilungen ist nur ausnahmsweise und unter besonderen Cautelen der Desinfection zu gestatten; dann kann Einschleppung fremder Contagien durch Fremde verhütet werden.

Uebertragung durch Gegenstände ist durch sorgfältige Desinfec-tion und strengste Reinlichkeit, die sich auf alle Gegenstände, wie Wäsche, Geschirr, Apparate und so weiter, zu beziehen haben wird, zu verhüten. Reichliche Anwendung antiseptischer Lösungen und Sterilisation durch strömenden Wasserdampf (Wäsche, Kleidungsstücke) eventuell Vernichtung durch das Feuer (Abfall, Nahrungsreste, Kehricht und so weiter) sind die Hilfsmittel, die Uebertragung zu verhindern.

III. *Verpflegung der Kranken.*

Die Verpflegung kranker Kinder ist weitaus schwieriger als diejenige der Erwachsenen, weil neben derjenigen Rücksicht, welche die Art und Schwere der Krankheit der Ernährungsart auferlegt, immer noch die Altersstufe der Erkrankten Berücksichtigung erheischt, überdies aber Gewöhnung und durch Erziehungsfehler geschaffenes Widerstreben der Kinder mehr als beim Erwachsenen zur Geltung gebracht wird; endlich beanspruchen einzelne Krankheitsformen besondere Ernährungsart.—Die Combinationen, welche für das erkrankte Kind nothwendig werden, sind also weit mannigfaltiger. Man wird bei sorglicher Berücksichtigung der erwähnten Momente zu folgenden Diätformen gelangen.

1. Diät für Reconvalescenten von schwerer Krankheit und für fieberlose, an zehrenden (chirurgischen) Affectionen Leidende.—Es wird einem Uebermass von Nahrungsbedürfniss zu genügen sein.

2. Diät für chronische, nicht fiebernde Kranke, mit gewöhnlichem physiologischen Nahrungsbedürfniss.

3. Diät für Kranke mit geringerem als physiologischem Nahrungsbedürfniss unter besonderer Berücksichtigung eines noch nicht völlig normal functionirenden Verdauungsvermögens. Es ist dies die Diät für mässig fiebernde oder kürzlich entfieberte Kranke im Beginne der Reconvalescenz.

4. Diät für hochfiebernde Kranke.—Fieberdiät, wesentlich in flüssiger Nahrung bestehend.

Es handelt sich also zunächst um Festsetzung von 4 Hauptdiätformen für alle Altersstufen. Lässt man nun die jüngste Altersperiode (Säuglingsalter selbst bis zur Mitte des zweiten Lebensjahres gerechnet) ausser Betracht, weil dieser Altersstufe durch hinreichende Milchzuführung unter Hinzufügung von relativ geringen Mengen von Amylaceen Genüge geleistet werden kann, so werden in einem Krankenhause, in welchem Kinder bis 12 eventuell selbst 14 Jahren verpflegt werden sollen, immer noch folgende Altersstufen besondere Berücksichtigung finden müssen.

a) Kinder im Alter vom 9. bis 12. eventuell 14. Jahr.

b) Kinder im Alter vom Anfang des 5. bis Ende des 8. Lebensjahres.

c) Kinder im Alter vom 1½—4 Jahren.

Es werden also jene oben erwähnten 4 Diätformen für jede dieser Altersstufen zu fixiren sein, so dass wir im Ganzen zu 4mal 3 Diätformen gelangen.

Nach den bisherigen, immerhin sehr wenig zureichenden Ermittelungen über das Nahrungsbedürfniss der Kinder in den verschiedenen Altersstufen ist es vielleicht gewagt, bestimmte fest begrenzte Nahrungsmengen zu fixiren, und es wird der empirischen Handhabung ein ziemlich weiter Spielraum belassen werden müssen, bis die fortschreitende Erfahrung auch hier sichere Normen kennen lehrt. Es muss dies namentlich aber für das erkrankte Kind in Geltung bleiben und es muss darauf hingewiesen werden, dass es eine der wichtigsten Aufgaben der modernen Kinderkrankenhäuser wird, die für gesunde Kinder inaugurirten Ernährungsstudien an Erkrankten und Reconvalescenten fortzusetzen.—Nach den vorliegenden Arbeiten von Forster, Camerer, Uffelmann u. A. wird man vielleicht wagen können, folgende Nahrungsmengen als die relativ richtigen für die erwähnten einzelnen Diätformen und relativen Altersstufen zu fixiren.

I. *Diätform.*

  a) (Altersstufe 9—12—14 Jahren). Bedürfniss pro Tag 88.0 g Eiweiss + 60 g Fett + 260 g Kohlenhydrate.

  b) (Altersstufe von 5—9 Jahren). Bedürfniss pro Tag 70.0 g Eiweiss + 50 g Fett + 200 g Kohlenhydrate.

  c) (Altersstufe von 1½—4 Jahren). Bedürfniss pro Tag 60 g Eiweiss + 45 g Fett + 150 g Kohlenhydrate.

II. *Diätform.*

  a) Bedürfniss pro Tag 70 g Eiweiss + 50 g Fett + 200 g Kohlenhydrate.

  b) Bedürfniss pro Tag 60 g Eiweiss + 45 g Fett + 150 g Kohlenhydrate.

  c) Bedürfniss pro Tag 52 g Eiweiss + 40 g Fett + 125 g Kohlenhydrate.

III. *Diätform.*

  a) Bedürfniss pro Tag 65 g Eiweiss + 50 g Fett + 165 g Kohlenhydrate.

  b) Bedürfniss pro Tag 55 g Eiweiss + 45 g Fett + 125 g Kohlenhydrate.

  c) Bedürfniss pro Tag 40 g Eiweiss + 40 g Fett + 100 g Kohlenhydrate.

IV. *Diätform.*

a) Bedürfniss pro Tag 60 g Eiweiss + 50 g Fett + 150 g Kohlenhydrate.

b) Bedürfniss pro Tag 50 g Eiweiss + 45 g Fett + 125 g Kohlenhydrate.

c) Bedürfniss pro Tag 42 g Eiweiss + 38 g Fett + 85 g Kohlenhydrate.

Man erkennt sofort, dass II *a*) sich fast deckt mit I *b*),

II *b*) " " " " I *c*),

so dass hier schon die Möglichkeit einer Reduction in der Zahl der
Diätformen sich ergibt und vielleicht werden noch weitere Ein-
schränkungen ohne Benachtheiligung sich möglich machen lassen:

Nach den König'schen Diättabellen wird es möglich, die vorgeschriebenen Werthe in solche Nahrungsmittel umzusetzen, welche
für die jeweilige Altersstufe und den jeweiligen, oben skizzirten
Zustand der Erkrankten passen.

Es wird hierbei darauf Bedacht zu nehmen sein, dass die jüngeren
Altersstufen ihren Eiweissbedarf in hervorragender Weise aus ani-
malischer Kost werden zu ziehen haben und dass das Gleiche auch
für die älteren Kinder gilt wenn es sich um Fieberzustände oder um
solche Zustände handelt, welche eine gewisse Rückständigkeit der
Verdauungsleistung voraussetzen lassen. Es wird dies insbesondere
für die Diätformen III und IV in Betracht zu ziehen sein.—Zwischen
Fetten und Kohlenhydraten wird, um einen etwas grösseren Wechsel
der Nahrung zu erzielen, in zwar nicht allzugrossem Massstabe,
indess immerhin bis zu einer gewissen Grenze nach Massgabe der
Calorien Vertretung stattfinden können; allerdings darf nicht ausser
Acht gesetzt werden, dass Kinder im Ganzen ein ziemlich reichliches
Bedürfniss nach Fettzufuhr haben.—Im Einzelnen wird die Vertheilung der Nahrungsmengen auf den Tag in den verschiedenen
Ländern nach Gewohnheit und Lebensweise verschieden sein. Für
Deutschland erscheint es zweckmässig, 5 Mahlzeiten anzunehmen,
davon sind 2 grössere, 3 kleinere, mit entsprechender Vertheilung
der Nahrungsmengen. In dem Masse als die Kinder fortgeschritt-
enen Altersstufen angehören und ihr Aufenthalt im Krankenhause in
fieberlosem Zustande sich verlängert, ist auf Wechsel in der Nahrung
Bedacht zu nehmen. Nur die Säuglinge vertragen die Monotonie
der Ernährung, da Milch das Nahrungsbedürfniss für lange Zeit bei
denselben deckt.

THE UTILITY, PECULIARITIES, AND SPECIAL NEEDS OF HOSPITALS FOR CHILDREN.

BY WILLIAM WALLIS ORD, M. D. Oxon., M. R. C. P. London.

Physician to Out-Patients at the Victoria Hospital for Children, Chelsea.
Physician to the West End Hospital for Nervous Diseases, London.

There has always been, both in the medical profession and out-side, a certain difference of opinion as to whether special hospitals can show a decided claim to a separate existence. In this country, certainly, most, if not all, of our special hospitals have originally been the outcome of individual benevolence, and it is still a moot-point whether in the present state of poverty of many of our great public charities any further advance in founding special institutions is advisable. Be this as it may, it is certain that many valuable insti-tutions of the kind exist in London and elsewhere, starting from small beginnings but in the end eventuating in great public boons.

> " Parva fuit, si prima velis elementa referre,
> Roma,"

may in truth be said of many of the hospitals of this land, and of none is it more true than of the special hospitals, and among them the hospitals for sick children are conspicuous instances. Many of these charities, started, as their histories tell us, in small and quite unsuitable tenements, have in the course of time become places world-wide in reputation not only as charities but as centers for research and the diffusion of knowledge. It has very truly been said that without special hospitals the rapid advance of science in the treat-ment of special diseases would have been seriously retarded. And this is most true with regard to children's hospitals. In most, if not all, of our great general hospitals in London there are departments for treating, and teaching on, diseases of the eye, the ear, the throat ; for the special diseases of women ; for the treatment of the severer forms of venereal disease. And yet with regard to the diseases of childhood, more, far more, important to the community at large than any of these, for we are all children once, how little is or indeed, I may almost say, can be done in these institutions. True it is that in many of our general hospitals there are special wards for children, into which a certain number of comparatively chronic cases are admitted yearly, and which serve more or less as a "show ward" when visitors are taken round the hospitals, but the amount of good that should be done in this direction is not to be measured in this way. In addition to the in-patient treatment we must bear in mind the exceedingly important out-patient department, and it is in this respect conspicuously that the general hospital fails. There is probably an out-patient department, which is open two or three times a week, under the care of a distinguished gynecologist, for the treatment of " women and children," but a single visit to one of these will show to what this admixture tends. The physician in charge is naturally anxious to obtain and impart knowledge in this particular line in which he is interested, and it comes about in process of time that this section of the out-patient department becomes the "department for women and children " with the children left out.

With regard to the treatment of children as in-patients in a general hospital we are at once confronted with serious difficulties. The special wards for women cannot, of couse, be filled with cases of hip disease and cholera infantum. If the hospital be fortunate enough to possess a special ward for children, cases requiring particular care—or operation—can, of course, be sent there. But even in such a case a children's ward in a general hospital is a focus of danger, and must necessarily be so. We shall see later how rife outbreaks of zymotic diseases are in special children's hospitals. It is just as true a fact here and causes, if possible, a greater upset of general routine. But if such a special ward do not exist, then the children have to be taken into the ordinary wards with the adult patients. This mode of procedure is open to three serious objections, from the point of view of the adult, from the point of view of the child, and from the point of view of the nurse. Nothing could, of course, possibly be worse than to have a squalling infant in a ward with a patient just coming round after a serious operation, or in the delirium of pneumonia or enteric fever. There are many people in health who cannot endure to be with children all the time. How much less then when they are afflicted with illness, acute or chronic? With regard to the children, too, it is evident that a certain number must be of an age to mark, learn and inwardly digest, and no less evident that, whether in the ordinary routine of the ward, or when, as they always do, they as convalescents become the pets of adult convalescents, they are exposed to the possibility of acquaintance with matters the knowledge of which it were at all events better to postpone. Thirdly, it is notorious that children require special care and special nursing, and it would be necessary not only to increase, but also to modify, existing nursing arrangements in the wards of general hospitals, should the admission thereto of child-patients exceed a certain proportion.

This, then, being a brief review of the method of treating children in general hospitals, let us turn to the other side of the question, and consider the advantages and disadvantages of special hospitals for children. The bugbear that meets us on the threshold is zymotic disease. If we take the history of one of our children's hospitals, we find that, in spite of the utmost care on the part of the staff, professional and nursing, we have from time to time serious outbreaks of infectious disease occurring within the walls. Whether children are congregated together, or whether they are distributed in a certain proportion among adults, these diseases are bound from time to time to make their appearance, but it is evident that the outbreaks must be more severe and more difficult to cope with in the former than in the latter case. Infection is introduced in various ways. The patient may be suffering from an intercurrent disorder, for which he is admitted, and may infect the ward before the specific nature of his ailment is recognized. There may be an error of diagnosis, pardonable enough, as I have had abundant means of knowing. But I am convinced that the greater proportion of infectious disease is introduced into the hospitals by the relations and friends, who may by the rules of the establishment visit them from time to time. The majority of outbreaks which I have come across in my own experience could be traced, by a process of exclusion, to this source.

That this is the case, the authorities of one of our largest London hospitals, which possesses a special ward for children, are so convinced, that relations and friends are not admitted as visitors to the ward in the ordinary way, but are only allowed in if the patient's life be in danger. It is a serious question in my mind whether this plan might not be with advantage adopted generally in the case of children's hospitals.

Another source of danger which can at all events in time be obviated, but which still exists in some of the children's hospitals in this country, which, as I have shown above, exists in buildings not originally intended for hospitals, but merely temporarily adapted for that purpose, is the existence of the out-patient department in the same building as the wards. Cases of infectious disease come to the out-patient department daily, of necessity, and, as they are bound to stay a certain time in the part of building set apart for them, are thus liable to infect the whole.

This danger of epidemics of infectious disease is really, as far as I know, the only argument against congregating children together in a hospital entirely devoted to their charge. Let us now examine the other side of the question, and see what advantages such institutions offer, both to the patients and the doctor.

I think there can be no doubt that children are happier in a ward by themselves than when mixed with adults. They see other children around them, a certain number able to sit up and play with their toys, and they thus soon learn to regard the hospital as a home, and to cease to pine after their relations. The discipline, too, is better. Children in a general ward nearly always are spoiled, by being made the pets of nurses and patients alike. This of course is obviated when all are children, and the consideration has no mean bearing upon their future life. In the second place, the nursing of children, especially those of tender years, is distinctly a branch by itself. Children require much more care in certain ways than adults, and the charge of them, though it may require for the moment a less amount of physical exertion, yet by the frequency and urgency of the calls renders the duty a most fatiguing and anxious one. With the nurse, as with the doctor, in a children's hospital, the fact that many of the patients cannot express their needs, sensations, or desires, induces a strain that is not felt with the majority of adult patients. There are numberless *petits soins* that are matters of daily routine in a children's ward, that would either be overlooked or a source of difficulty, and possibly of neglect, in another place. The matter of feeding alone may be adduced in support of this view. The sterilization and artificial digestion of food carried on as a matter of course in a children's ward, would be a still further tax on the already too multifarious duties of a nurse in a general ward.

From the point of view of the doctor, children's hospitals are a great boon. Apart from the fact that by their existence he has a particular set of cases congregated together, to be utilized as may be for the purpose of learning and teaching, we must face the fact that little or no teaching is done in this special line in the general hospitals, or at all events in the majority. There is one hospital in London where the most valuable and systematic teaching is given in this line in the wards, but in the majority it is neglected, mainly I think because those in charge of the out-patient departments do not "weed" the cases with discretion, their attention being naturally drawn to the more congenial points of adult disease, and hence it arises that the cases of disease in children admitted are, on the medical side, cases of extreme urgency, not available in the majority of cases for the purposes of clinical instruction, and are apt, on the surgical side, to be cases of chronic trouble which do not lend themselves attractively to the process of demonstration by the bedside; the number admitted in either case being of necessity comparatively small. Of clinical demonstration in the out-patient department there is, as I have said, little or none, and so the children's hospital becomes in consequence a happy hunting-ground to all who are possessed of the belief that a knowledge of the diseases which our flesh is heir to at the most critical time of our life is essential to one who aspires to become a physician or surgeon in the highest sense of the word. And let me say here that it is not in the wards alone, or even chiefly, but in the out-patient department, that this line of study can be carried out to the greatest advantage. It is unfortunately true that hitherto here in London the vast field of clinical material presented in the out-patient departments of our children's hospitals has been entirely neglected. But it is pleasant to learn that, under the extended curriculum now required by the General Medical Council, a certain amount of special attention to the diseases of children, both clinically and theoretically, is required, and I hope before long that our children's hospitals will take the place they should in our otherwise admirable system of clinical instruction in this country.

On coming to the question of peculiarities and special needs of children's hospitals, we are confronted at once by the great question of nursing. It is a commonly accepted dictum that the successful issue of a case of enteric fever depends more upon the nurse than the doctor. I think that with regard to the special case we have in view we may expand this statement and say, that in the treatment of all diseases of children, good and reliable nursing is of primary importance, and that our success largely depends on it. Not only do children, and particularly infants, require constant and careful supervision, but they require more than this. They require to have around them persons who, if they cannot on all occasions anticipate their wants and wishes, yet must be able, either by experience or natural aptitude, to recognize the signs and symptoms of wants and wishes which the patient in so many cases is unable to impart or explain. And in this respect the nursing of sick children is an arduous and anxious occupation. It is the practice, in this country at all events, to admit as nurses in children's hospitals women who would be disqualified by their youth from becoming nurses in general hospitals, and in the general hospitals themselves nurses are admitted as attendants in the children's ward, where it exists, at an earlier age than to the general wards. I suppose that this practice arose from the idea that a case of a child is, in colloquial nursing parlance, a "lighter case" than that of an adult, and that, the wear and tear of the system being consequently less, women of less mature age and development might be with safety employed. Now for my part I believe that this is a fallacy. Doubtless the actual physical exertion of lifting patients, or assisting them to rise, of making and rearranging beds, and of ministering to their periodical requirements, is much greater when adults than when children are in question. But on the other hand we must take into consideration that in the case of children the calls are more frequent and more urgent, and that the sense of responsibility which every nurse must feel is greatly increased in the latter case, and is a much greater strain mentally, and in a secondary manner corporeally, on a woman of 20 than on one of over 26 years of age. So that I think that in children's hospitals, nurses should not be admitted too young. I have seen many cases of breakdown, some of them serious, others only temporary, which could be referred, at all events in part, to the age of the nurse. With regard to the numbers of the nursing staff relative to the number of beds in the ward, it is the outcome of experience in this country that children's wards must be much more strongly nursed from a numerical point of view than adults' wards. This is a natural corollary of what has been said above with regard to the needs and requirements of child-patients. The large number of the nursing staff in a children's hospital naturally must cause a great increase in the annual expenses. It would be imagined, *a priori*, that the average cost per head per patient would be very much less, in a children's than in a general hospital. This is in reality the case, but the difference is so remarkably small as to be almost unappreciable. The average cost of each in-patient in ten of the largest London hospitals is £6 15s. 0d., in the six London children's hospitals £6 12s. 0d. approximately. Of course the children's hospitals, from the fact that the number of inmates is small as compared with the in-patients of a general hospital, would naturally have an increased cost per head, it being easier to treat a large number of patients at a less cost per head than a small number, but considering the saving that must necessarily be made in the way of food, dressings, etc., it is plain that there must be some source or sources of increased expenses in children's hospitals. This mainly arises from the absolute necessity, to which I have drawn attention above, of having a nursing staff proportionately larger than that of a general hospital. In fact, so much does the number of the necessary nursing staff increase the annual cost of the institution, that certain children's hospitals in this country do not admit as in-patients in the ordinary way children below the age of two years. How this extraordinary state of affairs came about originally I can hardly imagine. Certainly I have never heard any medical man express an opinion in its favor. That this is the most critical period of the child's life I think may be taken from the following facts, viz:—that in the annual report of the Victoria Hospital for Children for the year 1892 the total death-rate was 13.3 per cent, while the death-rate of children below the age of two years was 75 per cent. And yet unless a child is practically moribund it is not admitted to the hospitals above referred to, with the consequent result that a small death-rate and a diminished cost of working per head can be announced in the annual report. Not only, in my opinion, is such a regulation absolutely unjustifiable, but I consider, on the contrary, that special attention ought to be given to cases of this age, and that where possible a separate ward should be provided for infants, with a numerous and specially adapted nursing staff. As so many of these cases are of the nature of gastro-enteritis and the like, it is evident that ample and efficient means for attending to the special requirements are absolutely necessary for the safety and well-being of the hospital at large. But the difficulty must not be shirked by excluding them from the benefits of the institution, but rather the capacity of the latter must be extended to meet their needs.

With regard to the general construction of a children's hospital from an architectural point of view I have not much to say here, nor is it my province so to do. There is only one point which may be considered, and that is the number of cubic feet per bed. In the case of adults, the necessary cubic space is variously estimated from 1,200–2,000 cubic feet, but about 1,500 or 1,600 cubic feet are probably about the average. Of course the amount may be much lessened in the case of children, but it may be taken that in a children's hospital, where the age may vary from one day to 12 years, the minimum allowance should be 800 cubic feet per bed, and that 1,000 cubic feet would be more desirable. The following figures, extracted from Burdett's "Hospitals and Asylums of the World," give the cubic space per bed in some of the principal London children's hospitals:

Great Ormond Street Hospital. .... 919.92 c. f. per bed.
East London (Shadwell) Hospital...... 907.02 "   "   "
Victoria Hospital, Chelsea................ 833   "   "   "
Evelina Hospital, Southwark ... . 1096.2 "   "   "

while in the provinces and elsewhere the figures range from 1,683 per bed at Pendlebury to 715.55 at Aberdeen. It is extremely necessary that ample and rapid means of ventilation should be provided, as it is evident that, especially in summer, evil odors are inseparable from the cases, by reason of the nature of prevailing ailments, the proper dispersal of which is absolutely necessary. The wards should be of such construction that the principles of natural ventilation may obtain, but this is of course not always possible in the cases where the building has only been modified for hospital requirements and not specially built for that purpose.

I have here a few words to say, with regard to diet and cooking. The dietary of children of the varied ages indicated already must of necessity vary considerably. Consequently, the preparation of food must necessarily be more complex in a children's hospital. It is quite possible to prepare the bulk of the food in a general kitchen supplying the whole hospital. But the cooking, and especially the preparation by means of artificial digestion, of food for special cases is best carried out by the nurses in the ward kitchen, which should have all the necessary apparatus for this object.

Certain authorities, who are now taking the lead in bringing the process of hospital construction to a science, tell us that in all hospitals the out-patient department should be in an absolutely separate building from that in which the wards are situated. This proposition is naturally more true in the case of children's hospitals than of others, owing, of course, to the danger of the introduction of infectious disease from the out-patient department to the main hospital, when they are under the same roof. Of course, sheltered means of communication must exist between the two departments, but they should be practically isolated from one another. With regard to the out-patient department itself, there should be ample means therein to afford isolation to such cases as may require it. Every day cases of infectious disease come to the out-patient department of every children's hospital. Certain of these ailments of the less severe type, such as whooping-cough and varicella, should be at once, on recognition, segregated from the bulk of the cases, until the requisite medicines can be obtained, and they are removed by their friends. In the case of the more severe forms of infectious disease, such as scarlet fever or diphtheria, an absolutely isolated, well warmed, well ventilated and easily disinfected waiting-room must be provided for the accommodation of the case, until it can be removed in an ambulance either to a fever hospital, or in certain cases to its own home. Such a room should be so placed that while it is readily approached from the hospital, there is also ready communication with the street, so that in the process of conveyance to the ambulance, risk of spreading infection may be minimized.

With regard to infectious disease in the main hospital I am of opinion that in London at all events, with its special hospitals for the reception of cases of fever of all kinds, no case of infectious disease in its acute stage ought to be taken into a children's hospital, with one important exception, and that is diphtheria. For this disease there should be in every children's hospital a special ward, constructed for this purpose, and used for this disease alone. A lengthy experience as a resident medical officer and, since then, as a physician to a children's hospital, has shown me that a certain proportion of cases, varying according to the severity of the epidemic, must be treated within a very short time of the recognition of the disease, if any hope is to be entertained of their recovery, while in a certain smaller number removal to a fever hospital is practically, from the state of the patient, impossible. Such a ward must be ready for the reception of, and the necessary operations on, a case of diphtheria night and day. A few minutes' delay may mean death, a few minutes' gain by forethought and organization may mean safety. With regard to isolation-wards for the treatment of infectious diseases other than diphtheria there is, in London at all events, no necessity to provide them. They are bound to be in a way a source of danger, whatever proper precautions may be taken, and it is far better to send cases coming to the out-patient department or occurring in the wards to one of the recognized fever hospitals. It is, however, necessary to have a properly isolated ward into which surgical cases, which have been recently operated on, and which have contracted some acute specific fever, can be placed either until their surgical condition may admit of their removal to a fever hospital, or, in certain cases, until their complete convalescence from the fever. But such a ward must be used sparingly and with caution —only in cases of absolute necessity. I have heard it advocated that in children's hospitals there should be a separation-ward, in which cases of possible infectious disorder arising in the wards should be placed for a time until their exact nature is determined. I have seen such an experiment tried, and it was quite unsatisfactory. Cases of this kind must be settled at once, and delay in diagnosis only invites disaster. If once a habit is engendered among the resident medical officers of any hospital of regarding every case of rash as one of difficulty and doubt, farewell for the time to the efficiency of that hospital. Doubtful cases must of course arise from time to time. But in the majority of cases the symptoms are fairly prominent, and the diagnosis should be at once made. Proverbs are proverbially fallacious, but in the ordinary case of a suspicious rash the man who hesitates is lost.

Finally, there is one adjunct that is absolutely necessary to make an ideal children's hospital, at all events in the case of one situated in a great city, and that unfortunately is beyond the means of most of them to supply. I mean a convalescent home, situated either in the country, or better, at the seaside if possible. Such a home relieves the hospital wards in three ways. First it takes a certain number of cases from the out-patient room which are not progressing favorably under treatment, either from non-hygienic surroundings at home, or from want of proper care. Some of these cases would have to be admitted to the wards from time to time, and would increase the normal pressure. Secondly, cases of convalescence from medical and surgical diseases can be sent away to the convalescent home earlier than to their own homes, and with much more benefit to themselves. Thirdly, it is well known that a number of cases are admitted to the surgical wards the state of whose health precludes immediate operation. These can be sent to the home and prepared for the ordeal, thus rendering the ultimate result much more hopeful, both from the point of view of the patient and the surgeon.

The relief of pressure thus afforded to the parent hospital renders it a far more efficient agent for the treatment and relief of cases of urgency and danger than it could be possibly did it stand and work alone.

In conclusion I wish to thank you, sir, and through you the members of the Congress, for the great honor you have done me in allowing me to bring this paper before you.

CHILDREN'S HOSPITALS IN AMERICA.

By Miss Mary L. Rogers,

Superintendent Children's Hospital, Washington, D. C.

In attempting to fulfil the request for a paper on this subject, difficulty has been found in drawing a proper line between, first, institutions for children partly of hospital, partly of asylum or orphanage intent; second, those manifestly for children, yet admitting certain classes of adults, notably of gynæcological and obstetrical service; and third, the hospital exclusively for children : all of which are constantly broadly classed under the title children's hospitals. Each has its own merit and interest, but to treat of all would lead to confusion. It has been decided to speak only of the hospital designed for sick children alone, and with one exception (the San Francisco Children's) the hospitals referred to are strictly of this class.

These institutions have existed in America only during the last half of this century—indeed, have a history covering less than forty years. In 1850 appears almost the first literature upon the subject. A young dispensary physician in New York, writing under the title of Philopedos, sent out to the public an appeal for the lives of the children. He says that at this time there is no adequate place for the sick children in the general hospitals of the city, already overcrowded, and after a recital of their pitiful condition among the poorer classes, closes with a statement more emphatic than many pages of appeal, that in that year, of the entire city death-rate 81 per cent. were children under ten years.

To the ordinary mind statistics do not form interesting literature, but statistics such as this are impressive. And yet New York must have thought either that child-life was of little consequence, or that the building of hospitals was not the proper method for its preservation, for little was done there until the establishment of St. Mary's Free Hospital for Children twenty years later.

Philadelphia, in 1855, was the first to create such an institution for the exclusive care and treatment of sick children, and so little hold had it upon the public sympathy that it was opened with but twelve beds,—certainly a conservative number.

The history of each succeeding effort has been a repetition of this small beginning, until the very last one is instituted.

Boston came next in 1869, with the same service as Philadelphia, Washington in 1870 with six beds, and in the same year New York, already referred to, Albany in 1875 with two beds, San Francisco at the same time with four, Detroit in 1877 with twelve, and St. Louis in 1879 with ten. In New York the Laura Franklin was instituted seven years ago, and emboldened perhaps by the successful growth of its predecessors, opened with fifty beds, the only large beginning of which we have record. Canada has a representative hospital of this class in Toronto, built and conducted upon the most modern methods. Two years ago Louisville fell into line, representing in its hospital alone the entire work throughout the southwestern States.

The ensuing history of each is curiously similar. Under adverse conditions, with discouragements innumerable, the start was made. No large private endowments nor munificent public appropriations, such as so often lift other institutions of the kind beyond financial care, even in their infancy; only the hand-to-hand struggle of the few who recognized the need and the pity of any little child suffering from illness without proper care. Children's hospitals in America appear to be structures founded and finished by faith and pennies.

Another feature which strikingly presents itself, and which may very fittingly follow such a record, is that this has been in such large degree the work of women.

Physicians appear from the first to have advised and approved the establishment of these special hospitals. The boards of directors or managers may often be largely composed of men, but the earliest reports in nearly every instance show the names of women who provided the time, the zeal and the means for its establishment, and the latest reports as conclusively show that it is women who provide its yearly sustenance.

The character of work done is on one line, acute general medical and surgical service. In the large number of personal letters of information from hospitals of this class we gain, first, that there is no provision for admission of contagions. Of this feature of work it is only fair to say that it has not been merely disregarded by the various boards of trustees. The Philadelphia Children's Hospital, at great expense and infinite care, established a croup ward for admitting patients in the hope of successfully isolating and treating the malignant forms of throat disease, and were encouraged by most marked success, particularly in operative measures which would have been impracticable outside a hospital, owing to the lack of appliances for immediate emergency measures and of suitable after-care. After a short time, one or two years I think, the health board of the city ordered its discontinuance, much to the grief of the management. Others have spent much time and thought in attempting to arrive at a satisfactory arrangement, but with no permanent result, except perhaps in one or two instances where the work has been continued. Whether contagion can be safely handled continuously within the confines of a hospital with the highly susceptible class of patients we have to treat is still a mooted question. At best it is to be feared that until the same rigorous absolute isolation can be made to exist in all departments, with medical internes as with nurses and servants while engaged in its care, it is not too much to say that there is danger in it, and that the results of experiment will scarcely be such as to encourage boards of management to attempt it. Still, contagions form such an important feature in childhood diseases, they are so desperate in character in the large number of instances, they so particularly need the immediate, unceasing, unrelaxing care of both physician and nurse such as cannot be found elsewhere than in the hospital, that it is with reluctance that the withdrawal of this service from the children's hospital is looked upon, if any safe means can be devised for the reception and care of this class of patients. Perhaps a ward in the form of a separate establishment adjunct to the hospital, controlled by it, but at a considerable distance, connected when necessary by ambulance with the hospital proper, may be the solution. Such a plan has been discussed by one of these hospitals recently, and only discarded because of lack of funds. Again, there are no wards for chronic or incurable cases, although many of these last two classes are taken as an act of special mercy for a limited time. Yet again, one hospital only (the Detroit), in a list of twelve comprising the largest in the country, admits infants.

The outside age limit is from eighteen months to fourteen years, and in the greater number from two years to twelve.

Is there not food for reflection in these facts? In our cities, with the percentage they present of poor, whose conditions of life are those which foster these very chronic and incurable states in childhood, that no actual declared hospital provision is made for their amelioration, and that even more, infants, whose danger in illness is greatest, can actually not get in.

Will the child's hospital, as it now exists, grow broader in its line of work as its position becomes more assured, and eventually afford asylum for these now abjured classes, or is it destined, itself now a specialty, to subdivide its own little people into specialties each in its own institution? It is early to prognosticate futurities for this interesting work, but the shadowy signs of the times point to the second conclusion. New York, the center of advanced hospital methods, has even now for its children an institution for orthopedic surgery, and another for infants alone, both successfully managed and supported, even while there already exist two general hospitals of the class.

Whichever system may obtain, there is encouragement to believe that eventually all hospital care of children will be conducted in places designed for them alone.

To enter into the detailed plans of conducting all the work of these institutions would be beyond the scope of this paper, but a brief report of one department may be of interest to members of this Congress. Equally with other hospitals is the nursing growing to be regarded as of the greatest importance. At a superficial view there would seem to exist much less advance in this here than elsewhere, if lack of uniformity of method argues lack of advance. In truth, the nursing taken as a whole is in a somewhat chaotic state. No system has as yet been declared by general adoption as best. What this perhaps most truly argues is an appreciation of the peculiar nature of the work to be done, and the difficulty of fixing upon the best plan of conducting it.

To illustrate: one hospital employs a superintendent and head nurse (graduate nurses) who supervise, while the nursing is done by untrained assistants; and for serious cases trained nurses are temporarily employed. In another, one graduate nurse is regularly employed; a certain fixed number of pupil nurses from a training school of the same city are taken for one month each, and the remainder are untrained assistants. In another, the house physician is head nurse, with experienced not-trained nurses under him. The Boston Children's has recently established a school for nurses under a sisterhood. The Washington co-operates with another special hospital for its nursing, while the Children's of San Francisco comes out strongly in the sole ownership of a well appointed school of thirty nurses governed upon the lines of the large training schools.

Which system predominates? None. These hospitals are comparatively so few and the nursing methods so varied that we might say each is unique unto itself.

Which will predominate? It is only possible to say that no nursing requires more intelligence, more system, more comprehension of the work than this. Those who have lived and worked in the midst of a children's service will follow me with appreciation of its truth. Children in disease are more often non-committal than otherwise. Even pain, grave in its meaning, unless of acute character, is passed over unless the eye is always seeing and the judgment unerring. The error that may be made because the nurse does not see what the little patient cannot tell, is too often followed by grave results. Whatever method secures to the nurse more power to care with gentleness and with skill, quickens her perceptions of pain and danger, gives her most science to apply to her work, that method will predominate despite all difficulties. Twenty-five years ago a children's hospital which now stands pre-eminent in its broad ideas and advance of methods, offered a complete training and a certificate for sick-child nursing after a six months service in its wards, to girls not *under* sixteen years of age. It was preferred, although not compulsory, that the applicants should be able to read.

To-day we know that in child nursing we are undertaking one of the most delicate and difficult tasks of the profession, and that to do the work successfully the child's hospital must, at whatever cost, have the best system and the most capable nursing.

There is a question that is frequently repeated: Has this special hospital proved the best method of caring for the child, and are its advantages commensurate to the additional expense involved, over that of their treatment in the adult hospitals? In reply might we not ask: Does not the drawing together of the large number give opportunity for more comprehensive study of their diseases and of their best means of cure? Do we need more forcible argument than that from the small beginnings we have now hospitals averaging a hundred beds, each showing constant healthy growth; and that the reports of these institutions bear the names of the most distinguished men of the medical profession connected and identified with its work? Do we not know here may exist conditions advantageous to the special patient not to be acquired otherwise? In these days of exact science physicians take into account all things which may influence the patient's condition, when not merely the administration of drugs or the application of a surgical appliance is all that is considered in treatment of the sick. Children require certain surroundings and privileges with which to treat the adult would be unfavorable. The companionship of his kind does much to relieve home-sickness and the tedium of illness; the need of change in convalescence brings the playroom, the kindergarten, and the country home as adjuncts to the hospital. The child being the motive power, we study his particular needs, his wants and the conditions under which he seems most content in sickness and most rapidly improves, and supply them because it is our work to do this particular thing; until somewhere in the future the perfect sick home of the little child is formed,—a mosaic from the years of suggestions and trials and plans one by one conceived.

A larger number of patients who need hospital care are obtained, than would be in the adult hospitals with an equal number, taken all together, of beds to receive them. Repeatedly I have been told by mothers that "they would bring the child where so many other children were, because he would not be lonely, but would never take him to a 'big' hospital." The natural shrinking from transmitting the child to the care of strangers in the case of many parents, the ignorance and oftentimes sad indifference of others, must all be considered as factors in keeping the sick child at home, and whatever offers inducement to these to admit the child to the hospital cannot be too carefully considered. To have any work properly done, not cheaply done, is true economy.

There is one further point only of which I would speak: the children's hospital as a possible economic factor in the commonwealth. Our annual national expenditure for the care and protection of our physically afflicted children is a matter of national pride. Witness the asylums for the deaf and the blind, and the homes for the cripple, built upon magnificent lines, supported by individual charity, by church and by state. Some part of these inmates are suffering from avoidable conditions. A celebrated oculist in Washington told me that we are spending $15,000,000 every year to care for the blind, and that a large proportion of cases of blindness were preventable with proper and timely treatment; that his own experiences with neglected cases of ophthalmia neonatorum alone, resulting in total blindness, were the saddest part of all his work.

The hospitals mentioned in this paper are an almost complete list of those in the entire country. The Louisville children's hospital of twenty-four beds, which has been referred to, is the sole hospital service of this kind in seven States. While these are doing to their uttermost extent, they are entirely inadequate to the need. One in New York publishes in its annual report that many times there will be a list of ten waiting applicants for a bed in an operation ward. All state that the demand is generally in excess of the number of beds. Is it not wiser, considering these existing facts, to build more hospitals, if as a consequence less asylums of the other class would be required? From a purely utilitarian standpoint, can we not better afford hospitals to cure the ills of childhood, and prevent the later and more pitiful necessity of places of refuge for the little victims of neglect, through, oftentimes, long lives of helplessness and suffering?

TOKYO CHARITY HOSPITAL.

TOKYO, JAPAN, *May* 17, 1893.

DR. JOHN S. BILLINGS, *Chairman, Third Section.*

Dear Doctor:—The history of the country tells us that charity institutions had been from time to time established since the reign of the Kimmei Junto (thirteen centuries ago) down to the first year of Manyen (1860), by the order of the Imperial House and Tokugawa family, mostly attached to the Buddhist temples, but I do not think worth to mention the details of them,—in fact, impossible to get exact informations on them, from the want of minute records. Thirty-three years ago (1860) a hospital was established at Nagasaki according to an European model. It was, however, done so in paying system, and in late years, hospitals of a similar character have increased to several hundred. There was therefore no true charity hospital established till the year of 1882, when the Tokyo Charity Hospital has been instituted and is supported entirely by voluntary subscriptions.

I at first meant to prepare a paper including hospitals of every kind of descriptions in this country, but failed to get materials from various circumstances—hence my desire to send to you a short description of the Tokyo Charity Hospital alone.　　　　Yours very sincerely,

K. TAKAKI, F. R. C. S. Eng.,

President of the Tokyo Charity Hospital.

I. *Organization.* A hospital committee was formed in 1881, and has organized the hospital by obtaining one hundred and thirty-six subscribers, and opened it in August, 1882. The hospital is patronized by Her Majesty the Empress since the year 1886.

There is a committee consisting of ten ladies, specially appointed out of lady subscribers by Her Majesty the Empress, the president of which is the Princess Arisugawa.

There are twelve medical and surgical consulting members, appointed by Her Majesty the Empress.

The medical staff consists of ten members, with three house physicians and surgeons, all unpaid.

II. *Hospital Finance.* The hospital is kept up by the interest of the fund 120,000 yen, voluntary subscriptions, and the income of the work done by the ladies' committee, such as bazar, art exhibition, etc. Cost for an in-patient about fifty sen, that for an out-patient about five sen a day.

III. *Wards.* Two wards of two stories are built with bricks according to pavilion system, and subdivided into rooms which can accommodate one hundred and twenty-two beds, though only sixty beds are at present made use of.

IV. Practically no paying patients.

V. Two small wards are provided with six beds for contagious diseases.

VI. Hospital dietaries and kitchens entirely in the Japanese manner.

VII. An operating room built with wood.

VIII. All washing done outside of the hospital, and bedding, clothing, etc., used for contagious cases disinfected by sending to the government disinfecting house.

Table showing No. of in- and out-patients:

	In-patients.		Out-patients.		Daily average No. of in- and out-patients.
Years.	Number.	Treatment days.	Number.	Treatment days.	
1882	157	6,657	349	13,525	55
1883	211	8,907	862	33,662	116
1884	315	17,102	1,770	48,654	180
1885	315	17,828	2,659	46,850	177
1886	224	13,121	2,196	35,285	176
1887	368	18,645	3,645	51,148	191
1888	398	19,287	4,293	58,942	214
1889	439	20,162	7,564	79,132	272
1890	463	20,579	6,163	68,707	244
1891	504	19,363	7,568	95,340	314
1892	472	18,306	12,775	93,283	305

Tokyo Charity Hospital Training School for Nurses.

The school was established with a fund subscribed by volunteers in the year of 1885.

The course of study for students, two years and a half.

The subjects taught, elementary anatomy, physiology and nursing. In past eight years, one hundred and twenty-two students were admitted, of which forty-seven have finished their course of study and obtained certificate after written, *viva voce* and practical examinations, twenty-two still studying, and forty-eight fell off.

The trained nurses are well received by the public.

A SHORT SKETCH OF THE CHILIAN HOSPITALS.

By Louis Asta-Buruaga, M. D., Valparaiso, Chile.

The hospitals in Chile are public institutions, partly supported by the government and partly by private charity. They have, nevertheless, in their administrative organization, a semi-political and a semi-religious character, which can be best comprehended by having a knowledge of the form of government that rules this country. The information on this subject given by the following extract from a letter in the *New York Herald* of October 8th, 1883, will suffice for the purpose:

"To understand Chile as a political power it is needful to study it at Santiago, where two-thirds of the ruling families have palaces which they inhabit during the southern winter, spending the summer, after the adjournment of Congress, either on great estates in the country or in villas at Viña del Mar. Possessing wealth which makes it independent of toil for livelihood, this ruling class pursues politics as a profession. In every sense it is an aristocracy. It does not comprehend the practicability of a control of government by public opinion. There is no public opinion in Chile (unless it be on religious topics) except as it dictates."*

Having read this statement, it will be easy to understand the system of hospital general administration prevalent in Chile, which I shall now proceed to describe.

---

* Mr. Albert G. Browne's address to the American Geographical Society in 1885 on *The Growing Power of the Republic of Chile.*

According to a bill passed by the Chilian Congress in 1886, public charity in each department of the Republic was put in the hands of Boards of Charity, called *Juntas de Beneficencia*. The magnitude of the work that each Board or *Junta* has to perform can be calculated by a summary of the duties entrusted to its cares. These manifold duties are : to prescribe rules and regulations for the different institutions under its charge, viz. service of hospitals, hospices, pesthouses, orphan, foundling and lunatic asylums, cemeteries, maternities, dispensaries, etc., to determine the appropriate number of employees in said establishments, to fix their annual expenditures, to take charge of all moneys and properties of the corporation, to authorize the leasing, letting or selling of the real estate belonging to the same, to revise the general accounts, to accept or repudiate any legacies, donations and so forth with which charity is favored, to defend the interests of the corporation by going to law, to propose new buildings and approve their plans, to prescribe rules of hygiene, to organize a charity-treasury office and appoint clerks therefor, and several other items too long to enumerate.*

These Boards or *Juntas* are composed of members elected partly by the President of the Republic and partly by the city municipality, and of the hospital administrators (*administrador-es*) who, at first, were elected by the President of the Republic and subsequently by the departmental Boards of Charity.

Under such nomination one would naturally suppose that only influential political friends of the government or of the ruling class were elected members of the different boards and hospital administrators; and such is really the case. No special requirements of a technical kind or of scientific knowledge are needed to fulfil the membership duties of such boards, although there is a saying in Chile to the effect " that in order to become a member of a *Junta de Beneficencia* it is necessary to be old, rich and devout,"† and actually it appears that, according to its present organization, no other qualities are required. The names of a number of well-to-do lawyers, farmers, merchants, statesmen and other minor political personalities figure among the list of members; but strangely enough, and what is most extraordinary, not a single medical man

*Reglamentos para las Juntas de Beneficencia de la República. Santiago de Chile, 1886.
† Attributed to a celebrated physician in Santiago.

nor any other individual with scientific attainments is ever appointed to the board.*

On account of the mode of election and the peculiar composition of such managing boards, the vicissitudes of the political parties have much to do with the instability of hospital administration in Chile. When President Balmaceda was in power and had a strong opposition party against him, he discharged from their posts all such members of the Boards of Charity as well as all such hospital physicians as did not uphold his political views; and in turn, when the Revolutionists made their triumphal entry in the Chilian metropolis, one of the first things that the new government did was to sweep away with all the managers and doctors belonging to the presidential party, and even many of those who, having taken no active part in the civil strife, did not side with the revolutionary party. " The spoils for the victors !" was the cry, and managers, doctors, and even orderlies, were dismissed from the hospitals in order to make room for new men. Naturally, midst such changes, the patients were the worst sufferers.

Although charity in Chile is governed, in a great measure, by politics, religion has also a share in its government. All the hospitals are under the charge of Sisters of Charity of the Roman Catholic faith, and they generally direct the Administrator in hospital matters.

The Administrator visits the hospital, sometimes daily, sometimes weekly, and goes through its diverse departments accompanied by the head nun or religious matron. He is to see that everything is kept in good order, and all papers should be signed by him; his duties are not much above those incumbent upon a committee of inspection in an American hospital. His services are gratuitous.

The Sisters, on the other hand, have charge of the general accounts, of the purchase of provisions, of the paying of salaries, of the supervision of employees and the nursing staff, of the maintenance of discipline, of the work in the drug-store and the supply of the same, of the care of the surgical instruments, etc.; in one word, they have the entire control of all the hospital management, in the very same manner

* In fact, there is a special clause in the Regulations of the *Junta* that incapacitates hospital doctors from holding office as members of the board. The 5th article of the said Regulations, in which mention is made of all those who cannot become members of the board, says in its second clause, "All paid employees of the establishment." Whereas, all the most noted doctors in the country have hospital appointments and are paid for their services, none of them can become members of the Boards of Charity.

as they had in the Paris hospitals about a century ago. Consequent
with the aims of such religious congregations, they seem to attend
more to the spiritual needs than to the physical demands of the
patients. The very same abuses which led to the secularization of
the Parisian hospitals may be seen here in full play, thanks to the
unlimited authority vested upon the sisters.

Thus politics and religion predominate in the management of
Chilian hospitals, and science is very little or not at all consulted in
their behalf; the consequence of such a state of affairs being that the
hospitals in Chile are far below the standard reached by similar charitable institutions in Europe and in the United States.

The medical board is practically a dead body. Its advice is rarely
solicited, or not at all, in matters relating to the welfare of the hospital, and any suggestions in that line made by it are generally treated
with indifference and even contempt.

The medical staff is composed of several visiting or attending physi-
cian-surgeons and one resident medical officer for each hospital. They
are appointed by the Board of Charity, upon recommendation of the
Administrator.

As no classification of cases is carried out at the hospital (medical,
surgical, gynecological, puerperal and infectious cases being huddled
together in the same ward), the doctors practice indiscriminately both
branches of general medicine. Each visiting medical man has to
attend a ward-service of from 26 to 36 patients, and is not assisted
in his work by internes, as there are none, except the one just mentioned (resident medical officer), who, in some hospitals, has under
his charge six hundred patients during the greater part of the day
and all the night. The visiting physician-surgeon makes his rounds
in the morning, examining each case and prescribing accordingly.
He receives a monthly fee, ranging from 30 to 50 paper dollars. The
house medical officer is paid 250 paper dollars a month in the larger
hospitals.

No case-records are kept, outside of the statistical admissions and
discharges registered at the office, under the care of the clerk. Not
even in the hospital clinics is history-taking practiced.* Tempera-
ture-charts are a luxury not to be seen in Chilian hospitals.

---

* I claim to speak with authority on this subject, as I held the position, after
a competitive examination, of assistant to one of the medical clinics of the
University of Santiago. During the whole scholar year of 1890 I had the
greatest difficulty in persuading the students to write out the anamnesis of the
patients under their observation, and towards the end of the year I only suc-

The nursing is nominally done by the sisters, who are paid ten paper dollars a month for their services, and they really act as overseers of paid untrained orderlies and nurses. It is useless to mention that this department, so important in a well-managed hospital, could be vastly improved by the establishment of a training school for nurses.

The outlay and purchasing of drugs, as well as their compounding and the preparation of prescriptions, are placed in the hands of the sisters, as was formerly the custom in Paris. There are no titled apothecaries in the hospital service.

Finally, not a single hospital in Chile has a pathologist among its officers.

In 1891 there were seventy hospitals in all the Republic.* Many of them possess incomes of their own, and besides receive subsidies from the government. In fact, all of them are helped by the state with more or less funds, the total amount yearly being 478,000 dollars in paper money (one dollar of Chilian money being equivalent now-a-days to about 30 cents American gold). Ships contribute yearly ten cents per ton to the maintenance of the hospital of the port they enter. Charity also adds to the income of these hospitals.

All cases are received in the public hospitals free of charge ; in only one or two there are wards for pay-patients.

There are in existence throughout Chile, besides the above-mentioned hospitals, seventeen pest-houses, eight hospices, five foundling asylums, only one lunatic asylum and one maternity (both in Santiago), and ninety-one dispensaries, upon all of which the state spends annually 257,000 paper dollars.

Outside of the governmental hospitals and other state charities, a few private ones, mostly due to private enterprise, have been established, and thus in Valparaiso foreigners are treated in an English and a German hospital ; and furthermore, in Lota, a coal-mine district, a small hospital has been nicely fitted up by the mining company, in order to nurse therein the sick and wounded in their employ.

A lengthy description of each individual hospital of Chile, as well as being beyond the scope of the present paper, would be unnecessary, as a rough sketch of a few leading ones in Santiago and

---

ceeded in collecting some fourteen histories from about one-half that number of students, the class numbering over twenty-five.

* The accompanying data are taken from the *Sinopsis Estadistica y Geogrdfica de Chile* for 1891, an official publication founded by Mr. F. S. Asta-Buruaga, formerly Chilian Minister at Washington.

Valparaiso will suffice to give an idea of all others throughout the country.

Santiago, the capital of Chile, with 200,000 inhabitants, has four general hospitals, two of which are of comparatively modern construction.

The *San Juan de Dios* hospital was founded in 1556 by Pedro de Valdivia, the conqueror of Chile. It was destroyed by an earthquake in 1647 and was reconstructed in 1702. The two-story building with corridors which makes up its structure surrounds a square court. The wards contain from ten to thirty-six beds. The ventilation, which is effected by windows and ventilating outlets, is deficient, as the lower edge of the windows is at a high level and their upper edge does not reach the ceiling. The walls are whitewashed and the flooring is of pine wood. The wards have no service rooms, in regard to which commodity all Chilian hospitals are entirely destitute. No mess-room being at hand, the meals are accordingly distributed to the patients in their wards, in consequence of which the emanations from the food diffuse throughout the atmosphere of the sick-room. Although most of the hospitals boast of a general bath-house, in this one, as in all others, there is a total absence of baths in connection with the wards.

Only males are admitted to this hospital. On account of its central location a large number of the patients are casualty cases.

The following table, taken from the report of the Junta of Santiago for 1890–91,* gives an idea of the capacity and mortality of the institution:

	1890.	1891.
Discharged,	3314	5604
Died,	901	976
In hospital,	256	287
Total treated,	4471	6867
Mortality,	20.3 per cent.	15.6 per cent.

The *San Francisco de Borja* hospital for women was founded in 1772, and its general features are about the same as those of the former. The buildings are old, although they have received some modifications of late. There is a maternity service connected with it.

* *Memoria del Presidente de la Junta de Beneficencia*, correspondiente á 1890-91. Santiago de Chile, 1892.

The statistics for the hospital are as follows:

	1890.	1891.
Discharged,	7495	6089
Died,	1204	1102
In hospital,	509	469
Total treated,	9208	7650
Mortality,	13.7 per cent.	14.34 per cent.

The *San Vicente de Paul* hospital was inaugurated in 1874. It is built on the one-story pavilion plan, but the buildings are so close together that each pavilion throws its shadow upon its neighbor. Twenty pavilions of from twenty-six to thirty-six beds are distributed over a small lot of ground. The long axis of the wards runs from north to south. In the wards there is a lack of ventilation and of light, on account of the small total superficial area of windows, a very common defect in Chilian hospitals. At both extremities doors open to the exterior, but the entrance of the back one is blocked up by a huge altar; almost all hospitals, in fact, have altars instead of medicine-chests in the wards. The most expensive building in the hospital is the chapel, which approaches the dimensions of a city church and is a decided hindrance to ventilation.

Lately, six new brick wards have been constructed for clinical purposes, which will make the number of beds border on six hundred. Curiously enough, the axes of the new buildings run exactly in an opposite direction of the compass to those of the old pavilions. Why this innovation has been carried out is a problem difficult to solve, as the prevailing winds in this region come from the south and the climate is a temperate one.

The *San Vincente* is generally considered the best hospital in Chile, although it is somewhat hampered by its situation, as the southern wind reaches it after passing over the whole city, and, furthermore, the general cemetery lies north of it, and near-by there are a medical school and a pest-house, and the only lunatic asylum in the whole country.

In addition to its public character as a charity, this institution receives pay patients, it serves for clinical teaching, and is also a military hospital.

The records of the *San Vicente* hospital give a much lower death rate than the two former hospitals, as the accompanying figures show:

	1890.	1891.
Discharged,	5989	7004
Died,	726	598
In hospital,	535	558
Total treated,	7250	8160
Mortality,	10.1 per cent.	7.32 per cent.

The *Salvador* hospital. This is a new hospital in process of construction; but two wards have been opened to the public. It is situated in the outskirts of Santiago. I have not had an opportunity to visit this establishment, so that I cannot give a fair account of its construction. It is intended for incurables, such as cancer and tuberculous patients, although cases with acute diseases are also admitted.

The statistics of this hospital show a frightful mortality, when we compare them with those of hospitals abroad intended for the same purposes. The *Royal Chest* hospital in London gave for the years 1877, 1878 and 1879 the following death-rate respectively: 10.9, 12.7, and 11.9 per cent,[*] whereas in the *Salvador* hospital the mortality ranges between 27 and 30 per cent, as can be seen by the appended table:

	1890.	1891.
Discharged,	89	90
Died,	62	75
In hospital,	80	82
Total treated,	231	247
Mortality,	26.83 per cent.	30.3 per cent.

In Valparaiso, which has a population of 120,000 inhabitants, there is only one state hospital for both sexes, that of *San Juan de Dios.*

It consists of an agglomeration of buildings, old and new, in the midst of which there is a large chapel, situated at the foot of a hill, on the summit of which six wooden barracks for military patients are also clustered. The area of ground for the aggregate number of beds, which count almost six hundred, is very limited. About the same conditions hold in this hospital as in those of Santiago, with the exception that Valparaiso, as a seaport, being somewhat of a cosmopolitan city, is more prone to accept new ideas and put them in execution, as far as political and religious interests allow.

* Frederic J. Mouat : *Organization of Medical Relief in the Metropolis,* page 31 ; in Mouat and Snell's *Hospital Construction and Management.* London, 1883.

Thanks to the enterprise of one of the hospital administrators,* a gentleman of English extraction and educated abroad, a pavilion was erected with two finely built wards, which have service rooms and well-conditioned water-closets. The long axis of the building is from south to north, in the direction of the prevailing winds. The wood-work in the wards is excellent, the walls are painted, the sash-windows (which are seldom seen in Chile) give a large superficial area of light, as they reach near to the ceiling, and the ventilator inlets and outlets being ample, are well calculated to admit a sufficient supply of fresh air in relation to the total cubic space of the ward. Each infirmary contains thirty-six beds.

Another comparatively modern pavilion to be seen in this hospital is remarkable for the size of its wards. The dimensions of the upper one (there being two such wards, one over the other), which I took the pains to measure, are as follows:

Length,	63.60 meters.
Width,	8.10 "
Height,	4.55 "
Superficial area,	513. square meters.
Volume,	2336.60 cubic meters.

As the ward contains sixty-five beds, these figures give the following measurements for each bed:

Lineal wall space,	1.90 meter.
Floor space,	7.89 square meters.
Volume of air,	35.84 cubic meters.

There are seventeen windows on one side of the ward and thirteen windows and four doors that communicate with an open balcony on the other. At one end there is a door that leads into the scullery and to the water-closets. Erysipelas is endemic in these wards, which have not once been emptied or painted interiorly in six years.

The statistical record of the San Juan de Dios hospital of Valparaiso reads as follows:

	1890.	1891.
Discharged,	5245	5009
Died,	1001	1141
In hospital,	581	561
Total treated,	6827	6711
Mortality,	19 per cent.	22.79 per cent.

* Mr. Enrique Lyon, of Valparaiso.

A short time ago, owing to the munificence of a wealthy charitable lady, a new hospital on the pavilion plan was erected in this port, but as it generally happens in Chile, the professional element was not duly consulted in regard to its plans, and the consequence was that, after an expense of an enormous sum of money and the costly and monumental building having reached completion, it was found to be inadequate for the purpose of attending sick people. The building has been lately handed over to a religious congregation to serve as an orphan asylum.

In other Chilian cities the state hospitals are on more or less the same footing as those already described. Talca, a city in the interior, has a fairly well constructed hospital, with brick-built pavilions laid out in the form of an even-branched cross. The novelty which distinguishes these pavilions from other hospital buildings in Chile is that they are built slightly raised above the ground, permitting, thus, some circulation of air under the floor of the wards.

In Iquique, the principal saltpetre exporting port of the Republic, there is a small hospital composed of wooden huts.

Much more could be added to what I have already said about Chilian hospitals, but I am afraid the subject reads like ancient history, and thus is not worthy of exciting the interest of modern scientific men, whose main aims are to seek the best means obtainable and arrive at the most efficient manner of rendering help to the sick poor. In studying these hospitals, no new suggestions, no new lines of conduct can be elicited from their present organization and construction, and the only conclusion that can be formulated in regard to them is that they urgently need a total reform.

Allow me to state, in finishing up my remarks, that it would be most gratifying to me if some day I could see the hospitals in Chile based upon the same laws as the International Conference on Hospitals at Chicago may deem it proper to propose for the construction and management of charitable institutions.

VALPARAISO, *May* 1, 1893.

THE HOSPITAL CARE OF THE SICK AND THE TRAIN-ING OF NURSES AT AMSTERDAM.

BY EDWARD STUMPF,

Medical Director City Hospital.

If we limit the history of the origin of the hospitals at Amsterdam only to that which gave rise to the formation of the institutions now existing, we are obliged to go back even to the sixteenth century. We find mentioned in 1578 that the two hospitals existing at that time (the St. Peter and St. Mary hospitals) were removed to the nunneries of the "oude en nieuwe nonnen," the nuns being driven away from their homes for that purpose. These nunneries were therefore the first origin of the general city hospital called " Binnen Gasthuis," which is still to be found in the same place. Being considered for that time an extensive building, it was appropriated to males and females and to medical and surgical patients; it also contained, in addition to the necessary buildings for administration, an institution for the shelterless.

According to the municipal maps of Crommelin, the hospital was situated in the center of the city, and consisted of six buildings separated by gardens and canals. Each of these buildings was destined for different classes of the sick, and also for patients suffering from contagious diseases. This was, however, altered soon, for in 1630 a new foundation was built, about a quarter of an hour out of the town, which was exclusively designed for imbeciles and infectious patients. Both remained united under one management, a board of trustees assisted by a physician as general governor. Ever since this principle of management has been maintained, so that both these hospitals are managed by one board.

This management has to do only with general financial matters. The medical and nursing care of each of the institutions is entrusted to a medical director, who is assisted by a matron and house governor, respectively, as heads of nursing and administration. Although few alterations have been made in the management, many changes have been made in the building. If we compare their present plans with those of an earlier date, we find only a few subordinate parts which call to mind the former construction; everything else has disappeared. Not to mention improvements and rebuildings of a temporary nature, we see now the "Binnen Gasthuis" enriched in 1870 with an obstetric hospital for 50 persons; in 1875 with a surgical pavilion for 80 patients; in 1880 with a surgical barrack for 30 women; in 1881 with an extensive building for laboratories and post-mortems, and in 1890 with a large pavilion for 270 medical patients. Except the barrack for surgical females and the obstetric hospital, which are built according to the "corridor" system, all are built after the same principle, viz., buildings two or three stories high, with large wards at the end of each floor, while the middle wing is occupied by the smaller household apartments (bathrooms, tea-kitchens, nurse dwellings, etc.). The so called "Binnen Gasthuis" remained the longest unaltered. After being destroyed in 1730 by fire, it was rebuilt almost in accordance with the former plans, and not until 1889 was a new building erected. At this date, new pavilions, one for imbeciles, two for males and females. and three for infectious patients, were erected. The two city hospitals furnish altogether room for 1200 to 1300 patients. During the last hundred years we see, coincident with the extension of·the city hospitals, new foundations erected by private initiative. In 1804 the Dutch Hebrew Board of Charity bought a house in the street called Rapenburg, to use for their sick. They stayed there until 1820, then removed to a military hospital, thence to a new building which was opened in 1830, and which was again left in 1840, till at last in 1883 the present new institution was occupied. In 1834 the Portuguese Hebrew Board of Charity founded also a new hospital, to which only patients of the Hebrew religion were admitted. In 1839 the Roman Catholic Church erected the St. Bernardus institution, chiefly for the aged, but also available for nursing some patients.

In 1857 the "Vereeniging von Ziekenverpleeging," which had existed since 1844 (Association for Nursing), occupied a new building on the Prinsengracht, which in addition to being a home for the nurses was especially designed for the reception of patients. In 1865 the building of the Children's Hospital was opened, which, commencing with only 8 patients, extended steadily in the course of time, until there is at this moment room for more than 100 children.

In a short time Amsterdam saw several more institutions arise, viz., the "Inrichting voor Ooglyders" (Institution for Ophthalmic Patients). In 1874 the "Roomsch Katholike Verpleeging" (the Roman Catholic Hospital) in 1878; while, owing to the initiative taken by Dr. Berns, a paying hospital was opened in 1879, which soon becoming too small for the many applications, was left for a new building, the "Burgerziekenhuis," which is constructed according to the most modern requirements (pavilion-barrack system), and furnished room for 145 patients.

In 1889 Dr. Mendes de Leon opened his private hospital for women's diseases; in 1891 the "Vereeniging von gereformeerde Ziekenverpleeging" (the Association of Protestant Sisters) was established, like in 1892 the "Luthersche Diaconnessen Inrichting" (the Home for Lutheran Deaconesses), the Institution for Psychotherapeutics of Dr. Van Eden and Dr. van Renteghern, and the Institution for Pneumo- and Hydro-therapeutics of Dr. Arntzenius.

In this enumeration are not mentioned the military hospitals, because they do not profit the commune of Amsterdam, but are central government asylums.   Though all these institutions aim at the admitting of patients, the "Binnen Gasthuis," the "Buitengasthuis," the Children's Hospital, the Dutch Hebrew Hospital, the Institution for Ophthalmic Patients, the Association for Nursing, and the Roman Catholic Hospital, can only be considered as real hospitals, because the others either have very limited room or make their main business nursing outside the institution.

The management of the institutions differs.   All agree in one respect, that a board of guardians has the supervision, except at the private hospitals of Dr. Mendes de León and Dr. van Renteghern, which are managed absolutely by themselves, the difference being chiefly in the relation between the medical director and the board of guardians.   Undoubtedly we find the greatest power of this board in the Association for Nursing, the Roman Catholic Hospital, the Association of Protestant Sisters, and the Home for Lutheran Deaconesses, because there these boards have complete charge of the management, and because a medical director is wanting.   The Binnen Gasthuis, the Buitengasthuis and the Dutch Hebrew Hospital form the second class.   Here these boards are assisted by a medical director, who, participating with an advisory vote in the meetings, has the responsibility of the daily management, while the third class formed by the Burgerziekenhuis, the Institution for Ophthalmic Patients, and the Children's Hospital, where the medical director is a member of the board, and the whole management, including the financial part, is intrusted to him, but he is responsible to the board. As regards the means of support of these institutions, both the city hospitals and the Dutch Hebrew hospitals differ from the others.

The Binnen Gasthuis and Buitengasthuis are the two official city hospitals. Every expenditure which cannot be covered by the nursing rate is charged to the city, and this expenditure is considerable. As both the institutions are chiefly built for parish paupers, they are not proper for the admission of paying patients; so that the receipts are made up from patients who do not reside in Amsterdam, and by the payment of non-paupers who as accident cases are admitted in the hospitals, or for capital operations. That they are but a small proportion of the total number of patients is clearly indicated by the following table:

In 1881 the paying patients of the total number were 6.7 per cent.
" 1882   "   "   "   "   "   "   8.4   "
" 1883   "   "   "   "   "   "   6.3   "
" 1884   "   "   "   "   "   "   6.4   "
" 1885   "   "   "   "   "   "   7.6   "
" 1886   "   "   "   "   "   "   7.2   "
" 1887   "   "   "   "   "   "   8.8   "
" 1888   "   "   "   "   "   "   9.9   "
" 1889   "   "   "   "   "   "   6.9   "
" 1890   "   "   "   "   "   "   5.5   "
" 1891   "   "   "   "   "   "   5.2   "

The expenditures which were charged to the community of Amsterdam were:

In 1881 fl. 261,530   In 1887 fl. 374,832
 " 1882 " 273,660   " 1888 " 359,276
 " 1883 " 406,475   " 1889 " 373,589
 " 1884 " 423,115   " 1890 " 471,319
 " 1885 " 396,644   " 1891 " 509,226
 " 1886 " 387,869

Besides this expenditure the community is obliged to contribute to the expenses of the Hebrew hospitals. These institutions are chiefly for the nursing of poor Jews, and the community makes an annual contribution amounting to 65,000 florins. The other part of the expenditure of these hospitals is paid by the nursing receipts (9 per cent), legacies, donations, while the deficiency is paid by the Hebrew Board of Charity. In 1892 this parish subsidy amounted to fl. 30,000. These three are the only church hospitals enjoying subsidies from the community; all the others are maintained by donations, legacies, rents, and payments of the patients. Most of these institutions give opportunity for paid nursing at the following rates:

Burgerziekenhuis.			Association for Nurses.
1st class fl.	10		fl. 7.50
2d " "	7		" 5
3d " "	5		" 2
4th " "	1.50		

Institution for Ophthalmic Patients.			Gynæcological Hospital.	Roman Catholic Hospital.
1st class fl.	5		fl. 7.50	fl. 5
2d " "	3		" 5	" 3
3d " "	2		" 3	" 1.50
4th " "	1.25			free.

The Children's Hospital furnishes free beds. In the Roman Catholic Hospital 40 patients are nursed without payment from the community.

The construction of all these hospitals differs, partly owing to the influence of time, place and building, partly to the purposes for which they are used. The Buitengasthuis and the Burgerziekenhuis are the only ones which are built after both the pavilion and barrack systems. Similar to these are the two asylums where patients suffering from acute infectious diseases (scarlatina, variola morbilli, typhus, cholera, etc.) are nursed. The other hospitals cannot admit them, except the Children's Hospital, which has isolating wards for contagious diseases. Imbeciles are only cared for in the Dutch Hebrew Hospital and the Buitengasthuis, while the Roman Catholic Hospital excludes women in childbed and venereal patients. The Association for Protestant Sisters admits only medical patients, and finally, the Home for Lutheran Deaconesses only medical female patients. The special hospitals, as the Children's Hospital, the Institution for Ophthalmic Patients, and the Gynecological Hospital, are, as a matter of course, only accessible to patients suffering from the special diseases treated there. That frequent use is made of the different institutions is best shown by an enumeration of available beds compared with the total number of the days of nursing, each institution provides: Binnengasthuis, 600 to 700; Buitengasthuis, 500; Burgerziekenhuis, 27 first, second and third class, 97 fourth class, 21 isolating beds; Children's Hospital, 85 and 30 isolating beds; Dutch Hebrew Hospital, 110; Roman Catholic Hospital, 70; Hospital for Ophthalmic Patients, 5 first class, 8 second class, 45 third class; Association for Nursing, 17; Gynæcological Hospital, 12; Portuguese Hebrew Hospital, 21.

The number of days of nursing during the last ten years was annually:

	Binnengasthuis.	Buitengasthuis.	Burgerziekenhuis.	Children's Hospital. General.	Children's Hospital. Isolating.
1882	....	....	8,562	....	....
1883	159,036	95,011	9,959	16,529	1536
1884	174,473	111,416	10,247	17,061	4484
1885	172,243	95,760	9,955	13,887	3232
1886	171,786	116,593	10,868	16,583	3363
1887	178,376	118,169	10,936	17,817	2898
1888	166,382	130,541	10,341	19,076	2366
1889	168,400	137,821	11,520	17,507	3255
1890	206,305	150,755	11,766	18,363	3107
1891	227,553	167,380	15,635	14,632	3326
1892	236,013	160,386	26,689	21,559	2925

	Dutch Hebrew Hospital.	Roman Catholic Hospital.	Association for Nursing.	Hospital for Ophthalmic Diseases.	Portuguese Hebrew Hospital.	Gynæcological Hospital.
1882	21,498	10,158	3050			
1883	19,318	11,687	3021			
1884	21,628	14,191	3076			
1885	27,385	19,610	2047			
1886	25,440	19,625	2351	First class, 427.7. Second class, 659. Third class, 11,116. Average in the last 10 years:	Average in the last 10 years: 2655.	
1887	29,006	21,501	2974			
1888	25,410	22,271	2012			
1889	28,294	23,665	2480			
1890	33,111	23,497	2516			
1891	37,212	....	3147			2500
1892	35,536	....	4178			2500

Very different are the figures showing the length of residence per patient. We have thus:

	Binnengasthuis.	Buitengasthuis.	Burgerziekenhuis.	Children's Hospital. General.	Children's Hospital. Isolating.
1883	41 days	76.1	33	52	11
1884	34.79	74.3	35	51	15
1885	35.65	74.9	29	43	16
1886	35.18	69.5	26	45	15
1887	33.21	70.3	28	49	13
1888	34.32	69.8	30½	49	11
1889	36.64	61.7	29	45	13
1890	36.54	70.7	27½	45	9
1891	39.92	66.2	29	45	10
1892	39.21	62.2	36	40	11

	Dutch Hebrew Hospital.	Roman Catholic Hospital.	Hospital Ophthalmic Patients.	Portuguese Hebrew Hospital.	Gynæcological Hospital.
1883	33⅓ days	53			
1884	31½	54.3			
1885	33 9/10	46.8	Average: First class, 15.8. Second class, 13.3. Third class, 22.5.	Average, 49-50.	Average, 30-40.
1886	31¾	46.8			
1887	32¼	44.7			
1888	32¼	44.1			
1889	31⁴⁄₇	40.7			
1890	30⅝	43			
1891	35⅞				
1892	33¼				

The considerable numbers in columns 1, 2, 4 and 7 are partly caused by the fact that as the patients do not pay they show no desire to be discharged, and partly because the physician needs to exercise care in the discharge of patients, because they are often obliged to resume very fatiguing work. A bad feature also is the want of institutions where chronic patients and convalescents can be admitted (the incurable are in part admitted to the municipal almshouse). The long residence in the Buitengasthuis is partly due to these general causes, but must chiefly be attributed to the long residence of the neuropathics, who form there one-quarter to one-fifth of the total number of patients.

It is very difficult to compare the expenditure of the different hospitals. First of all, because the mode of calculation is so various. In the greater part of the institutions with class nursing, the medical side, the drugs, instruments, wine, etc., are paid separately, while in the hospital for parish paupers all expenses are reckoned in the per diem cost. It is a matter of course that in the large institutions, with extensive grounds, many pavilions, central warming and lighting, and the greater number of the subordinated staff, the administration and the expenses for maintenance are higher than in the smaller ones; that in the imbecile hospitals, where the patients work, a considerable saving of expenses is made in the cost for wages, maintenance and repairs, while also the nature of the diseases has an influence through the cost of drugs, bandages and instruments. There is in the hospitals of Amsterdam in this respect such a difference that any comparison is impossible. To show this I give here some figures indicating the average per diem cost: Binnengasthuis and Buitengasthuis, fl. 1.34-1.20; Dutch Hebrew Hospital, fl. 1; Burgerziekenhuis, fl. 1.12½-0.90 (only for food and medical assistance); Hospital for Ophthalmic Patients, fl. 1.74; Children's Hospital, fl. 1.03–1.40 (isolating bed, 1.27–2.20); Roman Catholic Hospital, fl. 0.75; Gynæcological Hospital, fl. 1.20.

Binnen Gasthuis.—We find the largest medical service in the Binnen Gasthuis. The hospital is united with the university, and the professors are charged with the medical treatment of a part of the patients. There are therefore four medical sections divided among the professors as consulting physicians and the medical director, two surgical with two consulting surgeons, one obstetric, one gynæcological, and one for syphilis and skin diseases, each under its respective professor. These eight chiefs of the sections are assisted by one or two assistant physicians, all graduate physicians, twelve in all, who are residents in the hospital and not allowed private practice. Besides these twelve physicians there are added to the staff two physicians in service of the first aid to the injured and one as prosector for the post-mortems. The latter works under the control of the professor of pathological anatomy. The twelve physicians who have charge of the treatment of the patients have each from 40 to 60 under their care. In the Buitengasthuis is a medical director who has the control over the treatment of all the patients, who are directly entrusted to four assistant physicians, also resident in the hospital. Each physician has charge of about 100, including the insane and the neuropathics.

Burgerziekenhuis.—For the 125 patients nursed there are two house physicians, while the control over the medical patients devolves upon the medical director, and a consulting surgeon has charge of the surgical section.

The Dutch Hebrew Hospital.—The medical director is resident in the hospital and head of the whole medical treatment, assisted by one non-resident assistant physician; while for consultation there are one surgeon, one ophthalmologist and one gynæcologist.

Hospital for Ophthalmic Patients.—The medical director (professor in ophthalmology at the university) is assisted in the treatment by four ophthalmologists, all non-resident in the hospital, while two assistant physicians are at the institution, of whom one is resident. Such a numerous staff is necessary here because of the great number of out-patients who are treated in the institution. In 1892, for instance, there were 10,229 out-patients.

Children's Hospital.—The treatment of the medical patients is entrusted to the medical director, that of the surgical to a surgeon.

Both have their residence next to the hospital. There are no other medical men.)

Gynæcological Hospital.—The medical director is resident in the hospital and assisted by one assistant physician, also resident in the hospital.

In all the other institutions there are no resident physicians, so that the patients are treated either by their private physician as in the Association for Nursing, or by the physicians who, though they are not resident, visit the institutions at regular times (for instance, the Roman Catholic Hospital, which has three physicians). To sum up we have thus:

	Consulting Physicians.		Medical Directors. Not resident.	Assistant Medical Directors.		Total Number of Beds.	Number of Beds per Medical Director resident in Hospital.
	Resident.	Not resident.		Resident.	Not resident.		
Binnengasthuis	I	7	..	12	..	700	55
Buitengasthuis	I	..	..	4	..	500	100
Burgerziekenhuis	..	2	..	2	..	145	70
Dutch Hebrew Hospital..........	I	3	..	I	I	110	55
Children's Hospital................	2	..	..	..	..	115	55
Hospital for Ophthalmic Patients..	..	I	4	I	I	58	58
Gynæcological Hospital ....,.....	I	..	..	..	..	12	12
Roman Catholic Hospital	..	..	3	..	..	70	..
Portuguese Hebrew Hospital	..	..	2	..	..	20	..

To compare the very different reports relating to nursing so as to give a good idea of them, it is necessary to distinguish between those institutions whose nurses nurse only in the hospital and those which furnish nurses outside the hospital.

To the first group, where all the nurses are for the service of the admitted patients, belong the Binnen Gasthuis, the Buitengasthuis, the Burgerziekenhuis, the Dutch Hebrew Hospital, the Hospital for Ophthalmic Patients, the Children's Hospital, and the Gynæcological Hospital. The above institutions agree in that they have exclusively lay-nursing,—in the first mentioned, mixed male and female nursing, while in the three last there exists only nursing by women. That at the present time all these institutions can supply a sufficient number of women of some cultivation and education, to satisfy the numerous demands for nurses without being obliged to resort to the Roman

Catholic Sisters or the Deaconesses, Amsterdam owes in great part to the Association of the " White Cross."

Since the " White Cross Association" began in the year 1878 to work to improve the hospital nursing, it fulfilled this voluntary duty so well, we can state with confidence that the hospitals in our city of Amsterdam possess an excellently trained nursing staff. If we limit our report to what prevails at present in Amsterdam, the arrangement is as follows : From the total number of applicants they take, as far as possible, women of cultivation who come as probationers to the four great hospitals. They reside there, receive all instruction free of cost, and are paid a moderate sum (about fl. 125). The medical director assisted by the matron has charge of the training. While the director in these institutions gives theoretical lectures—anatomy, physiology, hygiene, general nursing (special lectures on lung, heart and digestive diseases, nursing of contagious diseases of childbed and children, surgical nursing and aseptics, first aid to the injured, laying out corpses, etc.), the matron assisted by her staff nurses devotes herself to the practical training of the nurses. After having followed courses of lectures for about a year, the probationers are promoted to nurses, and after two or three years their training is considered to be finished. The nurses can then, after successful examination, leave the hospital to join one of the associations for private nursing.

The city of Amsterdam regards this training very favorably. The doctors of the four chief hospitals have united in a common standard of training and examination, so that in the course of time Amsterdam will possess a large number of excellently trained nurses who have had a uniform training. The condition has not long existed.

About ten years ago Dr. Van Deventer opened his first course of lectures, assisted by Dr. Blooker. Somewhat later, in 1884, Dr. Zegers followed with his lectures in the Binnen Gasthuis, while at last Dr. Stephan opened in 1892 the first regular course in the Burgerziekenhuis, and Dr. A. Courie one in 1892 in the Dutch Hebrew Hospital. In the other institutions mentioned above they have not these courses, because they get their nurses from among those trained in the four hospitals, and because the directors with their matrons can satisfactorily train the few women required for special nursing (children, ophthalmology, and gynæcology) in their institutions.

When nurses have been employed for a long time in the institution and distinguish themselves, they are promoted to be staff-nurses.

The general arrangement is to place a staff-nurse at the head of each section, to have charge of the nurses and the further practical education of the probationers.   All are inmates and have everything without payment, and receive fl. 125 to 525, according to their rank. The number of active nurses in the different institutions is as follows :

	Number of Beds.	Staff Nurses.	Nurses.		Proba- tioners.	Man Nurses and Male Servants.
			1st class.	2d class.		
Binnengasthuis,	700	11	10	39	35	23
Buitengasthuis,	500	3	6	23	25	8
Burgerziekenhuis,	145	3		28		2
Dutch Heb. Hospital,	110	2		9		5
Children's Hospital,	115	1		20		
Hos. for Ophth. Patients,	58			4		
Gynæcological Hospital,	12			3		
Portuguese Hebrew Hos.,	21			2		2

The nurses are commonly distributed as follows: In the Binnengasthuis there is 1 nurse for 8 adults or 6 children; Buitengasthuis, 1 nurse for 8 adults; Dutch Hebrew Hospital, 1 nurse for 17 adults; Children's Hospital, 1 nurse for 6 children; Burgerziekenhuis, 1 nurse for 6 adults; Hospital for Ophthalmic Patients, 1 nurse for 14 adults; Gynæcological Hospital, 1 nurse for 4 adults.

These numbers refer only to the day service.   The nurses in rotation are also charged with the night duty, lasting in the Binnengasthuis 12 hours, from 8.30 p. m. until 8.30 a. m.; in the Buitengasthuis, 12 hours, from 8.30 p. m. until 8.30 a. m.; in the Burgerziekenhuis, 11 hours; in the Dutch Hebrew Hospital, 10 hours, from 11 p. m. to 9 a. m.; in the Children's Hospital, 8 hours, from 10 p. m. to 6 a. m.

The Portuguese Hebrew Hospital and the Hospital for Ophthalmic Patients have no regular night service, as also the Gynæcological Hospital, but one of the nurses sleeps near the wards and can easily be called.

The term of night service of a nurse is in the Binnengasthuis 1 week and after that at least 2 weeks of day service; in the Buitengasthuis, 1 week and after that at least 2 weeks of day service; in the Burgerziekenhuis, 1 week and after that at least 5 weeks of day service; in the Dutch Hebrew Hospital, 1 week and after that at least 2 weeks of day service; in the Children's Hospital, thrice a week during 3 weeks of day service.

As has already been mentioned, there is, in addition to the nurses, a male nursing staff in the general hospitals, because all the patients are not nursed by women. The exceptions made are not the same in all the hospitals. The following are not nursed by women: In the Binnengasthuis, 1. the venereal males; 2. a part of the surgical males; 3. bathing of all the admitted males. In the Buitengasthuis, 1. the venereal males; 2. a part of the male imbeciles; 3. bathing of all the admitted males. In the Burgerziekenhuis, 1. bathing of all the admitted males; 2. assistance at some operations undergone by males.

In the Dutch Hebrew Hospital and the Portuguese Hebrew Hospital the women nurse only females and children under 12 years.

As indicated by the above mentioned, these hospitals agree in their requirements for nursing. They are absolutely different from those which, beside hospital nursing, furnish nurses outside the hospital. To this group belong from the hospitals mentioned in the beginning, the Association for Nursing, the Roman Catholic Hospital, the Association of Protestant Sisters, and the Association for Lutheran Deaconesses, and the St. Bernardus Hospital, while the "White Cross Association" and the Congregation of the Friars of St. John de Deo must also be added to it.

The nursing staff in these institutions belongs for the greater part to different clerical orders. We have thus in the Roman Catholic Hospital, the St. Bernardus Hospital, and the Congregation of Friars of St. John de Deo, Roman Catholic sisters and friars, in No. 4 Lutheran sisters. In No. 3 the sisters are under the clerical control of the Reformed Church. In No. 1 are only admitted sisters of Protestant religion, while the "White Cross" has lay-nursing. The exigencies of training differ very much. The "White Cross" resembles most nearly the first group. This association formerly gave its own courses of training, but has ceased to do so. The instruction given by the training schools in the hospitals being more complete, these separate courses had no reason to exist any longer. They were therefore given up, and the training of nurses was absolutely left to the hospitals. The committee of examination of this association is now formed of the directors of the hospitals at Amsterdam, so that the requirements are the same as in the hospitals; two or three years of hospital service and a scheme of instruction conforming to that of the Amsterdam hospital nurses are required. This association is in reality mainly composed of nurses formerly active in the four great hospitals.

Somewhat different from this is the education given in the Associ-ation for Nursing. Two physicians, Dr. Van Brakel and Dr. Waller, members of the board, give courses for the probationers, who after a year are promoted to nurses.

The Roman Catholic Sisters are trained in the nunneries at Maastricht, while the practical lectures at the sick-bed are given in the city hospital there by the medical director. The friars visit a training school in Germany, where the instruction is given partly by a physician, partly by the superior. This course lasts two and one-half years. The Lutheran Deaconesses go also to Germany; the elementary lectures, however, being given partly by one of the physicians in Amsterdam, Dr. Veltkamp, and partly by one of the clergymen here.

As these institutions employ their nurses mainly for private nursing, and hospital nursing is of minor importance, it is needless to mention along with the number of nurses the number of beds. The nursing staff amounts to: Association of Nursing, 30–40; Roman Catholic Hospital, 35; Friars of St. John de Deo, 19; The White Cross, 14; St. Bernardus Institute, 6; Lutheran Deaconesses, 9; Protestant Sisters, ?.

Besides the nurses employed in the hospitals, Amsterdam employs more than 100 nurses, not calculating the many nurses, most of them formerly employed in one of the hospitals, who nurse in private without joining one of the institutions. Most of them nurse one patient at a time, except the Protestant sisters, who divide their services among many families living in the same district. All the above-mentioned institutions furnish their nurses for separate day or night nursing and for continued service, the latter especially in cases of infectious diseases. All the institutions established for philan-thropic purposes furnish on request all aid free of expense. As they do not receive any subsidy from the community or the parish, they are mainly dependent on donations or legacies from grateful patients. That this private nursing is in great demand is proved by the following: Nurses of the "Witte Kruis" gave in 1887 3641 days of nursing, the number of which rose in 1891 to 4239 and in 1892 to 4336; 16 friars gave in 1891 4576 nights of duty; 17 friars in 1892 5685.

The night service lasts: Association of Nurses, from 10 o'clock p. m. till 9 o'clock a. m., 6 nights in succession, with 1 night's rest; Protestant Sisters, from 10 o'clock p. m. till 8 o'clock a. m., 5 nights in succession, with 1 night's rest; Witte Kruis, from 10 o'clock p. m. till 10 o'clock a. m., 6 nights in succession, with 1 night's rest.

Among the various points of difference between these associations and the hospitals the most beautiful is certainly that they all assume either complete provision for invalid nurses (Roman Catholic Hospital, Association of Nurses, Friars of St. John de Deo), or at a fixed age or in case of disease pay a pension (Witte Kruis).

It is deplorable that the resources of hospitals are not sufficient to assume this fair duty. Be the time not far away when a change can be made in this respect.

I finish this report wishing that the future may bring us a National Pension Fund for the nursing staff, assuring a lasting appreciation for services rendered.

THE MONTREAL GENERAL HOSPITAL; ITS ORGANIZATION, HISTORY AND MANAGEMENT.

With Plans of Surgical Pavilions and New Operating Amphitheater.

By W. F. Hamilton, M. D., C. M.,
Medical Superintendent.

In the year 1892 the Montreal General Hospital issued its seventieth annual report, and by the time this Congress will have closed seventy-one years will have passed since it was founded.

On January 30, 1823, in compliance with the petition of John Richardson, William McGillivray and Samuel Gerrard, Esquires, presented to the Legislative Council of Lower Canada on the 9th day of April, 1822, a charter was granted incorporating the society of the Montreal General Hospital, and enduing that society with the powers of such a body.

In 1859, after thirty-six years of operation, it was found that certain of the provisions of the original charter were, in practice, highly inconvenient, and therefore an amendment of that charter was asked for. This amended charter did not differ in any great degree from the original one, but made slight alterations with respect to property holding and alienating of property, the number, choice and qualification of the governors of the corporation, and the quorum of governors for transaction of business.

Before going farther into the history of this institution, it would be well to return to a period previous to 1823 and note the steps leading up to the petition for the royal charter.

We find, according to the writings of the late lamented Dr. R. Palmer Howard, that in the year 1819 a great need for increased hospital accommodations was felt. The city was rapidly increasing, a great influx of immigrants came, and cases of contagious fevers and other diseases so overcrowded those institutions which did receive them that four rooms were hired in a part of the city known as Chaboillez Square, and a temporary hospital was provided by a number of philanthropic persons, prominent among whom were the Rev. John Bethune, the Rev. Henry Esson and Staff-Surgeon Dr. Blackwood. From this small nucleus great things have come. The following year, 1820, April 25th, a meeting of subscribers was held in the courthouse for the establishment of a general hospital. These subscribers appointed various officers as president, vice-president, treasurer and secretary, medical attendants, etc., for the carrying on of the work contemplated, and indeed already begun.

Another and more convenient place was provided temporarily for the care of patients. The citizens of Montreal generously supported the early workers in so good a cause, and in 1820 the land upon which the hospital now stands was purchased, and over £2000 were subscribed to erect a suitable permanent building, to be called "The Montreal General Hospital." The institution was devoted to "the reception of patients of all diseases usually admitted into such hospitals in Great Britain, without distinction of religious denomination." This has always characterized the admission of patients to its wards.

We have said that in 1820 the present site was purchased. On the 9th of June of the following year the corner-stone of the present central building was laid, and in less than one year from that date it was ready for the reception of patients, of whom 70 were able to find accommodation at the same time. During the first year of its existence 421 were treated within its walls. The cost of site and building amounted to about $25,000.

During the next nine years the work of the institution made favorable progress. The building, at the end of this time, had become inadequate to the accommodation of the patients applying for relief. In this year also Hon. John Richardson, president of the governing body for the past ten years, died.

To perpetuate the memory of one who had rendered such invaluable service to the institution, it was decided to build a wing to the hospital. Accordingly the Richardson wing was promptly erected in 1831–32, and the capacity of the hospital increased.

The presidency of the hospital was now laid upon the Hon. John Molson, who held it until his death in 1835, when Samuel Gerrard, Esq., was made president. This office was thus faithfully held for twenty years. At the end of this period he resigned on the ground of advanced age, and the Hon. John Molson succeeded to this office in 1856. This officer held the presidential chair for three years only, when he was succeeded by Mr. John Redpath. It was in 1869 when this devoted member of the board of governors died, Mr. William Molson succeeded to the position of president.

In 1875 Peter Redpath was appointed to the presidency rendered vacant through the death of Mr. William Molson, one of the founders of the hospital, and on many occasions a munificent contributor to its funds.

In 1882 he was succeeded by Mr. Andrew Robertson. This officer resigned his position on account of ill-health at the end of seventeen years of devotion to the interests of the institution as treasurer, vice-president and president.

In 1889 the present president, Mr. John Stirling, was appointed, and many have been the improvements since that date.

Let us now take another glance over the history of the institution. We have touched upon the fact that the central building and Richardson wing have been erected.

In 1848–49 the Reid wing on the western portion was erected through the munificent gift of the much respected widow of the late Hon. Chief Justice Reid. Such an addition gave balance to the whole structure, greatly increased the capacity of the institution, and served not only as the noblest monument that could be erected to his memory, but as an appropriate realization of his oft-expressed wishes and sentiments.

In 1866, through the generosity of Messrs. Wm. Molson and J. G. McKenzie, a portion of property in front of the hospital was purchased. The buildings situated on it were removed, and a large open square in front of the institution was thus secured, adding much to the appearance and sanitary condition of the place. This open space still remains.

In 1868 more convenient and suitable provisions were made for

the treatment of contagious diseases, cases of which had hitherto
been cared for in the Reid wing without any proper isolation. A
building capable of receiving about 50 cases, constructed of red
brick, and at a cost of $10,674, was erected in the rear of the Rich-
ardson wing. About half the cost of this portion of the institution
was borne by Mr. William Molson.

The next addition to the hospital accommodation was that furnished by what is known as the Morland Wing, erected at a cost of
about $20,000. It was placed immediately in the rear of the Reid
wing, on St. Dominique street, as a monument to the memory of
the late Mr. Thos. Morland, whose zeal and activity in hospital
affairs were highly esteemed.

In 1889–90 the question of more suitable arrangements for accommodating the nurses was settled by the addition of a mansard story
to the central building and the two wings. Excellent bedrooms and
a large sitting-room, airy and well ventilated, were thus provided, at
a cost of upwards of $10,000.

In his report of 1882, the late lamented R. Palmer Howard, secretary of the Montreal General Hospital, in speaking of the overcrowded wards of this institution, asks: "Who amongst the merchant princes will contribute $100,000 to begin a wing of the new
hospital, which the governors have been for some years wishing to
erect, and which will be worthy of the largest and wealthiest city of
our Dominion?"

Two years after this report was published the question was fully
and satisfactorily answered. Lord Mount Stephen contributed
$50,000, and the bequest of the late David J. Greenshields swelled
the sum to $90,000. By the time that plans were made and settled
the sum exceeded the $100,000 asked for, and in June of 1891 the
work was begun on the site of the new surgical pavilions and operating room. The work on these new pavilions was not completed
until December, 1892, and on the 19th of that month the first patients
were admitted to these wards.

We will now turn to speak of the hospital site and buildings. The
Montreal General Hospital is situated in the midst of the city, and
occupies the most of a square between Dorchester and Lagauchetiere
streets. The original building and the Richardson and Reid wings
are built of Montreal building stone or limestone. It is of plainest
architecture, and no pretension to beauty or ornateness of design
has been made. The stone is for the most part smoothly cut, and

the lines of the building are straight. The Morland wing, of more recent construction, is of a more tasteful style, built of dressed limestone with embossed facings. Including basement and nurses' quarters, there are six floors in all. The basement is used as kitchen and laundry, store and furnace rooms, and beneath the Reid and Morland wings the outdoor department is situated. The first floor affords space for one large ward, accommodating fifteen patients; offices of medical superintendent and steward, the waiting-rooms, and rooms for the resident medical staff and lady superintendent. The second floor is devoted to wards for the patients, with a few private rooms. The third floor is also divided into wards, and in the Reid wing there is an operating amphitheater and lecture-room, with a southwestern aspect, affording accommodation for about one hundred and thirty students. We have already spoken of the uppermost flat, used by the nurses as dormitories, etc.

We have referred to the building and opening of two pavilions at the close of 1892. It is fitting at this point to enter more into detail of plan, etc., in speaking of this extension. The original part of the hospital is now long since out of date, and it is only the question of a few months when we hope that these old things will have passed away and we will have all things new, for the plans of remodeling are being arranged and will doubtless be executed in the near future.

The accompanying plans will serve to show the arrangement in the new portion of our institution.

Here are shown the three floors, basement, and first and second flats. The material of which these wings is constructed is red pressed brick. Each pavilion has two large wards containing twenty-four beds each. These wards are light and airy, with a large semicircular area or "bow-window" occupying the whole of the end of the ward. (We will speak later of the air space to each patient.)

In connection with each flat is a large lavatory, containing bath, hand basins, slop sink, porcelain washtub, and closets of most improved style, set up on tile floor; the lavatory is finished in marble.

In the lavatory, the antiseptic solutions, warming tins, bed pans and urinals are neatly put away on marble shelves especially arranged to receive them.

The kitchen contains dumb-waiter, sink, cupboards, refrigerator and gas stove and heater. In connection with each public ward there are two private wards. These apartments are lighted with incandescent lights of sixteen candle power each, with the exception of those two over the operating-room table, which are of fifty candles each.

The surgical amphitheater is sufficiently large to accommodate three hundred students. It is a bright and most convenient room, with a northwestern aspect. The glass of its main window is of cathedral ruby, while that of the others is of the plain variety. A large skylight, in addition to the main window, affords ample light for all operations. The accompanying plan will make clear the arrangement of rooms in the amphitheater building. The surgical supply room, and the anæsthetizing and instrument room, on the right, and surgeon's coat and preparatory rooms, with a recovery room, on the left.

The walls of the operating room are of finely finished white plaster. The semicircular portion in front of the students' seats, as well as the walls to a height of seven feet from the floor, are finished with marble. The floor is made of tiles.

Several months of experience in this amphitheater with a very active surgical service, enables us to speak very highly of the appointments in this department. The students see well. The light is good both by day and by night, and the facilities for entrance and exit of patients are in a high degree satisfactory.

Ventilation and Heating of New Pavilions.

In these days of improved and variously planned systems of ventilation and heating, it is of interest to know how so important matters are attended to in hospitals.

The description of these new pavilions would be quite incomplete without particular reference to this system now in operation here. It is what is known as the *plenum system of ventilation*, and I am deeply indebted to the architect, Alexander C. Hutchison, Esq., for the following description :

This system is one by which the air is forced into the wards, entering very close to the ceiling and passing out again at the floor, thence under the floor to a flue, into the open air.

For forcing the requisite volume of air into the wards, a pair of fans each six feet in diameter by three feet wide, made by Messrs. B. F. Sturtevant & Co., of Boston, were installed in the basement of the amphitheater building, and operated by a 28-horse power, high speed, automatic cut-off engine, the revolutions of the fan being arranged for 210 per minute.

From the fans, ducts made in brick work are carried along below the basement floor of each pavilion and of the amphitheater building, to vertical shafts leading to the several wards and rooms to be ventilated. In each of these large wards there are six of these shafts, while in the smaller wards and rooms, only one each. These shafts carry the air to the ceiling and there, through an ornamental iron casting, discharge it into the ward. To secure uniformity of temperature and a thorough mixing of air, these shafts, which are built in the external walls, have been placed so as not to be opposite each other.

The supply of air is taken through two windows, each 7 feet by 4 feet, from an open court removed from the dust of the street.

When the fans are in operation at a speed of 210 revolutions per minute, a large volume of air is forced into every room, an actual measurement showing the quantity to be 1,182,000 cubic feet per hour. At this rate the air in each room would be changed about four times every hour, while each patient would be supplied with 4000 to 5000 cubic feet per hour.

Extraction of the Air.—The air supply gains access to the wards near the ceiling. It then descends to the floor, thence it is carried away through gratings placed in the skirtings into ducts below the floors, to the extracting shaft in each section of the building, *i. e.*, each pavilion and the amphitheater section.

Each shaft has an area of one square foot to about each 5000 cubic feet in the building with which it is connected. They are built of brick, and rise about ten feet above the roof. At the bottom of each shaft a coil of steam pipes is fixed, and is especially intended for rarefying the air, creating a draught when the fans are not in operation.

Warming the Air.—There are no heated coils or radiators in the wards. The air is heated at two points (if necessary) in its course from the outside of the building to the inner part of the ward.

We have already spoken of the windows through which the air is drawn by the revolving fans. Between the windows and the fans is a hot-blast apparatus made by Messrs. B. F. Sturtevant & Co., of Boston. This apparatus consists of 7000 feet of one-inch iron pipe, arranged in a great number of sections, each section consisting of two upright pipes fixed in a cast iron base and connected together at the top by a cross pipe. The longest pipe in this apparatus is not more than 23 feet, and there is no danger from freezing, however rapid the condensation of steam.

The other point at which the air may be heated on its way to the wards is the reinforcing or supplementary heating chamber arranged in the basement for each vertical shaft.

In these chambers are placed cast iron radiators over which the air could be forced to flow, when it is found that the fans do not heat it sufficiently. These radiators so placed in the whole of the building, are equal to about 11,000 feet of one inch pipe, giving a total heating surface, including the piping in the hot-blast apparatus, of 5666 superficial feet. The flow of air through these chambers is under control of the engineer or nurse, who opens and closes the valve thereto, by handles worked in the ward, as occasion demands.

At this date we have passed through one of the coldest winters of our Canadian climate. At no time during this season has it been necessary to use the reinforcing chambers, nor have all the sections in the hot-blast apparatus been heated at the same time.

Notwithstanding these facts, the whole new department of the institution has been well heated, and the system affords general satisfaction. It appears, however, that the expenditure in this department has been far beyond the necessity of the case, for undoubtedly sufficient heat could have been secured without the reinforcing chambers—so far, at any rate, they are superfluous.

The objections to the system are few. That which suggests itself at first is the free motion of dust and smoke. This, however, may be reduced to a minimum by proper attention to the court, and in special rooms the insertion of gauze in the flues.

The great advantage of the system is, a free and constant ingress of fresh warm air, and the exit of vitiated air, and this without perceptible draughts.

Pay Patients in Hospitals.

One of the subjects for special consideration laid down by the committee of this Congress was that of pay patients in hospitals. This institution has such a class within its wards almost constantly. They may be divided into private pay patients and public pay patients. The former occupy single wards at a cost of two dollars per day. This does not include medical advice.

The latter are placed in the public wards and pay only fifty cents per day. Under this class come all citizens *able to pay*, while all strangers are *obliged* to pay this amount.

Immigrants to the city are admitted free when needing treatment in indigent circumstances.

The admission of sailors is made on recommendation of the Department of Customs, which guarantees the payment of ninety cents per day on presentation of the account to the Dominion Government.

It is a well-established fact that our terms for patients are too low if we would wish to be fully remunerated.

Neither in public wards nor private wards does the income cover the expenditure per patient, reckoning the whole current expenses on the number of patients treated.

The revenue from such cases is not large, about $7200 last year, while this year upwards of $8500 has been received.

The Numbers Treated Yearly.

To indicate the number of cases coming under treatment in the Indoor Department, the following figures may be found of interest:

Indoor :

For the year ending April 30, 1891, 2035 cases were treated.
" " " " 30, 1892, 2329 " " "
" " " " 30, 1893, 2359 " " "

Outdoor :

Consultations for year ending April 30, 1891, 30,074.
" " " " 30, 1892, 34,220.
" " " " 30, 1893, 34,100.

The Ambulance Service.

While reference is being made to the number of cases under treatment, it may be interesting to speak briefly of the ambulance service. Speaking generally it may be said that the service in this department is well rendered, both for promptness and efficiency. There are two well-equipped ambulances, and in cases of necessity a third can be placed upon the street.

We have spoken of the promptness of this service. Besides the readiness with which the ambulance carrying the surgeon may be got out, the highest rate of speed possible through crowded streets is secured and maintained, and thus the first aid to the injured in many cases is that given by an active, intelligent surgeon.

The Hospital Organization and Governing Bodies.

Under this division of our subject we include the board of governors, the committee of management, and the medical board. The board of governors consists at present of about four hundred members, a few of whom are ladies; they are either life or elected governors. Life governors are those who have paid a sum of one hundred dollars, and thereafter a yearly amount of twelve dollars. The number of elected governors is confined to twelve. There are six of these elected yearly. They are appointed by the board of governors and corporation for the term of two years. Each such member must pay twelve dollars per year.

Before leaving this part of the subject we will define in a word the term corporation mentioned above. Under this term is included that body of contributors whose yearly subscriptions are five dollars and upwards, whether any other amount has been subscribed or not.

It is quite impossible for so large a board of governors as that now contributing to this institution, to meet for the transaction of the business of the same. This board appoints what is termed the committee of management, consisting of president, vice-president and treasurer, and ten additional members, one of whom is a member of the consulting staff. This committee sits weekly, on afternoon of Monday, for the transaction of business in connection with the domestic economy of the house,—in a word, to oversee and control all matters connected with the management of the hospital At each meeting reports are made of the number of patients admitted during the week, and the number discharged; the average daily in the house, the number of those treated in the various outdoor departments, the number of deaths, with cause of same; and various other things incident to the management. The committee of management appoints from among its members three who act on what is known as the house committee. The function of this committee is implied in its name.

We come to speak next of the medical board. This board consists of the consulting staff, the physicians and surgeons, and the specialists who attend to patients in the hospital. The appointment of the members of this board is made by the governors. Any physician or surgeon who may have served the hospital in that capacity for twelve years is eligible to be elected on the consulting staff. The link between the last two and chief governing bodies is that afforded by the regulation that one member of the committee of management is selected from among the members of the medical board; he holds office on both boards.

In addition to the above outline, which indicates the chief governing bodies, which are external to the household, we must add a few words concerning the internal organization. This is directly under the supervision of the medical superintendent; each department, however, has a head. There are the various departments here. The nurses' department is directly governed by the lady superintendent. The domestic department is under the superintendence of the housekeeper and steward. The department of heating and ventilating, lighting, plumbing, etc., has a capable engineer at its head.

The resident house staff consists of medical superintendent, two house physicians, three house surgeons, one anæsthetist, and an apothecary. We have one non-resident clinical assistant, who acts in that capacity in the outdoor department of medicine and gynæcology and indoor gynæcology. The medical superintendent receives his appointment from the committee of management. The resident house officers are appointed by a vote of the board of governors.

Turning now to speak of the finances of this institution, we touch upon a subject the consideration of which cannot be indulged in without feelings of gratitude and pleasure. Ever since 1820, when this institution had its beginning, the citizens of Montreal have never failed to support its interests, and that liberality of spirit and gifts which at that time was manifested has flowed on in an ever-increasing degree. With the increase and extension of the work, the increasing need has been supplied—a fact not only satisfactory in itself, but most praiseworthy and commendable, speaking as it does of the place which the institution has in the hearts of the people.

The Montreal General Hospital is not a city or civic hospital. The support rendered by the municipality is small indeed. It is not a denominational institution, though most of its funds are subscribed by Protestants. One fact will show that in this sense it is general. Last year, 1891–92, the following were the divisions of religious bodies: Protestants 1309, Roman Catholics 943, other religions 77.

The hospital support is mainly derived from private sources. Each year collectors are appointed to solicit subscriptions throughout the various wards of the city. Then ordinary donations afford another source of revenue. The Provincial Government gives a grant of from two to five thousand dollars yearly.

The interest on capital invested, the revenue from patients, the fees of medical students, the rents, and contents of poor boxes, make up a yearly income of about fifty thousand dollars. This amount is not sufficient to defray the current expenses, which are yearly increasing,

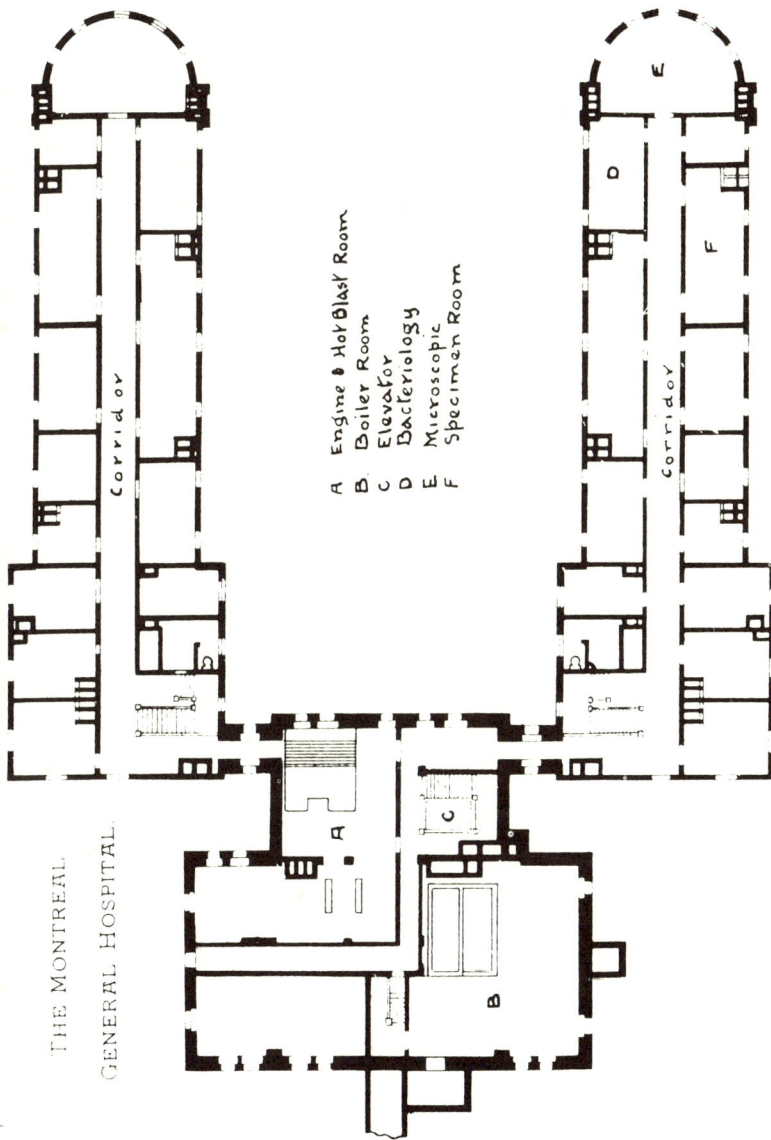

THE MONTREAL
GENERAL HOSPITAL.

A Engine & Hot Blast Room
B Boiler Room
C Elevator
D Bacteriology
E Microscopic
F Specimen Room

Corridor

Corridor

A

B

C

D

E

F

BASEMENT PLAN

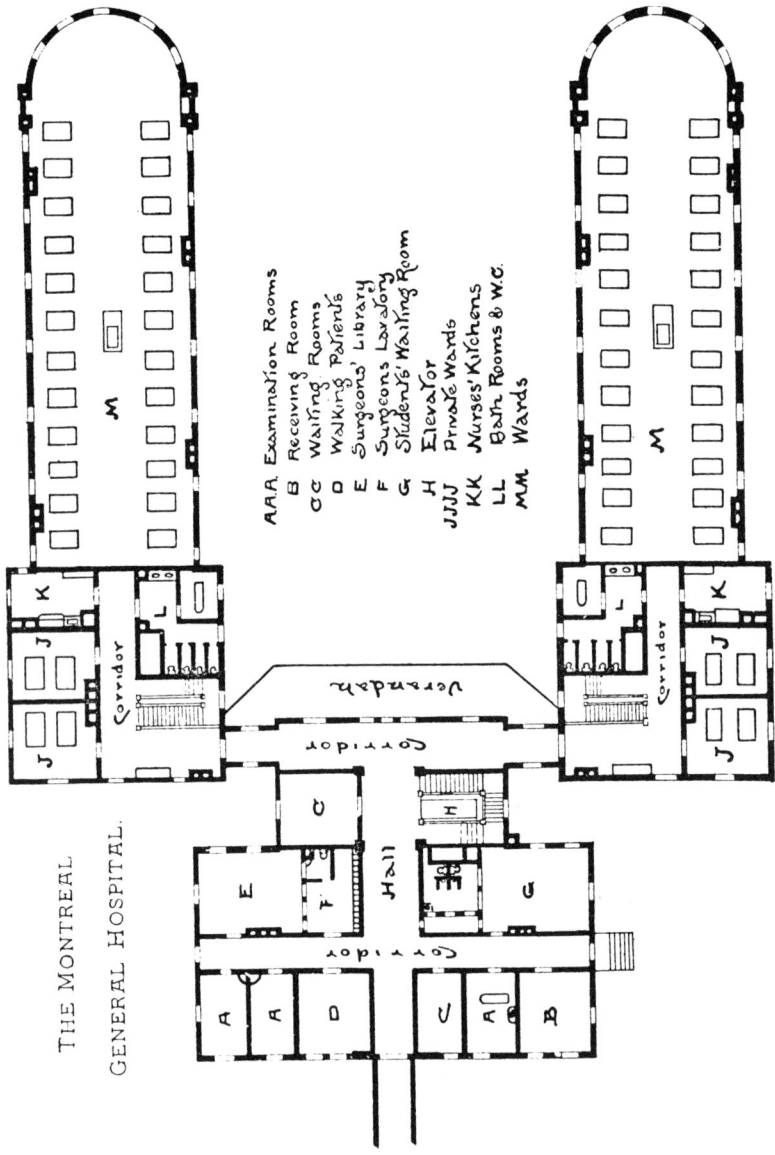

THE MONTREAL
GENERAL HOSPITAL.

AAA Examination Rooms
B Receiving Room
CC Waiting Rooms
D Walking Patients
E Surgeons' Library
F Surgeons' Lavatory
G Students' Waiting Room
H Elevator
JJJJ Private Wards
KK Nurses' Kitchens
LL Bath Rooms & W.C.
MM Wards

GROUND FLOOR PLAN

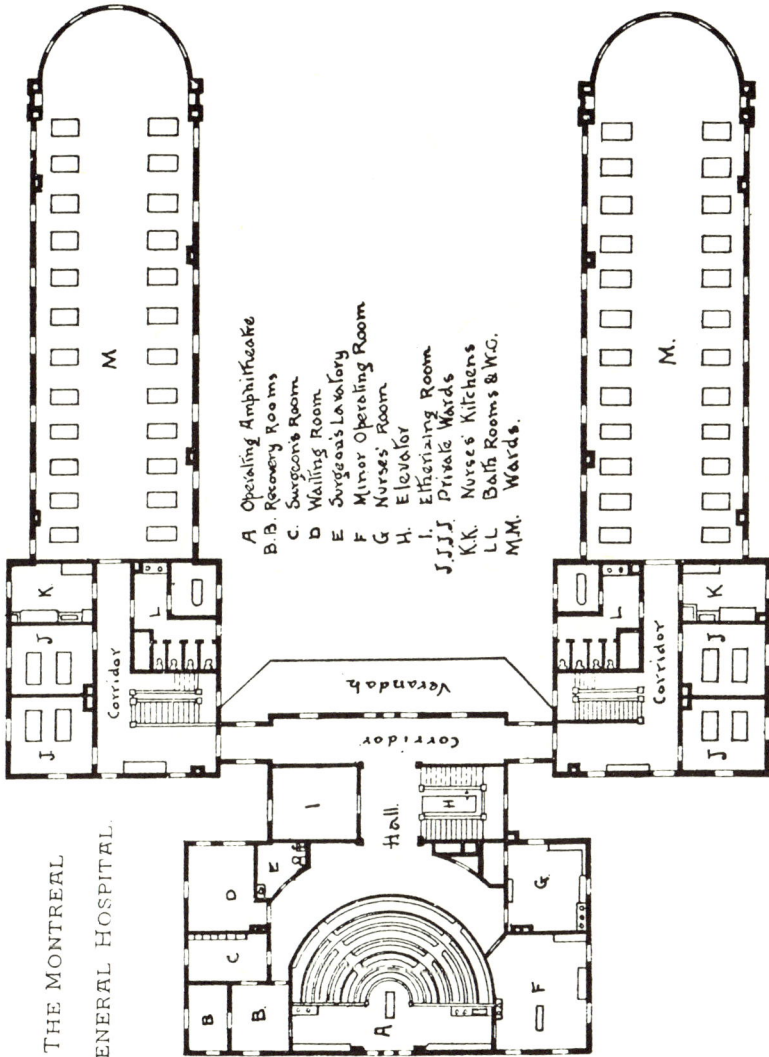

THE MONTREAL
GENERAL HOSPITAL.

SECOND FLOOR PLAN

A. Operating Amphitheatre
B.B. Recovery Rooms
C. Surgeon's Room
D. Waiting Room
E. Surgeon's Lavatory
F. Minor Operating Room
G. Nurses' Room
H. Elevator
I. Etherizing Room
J.J.J. Private Wards
K.K. Nurses' Kitchens
L.L. Bath Rooms & W.C.
M.M. Wards.

last year amounting to fifty-five thousand dollars, and upward, while this year it will find us with an expenditure of upwards of seventy thousand dollars to report.

We must now bring to a close this fragmentary paper, written as it has been in the midst of a most active and busy life within the walls of the institution. We have sought to present a few of the general points of interest concerning the history, organization, management and capacity of the institution, with plans of the new surgical pavilions. The writer's chief regret is the lack of time at his disposal; otherwise far more interesting and instructive matter would have been placed before this Congress of Charities, Correction and Philanthropy, and the Montreal General Hospital would have been seen through it more as it really is.

THE ROYAL VICTORIA HOSPITAL, MONTREAL.

By Jno. J. Robson, *Secretary.*

The accompanying illustration shows a front view of the hospital. The building is situated on the eastern slopes of Mount Royal, overlooking the city and the St. Lawrence river.

The institution owes its origin to the munificence of two distinguished Canadians, Lord Mount Stephen and Sir Donald Smith, K. C. M. G.

The buildings have been designed and the working drawings prepared by H. Saxon Snell, F. R. I. B. A., London, England, after consultation with, and receiving the final approval of the medical faculty of McGill University.

The narrowness of the site gave rise to much difficulty in designing the buildings, but a far greater problem had to be solved in consequence of the uneven nature and steepness of the ground, situated on a mountain (Mount Royal) which rises no less than 180 feet in its length and from 30 to 80 feet in its breadth; this difficulty, however, has been overcome by making the main entrance at the back midway up the slope on which the main building stands, thus permitting one floor of the various blocks to be reached on the same level.

The ward blocks are ranged along the northeast and southwest boundaries; between these is the administration block, in which are also the out-patients' department and receiving rooms. The entrance to this last building is approached by carriage and footways from Pine Avenue. The center portion contains, on the ground floor, the board room, secretary's office, medical officer's sitting and bed rooms, etc., and the entrance hall and porter's room and principal staircase. The upper floors contain a large number of bedrooms for the nurses, together with their common sitting and dining rooms, library, linen and bath rooms, lavatories, etc.

The lady superintendent's apartments are placed on the first floor. The general kitchen for the whole of the building is placed on the topmost floor of the center of the building, and also the scullery and accessory stores, larders, pantries, etc. The ward maids and other servants' rooms are in the adjoining roof floors. A service staircase and coal and food lifts communicate with all floors, so that the meals can be distributed to the wards in each and every block without difficulty or undue delay, or the necessity of ascending and descending staircases.

The rear extension of the block contains, on the basement floor, the stores and men's bedrooms, and on the ground floor the dispensary and also the medical officer's and lady superintendent's offices. On the upper are additional nurses' bedrooms. The two large projecting blocks on the southwest and northeast boundaries each contain three large wards, $123' \times 26'6''$ and $14'$ high, for the accommodation of 30 patients in each. The northeast block is devoted to medical and the southwest block to surgical patients. Attached to each large ward are four rooms comprising the ward-kitchens and day-room, separation ward and private ward. The bath-rooms and ward offices are contained in the round towers at the ends of the wards.

Adjoining each ward block is the staircase block containing a broad and easy-going staircase, patients' lift, patients' clothing and linen stores, etc.

In the center is the large ventilating shaft which draws the foul air from all the adjoining wards. Up the center of this is carried the smoke shaft from the boilers in the basement, which materially assists the draught power.

Beyond the staircase block in the southwest (surgical) side, are the wards for women and children, $28' \times 40'$ each.

The last block on this side is the surgical theater, which will seat 250 students; adjacent to which are the surgeons', nurses', anæsthetic and after-recovery rooms.

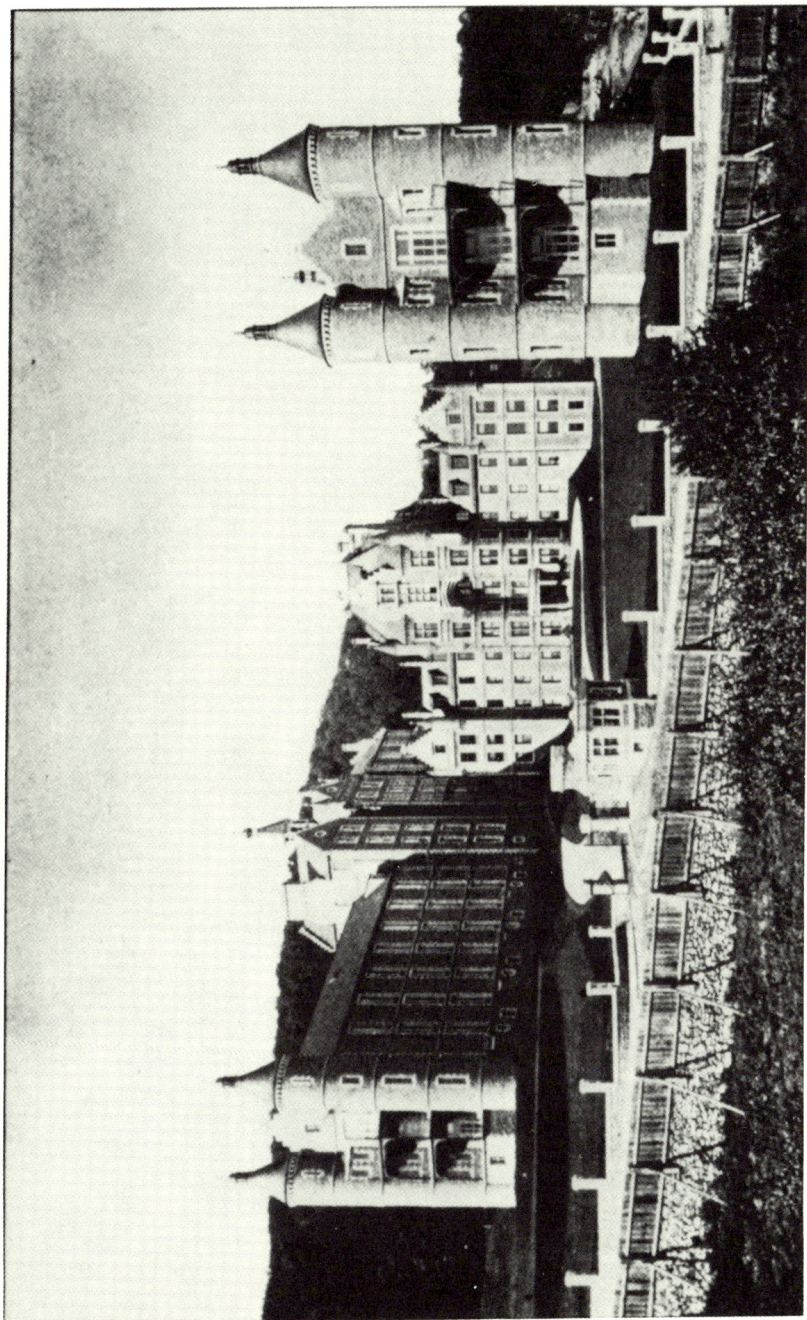

MEDICAL WING.

ADMINISTRATION BLOCK.

SURGICAL WING.

THE ROYAL VICTORIA HOSPITAL, MONTREAL.

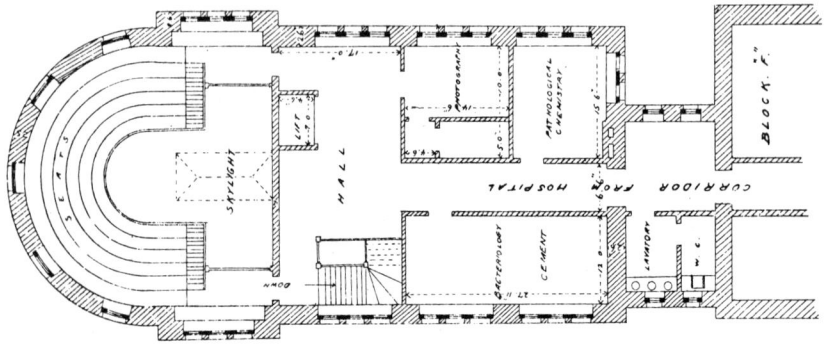

SECOND FLOOR PLAN

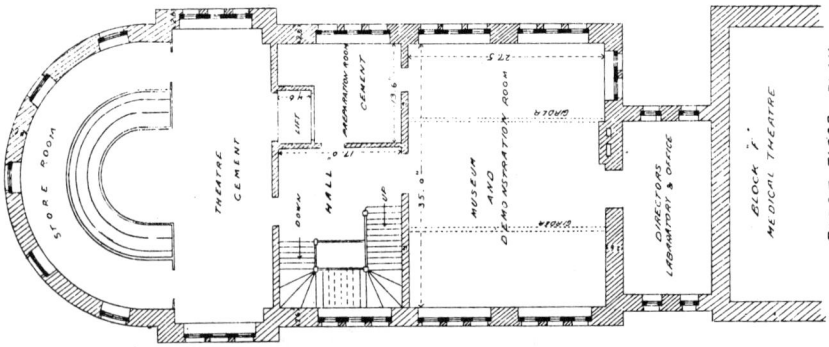

FIRST FLOOR PLAN

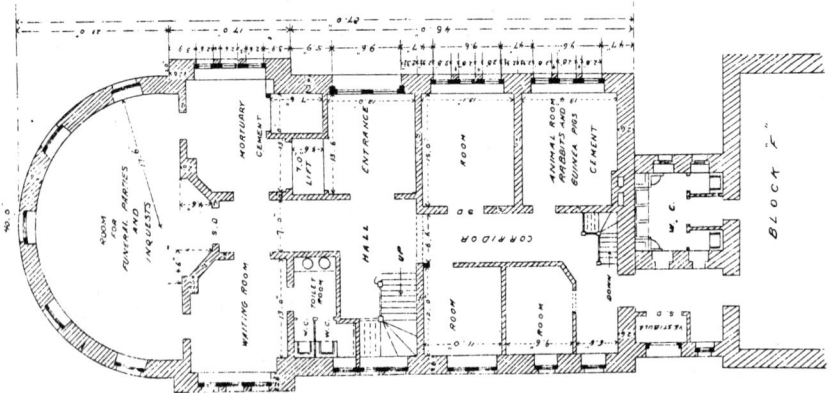

GROUND FLOOR PLAN

ROYAL VICTORIA HOSPITAL.   PATHOLOGICAL BUILDING.

Returning to the buildings on the northeast boundary (medical side), on the first floor of level of staircase block is a children's ward for 10 beds, and on the top floors are male and female erysipelas wards, comprising 4 male and 4 female wards, each for one bed, with ward kitchen and nurses' room adjoining.

The next block is the medical theater for 200 students; the adjoining professors' private room and patients' waiting-room being on ground floor of the staircase block.

Beyond the theater is the pathological block, 88' × 40' (see accompanying ground plans), containing on the ground floor inquest and waiting rooms, mortuary and working rooms. The second floor is occupied by the lower part of the demonstration theater, the preparation room, museum and director's office. The top floor, which connects with the main floor of the hospital, contains the upper part of the demonstration theater, bacteriology, photography and pathological chemistry rooms.

The drainage has been designed upon a carefully arranged system, with glazed earthenware pipes jointed in cement and laid on beds of cement concrete in trenches excavated in solid rock. Manholes and inspection pits, etc., have been liberally provided in accordance with the latest modern requirements.

HISTORY AND DESCRIPTION OF THE ROOSEVELT HOSPITAL.

By James R. Lathrop, *Superintendent.*

The Roosevelt Hospital is located on the block bounded by Fifty-eighth and Fifty-ninth streets and Ninth and Tenth avenues, in New York City. It owes its existence to the bequest of James H. Roosevelt, who was born in New York on November 10, 1800, and died on November 30, 1863, in the city of his birth. By will, executed on March 13, 1854, he provided, after making certain special bequests, that "all the rest and residue of his personal estate" should be employed "for the establishment in the city of New York of a hospital for the reception and relief of sick and diseased persons and for its permanent endowment." The execution of that trust was left to the direction of a board of nine trustees; five, *ex-officio*, by virtue of their being presidents of humane institutions in the city of New York, and four personal friends designated by name. The president of the hospital at this time is the only surviving member of the original board.

It is not known that Mr. Roosevelt ever had a very clear idea as to the character of the buildings which would form the group of the hospital structure. He was satisfied to leave that matter to the determination of the nine trustees whom he designated for the execution of his will.

In February, 1864, the Legislature of the State granted an act of incorporation to the hospital. The board of trustees was then duly organized; soon a building committee was appointed, and the principles of hospital construction, as they were then understood, were made the subject of earnest study by Dr. Stephen Smith, who was selected by the board for that purpose. The doctor visited many of the principal hospitals in this country and in Europe, and, as a result of careful deliberation, plans were adopted and the work of building began in 1869. The opening exercises, on November 2, 1871, were held in one of the wards of the building known as the Medical Pavilion, and located immediately east of the Administration Building, which was at that time unfinished. The purpose of the trustees was that the latter building should form the center of a group designed to eventually cover the block upon which the hospital stands. The funds at the disposal of the board enabled them, at the outset, to construct only the following:

(1) The *Administration Building*, in which are located, on the first floor, the executive offices, the apothecary's department, and a dining-room for the staff; on the second floor, the trustees' room, medical board room, superintendent's living apartments, and back of all the amphitheater for surgical uses and general clinical teaching ; on the third floor, six rooms and their accessories for private patients, and on the fourth floor a surgical ward for twelve women and fifteen children, the part for women being separated from that for children by an intervening corridor.

(2) The *Kitchen Building*, on the first floor of which are a general kitchen and scullery, a bakery, a store-room for kitchen and ward supplies, a laundry, and one dormitory for men ; on the second floor a dining-room for out-ward employes, a large sewing-room, and several sleeping-rooms for out-ward help, and in the basement an

ample vegetable store-room, a storage ice-house and refrigerator, and a coal and wood vault, and engineer's supply room; also back of these, the fresh-air duct separating them from the fan engine-room, main engine-room, and boiler-room.

(3) The *Medical Pavilion*, consisting of four stories: on the first floor, the gynæcological ward, now containing twenty-three beds; on the second floor, an active medical ward of twenty-eight beds for men; on the third floor, a convalescent ward of twenty-eight beds for men, and on the fourth floor an active medical ward of twenty-eight beds for women. The building extends nearly north and south, and has, on the southerly end, water-closets, bath-rooms, wash-rooms and linen-closets; and on the northerly end, dining-rooms, patients' clothes-rooms, nurses' sleeping-rooms and closets, as well as sleeping-rooms for members of the house staff and the apothecary.

(4) The *Surgical Pavilion*, a one-story structure, where thirty-six male patients are accommodated in a single ward of as many beds, and which lies directly east of the last-named building, and is fitted with rooms after the plan of the Medical Pavilion, except that the bath-rooms, water-closets and linen-closets for patients' use are located on the east side of the building near the center, instead of on the southerly end, the change in their position having been rendered desirable by reason of the unusual length of the ward. On the easterly side of this pavilion is a spacious exercise ground for convalescent male patients, and on the westerly side a similar exercise ground for convalescent female patients. All of the wards have the advantage of the morning and afternoon sunlight without the disadvantage of the trying rays of midday.

The only other building constructed at the outset was the *Dead House* and *Museum*, in which provision was also made for the *Pathological Laboratory*.

Until 1877, the buildings thus far mentioned accommodated the work of the hospital. It had by that time become apparent that an ambulance service was greatly needed, and on September 10th of that year it was established. A stable to accommodate it was built adjoining the Dead House and Museum, and it has served the needs of the hospital to the present date. An addition of two stories is now being constructed, the lower floor to be fitted for three horses, and the upper floor with sleeping-rooms for employees. The old stable will be utilized for ambulances alone.

The remarkable growth of the ambulance service is indicated by a comparison of the work done during the first full calendar year following its establishment, with that done in succeeding years.

In 1878 the number of calls was........................ 407
" 1882 " " " 734
" 1886 " " " 1,069

Since then the growth is shown by years :

In 1887...1,328
" 1888............... 1,415
" 1889.....................,..............................1,647
" 1890...2,220
" 1891...2,141
" 1892....,............................... 2,321

The next new departure for the hospital was the establishment of an *Out-patient Department*, which was opened in 1881. While the record of the first two years is incomplete, the number of cases treated annually is recorded as follows, the number of visits not being given :

In 1881......... 676
" 1882....,.. 3,620
" 1883.............. 5,520
" 1884...12,843
" 1885...................................... 13,493

On December 31, 1885, a new building was opened, especially adapted to the needs of the Out-patient Department, which until then had been insufficiently accommodated in the basement of the Administration Building. The public appreciation of the new quarters is evidenced by the record of the Out-patient Department since the opening of the new building.

In 1886 new patients treated, 18,254 ; new and old combined, 61,084
" 1887 " " " 20,828 ; " " " " 71,667
" 1888 " " " 20,271 ; " " " " 74,563
" 1889 " " " 20,834 ; " " " " 79,180
" 1890 " " " 23,229 ; " " " " 87,430
" 1891 " " " 25,948 ; " " " " 92,341
" 1892 " " " 25,484 ; " " " " 83,083

It will be observed that the attendance in 1892 was 9,258 less than in the preceding year. This may be partially accounted for by the fact that just before the opening of the year 1892 a new practice was instituted in the matter of collections for medicines, etc., with the result that the percentage of free prescriptions and dressings, which in

1891 was 31.1 per cent., fell in 1892 to 2.65 per cent. The number of *new* patients was only 464 less than the year before, and the gain to the hospital, in the matter of revenue derived from a charge of ten cents for each prescription and dressing, was nearly $4,000 for the year.

In December, 1890, the McLane Operating Room was used for the first time. It was constructed by Dr. James W. McLane (President of the College of Physicians and Surgeons and *ex-officio* trustee of this hospital) for the benefit of the gynæcological service, and as a memorial to his son, James W. McLane, Jr.

It is a model operating-room, and has been so pronounced by experts in the medical profession as well as by architects and others interested in hospital construction. It has subserved in a most satisfactory manner the purpose for which it was built.

The latest and most notable improvement has been the addition of "The Wm. J. Syms Operating Theater of the Roosevelt Hospital," rendered possible by the bequest of Mr. Syms, who left the sum of $350,000, and stipulated that $250,000, or as much thereof as the trustees might deem proper, should be expended in the erection of a building or buildings, on the site where it now stands, and that the residue should be invested by the board of trustees so as to yield an annual income for the maintenance of the building. He also provided that the building should be constructed as a surgical operating theater, under the especial care of Dr. Charles McBurney, the attending surgeon to the hospital. Much time and thought were given by the doctor to the consideration of the plans, in conjunction with the architect, Mr. W. Wheeler Smith, which resulted in the completion of the present building. It is worthy of note that the building was constructed and equipped throughout for the sum of $200,000, of the bequest and accumulated interest, so that the sum of $150,000 is left to provide a fund for its maintenance.

The structure is so unique that it seems worthy of special mention in this history. It may perhaps be best described by the following, prepared for publication by Dr. Edward Cowles, of Boston, Mass.:

"The Roosevelt Hospital in New York City presents the most remarkable structure of its kind that is now in existence. It is the Wm. J. Syms Operating Theater, a memorial building, for which the bequest was $350,000. It is two stories high in front and three in the rear. The amphitheater occupies the center of the building, and is lighted by a glass dome with a northern exposure, admitting the rays of light above and back of the audience, so that, so far as possible, the rays of light that illuminate the operating-table enter the room from behind the observer and nearly parallel with his line of vision, all cross rays being excluded.

" The architect was W. Wheeler Smith, but Dr. Charles McBurney was made responsible, in the will of the donor, for the construction and equipment of the building.

"The main entrance is on Fifty-ninth street, nearly opposite the College of Physicians and Surgeons. The broad vestibule has a marble mosaic floor and Italian marble trimmings, and stairway leading to the upper seats of the amphitheater, which has a seating capacity of 185. Three hundred and thirty, however, could be easily accommodated within the space of the amphitheater if it were desirable to admit that number of persons to a clinic. The seats, in six tiers, are of wood with wooden backs only ; they are supported by being fastened to iron standards. A wainscot of pure white marble, five feet high, encircles the room at the top of the amphitheater, while back of the operator an unbroken surface of marble rises from the pit to a line on a level with the top of the wainscot before referred to. Part of the pit extends backward within a recess lined with marble on every side, including its ceiling. The floor is of mosaic marble and its immediate surroundings are of marble and iron. The steps leading to the seats of the amphitheater are of slate. Under the seats the sloping surface is of asphalt over thin concrete on wire lath. At the top of the entrance stairway are two rooms, one for surgical records and the other for the house staff.

"A covered corridor leads from the hospital to the first floor of the building, all of which is laid in marble mosaic with angles rounded to meet a marble wainscot five feet high.

" Several of the most important rooms, where it is desirable to promote aseptic conditions, are fitted with doors of pure white Italian marble one-and-one-eighth inches thick, hung on massive metal hinges, a single slab in each case forming a door.

" The special operating-rooms for private cases and for septic cases are fitted with all conveniences, the interior and equipment being chiefly of marble, glass, and metal.

" The front part of the building rises to two stories and the central and rear portion to three stories above the basement. On the ground floor the outer rooms east and west are only one story high, and admit light by skylights as well as by large windows in the outer wall, which, from their situation, have to be fitted with semi-opaque glass. The rooms are carefully and ingeniously fitted for the use indicated in the plan; the instrument rooms, for example, have cases of metal frames with glass doors, sides and shelves which were imported especially for that purpose; and there are many devices for promoting asepsis.

"The amphitheater, as indeed every other part of the structure, is supplied with gas as well as electric lights, to insure the building never being without efficient means of lighting.

"An inclined plane has been provided, in place of an elevator, by which patients may be wheeled to the recovery rooms, four in number, on the second floor.

"The third floor is occupied by graduate nurses engaged in the special duties of that building.

"The warming is by steam; the air, taken at an elevation of twenty-two feet eight inches from the ground, passing over steam-pipes in great inlet ducts in the basement and being forced by fans throughout the building, one fan driving the air to the amphitheater alone, and a second fan to all other parts of the building.

"Fresh air, either hot or cold, as may be desired, is supplied to the amphitheater through one hundred four-inch iron inlets, commercially described as goose-necks, penetrating the inclined plane, from which it is aspirated, through a large register near the ceiling, into a heated chamber, which thence discharges its contents, at the highest point of the structure, to the outer air. In all other rooms of the building separate vent ducts rise directly upwards to their exit openings like chimney flues—a system which entails the risk of down drafts of cold air in some of them if a careful balance of the forcing and extracting power is not always maintained. Mention should be made of the sterilizing apparatus, occupying a room by itself and adding, in a marked degree, to the efficiency of the agencies employed to promote asepsis.

"The building is a most notable one in its elaborate perfection and practical fitness for carrying the work of operative surgery to the last degree of refinement."

Having described the buildings of the hospital in their inception and development, it may be of interest to refer to its relation to medical and surgical education. The immediate nearness of the College of Physicians and Surgeons affords a peculiar facility for convenient and frequent clinical instruction. At present weekly clinics are held on stated days in each of the three departments of the hospital, medical, surgical, and gynæcological. Opportunity is also afforded, to such of the students as desire it, to receive clinical instruction in the out-patient department. It may be observed that the helpful attitude of the hospital, in affording clinical instruction to the students of the College of Physicians and Surgeons, is becoming more marked with the growth of years. From the standpoint of the medical department of the hospital it is very natural, for the reason that with few exceptions the members of the medical board are connected with the faculty of the college or of the Vanderbilt clinic, which is tributary to the college. On behalf of the trustees, it may be said that with the location of the college, in the year 1887, in the immediate vicinity of the hospital, and appreciating the palpable advantage of hospital privileges for clinical instruction, they have extended all reasonable facilities to the faculty.

It may be doubted if the founder realized how important a factor the hospital, which he had conceived, was to become in the education of medical men. It is more likely that his only purpose was to ameliorate the ills to which humanity was subject, and with that conception he was probably content. The hospital has now had an existence of more than twenty-one years, having been opened on November 2, 1871, and the claim may fairly be made by its friends that it has not only happily realized the object of its founder, but it has become an important ally in the cause of medical education.

At the time of the founding of the Roosevelt Hospital no especial attention was given to the training of nurses for the care of patients. In more recent years a positive advance has been made in this direction, and the training of nurses for public and private requirements of the sick has become an important branch of hospital work. It will be noticed that no reference has been made, in this history, to a building for the instruction and accommodation of nurses. It is a seriously felt need which the trustees are earnestly considering the ways and means of supplying.

Changes,

to date (1893) in the members of the board of trustees and in the officers of the hospital since its organization; also in the medical board and the house staff.

Trustees.

1864.	George T. Trimble, *Pres. N. Y. Hospital.*	Died 1872.
"	Edward Delafield, *Pres. Coll. Phys. and Surg.*	Died 1875.
"	Thomas H. Taylor, *Pres. N. Y. Eye and Ear Infy.*	Retired 1866.
"	Frederic E. Mather, *Pres. Demilt Dispensary.*	Retired 1877.
"	Augustus Schell, *Pres. N. Y. Inst. for Blind.*	Died 1884.
"	James I. Roosevelt.	Resigned 1873.
"	Edwin Clark.	Died 1878.
"	John M. Knox.	
"	Adrian H. Muller.	Died 1886.
1866.	Royal Phelps, *Pres. N. Y. Eye and Ear Infy.*	Retired 1883.
1872.	John C. Green, *Pres. N. Y. Hospital.*	Died 1875.
1873.	James A. Roosevelt.	
1875.	Alonzo Clark, M. D., *Pres. Coll. Phys. and Surg.*	Retired 1883.
"	Robert Lenox Kennedy, *Pres. N. Y. Hospital.*	Retired 1882.
1877.	Joseph W. Patterson, *Pres. Demilt Dispensary.*	Died 1881.
1878.	John H. Abeel.	
1881.	Charles H. Tracy, *Pres. Demilt Dispensary.*	Died 1885.
1882.	William H. Macy, *Pres. N. Y. Hospital.*	Died 1887.
1884.	John C. Dalton, M. D., *Pres. Coll. Phys. and Surg.*	Died 1889.
"	Benjamin H. Field, *Pres. N. Y. Eye and Ear Infy.*	Died 1893.
"	Robert S. Hone, *Pres. N. Y. Inst. for the Blind.*	Retired 1889.
1886.	Charles C. Savage, *Pres. Demilt Dispensary.*	
"	W. Irving Clark.	
1887.	James M. Brown, *Pres. N. Y. Hospital.*	Died 1890.
1889.	James Woods McLane, M. D., *Pres. Coll. Phys. and Surg.*	
"	James M. McLean, *Pres. N. Y. Inst. for the Blind.*	Died 1890.
1890.	Robert J. Livingstone, *Pres. N. Y. Hospital.*	Died 1891.
"	John Treat Irving, *Pres. N. Y. Inst. for the Blind.*	
1891.	Merritt Trimble, *Pres. N. Y. Hospital.*	

By Charter. (margin)

Officers.

Presidents.

1864. James I. Roosevelt.	1875. Adrian H. Muller.
1867. Edward Delafield.	1886. John M. Knox.

Vice-Presidents.

1864. Edward Delafield.	1884. John M. Knox.
1867. Adrian H. Muller.	1886. John H. Abeel.
1875. John C. Green.	1887. James A. Roosevelt.
1875. Royal Phelps.	

Secretaries.	Treasurers.
1864. John M. Knox.	1864. George Trimble.
1877. James A. Roosevelt.	1872. Merritt Trimble.
1887. W. Irving Clark.	1891. Richard Trimble.

Pathologists.

1871.	Francis Delafield, M. D.	Resigned 1890.
1890.	Eugene Hodenpyl, M. D.	

Out-patient Department.

Attending Physicians.

1883.	J. West Roosevelt, M. D.	Resigned 1887.
1887.	Frank W. Jackson, M. D.	

Attending Surgeons.

1883.	William S. Halsted, M. D.	Resigned 1886.
1886.	Richard J. Hall, M. D.	Resigned 1888.
1888.	Frank Hartley, M. D.	

Attending Gynæcologists.

1884.	George M. Tuttle, M. D.	Resigned 1888.
1888.	Edwin B. Cragin, M. D.	

Assistants.

Assistants to the Attending Surgeon.

1883.	William S. Halsted, M. D.	Resigned 1886.
1886.	Richard J. Hall, M. D.	Resigned 1888.
1886.	Frank Hartley, M. D.	
1887.	George S. Huntingdon, M. D.	Resigned 1890.
1890.	Alexander B. Johnson, M. D.	
1892.	Lucius W. Hotchkiss, M. D.	

Assistant Pathologists.

1875.	Henry N. Heineman, M. D.	Resigned 1882.
1882.	J. West Roosevelt, M. D.	Resigned 1890.

Curators.

1873.	Edward K. Henschel, M. D.	Resigned 1876.
1876.	Robert Abbe, M. D.	Resigned 1880.
1880.	Henry N. Heineman, M. D.	Resigned 1882.
1882.	J. West Roosevelt, M. D.	Resigned 1888.
1888.	Eugene Hodenpyl, M. D.	Resigned 1890.

Museum transferred to College of Physicians and Surgeons in 1890.

House Staff.

House Physicians.		House Surgeons.
1871, Nov.	William D. Schuyler, M. D.	
1872, Apl.	Nelson B. Sizer, M. D.,	Wm. T. Bacon, M. D.
Oct.	Coert Dubois, M. D.,	William S. Reynolds, M. D.
1873, Apl.	Samuel I. North, M. D.,	Edward K. Henschel, M. D.
Oct.	Allan C. Hutton, M. D.,	Louis A. La Garde, M. D.
1874, Apl.	George L. Peabody, M. D.,	Gerrit V. Blauvelt, M. D.
Oct.	Edward H. Maynard, M. D.,	Joseph Fewsmith, M. D.

1875, Apl.	Henry N. Heineman, M. D.,	Wm. W. Wendover, M. D.
Oct.	Frank B. Green, M. D.,	Charles H. Knight, M. D.
1876, Apl.	John B. Knapp, M. D.,	J. Warren Rice, M. D.
Oct.	Stephen S. Burt, M. D.,	Samuel W. Budd, M. D.
1877, Apl.	George E. Twiss, M. D.,	John Jos. Crane, M. D.
Oct.	Etienne Evetzky, M. D.,	Wm. B. Berry, M. D.
1878, Apl.	George A. Church, M. D.,	Charles T. Buffum, M. D.
Oct.	Luther D. Woodbridge, M. D.,	H. Ashland Clay, M. D.
1879, Apl.	Isaac Weil, M. D.,	Richard J. Hall, M. D.
Oct.	Wm. P. Northrup, M. D.,	Ellsworth E. Hunt, M. D.
1880, Apl.	Frank W. Jackson, M. D.,	John W. Hopper, M. D.
Oct.	Nelson H. Henry, M. D.,	Augustus M. Hurlbutt, M. D.
1881, Apl.	J. West Roosevelt, M. D.,	William A. Hume, M. D.
Oct.	John B. McMahon, M. D.,	George D. Parmly, M. D.
1882, June,	Henry Ling Taylor, M. D.,	Edgar T. Weed, M. D.
Dec.	Wm. T. Van Vredenburgh, M. D.,	Morris L. King, M. D.
1883, June,	J. Duncan Emmet, M. D.,	Frank H. Harrison, M. D.
Dec.	Edgar B. Doolittle, M. D.,	Harry A. Henriques, M. D.
1884, June,	Jas. E. Newcomb, M. D.,	Wm. G. LeBoutillier, M. D.
Dec.	Walter B. James, M. D.,	
1885, June,	Henry S. Upson, M. D.,	Jas. H. Montgomery, M. D.
Dec.	William B. Gilmer, M. D.,	George S. Huntington, M. D.
1886, June,	Louis Asta-Buruaga, M. D.,	George Woolsey, M. D.
Dec.	Clarkson S. Mead, M. D.,	Frank T. Hopkins, M. D.
1887, June,	Edwin B. Cragin, M. D.,	Edward V. Silver, M. D.
Dec.	Charles N. Dowd, M. D.,	George A. Tuttle, M. D.
1888, June,	Allan M. Butler, M. D.,*	William H. Park, M. D.
Dec.	Alexander H. Travis, M. D.,	Frederick J. Brockway, M. D.
1889, June,	L. Olmsted Wiggins, M. D.,	Calvin L. Harrison, M. D.
Dec.	William K. Draper, M. D.,	Robert Alfred Sands, M. D.
1890, June,	Robert G. Cook, M. D.,	Sinclair Tousey, M. D.
Dec.	Angier B. Hobbs, M. D.,	Robt. Coleman Kemp, M. D.
1891, June,	Henry F. Adams, M. D.,	Otto Henry Schultze, M. D.
Dec.	Henry B. Carpenter, M. D.,	John M. Macdonald, M. D.
1892, June,	Douglass Ewell, M. D.,	Edward G. Blair, M. D.
Dec.	James Ewing, M. D.,	Howard C. Taylor, M. D.

House Gynæcologists.

1888, Dec.	William H. Park, M. D.	1891, June,	Eugene C. Savige, M. D.
1889, June,	Hersey G. Locke, M. D.	Dec.	Alvah M. Newman, M. D.
Dec.	George W. Jarman, M. D.	1892, June,	Edward W. Peet, M. D.
1890, June,	Gustav W. Bratenahl, M.D.	Dec.	Eugene P. Mallett, M. D.
Dec.	Eden V. Delphey, M. D.		

* Dr. Butler died in the service, just before entering upon his term as House Physician, following an operation for appendicitis, and Dr. Charles N. Dowd was retained for an additional six months as House Physician.

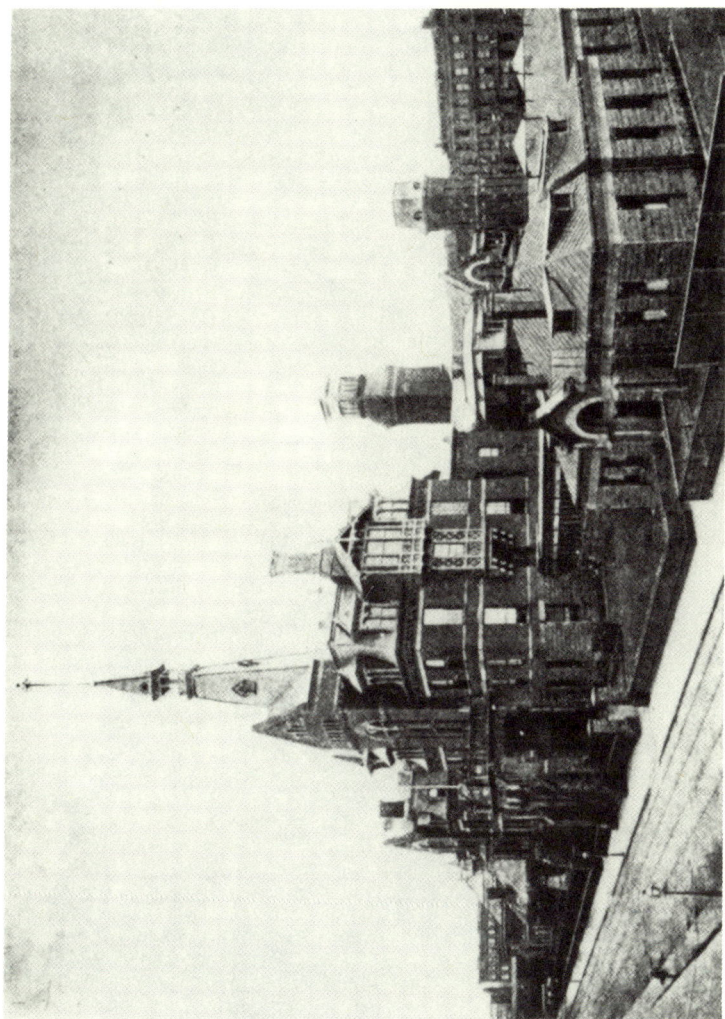

View of Hospital from north-west.

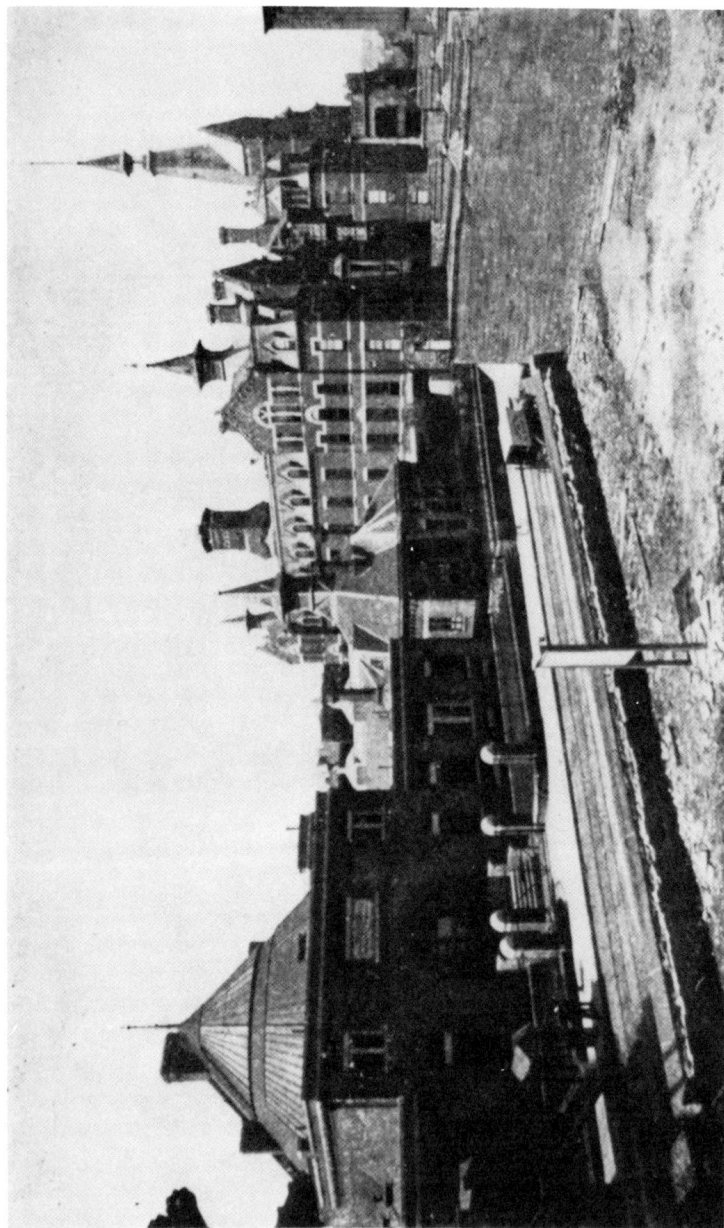

View of Hospital from north-east — Syms Operating Building in the foreground.

Plot Plan of the Hospital Block.

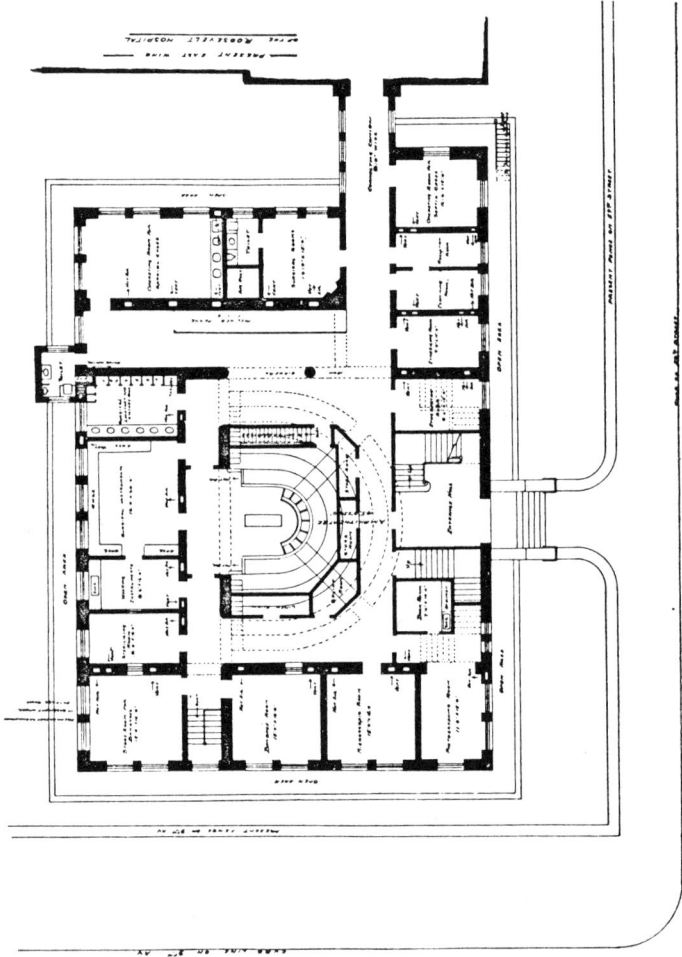

:FIRST STORY PLAN:

Syms Operating Building.

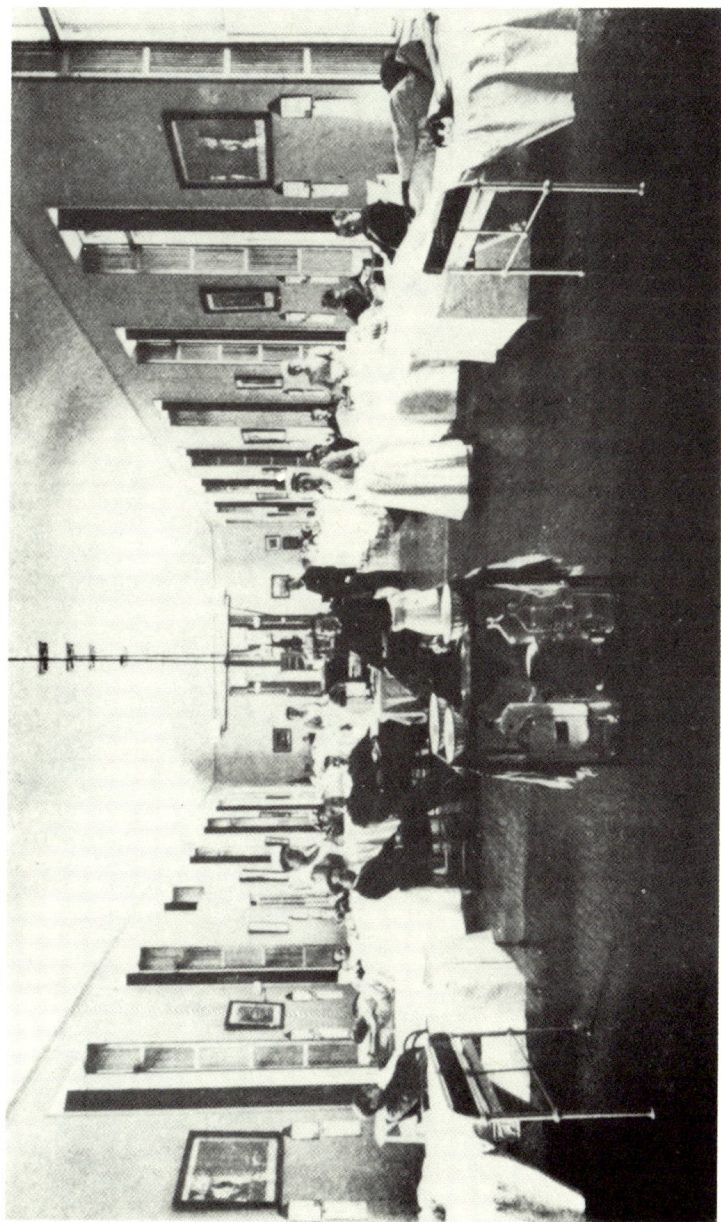

Active Surgical Ward for Men.

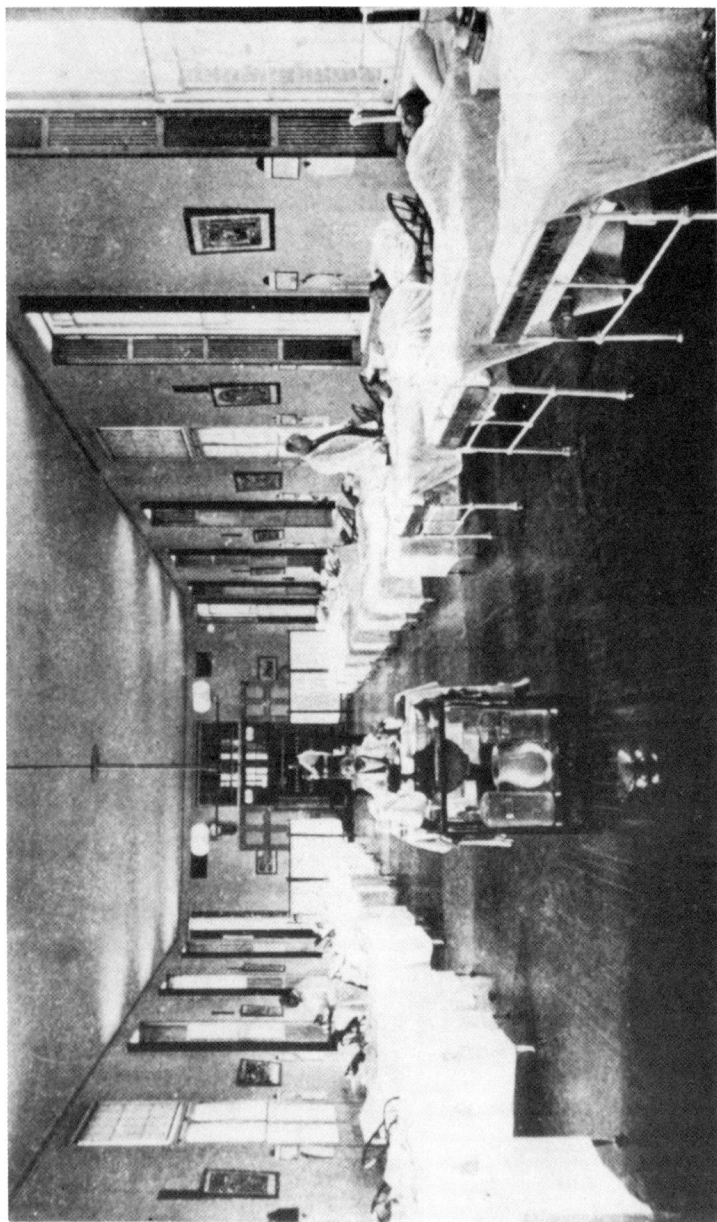

Active Medical Ward for Men.

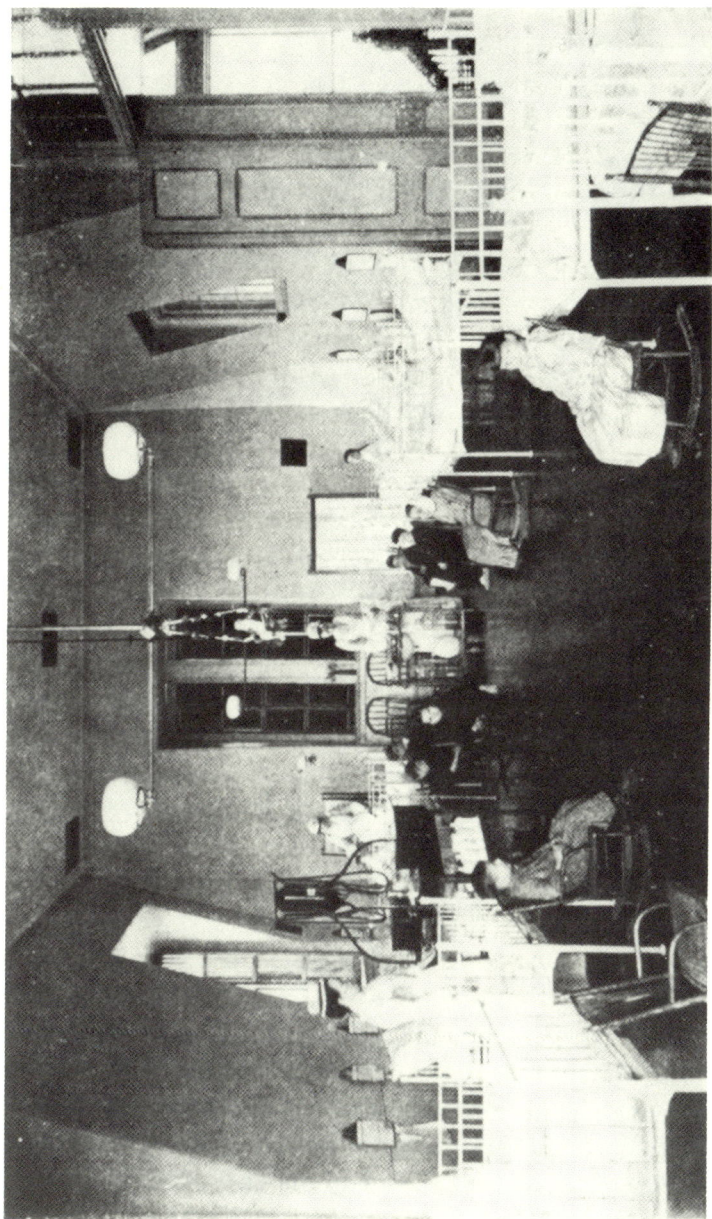

Surgical Ward for Children.

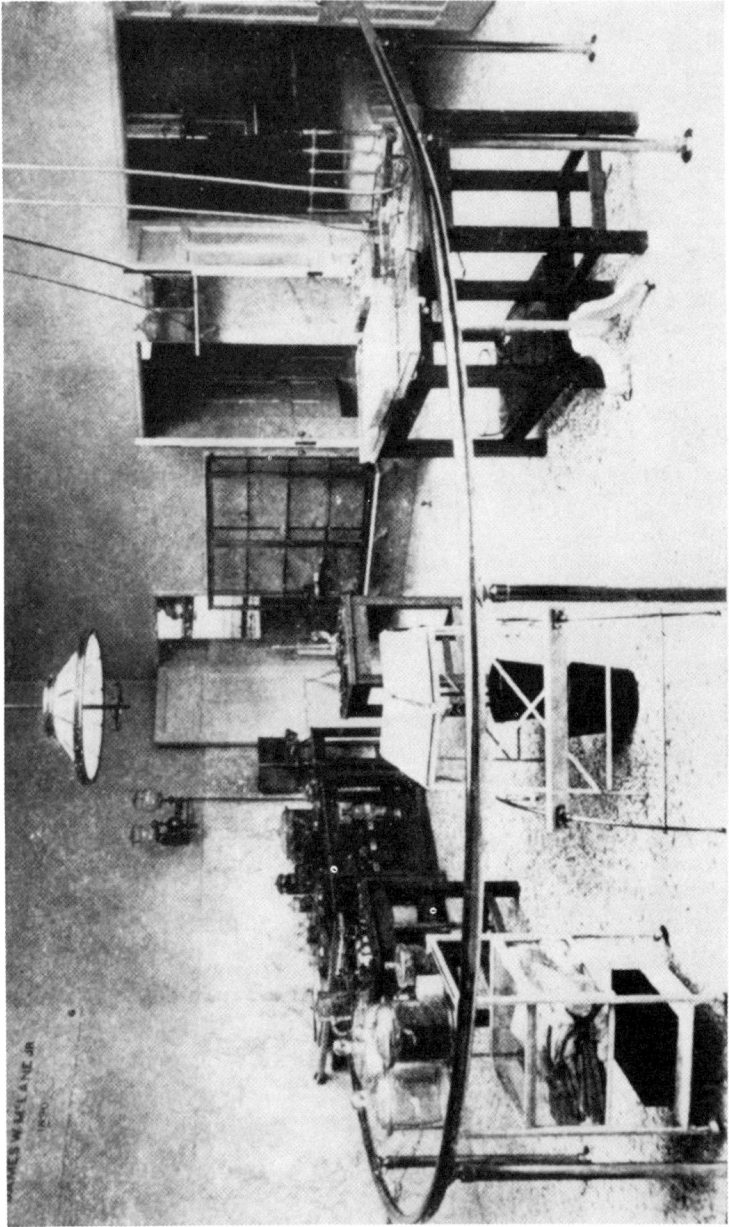

McLane Operating Room for the Gynæcological Service.

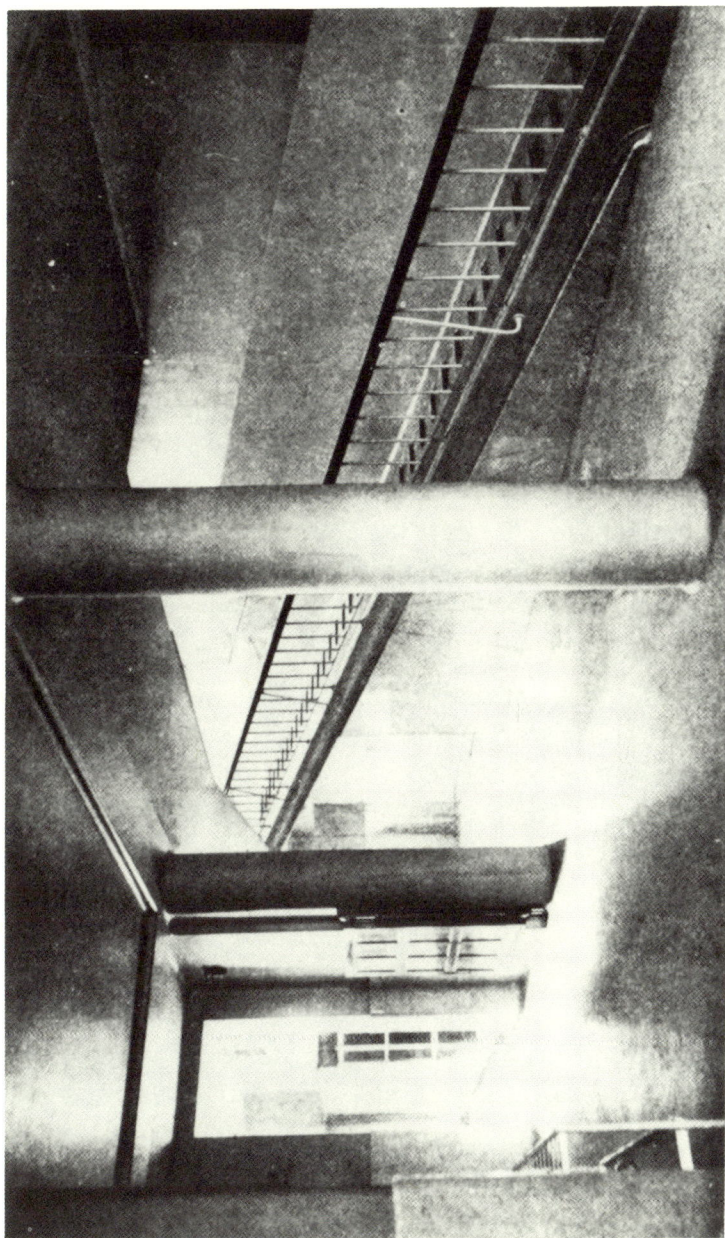

Syms Building — Inclined Plane leading to floor of Recovery Rooms.

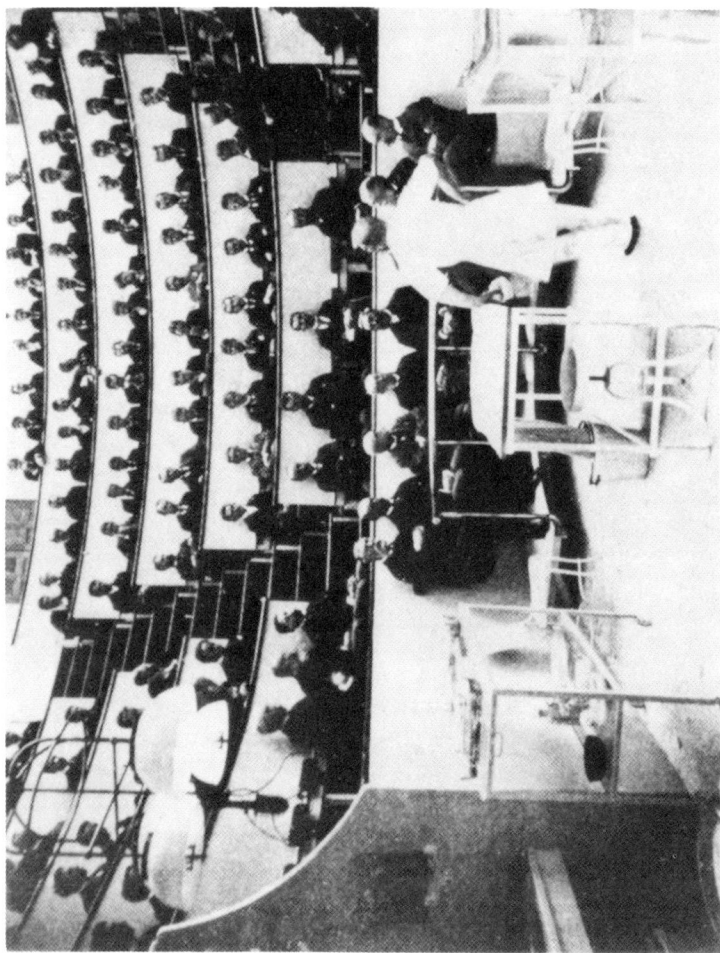

Syms Operating Building—Main Amphitheatre on occasion of First Public Clinic, Nov. 5th, 1892.

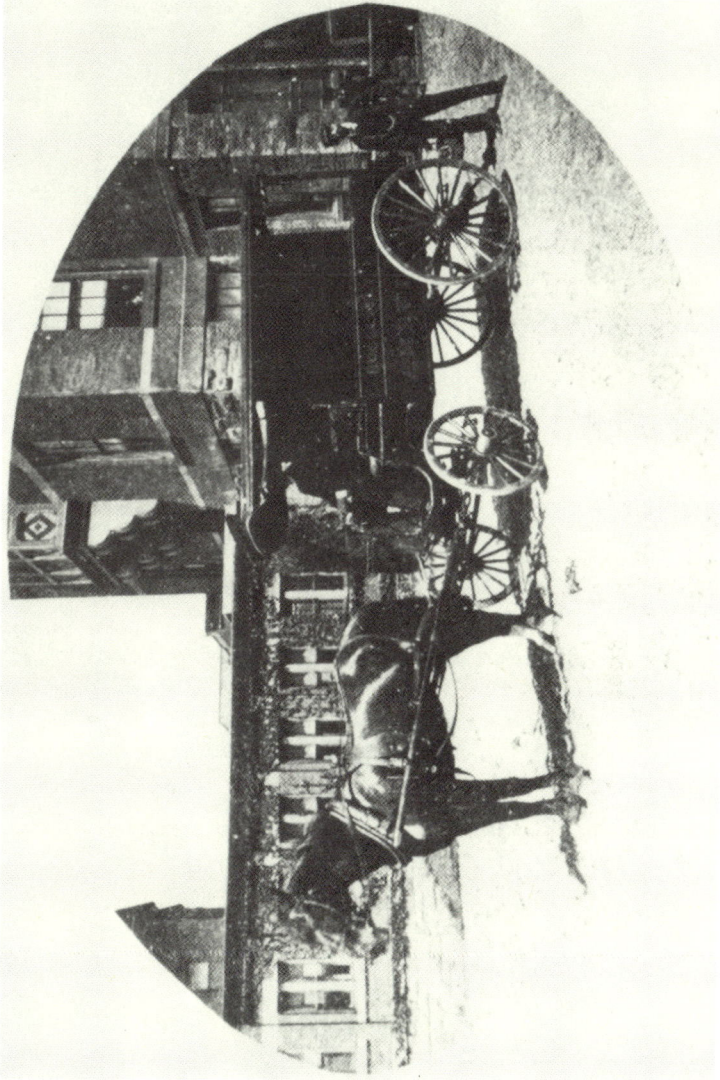

Ambulance returning from a Call.

DESCRIPTION OF THE JOHNS HOPKINS HOSPITAL, BALTIMORE, MD.

By Henry M. Hurd, M. D.,

Superintendent of the Johns Hopkins Hospital.

In 1873 Johns Hopkins, a retired merchant of Baltimore, placed in the hands of trustees a large sum of money for the erection of a hospital. In a subsequent letter he gave specific directions as to its location and general arrangement. Upon his death the trustees, after consultation with many eminent hospital men in this country and Europe, selected Dr. John S. Billings, surgeon of the United States Army, to act as their medical adviser in the perfection of plans and the erection of the buildings. The work upon the grounds was commenced in 1875, and the buildings were finally completed in 1889. The wards were formally opened for the admission of patients in May, 1889.

The grounds upon which the hospital is built are located in East Baltimore, between Broadway and Wolfe streets on the west and east, and between Monument and Jefferson streets on the north and south, and include an area of about 14 acres, measuring about 856 feet from east to west, and 708 feet from north to south. The grounds are on the side of a hill, near its summit, sloping toward the southwest, the lowest point being at the southwest corner, 87 feet 6½ inches above mean tide; and the highest at the northeast corner, 115 feet 6 inches above mean tide. The subsoil is clay, with layers of sand for a depth of 20 feet, with sand pockets at irregular intervals.

The west front of the buildings is shown in Plate I, where a view is given of the administration building and the two pay wards. In Plate II a rear view of the hospital is given. Here, in order from the left, are the nurses' home, the female pay ward, the gynecological operating-room, the administration building, the male pay ward, the octagon ward, three common wards, a double ward for colored patients, and the isolating ward for contagious diseases. All the buildings mentioned are connected by a covered corridor, in the basement of which the hot and cold water, steam, soil, and drainage pipes are carried in what has been termed the "pipe-tunnel." Upon the first floor a covered corridor extends as a passage-way from the different wards. Upon the top of this corridor an open terrace walk, on a level with the ward floors, at a uniform level of 124 feet above mean tide, is provided. In addition to the buildings shown in the rear view, there are shown upon the block plan (Plate III) a bath house, kitchen building, clinical amphitheater, dispensary, stable, pathological laboratory, and autopsy building, and laundry.

The capacity of the hospital is three hundred and ten beds. When completed according to the original plan, it will contain four hundred beds.

Construction.

The buildings are constructed of brick, with trimmings of sand-stone and of molded terra cotta. The foundations of the principal buildings consist of a solid concrete base; of the other buildings, broad flags of granite. All foundation and interior walls are of hard brick laid in Cumberland cement below the ground level, at which point they are covered by a layer of heavy slate. Lines of drain tile are laid around the foundations, and for all the buildings having cellars or half-basements, the outer surface of the walls beneath the ground is sheathed with overlapping slates. Above the horizontal layers of slate at grade the walls are hollow, with a 2-inch air space 9 inches from the inner surface. All pitched roofs are covered with carefully selected slate, laid on English asphalt felt, and secured with copper nails. The comparatively flat portions of the roofs are covered with copper, which is also used for all gutters, flashings, and down spouts. The floors of the principal buildings and of the corridor are formed of molded hollow blocks of hydraulic lime of Teil laid upon iron beams of suitable size and covered with wood, concrete, or asphalt. The floors of the basements are of artificial stone laid in large blocks, and underneath all heat coils is placed a heavy coat of asphalt to prevent the passage of ground air up through the heating coils. The floors of the pipe-tunnel and kitchen are of concrete. The floors of the corridor and of the bath-house are composed of cement and ground granite laid in blocks of suitable size, which form a very hard, smooth, and durable covering, easily cleaned. The floors of the bath-rooms, water-closets, and lavatories are of asphalt. The floors of the main kitchen, and of all tea kitchens, are of concrete. The floors of all wards and rooms for the sick are of edge grain Georgia pine, 1½ inches thick. All walls are plastered in three coats, and for the most part finished with a hard

troweled sand finish. The stairways in the wards are of iron with a
layer of asphalt in the treads. In all wards and rooms occupied by
the sick, woodwork is very sparingly used. Window sills are of
slate. The woodwork is of ash, with plain beveled and rounded
moldings, which may easily be cleaned with a damp cloth. The
windows are finished with plain half-round heads and moldings.
The wards are supplied with outside shutters so constructed that
they can be opened above and below in the ordinary manner, or the
lower half of the shutter can be turned outward to form a sort of
awning, promoting free admission of air and excluding light. The
roofs are high pitched, giving an ample space above the ceilings,
which space is ventilated so that the heat of the sun upon the slate
roofs during the hot season does not affect the wards. The walls of
the wards are painted in oil of a French gray color. All hard wood
is finished in hard oil.

Heating and Ventilating.

The general heating plans, with sections, are given upon Plate IV.
All the wards are heated mainly by a system of circulation through
iron pipes of hot water of comparatively low temperature and
pressure, the heat being furnished by boilers in the basement of the
kitchen and nurses' home. In many of the rooms fireplaces are also
provided. The hot water boilers for heating are six in number.
Each boiler is 5 feet in diameter and 16 feet long. From the boilers
the heated water passes into the great outflow main, which is a cast-
iron pipe 26 inches inside diameter, hung on rollers from the ceiling
of the pipe-tunnel and provided with expansion joints, to guard
against a breakage of the pipe from expansion and contraction.
From this main flow pipe, pipes are given off at each building, and
from these smaller mains the pipes in the heating coils are supplied.
From these heating coils the cooled water returns by a similar
system of pipes and mains to the boilers. The circuit is practically
a closed one, none of the water being drawn off or used at any
point, so that there is very little loss. The force which produces
this circulation is a small one, being the difference between the
weight of a column of heated water and that of a similar column of
water at a temperature from 8° to 15° F. lower, each column being
about 29 feet high, this being the difference in level between the
water in the boilers and that of the top of the heating coils. By
means of valves on all mains, and on the supply and discharge pipe

to each coil, the rapidity of the circulation can be controlled for each building and each coil, thus giving a corresponding control over the temperature of the coils themselves, since this is dependent on the amount of water of a given temperature which passes through the coil in a given time. The entire system of hot water heating contains about 175,000 gallons of water, and practical trial has shown that it produces an equable, agreeable temperature in all the buildings to which it is applied, in all conditions of cold weather and with the fullest ventilation desired. To prevent loss and waste of heat from the mains in the pipe-tunnel, and in the basements of the several buildings, these pipes are covered with felt enveloped in asbestus paper, and the whole is inclosed with stout canvas thoroughly painted. The effect of this protection is marked and satisfactory, very little heat is lost, as is shown by the low temperature in the pipe-tunnel, and a great saving of fuel is thus effected. With a temperature of 92.6° F. in the flow-pipe, and 85.4° F. in the return, the rate of flow of water in this apparatus is 13.5 feet per minute. With a temperature of 134.8° F. in the flow-pipe, and 129.7° F. in the return, the velocity of the water is 16 feet per minute.

In the wards the flues, registers, and heating surfaces have been arranged to supply 1 cubic foot of fresh air per second for each person in the ward, with the possibility of doubling this supply for a short time should it become necessary to flush the ward with fresh air. In the isolating ward, designed for cases giving rise to offensive odors, or in which a large amount of organic matter is thrown off, the air supply is fixed at 2 cubic feet per second per person. Three rooms in the isolating ward are arranged with perforated floors to supply 4 cubic feet of air per second per person, with the ability to double it, if desired. All the air in cold weather is warmed before it is admitted to the wards. The fresh-air registers are placed in the piers in the outer walls at a height of 9 inches from the floor, one register being allowed to each pair of beds. Besides these there are registers beneath the windows in the wards, which are used in cold weather to check the down drafts produced by the chilling of the air from contact with the glass of the windows. The chief register in the pier between each pair of beds is so arranged that the nurse, by turning the iron arm upon its face, can reduce the temperature of the incoming air nearly to that of the external air, or can increase it to the maximum which the heating coil affords, but without changing the quantity of the air admitted. In other words, the supply of fresh air cannot be shut off whenever it becomes necessary to reduce the temperature of a ward.

Sewage Disposal and Drainage.

The foul water from the various buildings, the water-closet and ward sink sewerage are kept distinct from the water discharged from the kitchen sinks, wash basins, etc. All pipes, whether soil or drainage, are placed so as to be readily accessible and fully exposed to view. All fixtures have separate traps placed as close to the fixture as possible. All traps have back ventilation, and all perpendicular soil pipes extend upward through the roof full size and open freely to the outer air. The water-closets are washout closets. The bath-tubs are of iron, not inclosed with woodwork, and are movable from place to place, being unconnected with the plumbing. The sinks are of porcelain. Those for the use of the ward nurses and housemaids have an all-around flushing rim, as well as a central flush. All pipes and traps are either fully exposed to view or are readily accessible by opening a door. In all the wards the perpendicular soil and trap vent pipes are placed in a large ventilating shaft, which extends above the roof and has in it an accelerating steam coil to secure a constant upward current. Into this shaft pass ventilating pipes from the water-closets and urinals.

The Octagon Ward.

This ward has two stories, besides the usual basement for heating apparatus. The exterior view of it is shown in Plate V, an interior view in Plate VI. The diameter of this ward is 57 feet 8 inches; the length of each face on the inner surface is 23 feet 10 inches. The height at the center against the central chimney is 16 feet, the height at the walls is 15 feet. The average wall area per bed is 120 square feet. The number of square feet of floor area per bed is 114.9, and the number of square feet per bed is 1,760.8. The cubic capacity of the whole ward, including the bay window, is 42,160.8 feet.

The heating of the ward is effected by hot water coming from the mains in the pipe tunnel, and passing through coils of 3-inch cast-iron pipe, arranged in stacks in the basement against the outer walls. Under ordinary circumstances in cold weather, the average temperature in these coils is 150° F., but this temperature may be lowered by lessening the velocity of the current of water passing through the pipes. The fresh air supply is admitted through openings in the exterior walls of the basement of the ward, coming from over the green lawn surrounding it. This opening in the wall is protected by wire netting, and communicates with a galvanized-iron flue which passes downward to open in the chamber beneath the heating coil, and also upward directly to the fresh-air register in the ward. In this flue opposite the external opening is a cast-iron valve or damper, operated from the ward above, by means of which the incoming air can be either directed wholly downward so that it must all pass through the heating coil, or wholly upward so that it passes directly to the ward without being heated, or partly upward and partly downward so as to produce a mixture of any desired temperature. The heating coils are inclosed in brick chambers which have at the top in front of the coils a large plate composed of two sheets of galvanized iron with felt between. These plates or doors fit tightly, but can be readily removed to give access to the pipes for the purpose of cleansing or repair.

Ventilation.—Rising through the center of the ward is an octagonal brick chimney 8 feet in diameter internally, and with walls 2 feet 6 inches thick, making a total external diameter of 13 feet. Upon each face of this chimney are two openings from the ward, one near the floor, the other near the ceiling, each measuring 20 by 26 inches. Those in the lower ward open directly into the central shaft. Within this brick chimney is set a boiler-iron tube 5 feet 9 inches in diameter, rising on a projecting cast-iron base built into the walls, which tube extends from the floor of the lower ward to above the ceiling of the upper one. Into the space between this boiler-iron flue and the outer chimney the openings from the upper ward enter. Just above the top of the boiler-iron flue is placed an accelerating coil of steam pipe. Through the center of the chimney rises a cast-iron pipe 12 inches in diameter, which serves as a smoke flue for the open fireplaces to be placed in the wards against the central chimney, should they be found necessary.

In the wards the general direction of the air currents is from the circumference toward the central shaft. In cold weather the air passes either entirely or in part through the heating coils, and is allowed to escape through openings near the floor in the central shaft in order to secure a uniform diffusion of fresh air and to diminish the loss of heat. During the warm weather or when it is desired to rapidly change the air of the ward, the upper registers in the central shaft near the ceiling are opened in addition to the lower ones.

Next to the ward at the north end are the nurses' closet, the bath-room, lavatory, and water-closets, while on the other side of the corridor are the tea-kitchen, the dining-room, two wards for one or two beds each, and the clothing and linen closets. The nurse has neither sleeping nor sitting-room, but resides in the adjacent nurses' home. The tea-kitchen is provided with a small gas range and a steam table. In the nurse's closet is a drying closet heated by steam. The bath-tub is movable, and can be raised on a truck and carried to any bedside, if desired.

The ground plan of the octagon ward is given in Plate VII. A longitudinal section of the building from north to south is given in Fig. 1, Plate VIII; a cross section from east to west is given in Fig. 2, Plate VIII.

The Common Ward.

The longitudinal pavilions, known as the common wards, are three in number. The exterior view from the southeast is given in Plate IX. An interior view is given in Plate X. The main floor plans and sections showing ventilation and arrangement of rooms, are shown upon Plate XI. The basement and attic floor plans are given upon Plate XII. The longitudinal section from north to south is given upon Plate XIII. The axes of all the wards run directly north and south, so that the windows generally face east and west. The least distance between any two pavilions is 60 feet.

The main ward is a room 99 feet 6 inches long, 27 feet 6 inches wide, 15 feet high at the side walls, and 16 feet high in the clear in the center. It is intended to contain twenty-four beds. Each bed has a wall space of 7 feet 6 inches, a floor area of 106.9 square feet, and a cubic air space of 1,768.9 feet. At the south end of the ward is a large bay window, which forms a sun room. Right angles in the ward are avoided as far as possible; all corners are rounded. The junction of the ceiling with the walls forms a quarter circle, and also the junction of the walls with the floor. The method of heating is similar to that described in the octagon ward.

Ventilation.—Two systems of exhaust flues are provided to remove foul air from the ward. The first consists of a series of circular openings in the floor of the ward, one beneath the foot of each bed. These openings are 12 inches in diameter, and are each covered with a nearly hemispherical dome of wire netting to prevent the accumulation of rubbish in the flues beneath. Each opening communicates with a galvanized-iron tube, 12 inches in diameter, which passes obliquely on the ceiling of the basement to enter the lower foul air duct, which runs longitudinally beneath the ward floor and enters the ventilating chimney. The main longitudinal foul air duct is constructed of wood, lined with galvanized iron. At the end most remote from the chimney it measures internally 1 foot 10 inches by 1 foot 3 inches, and from this point it gradually enlarges to provide for the additional flues which enter it, until at the point where it enters the ventilating chimney it measures 4 feet 4 inches by 2 feet 10 inches. The ventilating chimney is 4 feet 2 inches in diameter and 75 feet high. The upper system for the escape of foul air consists of six openings in the center of the ceiling of the ward, each measuring 2 feet by 2 feet and placed 13 feet apart. These open into the upper foul air duct running longitudinally in the attic above the ceiling of the ward to the ventilating chimney and corresponding to the lower duct. The ceiling of the ward is 1 foot higher in the center than at the sides. The openings in the ceiling leading into the upper foul air duct are controlled by shutters, which can be raised or lowered by moving an iron lever in the ventilating chimney. In the main ventilating chimney or aspirating shaft, a coil of steam pipe, heated by high pressure steam, is placed to increase the velocity of the upward current of air in the chimney. Under ordinary circumstances the downward ventilation alone is used. Whenever the ward becomes heated, however, or it is desired to pass a large quantity of air through it, the ceiling registers are opened. In moderate and warm weather both sets of registers are open. In addition to these methods of producing air currents, a propelling fan is placed in the basement at the south end. This fan, which is propelled by steam-power, is 4 feet in diameter. It is placed in the mouth of a duct communicating with each coil-chamber at the floor. By means of this fan a very large amount of fresh air can be forced into the ward to secure a thorough flushing and the removal of unpleasant odors. The whole system of ventilation is designed to secure 1 cubic foot of fresh air per second for each of the twenty-four beds in the room. This amount can be doubled, should it become desirable to do so.

Double Ward.

A pavilion for colored patients is in process of erection. This ward building, from the necessity of providing at least four classifications, has been arranged to be of two stories, with two wards upon each fl)or, north and south respectively from a central service building. This service building contains a common dining-room and tea-kitchen, two private wards, bath-room, lavatory, nurses' closet, clothes room and storeroom. At the south end of the south wards are large sun-rooms, and upon the east side of the building commodious porches for those patients who can go into the open air. The building is heated by hot water, and the system of ventilation resembles that of the octagon ward, being effected by a central shaft into which openings have been provided at the floor and ceiling level, the fresh air inlets being through mixing valves as in the other buildings. Each ward provides accommodations for eighteen patients. The location of the ward upon a line with the other wards at the eastern side of the grounds, renders it practicable to extend to it the present hot water flow and return pipes. The pavilion is connected with the others by a low corridor, in the basement of which the heating apparatus is carried, and upon the main floor a covered way connects it with the buildings already constructed. The building corresponds in construction, general arrangement and architectural details with those already built upon the grounds.

The Isolating Ward.

An exterior view from the northeast is shown upon Plate XIV. A longitudinal section from north to south and details are shown upon Plate XV.

The essential feature of this pavilion is that the central corridor is freely open to the external air at either end, and rises through the building in a clerestory at the top, the sides of the clerestory being fitted with movable glass louvers.

The walls of this corridor are practically double, and it is necessary to pass through a vestibule with two sets of doors to enter a patient's room. Each room measures 11 feet by 13 feet 1 inch. It has an open fireplace with a separate chimney flue placed in the center of the inner wall of the room. At one side of this chimney and fireplace is an entrance to the room from the corridor, through the vestibule mentioned above. On the other side of the chimney is a small closet to contain a commode, access to which is gained from the outside through an opening in the wall. This closet is lined with galvanized iron and has a separate exit flue, provided with an accelerating steam coil. The door of the closet is arranged for free access of air, and the exit of foul air from the room takes place mainly through the special flue of this closet. The whole of the closet and its exit flue can be readily cleansed with flame. This arrangement is made so that every patient taken to this ward can be isolated not only from the rest of the hospital, but also from all other patients in the ward. There is no common water-closet or bathroom, and no possibility of the passage of air from one room to another by means of the common corridor, because this is practically an open-air passage. Fresh air enters these rooms through registers in the outer wall, the arrangements for heating and regulating the temperature of the incoming air being substantially the same as those described for the common ward pavilion. The amount of heating surface, however, is greater, being calculated for a constant supply of 2 cubic feet per second per person. The chamber utensils containing excreta when removed from the commodes are taken to a sink inclosed by glass doors with special ventilation and air supply, so that the excreta can be thoroughly disinfected and disposed of.

Three of the rooms marked I on the plan shown in Fig. 1, Plate XVI, are larger than the others, and in these rooms the fresh incoming air, instead of entering through a register in the side walls, enters through the floor which, for a distance of 7 feet from the outer wall, is perforated with one-fourth inch holes, giving more than 94 square feet of floor with fifty holes to the square foot. These holes are slightly funnel shaped, and twenty of them are estimated to be equal to 1 square inch of inlet. The object is to supply a large amount of air, about 4 cubic feet per second to each inmate, and to have this air pass constantly upward so that no portion of it shall be rebreathed or come a second time in contact with the patient, thus placing him in the condition of being out of doors in a gentle current of air.

In order to secure as little communication as possible between this ward and the rest of the hospital, arrangements are provided that the nurses on duty in this building shall remain for considerable periods of time, and accordingly two bedrooms are provided for nurses, each room to contain two beds. The bath-tub in this building is provided with a truck which can be readily wheeled into any room.

The Administration Building.

The administration building contains three floors besides the cellar, and finished attic story, and is crowned with a dome and spire in the center. It also has an annex in the rear which contains water-closets and bathrooms. The cellar or half-basement is 14 feet in the clear, is floored with concrete, and contains the hot water coils for heating the building. The main or first floor contains a large rotunda opening through the entire building to the central dome, the offices, library, reception, examination, and board rooms. The second floor is devoted to the living rooms of the superintendent and resident physicians, and the third floor is intended for bedrooms for the resident students. All water and soil pipes are confined to the rear annex building, on the upper floor of which are three boiler-iron water tanks, which hold 31,843 gallons of water.

Immediately in the rear of the administration building, separated from it by a covered corridor, is the apothecary's building so-called, which contains a pharmacy, with waiting room and bedrooms for the apothecary and his assistant; also a large general dining-room for the officers of the hospital. The second and third stories contain rooms for female employés, with bathrooms and water-closets. The cellar of the building contains rooms for the storage of drugs, and a room with a furnace, smoke chimney, and ventilating chimney, for the manufacture of pharmaceutical products.

The Pay Wards.

The pay wards are two in number, the north one being devoted to general medical and surgical cases, the south one to gynecological cases. Each ward is 130 feet long, 49½ feet wide, and two stories high, with a cellar; also a rear projection in the center, containing bathrooms, water-closets, staircases, etc. Each floor contains a series of rooms situated upon each side of a central corridor, which runs north and south, opening at either end upon a veranda. The rooms for patients are each 15 feet 5 inches long, and from 12 to 13 feet in width. Each has an open fireplace in the corner next the corridor. The fresh air is brought in through a register near the floor in the external wall. Besides the open fireplace and chimney flue each room has an exit flue 9 by 16 inches in the inner or corridor wall next the fireplace. These flues pass upward to the attic, where they are gathered into a single galvanized iron flue which passes to the center of the building, where it enters a perpendicular shaft in which is an accelerating steam coil. The buildings are finished in ash, and are plainly but comfortably furnished. Each bed has over it an iron crane or swinging bracket, from which is suspended a strong leather strap, so that a patient can assist himself to turn or rise in bed.

Gynecological Operating Room.

Upon the opening of the hospital, arrangements were made to use a large room in the private ward for an operating room. This arrangement was satisfactory at first when the number of serious operations was comparatively small and its use was infrequent, but a rapid and unprecedented increase in the amount of operative work soon suggested a change. It was accordingly decided in the spring of 1891 to erect a building to be used exclusively for operative work. The site selected was that which had previously been set apart for the general bath-house for women, adjacent to the projected row of pavilions for female patients. The building comprises a large operating room, 25.8 × 25.9, the floor of which is covered with Sinsig tile laid upon lime of Teil arches, and the walls are wainscoted to the height of four feet with Tennessee marble. The walls are plastered with King's cement, which furnishes a hard, smooth and non-absorbent surface with little opportunity for the lodgment of infectious germs. Adjoining the operating room is an etherizing room, 10 × 12 feet. Communicating with this is a recovery room, of the same size, with an adjoining bath-room and water-closet. The building also has a supply closet, dressing-room and photographic room. It is heated by low steam and ventilated by a shaft. The floor of the building is on a level with the floor of the main corridor, and the building is one story in height. The operating room is lighted by two windows looking west, a large double window looking north and a large skylight. The windows and skylight are of obscure glass, so that the light which enters is thoroughly diffused, and strong and annoying cross-lights are prevented. The interior lighting is both by gas and electricity. The structure is of brick, with a slate roof, and corresponds in general appearance with the other buildings upon the grounds. The only departure from the method of heating adopted in the remainder of the buildings was in the location of the heating flues at a height of six feet from the floor, it having been found by experience that this arrangement prevents annoying drafts of air upon patients. (See views and ground plan.)

The Kitchen.

The kitchen building is 75 feet square and three stories in height. The main floor is on a level with the floor of the corridor, into which it opens on the south. It contains a kitchen, scullery, refrigerating rooms, store-room, and employés' dining-room. The second floor contains rooms for the housekeeper and cooks, the dining-rooms for the servants and employés of the hospital. The basement floor contains a bakery, bread store-room, training-school kitchen, and cold rooms. In the basement are boiler vaults, containing hot water and steam boilers, also water-filters for the entire hospital. Immediately adjacent and under the sidewalk are vaults for the storage of fuel.

The Nurses' Home.

The nurses' home is a square building measuring 90 feet on each side, four stories in height above the cellar, with a central clerestory. The cellar of this building contains hot-water boilers, fuel vaults and store-room. The basement contains the nurses' dining-room, a small kitchen, a large pantry, a lecture-room, dormitories, and storerooms. The main floor, which is on a level with the corridor floor, contains a large main hall, the nurses' parlor, and library, apartments for the superintendent of nurses, rooms for the head nurses, etc. The two upper floors contain rooms for the pupil and night nurses. The building is in reality a square central tower surrounded by corridors on all sides with an external shell of living rooms. The central tower contains a large ventilating chimney, the stairway, water-closets, and bathrooms. All water and soil pipes are in the central tower, and two large shafts for air and light are also carried up through it. The building is heated by hot water, radiating coils being in the cellar for all living rooms. The nurses' home is an entirely independent building.

Amphitheater and Dispensary.

The amphitheater is a one-story building with a cellar, measuring 91 by 75 feet, and is connected with the hospital by an inclosed corridor. It contains a large amphitheater, measuring 52 by 47 feet, with a seating capacity for about two hundred and eighty persons, a special operating room, measuring 18 by 24 feet, well lighted from the south and by a large bay window on the east, an etherizing room, recovering room, a surgeon's room, a small special ward for three beds, and an accident reception room containing two beds. The heating of the amphitheater is effected by steam coils placed in the space below the seats, the fresh warm air entering through the risers. The foul air is drawn off into a ventilating chimney 6 feet square, which is in the center of the building. The amphitheater is lighted by a large skylight, and also by a window on the north side.

The dispensary, which is situated east of the amphitheater and connected with it by a covered corridor, is a brick building of one story, measuring 91 by 75 feet. It contains a large central waiting room 52 feet square, on the east and west sides of which are rooms for the physicians, surgeons, and specialists, who have charge of this service. It is heated by steam coils in the cellar, the fresh warm air being delivered through the risers and backs of the benches. The foul air is extracted by a large ventilating shaft on the south of the general waiting room, this shaft being 6 feet square internally. The foul air may enter this through a large opening near the floor level, or through a large duct communicating with the skylight. The general waiting room is lighted by a large central skylight, the other rooms by side windows. Medicines are dispensed from the pharmacy, which is on the south side of the waiting room.

The Pathological Building.

The pathological building is situated on the northeast corner of the hospital grounds, and is disconnected from all other buildings. It is a four-story building, measuring 58 by 78 feet. On the lower or ground floor is a morgue, a waiting room, an autopsy theater, a room for those engaged in private research, and rooms for bacteriological work. On the second floor is the director's laboratory, a laboratory for pathological histology, one for experimental pathology, a pathological museum, and a photograph room. The morgue measures 17 by 29 feet. It is not heated, and is ventilated so that no communication exists between the air of this and any other room in the building. The floor is of asphalt. The autopsy theater measures 29 by 38 feet, and extends through both stories of the building. It is so arranged that observers can stand upon elevated tiers arranged semicircularly around the autopsy table. The floor is of asphalt. The room is ventilated by a ventilating shaft 3 feet by 3 feet 6 inches. The third and fourth floors of the building are occupied temporarily by the Medical School of the Johns Hopkins University.

The Laundry.

The laundry is situated on the southeast corner of the hospital grounds, at a point so far removed from the other buildings that no offense may arise from it. It is a brick building measuring externally 115 by 56 feet, and is one story high, with a basement and cellar. The basement contains the steam boilers, storage vaults for

Plate I.

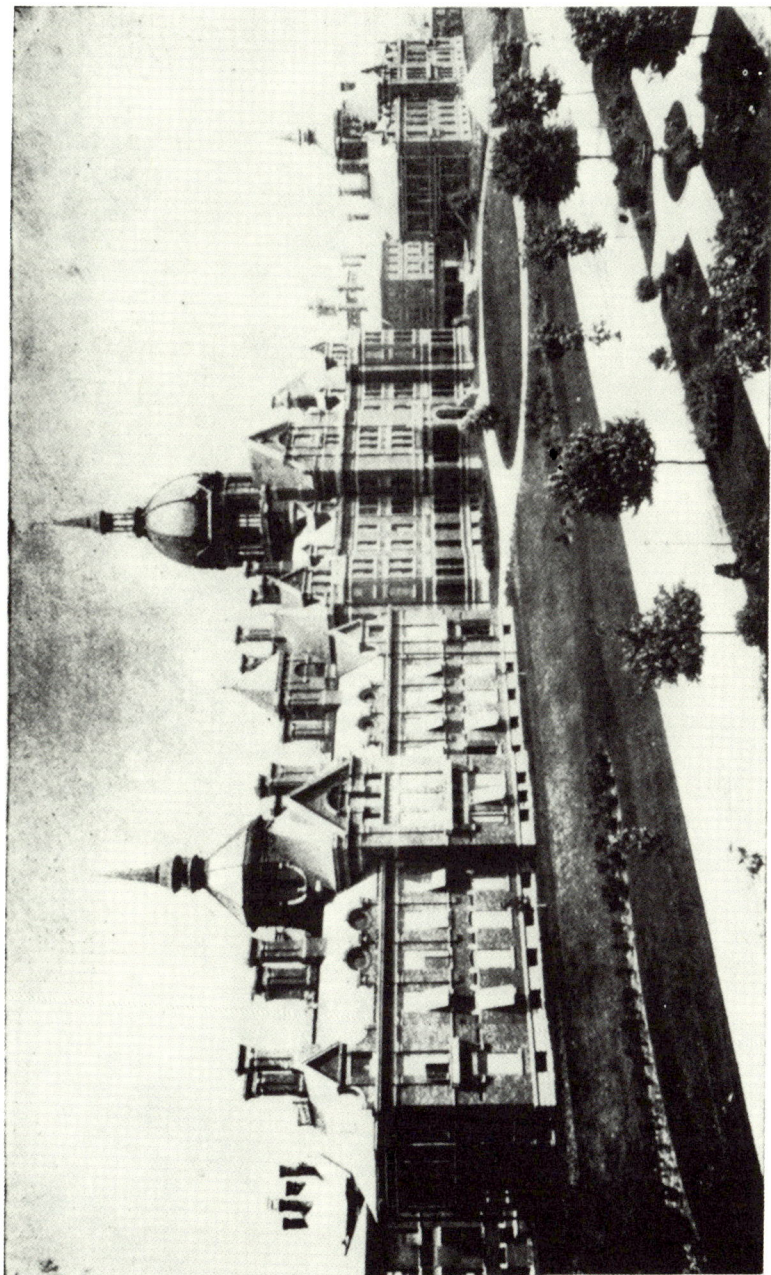

The Johns Hopkins Hospital — Front View.

Plate II.

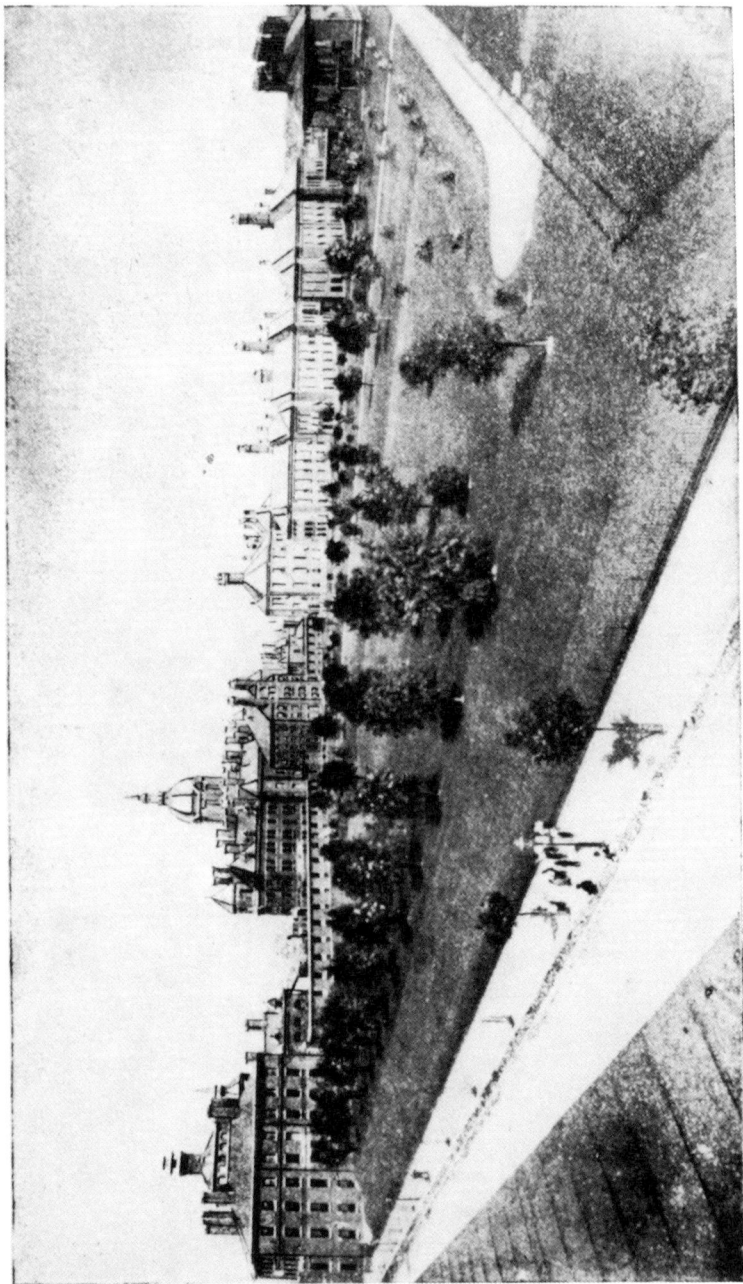

The Johns Hopkins Hospital — Rear View.

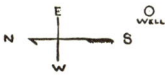

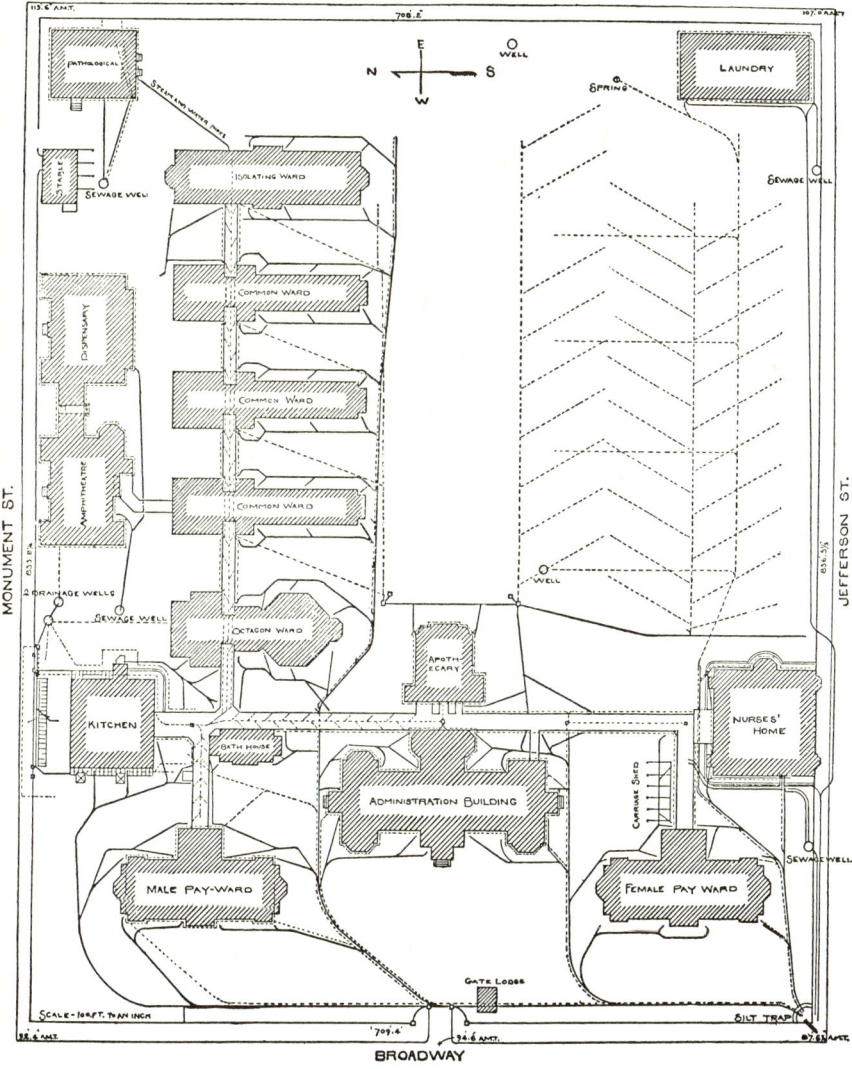

The Johns Hopkins Hospital — Block Plan.

Plate IV.

The Johns Hopkins Hospital — Heating Plans.

PLANS AND SECTIONS.

A	Administration building.	I	Isolating ward.	R	Pathological building.	T	Gate lodge.

A   Administration building.   I   Isolating ward.   R   Pathological building.   T   Gate lodge.
X   Apothecary's building.   O   Dispensary.   K   Kitchen.   S   Stable.
B and C Pay wards.   U   Amphitheatre.   L   Laundry.   HW   Hot-water boilers.
D, E, F, G, and H Wards.   N   Nurses' home.   Y   Bath house.   SB   Steam boiler.

FIG. 1. Section of corridor at *a-b*, looking east.
FIG. 2. Section of corridor at *b-c*, looking north.

FIGS. 3 and 4. Detail of cut-off valve V.
FIG. 5. Switch for testing the velocity of water in heating pipes.

Plate V.

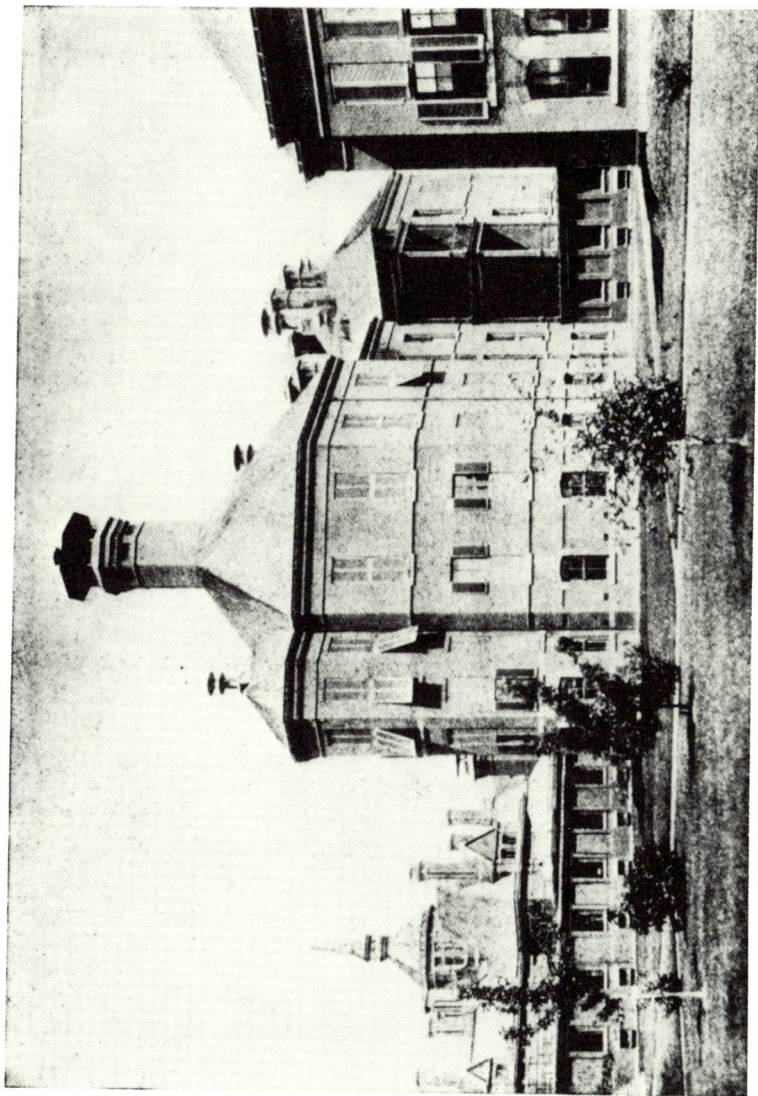

The Johns Hopkins Hospital—Octagon Ward.

Plate VI.

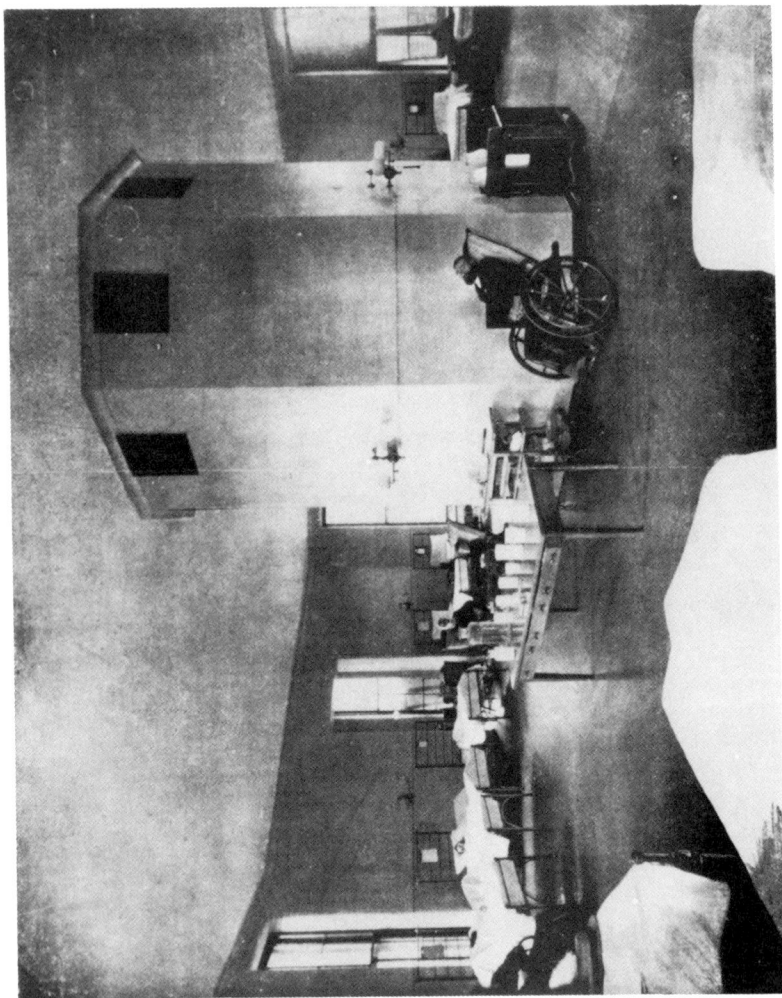

The Johns Hopkins Hospital — Octagon Ward, Interior.

Plate VII.

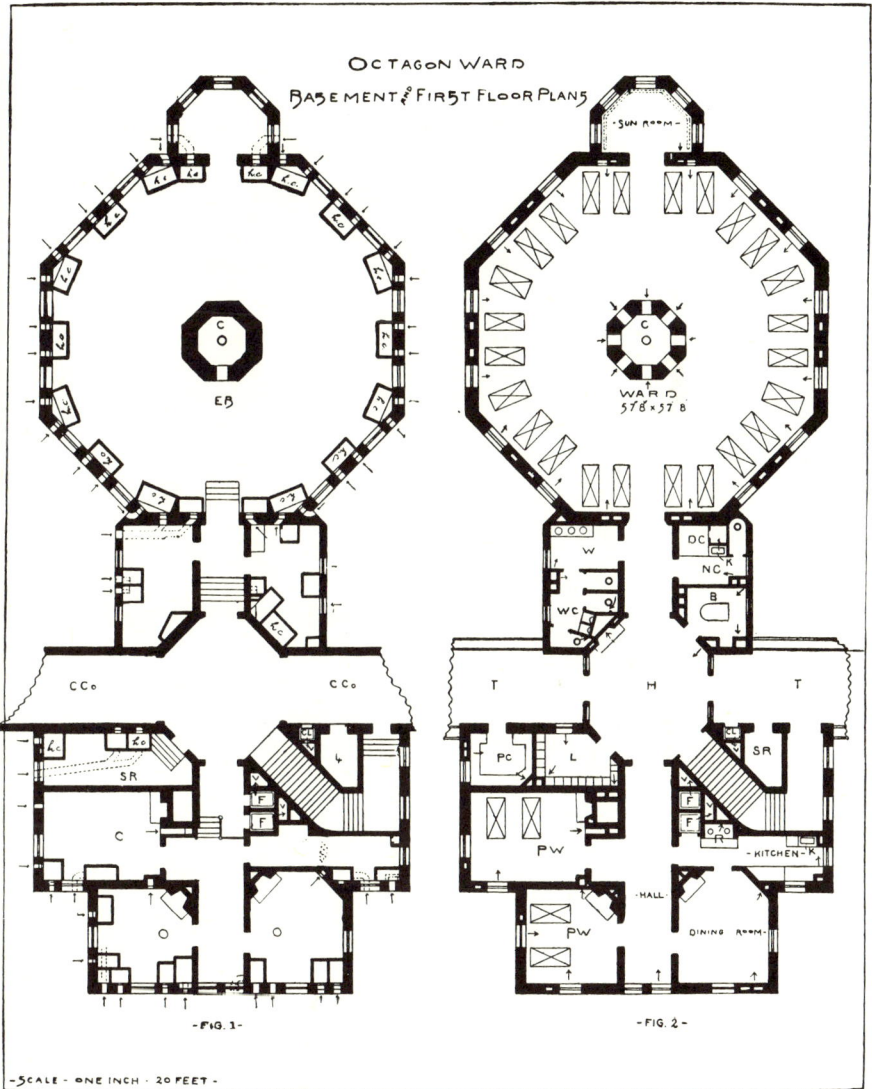

OCTAGON WARD

BASEMENT AND FIRST FLOOR PLANS

- FIG. 1 -

- FIG. 2 -

- SCALE - ONE INCH · 20 FEET -

The Johns Hopkins Hospital — Octagon Ward.

BASEMENT AND FLOOR PLANS.

FIG. 1. Basement plan.

		SR	Store room.	hc	Heat coils.	V	Ventilating shaft for lift.
C	Central ventilating chimney.	O	Orderlies.	L	Closet.	F	Food lift.	CL	Coal and soiled-clothes lift.
EB	Empty basement.	CCo	Covered corridor.						

FIG. 2. Main floor plan.

C	Central ventilating chimney.	W	Lavatory.	L	Clean linen closet.	R	Range.	DC	Drying closet.
V	Ventilating shaft for lift.	B	Bathroom.	NC	Nurses' closet.	F	Food lifts.	SR	Storeroom.
H	Central hall.	WC	Water-closets.	CL	Coal and soiled-clothes lift.	K	Sink	T	Open terrace over corridor.
PW	Private wards.	PC	Patients' clothing.						

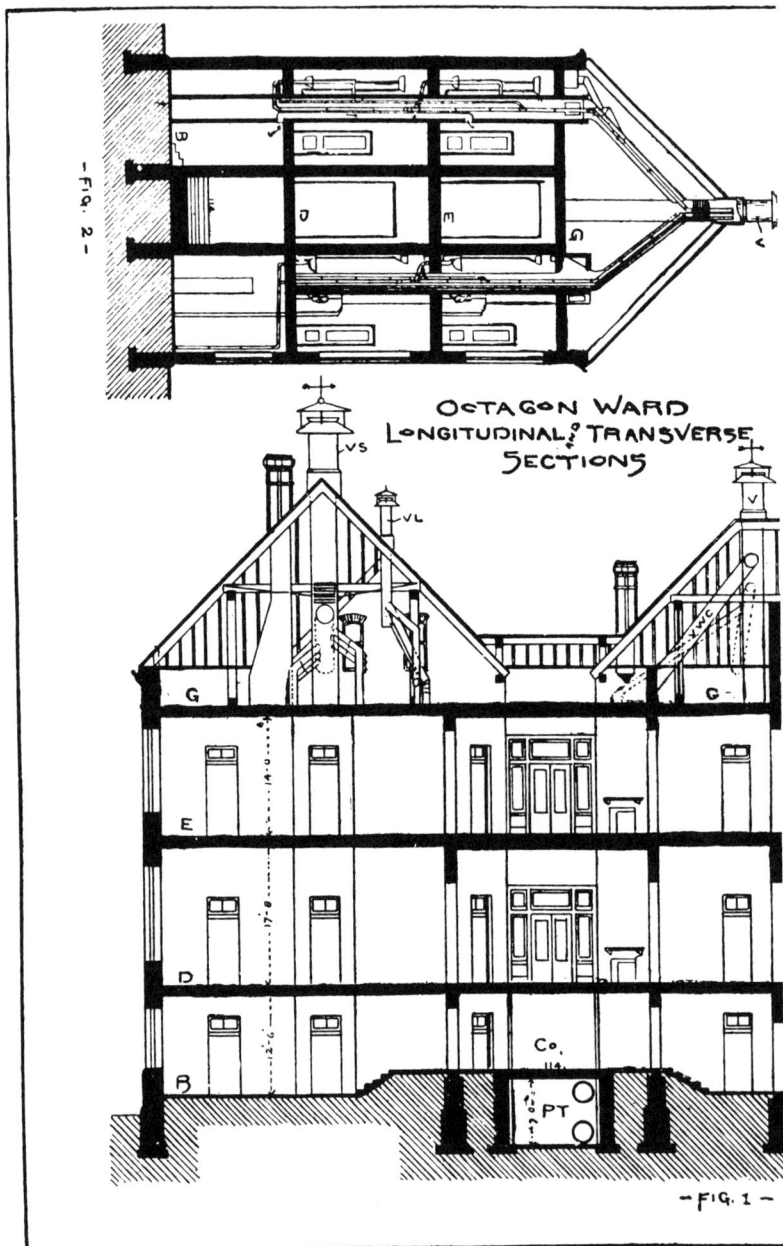

OCTAGON WARD
LONGITUDINAL & TRANSVERSE
SECTIONS

- FIG. 2 -

- FIG. 1 -

- SCALE - 20 FT. TO AN INCH -

The Johns Hopkins Hospital — Octagon Ward.

FIG. 1. Longitudinal section, north and south.

C	Central ventilating chimney.		V	Ventilator for water-closet, bath-room, and lavatory.
BC	Boiler-iron cylinder.			
AC	Accelerating steam coils.		VS	Ventilator for special wards.
VWC	Vent pipe from water-closet.		VL	Ventilator for linen closet and clot[

FIG. 2. Transverse section through water-cl[
V Ventilator for water-closet, bath-room, and lavatory.   B Basement floor.
FIG. 3. Section of ventilating chimney, showing damper.

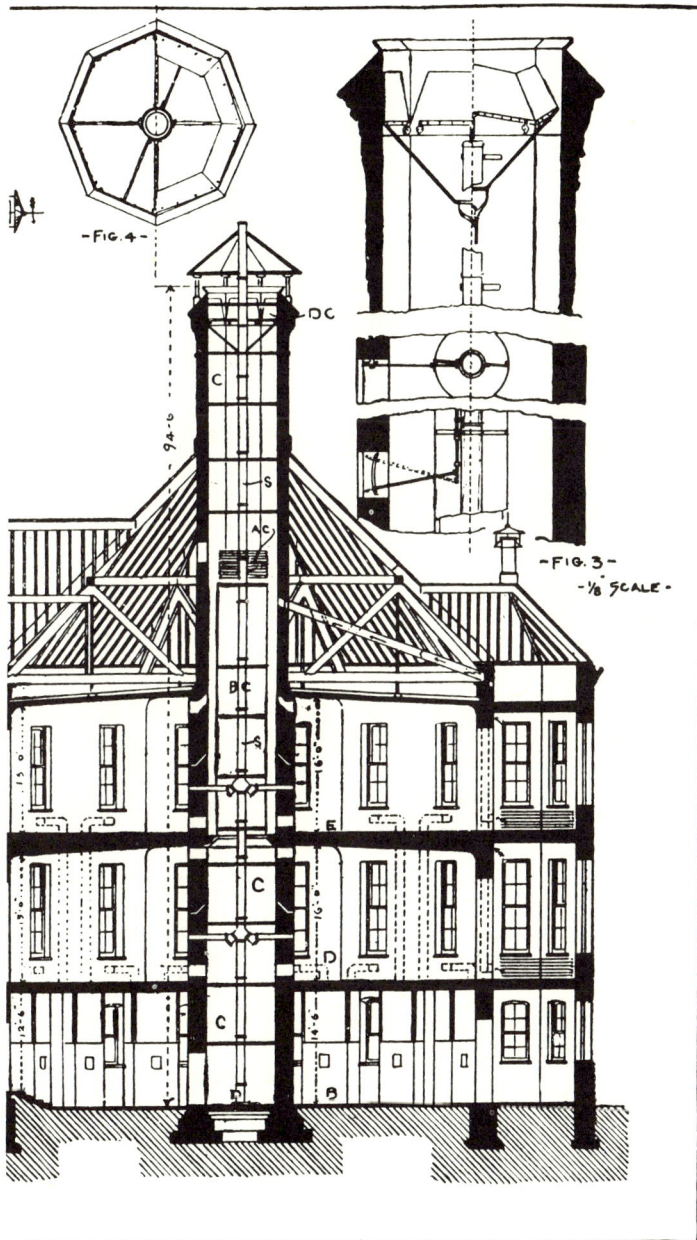

-FIG.4-

-DC

-FIG.3-
-⅛ SCALE-

Longitudinal and Transverse Sections.

Co	Corridor.		E	Second floor.
PT	Pipe tunnel.		G	Attic floor.
B	Basement floor.		DC	Chimney damper.
D	Main floor.		S	Smoke pipe.

ies room.

sets, lry closets, etc., east and west.

D Main floor.   E Second floor.   G Attic floor.

FIG. 4. Plan of chimney damper.

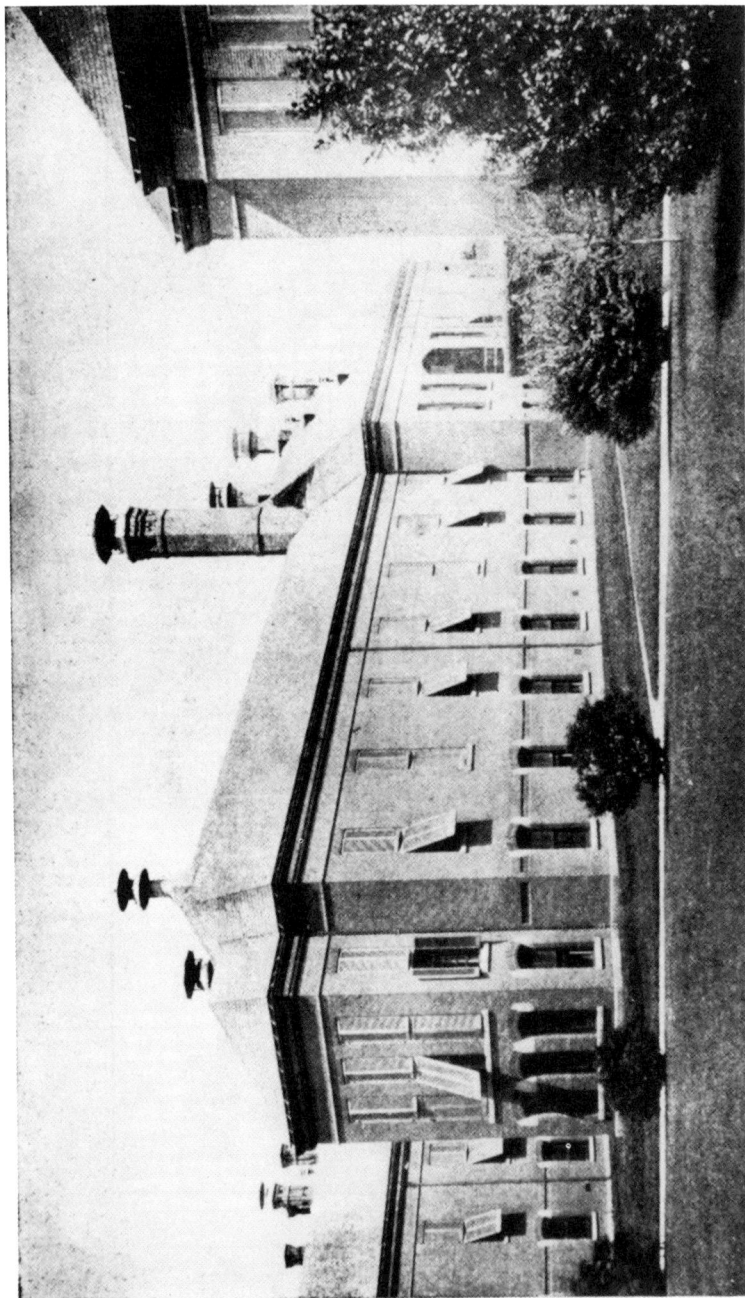

Plate IX.

The Johns Hopkins Hospital — Common Ward.

Plate X.

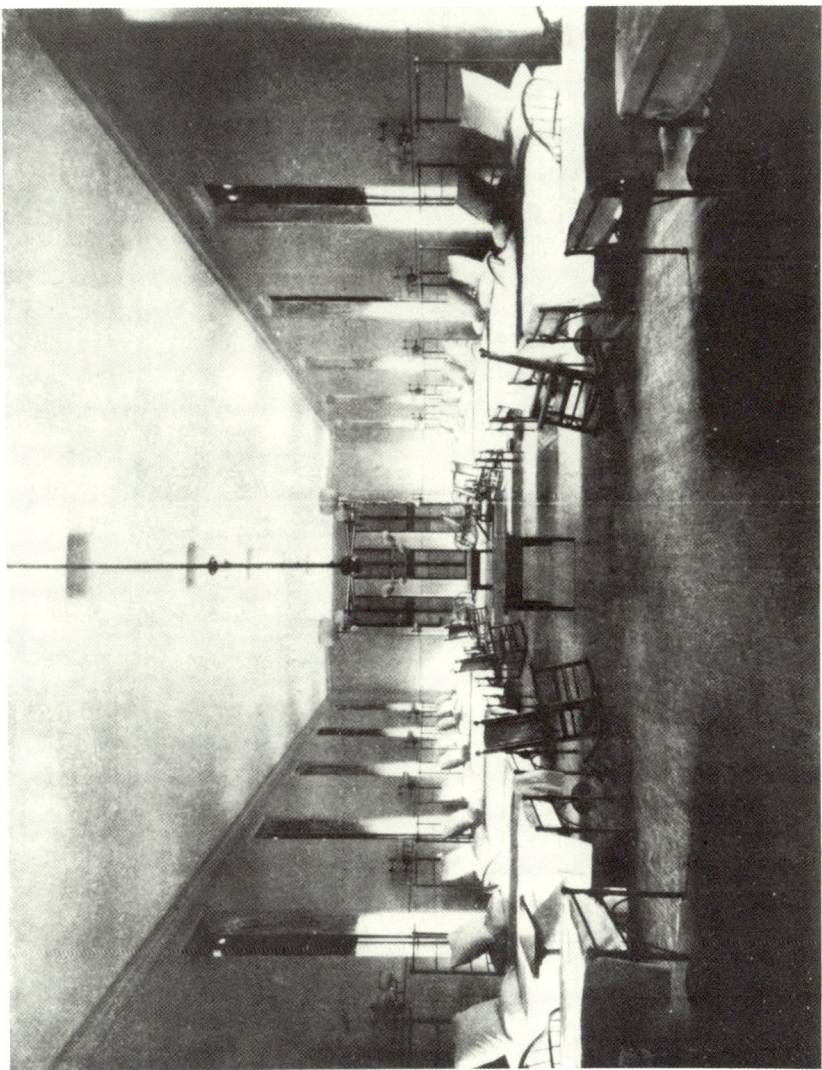

The Johns Hopkins Hospital — Common Ward

Plate XI.

COMMON WARD
MAIN FLOOR PLANS & SECTIONS

FIG. 3

- SUN ROOM -

WARD 27'6"×91'8"

W

WC

NC

B

OPEN TERRACE OVER CORRIDOR

H

OPEN TERRACE OVER CORRIDOR

PC

L

PW

KITCHEN

PW

- DINING ROOM -

FIG. 1.

- SCALE · ONE INCH · 20 FEET -

FIG. 2.

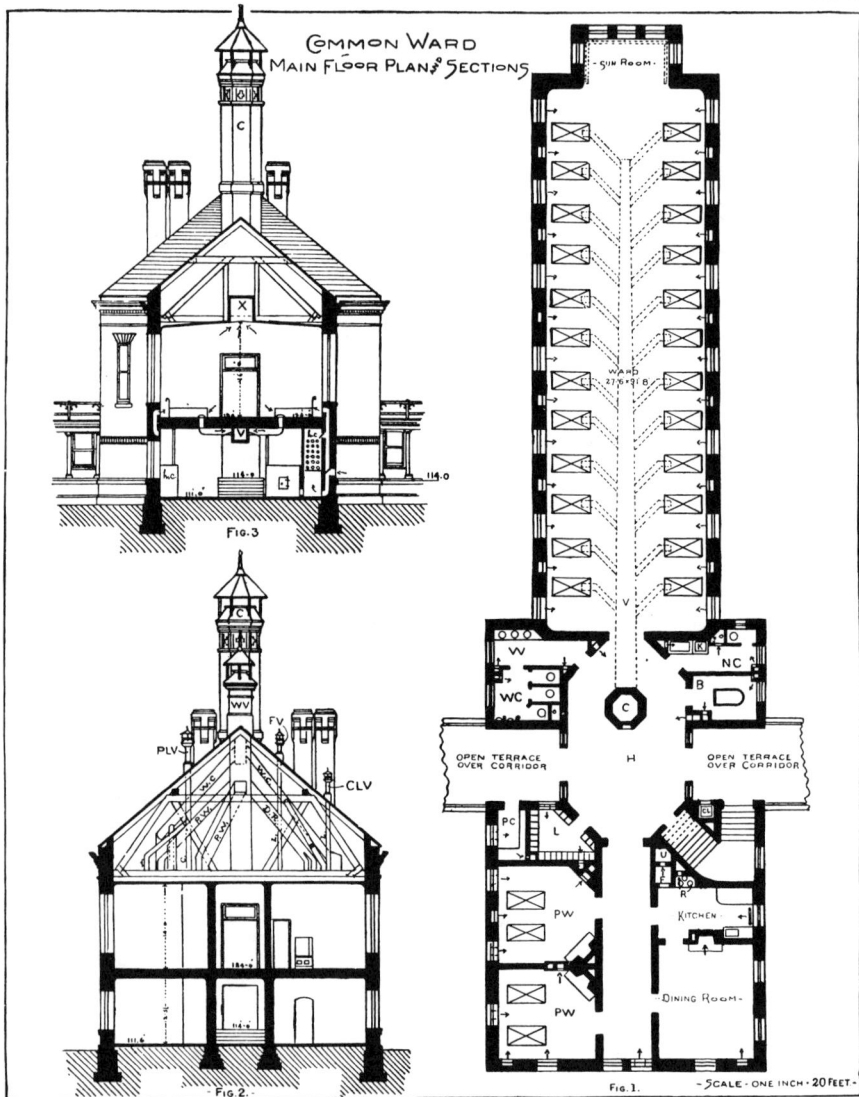

The Johns Hopkins Hospital — Common Ward.

MAIN FLOOR PLAN AND SECTIONS.

FIG. 1. Plan of ward floor.

C Central ventilating chimney.	H Central hall.	B Bathroom.	L Clean-linen closet.	R Range.
V Exit of ventilating ducts.	PW Private wards.	WC Water-closet.	NC Nurses' closet.	F Food lift.
U Ventilating shaft for lift.	W Lavatory.	PC Patients' clothing.	CL Coal and soiled-clothes lift.	K Slop sink.

FIG. 2. Transverse section of service building through kitchen.

C Central ventilating chimney.	WC Ventilation for water-closets.	DR Ventilation for dining room.	FV Food-lift vent.
VW Ventilating shafts for water-closets.	PW Ventilation for private wards.	CLV Coal and soiled-clothes lift vent.	PLV Patients' clothing and clean-linen vent.

FIG. 3. Transverse section through ward.

C Central ventilating chimney.	X Foul-air duct in attic.	V Foul-air duct in basement.
		hc Heating coil.

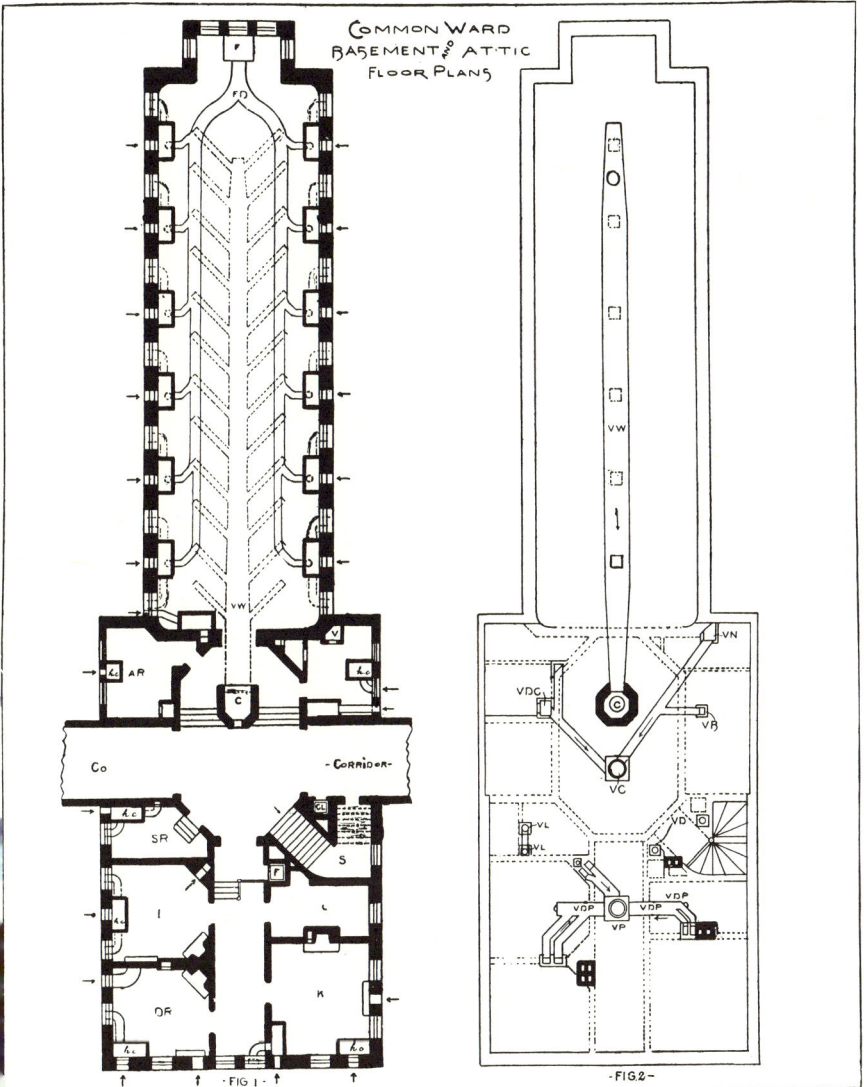

Plate XII.

The Johns Hopkins Hospital — Common Ward.

BASEMENT AND ATTIC FLOOR PLANS.

FIG. 1. Basement.

C	Central ventilating chimney.	AR	Airing room for blankets, beds, etc.	S	Stairway.
VW	Ventilating duct from ward floor.	hc	Heating coils.	I, K, and L Clinical laboratory.
V	Vent shaft to water-closet and nurses' closets.	FD	Fan duct.	DR	Directors' room.
		F	Fan.	Co	Corridor.

SR Storeroom.
CL Coal and soiled-clothes lift.
F Food lift.

FIG. 2. Plan of attic story.

C	Central ventilating chimney.
VW	Vent to ward ceiling.
VP	Vent shaft, private wards.

VDP Vent ducts, private wards.
VC Vent shaft to water-closets, baths, etc.
VD Lift vent.

VDC Vent ducts to water-closets.
VN Vent to nurses' closet, slop hopper, water-closets, and dry closets.

VB Vent to bathroom.
VL Vent to linen room and patients' clothes room.

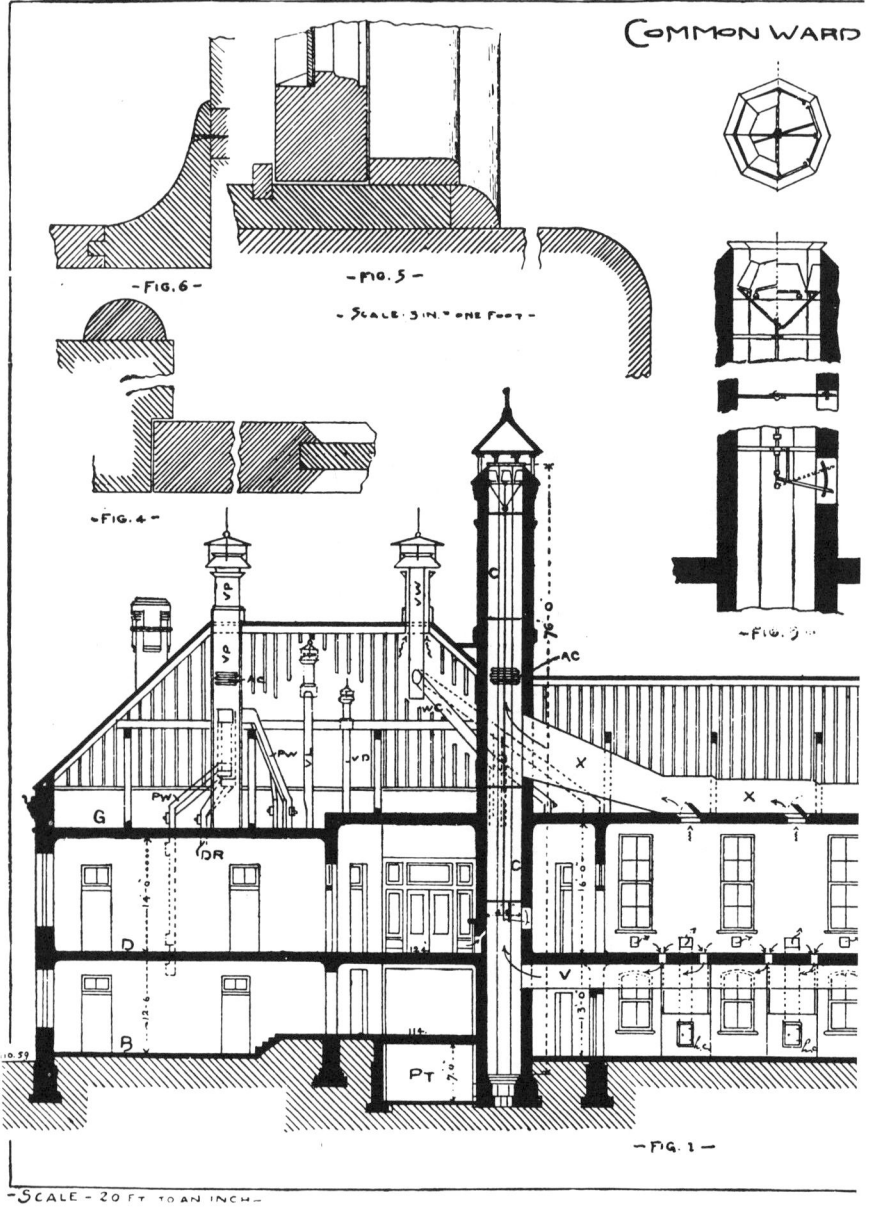

COMMON WARD

- FIG. 6 -

- FIG. 5 -

- SCALE · 3 IN · = ONE FOOT -

- FIG. 4 -

- FIG. 3 -

- FIG. 1 -

- SCALE - 20 FT TO AN INCH -

The Johns Hopkins Hospital — Common Ward. Longitudinal

B   Basement floor.
D   Main floor.
G   Attic floor.
PT   Pipe tunnel.

C   Central ventilating chimney.
AC   Accelerating steam coils.
X   Foul-air duct in attic.
V   Foul-air duct in basement.

FIG. 2.   Section of heating coil chamber.
FIG. 3.   Section and plans of ventilating chimney, showing damper.
FIG. 6.   Section of washboard.

FIG. 1.   Longitudinal section of ward.
VW   Ventilating shaft for water-
        closets.
WC   Vent pipe from water-closets.
DR   Vent pipe from dining room.

-Longitudinal Section North & South

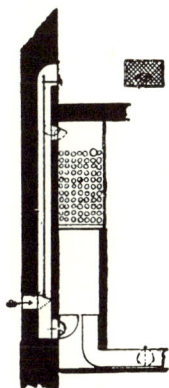

-FIG. 2-
- ⅛ scale -

GV

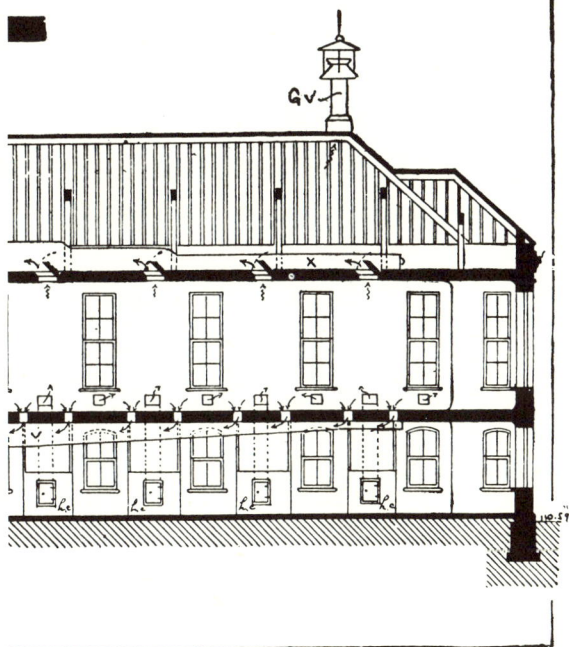

Section, North and South.

PW Vent pipe from private
       wards.
GV Attic ventilation.
V Lift vent.
    FIG. 4. Plan of doors, showing finish.
    FIG 5. Plan of windows, showing finish.

VL Vent to linen and patients'
       clothes rooms.
VP Vent shaft, private wards.
hc Heat coils.

Plate XIV

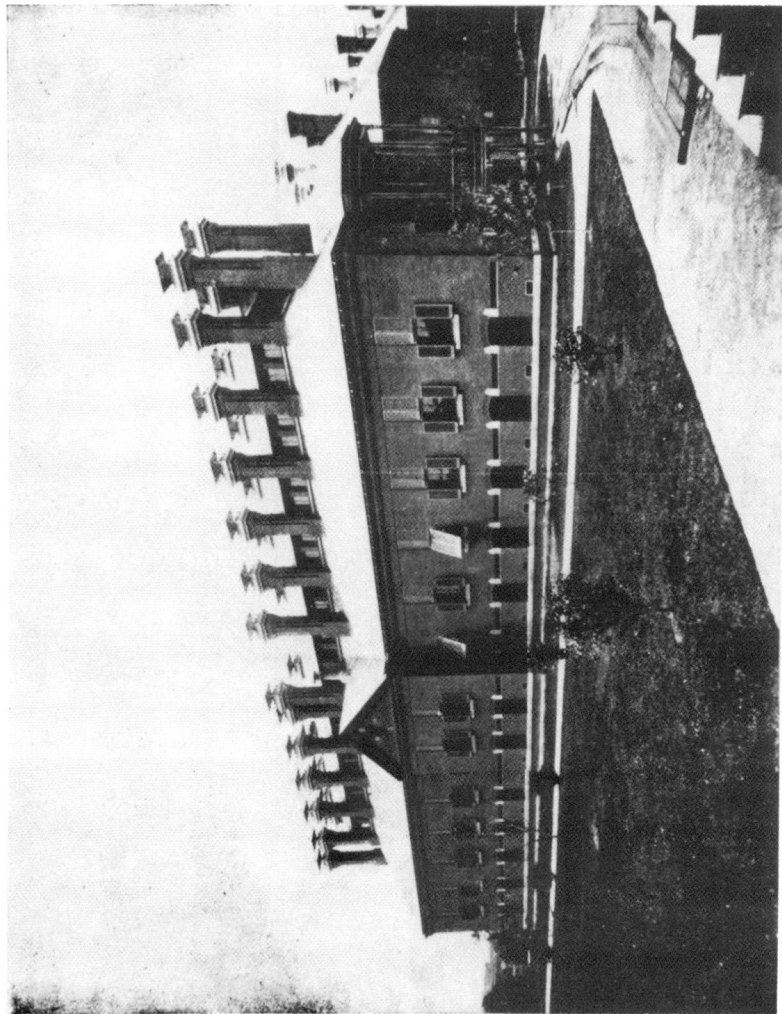

The Johns Hopkins Hospital — Isolating Ward

Plate XV.

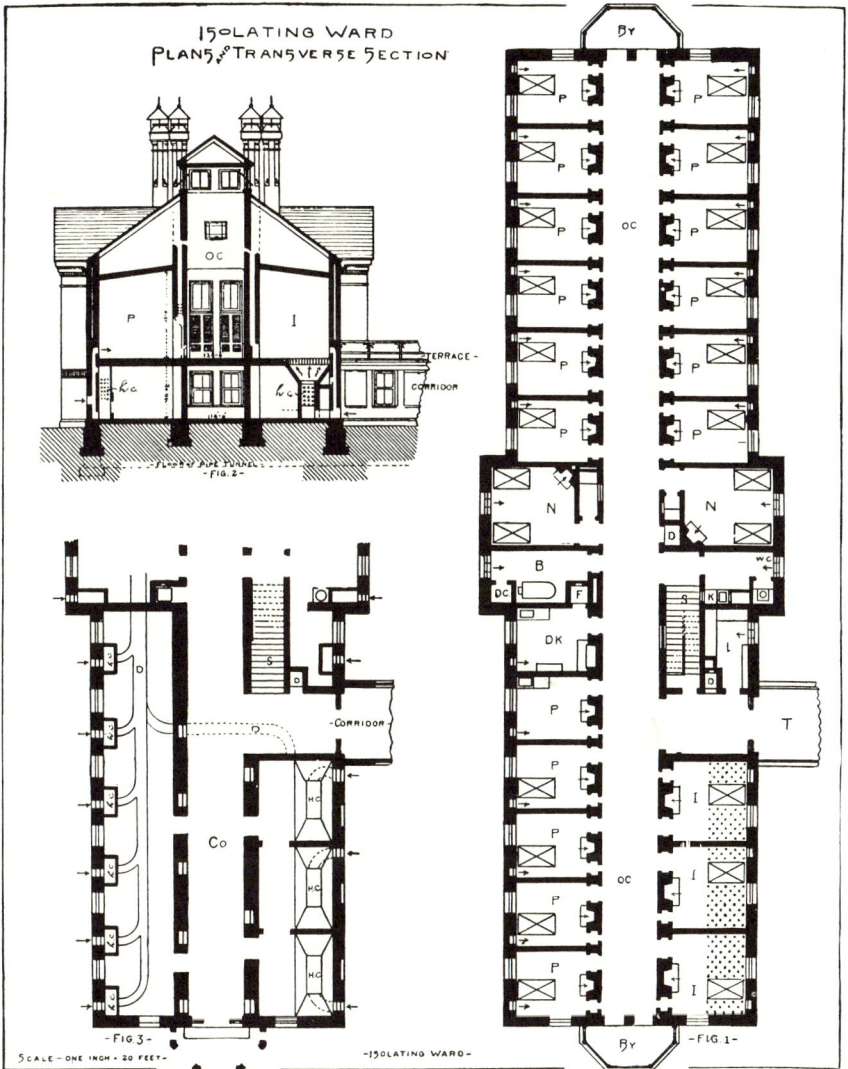

ISOLATING WARD
PLANS & TRANSVERSE SECTION

- FIG. 2 -

- FIG. 3 -

SCALE - ONE INCH = 20 FEET -

- ISOLATING WARD -

- FIG. 1 -

The Johns Hopkins Hospital — Isolating Ward.

PLANS AND TRANSVERSE SECTION.

FIG. 1. Plan of ward floor.

OC Open-air corridor.	DK Diet kitchen.	DC Dry closet.	By Balcony.
P Patients' rooms.	F Food lift.	WC Water-closet.	D Lift.
I Rooms with perforated floors.	B Bathroom.	T Open terrace over corridor.	S Stairs.
N Nurses' rooms.	L Linen closet.	K Sink.	

FIG. 2. Transverse section.

OC Open air corridor.   P Patients' rooms.   I Rooms with perforated floors.   he Heating coils.

FIG. 3. Plan of north end of basement.

Co Corridor.   S Stairs.   D Fan duct.   he Heating coils.

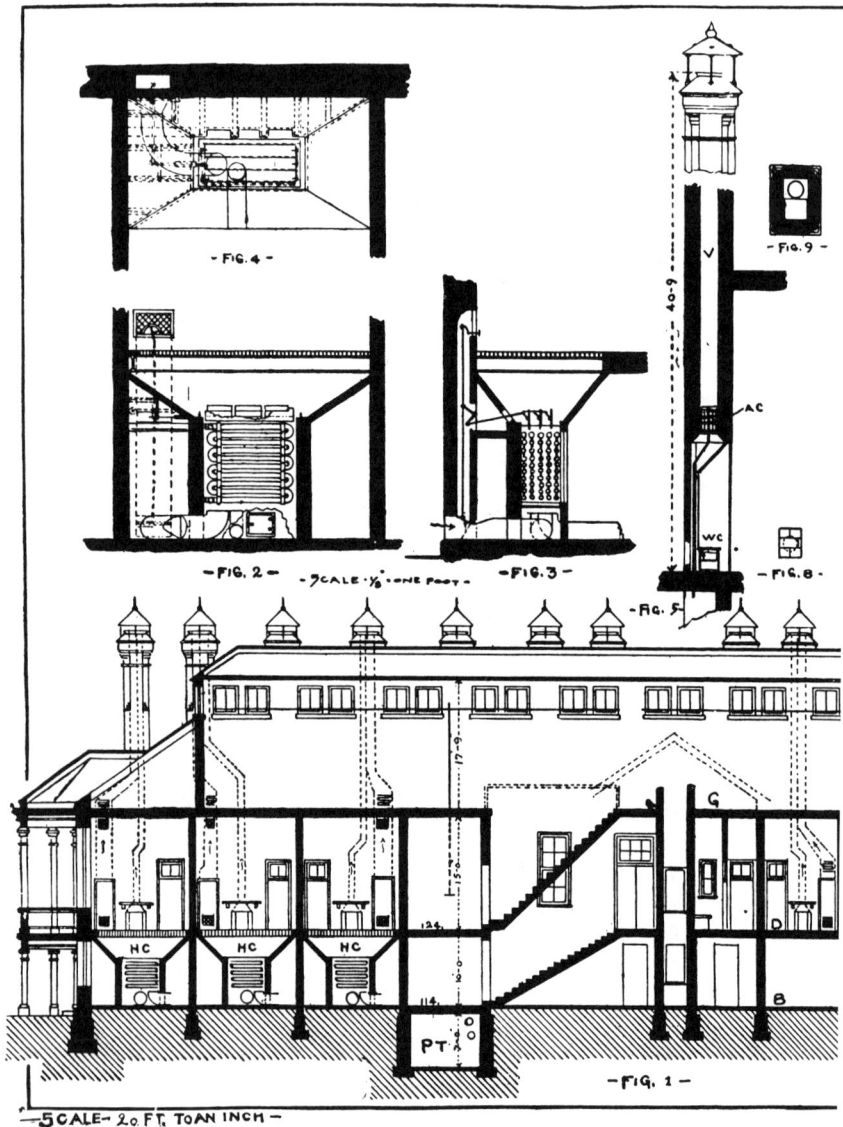

The Johns Hopkins Hospital — Isolating Ward. Longitudinal Section.

B Basement floor. D Main floor. G Attic floor. HC Heat chambers for

Fig. 1. Longitudinal section, north and south.

Fig. 2. Longitudinal section of heat chamber of rooms with perforated floors. Fig. 3. Transverse

Fig. 5. Transverse section of commode.

V Ventilating flue. AC Accelerating steam coil.

Fig. 6. Longitudinal section of commode and fireplace.

V Ventilating flue from commode. S Smoke flue from fireplace.

Fig. 7. Plan of fireplace and commode. Fig. 8. Commode stand.

ISOLATING WARD
LONGITUDINAL SECTION

- FIG. 7 -

- FIG. 6 -

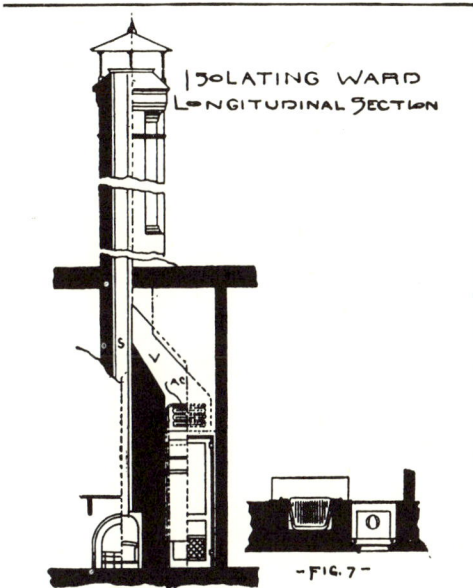

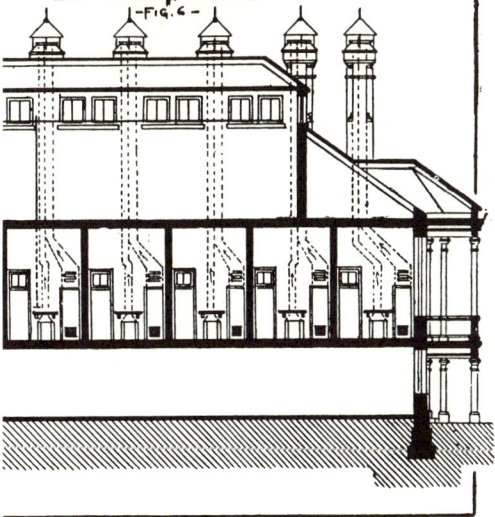

rooms with perforated floors.
section of heat chambers.

PT   Pipe tunnel.
FIG. 4.   Plan of heat chambers.

WC   Commode.

AC   Accelerating steam coil.
FIG. 9.   Plan of chimney, showing vent and smoke flue.

PLATE XVII.

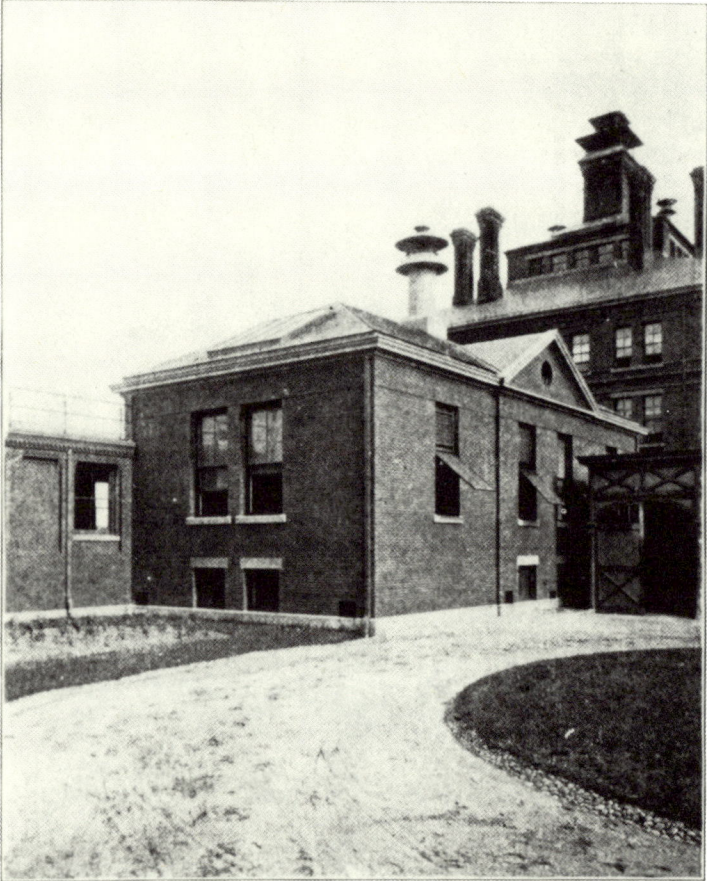

GYNAECOLOGICAL LABORATORY, JOHNS HOPKINS HOSPITAL.

PLATE XVIII.

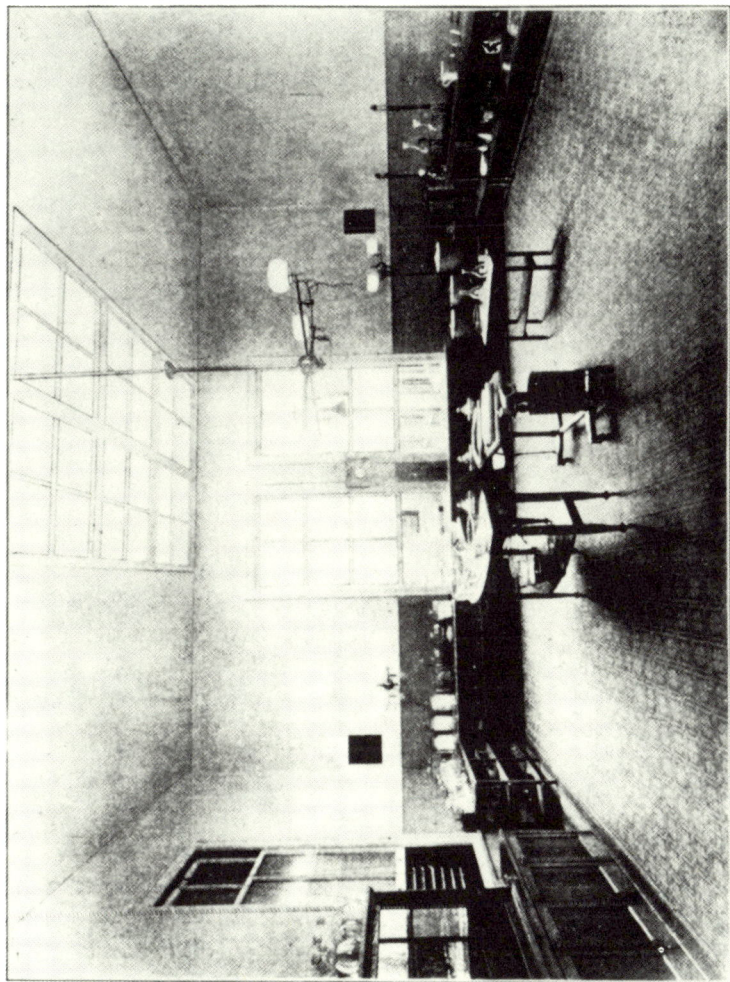

GYNAECOLOGICAL OPERATING ROOM, JOHNS HOPKINS HOSPITAL.

PLATE XIX.

GYNAECOLOGICAL OPERATING ROOM

FOR

THE JOHN'S HOPKINS HOSPITAL BALTIMORE, MD.

SCALE.

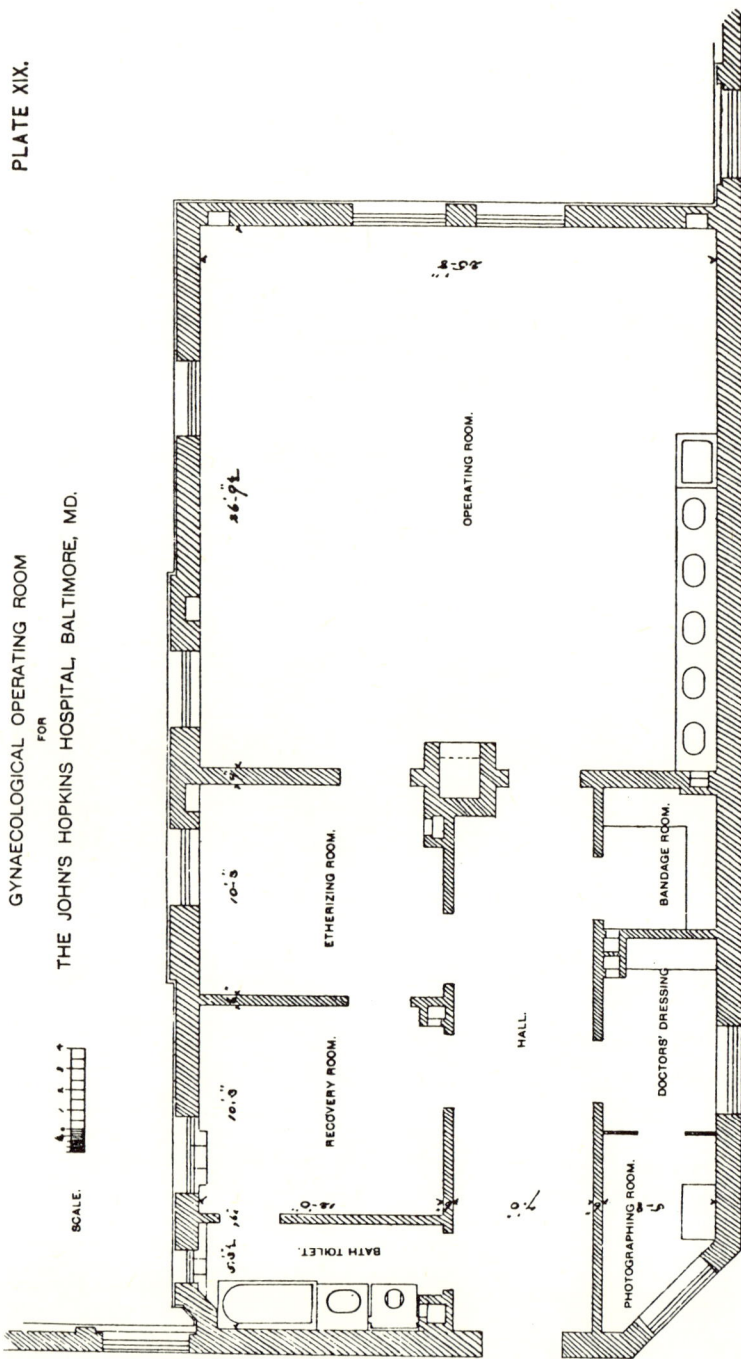

OPERATING ROOM.

ETHERIZING ROOM.

RECOVERY ROOM.

HALL.

BATH TOILET.

BANDAGE ROOM.

DOCTORS' DRESSING

PHOTOGRAPHING ROOM.

PLAN.

coal, the steam-engine, and disinfecting chamber. The disinfecting chamber is made of boiler-iron, and has a double shell, into the space between which steam is forced. Live steam can also be admitted into the interior chamber. It is elliptical in shape, the longer diameter being perpendicular. The chamber is 7 feet 2 inches long, 7 feet 5 inches high, and 5 feet 4 inches wide. There is also a large iron kettle of a capacity of 90 gallons, double jacketed, heated by steam, in which articles of clothing or bedding can be steamed or boiled, should occasion require. The main floor of the laundry contains rooms for the washing and drying of the bedding and clothing from patients, and similar rooms for the laundry work of the officers and employés. The vapor from the washing machines is carried off through copper pipes 4 inches in diameter into a ventilating shaft. The top of the laundry has a flat roof, and is provided with lines for hanging clothing in the fresh air and sunshine whenever the weather will permit, the clothing being conveyed by a steam lift to and from the roof.

III.

NURSING OF THE SICK.

SICK NURSING AND HEALTH NURSING.

By Florence Nightingale.

I. A new art and a new science has been created since and within
the last forty years. And with it a new profession—so they say ; we
say, *calling*. One would think this had been created or discovered
for some new want or local want. Not so. The want is nearly as old
as the world, nearly as large as the world, as pressing as life or death.
It is that of sickness. And the art is that of *nursing the sick*. Please
mark—nursing the *sick ; not* nursing sickness. We will call the art
nursing proper. This is generally practised by women under scientific heads—physicians and surgeons. This is one of the distinctions
between nursing proper and medicine, though a very famous and
successful physician did say, when asked how he treated pneumonia,
" I do not treat pneumonia, I treat the person who has pneumonia."
This is the reason why nursing proper can only be taught by the
patient's bedside, and in the sick room or ward. Neither can it be
taught by lectures or by books, though these are valuable accessories, if used as such; otherwise, what is in the book stays in the
book.

II. But since God did not mean mothers to be always accompanied
by doctors, there is a want older still and larger still. And a new
science has also been created to meet it, *but not* the accompanying
art, as far as households are concerned, families, schools, workshops;
though it is an art which concerns every family in the world, which
can only be taught from the home in the home.

This is the art of health, which every mother, girl, mistress,
teacher, child's nurse, every woman ought practically to learn. But
she is supposed to know it all by instinct, like a bird. Call it *health
nursing* or *general nursing*—what you please. Upon womankind
the national health, as far as the household goes, depends. *She*

must recognize the laws of life, the laws of health, as the nurse proper must recognize the laws of sickness, the causes of sickness, the symptoms of the disease, or the symptoms, it may be, not of the disease, but of the nursing, bad or good.

It is the want of the art of health, then, of the cultivation of health, which has only lately been discovered ; and great organizations have been made to meet it, and a whole literature created. We have medical officers of health ; immense sanitary works. We have not nurses, " missioners " of health-at-home.

How to bring these great medical officers to bear on the families, the homes and households, and habits of the people, rich as well as poor, has not been discovered, although family comes before Acts of Parliament. One would think " family " had no health to look after. And woman, the great mistress of family life, by whom everybody is born, has not been practically instructed at all. Everything has come before health. We are not to look after health, but after sickness. Well, we are to be convinced of *error* before we are convinced of *right;* the discovery of sin comes before the discovery of righteousness, we are told on the highest authority.

Though everybody *must* be born, there is probably no knowledge more neglected than this, nor more important for the great mass of women, viz., how to feed, wash and clothe the baby, and how to secure the utmost cleanliness for mother and infant. Midwives certainly neither practise nor teach it. And I have even been informed that many lady doctors consider that they have " nothing to do with the baby," and that they should " lose caste with the men doctors " if they attempted it. One would have thought that the ladies " lost caste " with themselves for *not* doing it, and that it was the very reason why we wished for the " lady doctors," for them to assume these cares which touch the very health of everybody from the beginning. But I have known the most admirable exceptions to this most cruel rule.

I know of no systematic teaching for the ordinary midwife or the ordinary mother, how to keep the baby in health, certainly the most important function to make a healthy nation. The human baby is not an invalid, but it is the most tender form of animal life. This is only one, but a supremely important instance of the want of health-nursing.

III. As the discovery of error comes before that of right, both in order and in fact, we will take first: (*a*) Sickness, nursing the sick ;

training needful; (*b*) Health, nursing the well at home; practical teaching needful. We will then refer (IV) to some dangers to which nurses are subject; (V) the benefit of combination; and (VI) our hopes for the future.

What is sickness? Sickness or disease is nature's way of getting rid of the effects of conditions which have interfered with health. It is nature's attempt to cure. We have to help her. Diseases are, practically speaking, adjectives, not noun substantives. What is health? Health is not only to be well, but to be able to use well every power we have. What is nursing? Both kinds of nursing are to put us in the best possible conditions for nature to restore or to preserve health—to prevent or to cure disease or injury. Upon nursing proper, under scientific heads, physicians or surgeons must depend partly, perhaps mainly, whether nature succeeds or fails in her attempts to cure by sickness. Nursing proper is therefore to help the patient suffering from disease to live—just as health nursing is to keep or put the constitution of the healthy child·or human being in such a state as to have no disease.

What is training? Training is to teach the nurse to help the patient to live. Nursing the sick is an art, and an art requiring an organized, practical and scientific training; for nursing is the skilled servant of medicine, surgery and hygiene. A good nurse of twenty years ago had not to do the twentieth part of what she is required by her physician or surgeon to do now; and so, after the year's training, she must be still training under instruction in her first and even second year's hospital service. The physician prescribes for supplying the vital force, but the nurse supplies it. Training is to teach the nurse how God makes health, and how He makes disease. Training is to teach a nurse to know her business, that is, to observe exactly in such stupendous issues as life and death, health and disease. Training has to make her, not servile, but loyal to medical orders and authorities. True loyalty to orders cannot be without the independent sense or energy of responsibility, which alone secures real trustworthiness. Training is to teach the nurse how to handle the agencies within our control which restore health and life, in strict, intelligent obedience to the physician's or surgeon's power and knowledge; how to keep the health mechanism prescribed to her in gear. Training must show her how the effects on life of nursing may be calculated with nice precision, such care or carelessness, such a sick rate, such a duration of case, such a death-rate.

What is discipline? Discipline is the essence of moral training. The best lady trainer of probationer nurses I know says, " It is education, instruction, training—all that, in fact, goes to the full development of our faculties, moral, physical, and spiritual, not only for this life, but looking on this life as the training ground for the future and higher life. Then discipline embraces order, method ; and as we gain some knowledge of the laws of nature ('God's laws'), we not only see order, method, a place for everything, each its own work, but we find no waste of material or force or space ; we find, too, no hurry, and we learn to have patience with our circumstances and ourselves ; and so, as we go on learning, we become more disciplined, more content to work where we are placed, more anxious to fill our appointed work than to see the result thereof. And so God, no doubt, gives us the required patience and steadfastness to continue in our ' blessed drudgery,' which is the discipline He sees best for most of us."

What makes a good training school for nurses? The most favorable conditions for the administration of the hospital are :

First. A good lay administration with a chief executive officer, a civilian (be he called treasurer or permanent chairman of committee), with power delegated to him by the committee, who gives his time. This is the main thing. With a consulting committee, meeting regularly, of business men, taking the opinions of the medical officers. The medical officers on the committee must be only consulting medical officers, not executive. If the latter, they have often to judge in their own case, which is fatal. Doctors are not necessarily administrators (the executive), any more than the executive are necessarily doctors. Vest the charge of financial matters and general supervision, and the whole administration of the hospital or infirmary, in the board or committee acting through the permanent chairman or other officer who is responsible to that board or committee.

Secondly. A strong body of medical officers, visiting and resident, and a medical school.

Thirdly. The government of hospitals, in the point of view of the real responsibility for the conduct and discipline of the nurses, being thrown upon the matron (superintendent of nurses), who is herself a trained nurse, and the real head of all the female staff of the hospital. Vest the whole responsibility for nursing, internal management, for discipline and training of nurses in this one female head of the nursing staff, whatever called. She should be herself responsible directly to the constituted hospital authorities, and all her nurses and servants should, in the performance of their duties, be responsible in matters of conduct and discipline, to her only. No good ever comes of the constituted authorities placing themselves in the office which they have sanctioned her occupying. No good ever comes of any one interfering between the head of the nursing establishment and her nurses. It is fatal to discipline. Without such discipline, the main object of the whole hospital organization, viz. to carry out effectively the orders of the physicians and surgeons with regard to the treatment of the patients, will not be attained.

Having then, as a basis, a well organized hospital, we require as further conditions:

(1) A special organization for the purpose of training, that is, where systematic technical training is given in the wards to the probationers; where it is the business of the ward "sisters" to train them, to keep records of their progress, to take "stock" of them; where the probationers are not set down in the wards to "pick up" as they can.

(2) A good "home" for the probationers in the hospital where they learn moral discipline—for technical training is only half the battle, perhaps less than half—where the probationers are steadily "mothered" by a "home" sister (class mistress).

(3) Staff of training school. (a) A trained matron over all, who is not only a housekeeper, but distinctly the head and superintendent of the nursing. (b) A "home" sister (assistant superintendent)—making the "home" a real home to the probationers, giving them classes, disciplining their life. (c) Ward sisters (head nurses of wards) who have been trained in the school—to a certain degree permanent, that is, not constantly changing. For they are the key to the whole situation, matron influencing through them nurses (day and night), probationers, ward-maids, patients. For, after all, the hospital is for the good of the patients, not for the good of the nurses. And the patients are not there to teach probationers upon. Rather, probationers had better not be there at all, unless they understand that they are there for the patients, and not for themselves.

There should be an *entente cordiale* between matron, assistant matrons, "home" sister, and whatever other female head there is, with frequent informal meetings, exchanging information, or there can be no unity in training.

Nursing proper means, besides giving the medicines and stimu-, lants prescribed, or the surgical appliances, the proper use of fresh air (ventilation), light, warmth, cleanliness, quiet, and the proper choosing and giving of diet, all at the least expense of vital power to the sick. And so health-at-home nursing means exactly the same proper use of the same natural elements, with as much life-giving power as possible to the healthy.

We have awakened, though still far from the mark, to the need of training or teaching for nursing proper. But while a large part of so-called civilization has been advancing in direct opposition to the laws of health, we uncivilized persons, the women, in whose hands rests the health of babies, household health, still persevere in think-ing health something that grows of itself (as Topsy said, "God made me so long, and I grow'd the rest myself"), while we don't take the same care of human health as we do of that of our plants, which, we know very well, perish in the rooms, dark and close, to which we too often confine human beings, especially in their sleeping rooms and workshops.

The life duration of babies is the most "delicate test" of health conditions. What is the proportion of the whole population of cities or country which dies before it is five years old? We have tons of printed knowledge on the subject of hygiene and sanitation. The causes of enormous child mortality are perfectly well known; they are chiefly, want of cleanliness, want of fresh air, careless dieting and clothing, want of whitewashing, dirty feather-beds and bedding—in one word, want of household care of health. The remedies are just as well known; but how much of this knowledge has been brought into the homes and households and habits of the people, poor or even rich? Infection, germs, and the like are now held responsible as carriers of disease. "Mystic rites," such as disinfection and anti-septics, take the place of sanitary measures and hygiene.

The true criterion of ventilation, for instance, is to step out of the bedroom or sick-room in the morning into the open air. If on returning to it you feel the least sensation of closeness, the ventila-tion has not been enough, and that room has been unfit for either sick or well to sleep in. Here is the natural test provided for the evil.

The laws of God—the laws of life—are always conditional, always inexorable. But neither mothers, nor school-mistresses, nor nurses of children are practically taught how to work within those laws, which God has assigned to the relations of our bodies with the world

in which He has put them. In other words, we do not study, we
do not practise the laws which make these bodies, into which He
has put our minds, healthy or unhealthy organs of those minds; we
do not practise how to give our children healthy existences.

It would be utterly unfair to lay all the fault upon us women,
none upon the buildings, drains, water-supply. There are millions
of cottages, more of town dwellings, even of the rich, where it is
utterly impossible to have fresh air.

As for the workshops, work-people should remember that health
is their only capital, and they should come to an understanding
among themselves not only to have the means, but to use the means
to secure pure air in their places of work, which is one of the prime
agents of health. This would be worth a "Trades Union," almost
worth a strike.

And the crowded National or Board School—in it how many
children's epidemics have their origin! And the great school dormitories! Scarlet fever and measles would be no more ascribed to
"current contagion," or to "something being much about this year,"
but to its right cause; nor would "plague and pestilence" be said to
be "in God's hands," when, so far as we know, He has put them
into our own.

The chief "epidemic" that reigns this year is "folly." You must
form public opinion. The generality of officials will only do what
you make them. *You*, the public, must make them do what you
want. But while public opinion, or the voice of the people, is somewhat awake to the building and drainage question, it is not at all
awake to teaching mothers and girls practical hygiene. Where,
then, is the remedy for this ignorance?

Health in the home can only be learnt from the home and in the
home. Some eminent medical officers, referring to ambulance
lectures, nursing lectures, the fashionable hygienic lectures of the
day, have expressed the opinion that we do no more than play with
our subject when we "sprinkle" lectures over the community, as
that kind of teaching is not instruction, and can never be education;
that as medicine and surgery can, like nursing, only be properly
taught and properly learnt in the sick-room and by the patient's
side, so sanitation can only be properly taught and properly learned
in the home and house. Some attempts have been made practically to realize this, to which subsequent reference will be made.

Wise men tell us that it is expecting too much to suppose that we shall do any real good by giving a course of lectures on selected subjects in medicine, anatomy, physiology, and other such cognate subjects, all "watered down" to suit the public palate, which is really the sort of thing one tries to do in that kind of lectures.

It is surely not enough to say, "The people are much interested in the lecture." The point is, Did they practise the lecture in their own homes afterwards? did they really apply themselves to household health and the means of improving it? Is anything better worth practising for mothers than the health of their families?

The work we are speaking of has nothing to do with nursing disease, but with maintaining health by removing the things which disturb it, which have been summed up in the population in general as "dirt, drink, diet, damp, draughts, drains."

But, in fact, the people do not believe in sanitation as affecting health, as preventing disease. They think it is a "fad" of the doctors and rich people. They believe in catching cold and in infection, catching complaints from each other, but not from foul earth, bad air, or impure water. May not some remedy be found for these evils by directing the attention of the public to the training of health-nurses, as has already been done with regard to the training of sick-nurses?

The scheme before referred to for health-at-home nursing has arisen in connection with the newly-constituted administration of counties in England, by which the local authority of the county (County Council) has been invested by Act of Parliament with extended sources of income applicable to the teaching of nursing and sanitary knowledge, in addition to the powers which they already possessed for sanitary inspection and the prevention of infectious diseases. This scheme is framed for rural districts, but the general principles are also applicable to urban populations, though, where great numbers are massed together, a fresh set of difficulties must be met, and different treatment be necessary.

The scheme contemplates the training of ladies, so-called health missioners, so as to qualify them to give instruction to village mothers in: (1) The sanitary condition of the person, clothes and bedding, and house. (2) The management of health of adults, women before and after confinement, infants and children. The teaching by the health missioners would be given by lectures in the villages, followed by personal instruction by way of conversation with the mothers in their own homes, and would be directed to: (1) The condition of the homes themselves in a sanitary point of view; (2) the essential principles of keeping the body in health, with reference to the skin, the circulation, and the digestion; and (3) instruction as to what to do in cases of emergency or accident before the doctor comes, and with reference to the management of infants and children.

In the addendum to this paper will be found a scheme for training health-at-home missioners, a syllabus of lectures given by the medical officer to the health missioners, and a syllabus of health lectures given by the health missioners to village mothers.

IV. Dangers. After only a generation of nursing arise the dangers: (1) Fashion on the one side, and its consequent want of earnestness. (2) Mere money-getting on the other. Woman does not live by wages alone. (3) Making nursing a profession, and not a calling.

What is it to feel a *calling* for anything? Is it not to do our work in it to satisfy the high idea of what is the right, the best, and not because we shall be found out if we don't do it? This is the "enthusiasm" which every one, from a shoemaker to a sculptor, must have in order to follow his "calling" properly. Now, the nurse has to do not with shoes or with marble, but with living human beings.

How, then, to keep up the high tone of a calling, to "make your calling and election sure"? By fostering that bond of sympathy (*esprit de corps*) which community of aims and of action in good work induces. A common nursing home in the hospital for hospital nurses and for probationer nurses; a common home for private nurses during intervals of engagements, whether attached to a hospital, or separate; a home for district nurses (wherever possible), where four or five can live together; all homes under loving, trained, moral, and religious, as well as technical superintendence, such as to keep up the tone of the inmates with constant supply of all material wants and constant sympathy. Man cannot live by bread alone, still less woman. Wages is not the only question, but high home-helps.

The want of these is more especially felt among private nurses. The development in recent years of trained private nursing, *i. e.* of nursing one sick or injured person at a time at home, is astonishing. But not less astonishing the want of knowledge of what training is, and, indeed, of what woman is. The danger is that the private nurse may become an irresponsible nomad. She has no home. There can be no *esprit de corps* if the "corps" is an indistinguishable mass of hundreds, perhaps thousands, of women unknown to her, except, perhaps, by a name in a register. All community of feeling and higher tone absents itself. And too often the only aim left is to force up wages. Absence of the nursing home is almost fatal to keeping up to the mark. Night nurses even in hospitals, and even district nurses (another branch of trained nursing of the sick poor without almsgiving, which has developed recently), and above all, private nurses, deteriorate if they have no *esprit de corps*, no common home under wise and loving supervision for intervals between engagements. What they can get in holidays, in comforts, in money, these good women say themselves, is an increasing danger to many. In private nursing the nurse is sometimes spoilt, sometimes "put upon," sometimes both.

In the last few years, private trained nursing, district trained nursing, have, as has been said, gained immeasurably in importance, and with it how to train, how to govern (in the sense of keeping up to the highest attainable in tone and character, as well as in technical training), must gain also immeasurably in importance, must constitute almost a new starting-point. Nursing may cease to be a calling in any better sense than millinery is. To have a life of freedom, with an interesting employment, for a few years—to do as little as you can and amuse yourself as much as you can, is possibly a danger pressing on.

(4). There is another danger, perhaps the greatest of all. It is also a danger which grows day by day. It is this: as literary education and colleges for women to teach literary work start and multiply and improve, some, even of the very best women, believe that everything can be taught by book and lecture, and tested by examination—that memory is the great step to excellence.

Can you teach horticulture or agriculture by books, *e. g.* describing the different manures, artificial and natural, and their purposes? The being able to know every clod, and adapt the appropriate manure to it, is the real thing. Could you teach painting by giving *e. g.* Fuseli's Lectures? Fuseli himself said, when asked how he mixed his colors, "With brains, sir"—that is, practice guided by brains. But you have another, a quite other sort of a thing to do with nursing; for you have to do with living bodies and living minds, and feelings of both body and mind.

It is said that you give examinations and certificates to plumbers, engineers, etc. But it is impossible to compare nurses with plumbers, or carpenters, or engineers, or even with gardeners. The main, the tremendous difference is that nurses have to do with these living bodies and no less living minds; for the life is not vegetable life, nor mere animal life, but it is human life—with living, that is, conscious forces, not electric or gravitation forces, but human forces. If you examine at all, you must examine all day long, current examination, current supervision, as to what the nurse is doing with this double, this damaged life entrusted to her.

The physician or surgeon gives his orders, generally his conditional orders, perhaps once or twice a day, perhaps not even that. The nurse has to carry them out, with intelligence of conditions, every minute of the twenty-four hours.

The nurse must have method, self-sacrifice, watchful activity, love of the work, devotion to duty (that is, the service of the good), the courage, the coolness of the soldier, the tenderness of the mother, the absence of the prig (that is, never thinking that she has attained perfection or that there is nothing better). She must have a three-fold interest in her work—an intellectual interest in the case, a (much higher) hearty interest in the patient, a technical (practical) interest in the patient's care and cure. She must not look upon patients as made for nurses, but upon nurses as made for patients.

There may also now—I only say *may*—with all this dependence on literary lore in nurse training, be a real danger of being satisfied with diagnosis, or with looking too much at the pathology of the case, without cultivating the resource or intelligence for the thousand and one means of mitigation, even where there is no cure.

And never, never let the nurse forget that she must look for the fault of the nursing as much as for the fault of the disease, in the symptoms of the patient.

(5). Forty or fifty years ago a hospital was looked upon as a box to hold patients in. The first question never was, will the hospital do them no harm? Enormous strides have had to be made to build and arrange hospitals so as to do the patients no sanitary or insanitary harm. Now there is danger of a hospital being looked upon as a box to train nurses in. Enormous strides must be made not to do them harm, to give them something that can really be called an " all-around " training.

Can it be possible that a testimonial or certificate of three years' so-called training or service from a hospital—*any* hospital with a certain number of beds—can be accepted as sufficient to certify a nurse for a place in a public register? As well might we not take a certificate from any garden of a certain number of acres, that plants are certified valuable if they have been three years in the garden.

(6). Another danger—that is, stereotyping, not progressing. "No system can endure that does not march." Are we walking to the future or to the past? Are we progressing or are we stereotyping? We remember that we have scarcely crossed the threshold of uncivilized civilization in nursing; there is still so much to do. Don't let us stereotype mediocrity.

To sum up the dangers:

i. On one side, fashion, and want of earnestness, not making it a life, but a mere interest consequent on this.

ii. On the other side, mere money-getting; yet man does not live by bread alone, still less woman.

iii. Making it a profession, and not a calling. Not making your "calling and election sure"; wanting, especially with private nurses, the community of feeling of a common nursing home,* pressing towards the "mark of your high calling," keeping up the moral tone.

iv. Above all, danger of making it book-learning and lectures—not an apprenticeship, a workshop practice.

v. Thinking that any hospital with a certain number of beds may be a box to train nurses in, regardless of the conditions essential to a sound hospital organization, especially the responsibility of the female head for the conduct and discipline of the nurses.

vi. Imminent danger of stereotyping instead of progressing. "No system can endure that does not march." Objects of registration not capable of being gained by a public register. Who is to guarantee our guarantors? Who is to make the inquiries? You might as well register mothers as nurses. A good nurse must be a good woman.

V. The health of the unity is the health of the community. Unless you have the health of the unity there is no community health.

Competition, or each man for himself, and the devil against us all, may be necessary, we are told, but it is the enemy of health. Combination is the antidote—combined interests, recreation, combination to secure the best air, the best food, and all that makes life useful,

---

* In the United States it is probable that private nurses are of higher education than in England. On the other hand, they have the doubtful dignity of graduates.

healthy and happy. There is no such thing as independence. As far as we are successful, our success lies in combination.

The Chicago Exhibition is a great combination from all parts of the world to prove the dependence of man on man.

What a lesson in combination the United States have taught to the whole world, and are teaching!

In all departments of life there is no apprenticeship except in the workshop. No theories, no book-learning can ever dispense with this or be useful for anything, except as a stepping-stone. And rather more, than for anything else, is this true for health. Book-learning is useful only to render the practical health of the health-workshop intelligent, so that every stroke of work done there should be felt to be an illustration of what has been learned elsewhere—a driving home, by an experience not to be forgotten, what has been gained by knowledge too easily forgotten.

Look for the ideal, but put it into the actual. "Not by vague exhortations, but by striving to turn beliefs into energies that would work in all the details" of health. The superstitions of centuries, the bad habits of generations, cannot be cured by lecture, book, or examination.

VI. May our hopes be that, as every year the technical qualifications constituting a skillful and observing nurse meet with more demands on her from the physicians and surgeons, progress may be made year by year, and that not only in technical things, but in the qualifications which constitute a good and trustworthy woman, without which she cannot be a good nurse. Examination papers, examinations, public registration, graduation, form little or no test of these qualifications. The least educated governess, who may not be a good nurse at all, may, and probably will, come off best in examination papers, while the best nurse may come off worst. May we hope that the nurse may understand more and more of the moral and material government of the world by the Supreme Moral Governor—higher, better, holier than her "own acts," that government which enwraps her round, and by which her own acts must be led, with which her own acts must agree in their due proportion, in order that this, the highest hope of all, may be hers; raising her above, *i. e.*, putting beneath her, dangers, fashions, mere money-getting, solitary money-getting, but availing herself of the high helps that may be given her by the sympathy and support of good "homes"; raising her above intrusive personal mortifications, pride in her own proficiency (she may have a just pride in her own doctors and training-school), sham, and clap-trap; raising her to the highest "grade" of all—to be a fellow-worker with the Supreme Good, with God! That she may be a "graduate" in this, how high! that she may be a "graduate" in words, not realities, how low!

We are only on the threshold of nursing.

In the future, which I shall not see, for I am old, may a better way be opened! May the methods by which every infant, every human being, will have the best chance of health—the methods by which every sick person will have the best chance of recovery, be learned and practised! Hospitals are only an intermediate stage of civilization, never intended, at all events, to take in the whole sick population.

May we hope that the day will come when every mother will become a health nurse, when every poor sick person will have the opportunity of a share in a district sick-nurse at home! But it will not be out of a register; the nurse will not be a stereotyped one. We find a trace of nursing here, another there; we find nothing like a nation, or race, or class who know how to provide the elementary conditions demanded for the recovery of their sick, whose mothers know how to bring up their infants for health.

May we hope that, when we are all dead and gone, leaders will arise who have been personally experienced in the hard, practical work, the difficulties and the joys of organizing nursing reforms, and who will lead far beyond anything we have done! May we hope that every nurse will be an atom in the hierarchy of the ministers of the Highest! But then she must be in her place in the hierarchy, not alone, not an atom in the indistinguishable mass of the thousands of nurses. High hopes, which will not be deceived!

Addendum.

District Nursing.

It is necessary to say a word about district nursing, with its dangers like private nursing, and its danger of almsgiving.

District nurses nurse the sick poor by visiting them in their own homes, not giving their whole time to one case, not residing in the house. They supply skilled nursing without almsgiving, which is incompatible with the duties of a skilled nurse, and which too often pauperizes the patient or the patient's family. They work under the doctor, who, however, rarely comes more than once a day, if so often. The district nurse must be clinical clerk, and keep notes for him, and dresser as well as nurse. She must, besides, nurse the room—often in towns, the family's only room—that is, put it in good nursing order as to ventilation, cleanliness, cheerfulness for recovery; teach the family, the neighbor, or the eldest child to keep it so; report sanitary defects to the proper authority. If the patient is the wage-earner, and the case is not essentially one for the hospital, she often thus prevents the whole family from being broken up, and saves them from the workhouse. If essentially a case for the hospital, she promotes its going there.

Though the district nurse gives nothing herself, she knows, or ought to know, all the local agencies by whom indispensable wants may be supplied, and who are able to exercise a proper discrimination as to the actual needs.

Having few or no hospital appliances at her disposal, she must be ingenious in improvising them.

She must, in fact, be even more accomplished and responsible than a nurse in a hospital.

She may take, perhaps, eight cases a day, but must never mix up infectious or midwifery nursing with others.

She must always have the supervision of a trained superior. She should, whenever possible, live in a nursing home with other district nurses, under a trained superintendent, not in a lodging by herself, providing for herself, and so wasting her powers and deteriorating. This is, of course, difficult to manage in the country, and especially in a sparsely populated country, *e. g.* like Scotland. Still approximations may be made; *e. g.*, periodical inspection may take the place of continuous supervision. She also should be a health missioner as well as a sick nurse.

Health Nurse Training.

The scheme for health-at-home training and teaching to health missioners may be summarized as follows:

1. A rural medical officer of health selected by the proper local authority for his fitness and experience.

2. Lectures to be given by the rural officer of health to ladies desirous of becoming health missioners, and others. This course, not less than fifteen lectures, to include elementary physiology, that is, an explanation of the organs of the body, how each affects the

health of the body, and how each can be kept in order,—a summary in fact, of the science of hygiene, framed to give the scientific basis on which popular familiar village teaching is to be founded.

3. Further instruction by the lecturer to those who wish to qualify themselves as health missioners, both by oral instruction and papers.

4. Instruction by the medical officer to those who attend the classes, by taking them into the villages to visit the cottages, and showing them what to observe and how to visit.

5. Selection by the medical officer of a certain number of candidates as qualified to be examined for health missioners. These qualifications are—good character, good health, personal fitness for teaching, and tact in making herself acceptable to the village mothers.

6. Examination of the candidates by an independent examiner appointed by the local authority ; one who is familiar with the conditions of rural and village life, who then, in conjunction with the medical officer, recommends the candidates who have satisfied them both to the local authority, and the latter appoints as many as are required.

7. The health missioners are appointed to districts consisting each of a number of small villages grouped with a larger one, or the market town. Over these there is a district committee, which is represented on the local authority. Each village has a local committee, represented on the district committee. The local committee makes arrangements for the lectures by the health missioner, and makes the necessary arrangements for receiving her.

8. The health missioner works under the supervision of the medical officer of health, who as often as possible introduces her to the village in the first instance, and he makes it his business to inquire into the practical results of her work.

9. The lectures are delivered in simple, homely language. The lecturer aims at making friends with the women, and by afterwards visiting them at their own homes, endeavors practically to exemplify in their houses the teaching of the lectures.

10. After a health missioner has become settled in a district she will then be able to receive a probationer, who, while attending the medical officer's lectures and classes, will find time to accompany the health missioner in her round of visiting.

Syllabus of Lectures to Health Missioners.

I. Sanitary condition of the (1) Person ; (2) Clothes and Bedding ; (3) House.

II. Management of Health of (1) Adults ; (2) Women before and after Confinements ; (3) Infants and Children.

I. Sanitary condition of :

(1) *Person.* Care of the whole body ; cleanliness of the skin ; hair and hairbrushes ; teeth and tooth-brushes ; simplest appliances sufficient, with knowledge ; large vessels and much water not indispensable for daily cleansing (though in some cases a bath and much scrubbing with soap are absolutely necessary) ; advantages of friction of the skin ; the body the main source of defilement of the air, and the most essential thing to keep clean.

(2) *Clothes and bedding.* Clothes to be warm, light, and loose, no pressure anywhere ; danger of wearing dirty clothes next the skin ; re-absorption of poison cast out by the body ; danger of wearing the same underclothing night and day ; importance of airing clothes and bedding ; hanging out non-washing clothes in sunshine ; infection stored up in old clothes and bedding ; danger of using damp sheets and damp underlinen ; bed reform ; feather beds should be picked, and the tick washed every year.

(3) *House.* How to choose a healthy dwelling—aspect, situation, not to be in a hole ; fogs in valleys ; good foundations ; value of sunshine and wind; look after water and air and all that poisons them ; you must swallow the air in your house ; fresh air will do, even with poor food (well cooked), but the best food will not make up for the absence of fresh air. What sanitary authorities to appeal to in the country about drains, water, sewage, privies, etc., plumbing, traps, what shows a trap to be unsafe ; best disinfectants—cleanliness, clean hands, fresh air.

Ventilation in bedrooms ; poisonous air in close bedrooms at night ; bad smells as danger signals ; danger of overcrowding sleeping rooms ; danger of dust, dirt and damp ; how to make the beds ; how to clean the floors, walls, bedroom crockery, kitchen pots and pans ; foul floors a source of danger; bricks porous ; interstices between boards may become filled with decaying matter ; dangerous to sluice with much water, wipe with a damp cloth, and rub with a dry one ; clean wall papers, not put up over old dirty ones ; merits of whitewash ; effect of direct sunlight ; danger of uninhabited rooms ; the genteel parlor, chilling to the bone, kept for company ; danger of dirty milk pans and jugs, kitchen tables, chopping blocks, etc. ; water, hard and soft—see that it is water, not water plus sewage ; that milk is milk—not milk plus water, plus sewage.

II. Management of Health of :

(1) *Adults.* Diet ; influence of sex, age, climate, occupation, variety ; animal food, vegetable food ; milk, butter, cheese, eggs, etc. ; effects of insufficient food, of unwholesome food, food insufficiently cooked ; danger of diseased meat, of decaying fish, meat, fruit, and of unripe fruit and vegetables ; spread of disease through milk ; chills, constipation, diarrhœa, indigestion, ruptures, rheumatism, gathered fingers, etc,

(2) *Women before and after Confinements.* Diet, fresh air, cheerfulness; danger of blood-poisoning by lying-in on dirty feather beds.

(3) *Infants and Children.* Nursing, weaning, hand-feeding; regular intervals between feeding; flatulence, thrush, convulsions, bronchitis, croup; simple hints to mothers about healthy conditions for children; cleanliness; food; what to give to prevent constipation or diarrhœa; danger of giving children alcohol or narcotics; danger of a heavy head covering to a child while bones of skull still open; deadliness of soothing syrups; how to recognize the symptoms of coming illness in body and mind—fever, hip disease, curvature of the spine, indigestion, sleeplessness, drowsiness, headache, peevishness, etc. *What to do till the Doctor comes.*—If clothes catch fire, or for burns, scalds, bites, cuts, stings, injuries to the head; swallowing fruit-stones, pennies, pins, etc. *After the Doctor has left.*—How to take care of convalescents; how to feed; danger of chills; overwork at school, etc.

Syllabus of Health Lectures given by the Health Missioners to Village Mothers.

I. Our Homes.
   1. The Bedroom.
   2. The Kitchen and Parlor.
   3. The Back Yard and Garden.

II. Ourselves.
   4. The skin, and how to keep the body clean—washing.
   5. The circulation, and how to keep the body warm—clothes.
   6. The digestion, and how to nourish the body—food.

III. Extra Lectures.
   7. What to do till the doctor comes, and after the doctor has left.
   8. Management of Infants and Children.

Lecture I.—The Bedroom.

(a). *Introductory.*—Busy life of cottage mothers; why they should come to classes; preventable illnesses; the mothers should ask questions, and help the lecturers by relating their own experiences; proposed plan of the lecturers.

(b). *Bedroom.*—What we want to get into a bedroom; what we want to get out of a bedroom; sunshine—its effect on health; fresh air—difference between clean air and foul air; an unaired bedroom is a box of bad air; ventilation near the ceiling; fireplace—no chimney boards.

(c). *Furniture of Bedroom.*—The bed and bedding; walls; carpets; airing of room during the day; cleansing of bedroom crockery; danger of unemptied slops; how to get rid of dust—washing of floors; vermin; damp; lumber; fresh air and sunshine in the bedroom by day promote sleep by night.

Lecture II.—The Kitchen and Parlor.

Kitchen.—Danger from refuse of food; grease in all the rough parts of kitchen table and chopping block—crumbs and scraps in interstices of floor—

remains of sour milk in saucepans, jugs ; all refuse poisons the air, spoils
fresh food, and attracts vermin, rats, beetles, etc.; bricks porous; dangerous
to sluice with too much water; water for cooking, whence obtained—often
water plus sewage ; milk easily injured—often milk plus water plus sewage ;
how to clean kitchen table, crockery, pots and pans ; how to keep milk cool ;
danger of dirty sink.

Parlor.—Danger of uninhabited rooms without sunlight and fresh air ; genteel parlor chilling to the bone ; clean papers not to be put over dirty ones ;
tea-leaves for sweeping carpets.

Lecture III.—The Back Yard and Garden.

Back Yard.—Where are slops emptied? slops to be poured slowly down a
drain, not hastily thrown down to make a pool around the drain ; gratings of
drain to be kept clean, and passage free ; soil around the house kept pure,
that pure air may come in at the window ; danger of throwing bedroom slops
out of window ; no puddles allowed to stand around walls ; privy refuse to be
got into the soil as soon as possible ; danger of cesspools ; well and pump ;
wells are upright drains, so soil around them should be pure ; bad smells
danger-signals ; pigsties, moss-litter to absorb liquid manure cheap and profit-
able ; danger from pools of liquid manure making the whole soil foul.

Lecture IV.—The Skin, and how to keep the Body clean.

The Skin.—Simple account of functions of skin : as a covering to the body ;
beauty dependent on healthy state of skin ; use of the skin as throwing out
waste matter ; dangers of a choked skin ; how and when to wash ; care of
whole body ; teeth—sad suffering by their neglect ; hair and hair-brushes ;
large vessels and much water not indispensable for daily cleansing ; advantages of a bath ; friction of the skin ; not babies only, but men and women,
require daily washing ; the body the source of defilement of the air.

Lecture V.—The Circulation, and how to keep the Body warm.

Clothes.—Simple account of how the heart and lungs act ; clothes to be warm
and loose, no pressure ; test for tight-lacing if measurement round the waist is
more with the clothes off than when stays are worn ; danger of dirty clothes
next the skin—re-absorption of poison ; danger of wearing the same clothes
day and night ; best materials for clothing ; why flannel is so valuable ; danger of sitting in wet clothes and boots ; too little air causes more chills than
too much ; the body not easily chilled when warm and well clothed.

Lecture VI.—The Digestion, and how to nourish the Body.

Food.—Simple account of how food is digested and turned into blood—
worst food (well cooked) and fresh air better than best food without fresh air ;
diet, not medicine, ensures health ; uses of animal and of vegetable food ; danger of all ill-cooked and half-cooked food ; nourishing value of vegetables and
whole-meal bread ; danger of too little food and too much at the wrong times ;
dangers of uncooked meat, especially pork, diseased meat, decaying fish,
unripe and overripe fruit, and stewed tea ; vital importance of cooked fruit

for children, stewed apples and pears, damsons, blackberries ; value of milk as food ; influence of diet upon constipation, diarrhœa, indigestion, convulsions in children ; small changes of diet promote appetite and health.

Lecture VII.— What to do till the Doctor comes, and after the Doctor has left.

Small Treatment.—Grave danger of being one's own doctor, of taking quack medicines, or a medicine which has cured some one else in quite a different case ; liquid food only to be given till the doctor comes ; danger-signals of illness, and how to recognize them, hourly dangers of ruptures if not completely supported by trusses ; what to do if clothes catch fire ; and for burns, scalds, bites, cuts, stings, injuries to the head and to the eye, swallowing fruit-stones, pins; etc.; simple rules to avoid infection. *After the Doctor has left.* How to take care of convalescents ; how to feed ; when to keep rooms dark, and when to admit plenty of light ; danger of chills.

Lecture VIII.—Management of Infants and Children.

Infants and Children.—Nursing, weaning, hand-feeding, regular intervals between feeding ; flatulence, thrush, convulsions, bronchitis, croup ; simple hints to mothers about healthy conditions for children ; baths ; diet; how to prevent constipation and diarrhœa ; what to do in sudden attacks of convulsions and croup ; deadly danger of giving soothing syrups or alcohol ; headache often caused by bad eyesight ; symptoms of overwork at school—headache, worry, talking in the sleep; danger to babies, and to little children of any violence, jerks, and sudden movements, loud voices, slaps, box on the ear ; good effects upon the health of gentleness, firmness, and cheerfulness ; no child can be well who is not bright and merry, and brought up in fresh air and sunshine, surrounded by love—the sunshine of the soul.

ON NURSING.

By the Hon. Mrs. Stuart Wortley.

To give a full statement of the entire range of this subject would far exceed the possibilities of such a paper as the present one ; but an attempt is here made to give a short survey of the rise and actual condition of Nursing as a profession as it exists in England.

It seems needless here to recapitulate what the world owes to the great pioneer of nursing, Miss Nightingale, who, long before the Crimean War gave her a European reputation, left the joys of home and the pleasures of the best society, which she was in a position to command and adorn, to undertake the care of a Home for Diseased Gentlewomen. It was her great spiritual and moral force that convinced the public that to leave helpless human beings in the hour of suffering to ignorant, untrained supervision was a disgrace to the intelligence of the nineteenth century. Simultaneously, the inimitable works of Dickens presented the reverse of the picture; and, not without controversy and some misgiving in headquarters, Mr. Sidney Herbert succeeded in despatching, for the first time in the world's history, a woman to take a definite place in the operations of an army in the field. How she sped is now a matter of universal knowledge, and nobly have her pupils and sisters in the military service followed her footsteps. On the return of Miss Nightingale after the war, the gratitude of the English nation took expression in a large contribution placed at her disposal. This was devoted by her to the foundation of the Nightingale Training Institution for Nurses, in St. Thomas's Hospital, which, by introducing the best kind of nursing into hospitals, established a right standard of practice, and led to the foundation of schools of nursing in connection with almost all the large hospitals throughout the kingdom.

The military and naval services have been the great nurseries and pioneers of good nursing, and in a return kindly supplied to me by the War Office I find a list of no less than thirty-four nurses, all decorated for good service, who have been employed in the recent wars in India, Egypt, Burmah, and elsewhere. Their distinction can only be equaled by their modesty, and I have not found it easy to obtain any details of the work done. But something is known of what Miss Florence Lees, now Mrs. Dacre Craven, underwent in 1870 in the Franco-German War, when the Empress Frederick and Princess Alice sent her to the front, and she spent eight weeks in the hospital for typhus cases before Metz. There, in the midst of the raging infection, she nursed a building containing eighty beds, which, on her arrival, was destitute of every special accommodation for patients. She found only the wards, the beds, and the same rough food supplied as would be served out to the same men in the field if in health. There were absolutely no cups or vessels for use of any description, but one pail. She had two other nurses with her, and they subsequently had to be repeatedly relieved; but this heroic woman went on with her life in her hand for the whole eight weeks, more than once in additional danger from the poor fellows when in violent delirium, who could only be restrained by the assistance of convalescent inmates, trained by her into hospital orderlies.

Before Miss Nightingale's school had quite developed, an import-

ant move forward was made by religious sisterhoods; and for a considerable time the best nursing work then to be had emanated from
the St. John's House, Norfolk street, Strand, followed closely by the
All Saints' Sisterhood in Margaret street, by the East Grinstead
Sisters, and the Sisters of St. Peter. I might append here a long
list of sisterhoods, most of which include some nursing of the poor
among the different objects of their work. Their devoted spirit has
been invaluable in teaching the world how noble a thing good
nursing is. Though all did not attain to the highest standard of
professional training, the All Saints' and St. John's Sisterhoods are
still among the heads of the profession and in the first rank of those
who give their services to the poor. These last-named bodies provided nurses for hospitals (King's College and Charing Cross), and
also supplied nurses to private cases that could pay for them. But
the first attempt to supply nurses to the poor was in Liverpool in
1859, where a beginning was made with one single nurse, whose
energy and success rapidly led to the establishment of a nursing
home, and a place for training nurses to visit the sick poor in their
own homes, in Liverpool.

During the great cholera epidemic of 1866 in London much
admirable work was done by the sisters, and the highest testimony to their efficiency and devotion was given by Bishop (afterwards Archbishop) Tait, and by Mrs. Gladstone, who daily visited
the London Hospital during the worst days of that awful scourge.

It was that same visitation which led to the formation of the East
London Nursing Society, the first of the London societies organized
for the sole benefit of the poor. That society places a trained nurse
in each parish, obtains her lodging from the local funds, and supplies
fully trained nursing superintendence from matrons living in the
immediate neighborhood. There are twenty-nine nurses now established, one residing in each parish, under four matrons; and they
have an efficient plan for the supply of necessary diet and comforts
for the patients. The value of these services in the deep poverty of
the East End is incalculable.

Developments followed quickly in the form of a really grand
scheme for training and giving the highest form of nursing to the
poor, initiated by the Duke of Westminster, who, in 1870, founded
the Metropolitan and National Nursing Association, with a central
training-home in Bloomsbury Square. It is composed almost
entirely of ladies, who are trained by Mrs. Dacre Craven, whose

exploits have already been referred to. This institution is now divided into a great number of branches, and the central training-home in Bloomsbury continues to stand out as the highest for completeness and efficiency. But among the efforts to comfort poor people few exceed in value the Association for Providing Trained Nurses to Workhouses, which followed closely after the kindred institutions for the poor in their own homes.

The establishment of schools for trained nurses in almost every large hospital is now an accomplished fact. The nurses to private cases who receive full payment greatly benefit the institutions to which they belong; among the earliest was the Westminster training-school, founded by the late Lady Augusta Stanley. Our space makes a mention of all impossible, but they are usually all on the same system, viz. to train nurses for private cases, reserving a few for the poor.

The movement recently instituted by H. R. H. the Princess Christian, to consolidate the general nursing profession by giving a certificate under royal charter to all who have received three years' full training, is expected to assist the value of their work by consolidating their social status. But Her Majesty Queen Victoria stands pre-eminent among the supporters of this great duty of providing nurses for the sick poor, and by her action has made this movement a national one. By her appointment, the Duke of Westminster, Sir Rutherford Alcock and Sir James Paget were made trustees, and from information obtained by them it appears that beside the work done in London and Liverpool, there are district nursing organizations in Derby, Bristol, Brighton, Manchester, Worcester, Leeds, Oxford, Newcastle, Maidstone, Edinburgh, Glasgow, Belfast, Dublin, and many other towns. These nursing organizations are exclusive of the institutions for providing nurses to the rich, and are far more effectual for the poor than those on the mixed system; though it cannot be denied that the latter are very beneficial. In January, 1888, the trustees recommended that the bulk of the Jubilee Fund, amounting to £70,000, should be applied for the training of nurses for the poor. Her Majesty finally approved a scheme for uniting this fund with the ancient charity of St. Katherine's Hospital, founded in 1148 by Queen Matilda, wife of King Stephen, chartered in 1273 by Queen Eleanor, widow of Henry III, when the duty of visitation of the sick poor was expressly imposed. As soon as the necessary arrangements for the adjustment of its revenues are completed, this ancient foundation will have increased funds at its disposal. The committee made it its first duty to develop training-schools in London, Edinburgh, and Dublin, and in Edinburgh the energy of the late Lady Rosebery rapidly formed a center, extending to Glasgow, Aberdeen and other important places. In Dublin a commencement has been made, and throughout England associations have come forward to accept the conditions of affiliation. A noble gift from Mr. Tate has greatly assisted the work. But although the positions occupied by the above foundations are the first in importance, both by intrinsic merit and official sanction, full justice cannot be done to the interest felt in the subject of nursing, especially on behalf of the poor in Great Britain, without mentioning some very leading institutions which have made this work an integral portion of their plan. Among these, the institution founded by the late Mrs. Ranyard to send "Bible women" to the poor is doing good nursing work, and has nearly one hundred nurses employed in various poor parishes in London. The nursing branch is under the direction of Mrs. Selfe-Leonard, and the institution gives its nurses three months' hospital training. These nurses are selected with extreme care, and though they could not be certified as fully trained nurses, have done very valuable work.

The institution known as the Mildmay Deaconesses also has a branch for nurses and employs them in the homes of the poor. The Sisters of St. John the Divine, formerly a part of the Norfolk street institution, have now established themselves in Poplar, and give efficient help to the poor.

It is difficult to decide whether maternity work should be classed as nursing, and therefore included among the undertakings described in this paper, or classed among the strictly medical charities. If it is regarded as women's work for women, we may mark its progress with approbation. A very decided effort is now being made to provide well-trained midwives for the poor, and though inadequate to the wants of the ever-growing population of London, there is a nucleus of excellent work in the East End Mothers' Home, which trains midwives; and a very remarkable effort to promote good work of this kind should be noticed in the Maternity Hospital at Clapham, in which there is a school for midwives, and the whole machinery of the medical and nursing staff is entirely composed of women.

The institutions here indicated mostly concern London only, or
have their centers there ; but there is a very active general movement
to supply nurses throughout the country districts in England, which
is taking form in various ways.

The Cottage Nursing Association, of which the center is in Gloucestershire, gives the best nursing by fully trained nurses and midwives and deserves the highest praise. The same or a kindred plan,
also supplying highly trained nurses, is established at West Malling,
in Kent. All the institutions named previously as having centers in
towns, of course, also supply fully trained nurses. A very large
number of single nurses, with different degrees of training, is
employed by ladies ; one or perhaps two nurses being placed in a
parish, though in some cases they come from the organization provided for cottage hospitals. But in the remote country districts
those who would wish thus to assist poor people find themselves
much hindered by the unwillingness of the peasant poor to admit
very highly trained nurses into their houses. Their remoteness
makes daily visits of a single hour or more (without residence)
unattainable ; and they will not accept the services of any nursing
attendant who does not undertake to assist, or even to fulfil, all the
necessary household duties, and supply whatever is wanted for the
general comfort of the family as well as care of the patient. Now it
does seem an injustice to compel fully trained nurses, who have
sacrificed much time and money to the attainment of the delicacy of
touch needed for the highest surgical work, to undergo the risk of
spoiling their hands by housework. And it is very unusual that the
severest surgical cases are ever attended at home. These (mostly
accidents) are usually removed at once to the great hospitals in the
nearest towns. I am far from intending to imply that fully trained
nurses are not always the most valuable ; but the difficulty above
indicated is a very real one, and can only be met by supplying a
nurse of less ambitious quality. Another difficulty arises from the
fact that a fully trained nurse placed alone in a remote country parish
often finds that there is not work enough to employ her time.
These impediments have been best overcome by the Ockley system,
suggested by Miss Broadwood, a lady residing near Horsham, in
Surrey. The plan here is to employ well selected women from the
district, and give them three or four months' training at the hospital
at Plaistow. They are distributed as asked for by the different
parishes belonging to groups arranged in various neighborhoods.

By a very excellent adoption of the "benefit" principle, funds for these nurses are provided by a settled contribution from each parish calculated in proportion to the amount of its population. It is found that a subscription at the rate of twenty-five or twenty-seven shillings for every hundred persons annually will, if there is a large group of parishes, supply the wages of the nurses. The patients pay a weekly fee on a graduated scale according to their social position, viz. two shillings weekly for the poor of the neighborhood, five shillings for artisans and small farmers, seven and sixpence for substantial tradesmen, and one pound for the gentry and wealthy inhabitants. An annual subscription is expected, of the same amount as their weekly fee. Evidently the plan suited the wishes of the poor, for it was rapidly adopted in twenty parishes round Horsham, and, with various modifications, is being established in many other places, such as Battle, Rye, the neighborhood of Grantham, etc. These nurses, though not fully trained, have learned the primitive principles of sanitation and the necessary obedience to doctors; the medical men who have tried them (some very eminent ones) value them highly, and there can be no doubt that the future establishment of a complete network of fully-trained nursing is likely to be greatly forwarded by the growth of this humble but very useful beginning. As there has been some controversy on the point, it is right to add here that no want of devotion or sacrifice has been perceived on the part of the highly trained nurses who in many village epidemics have occasionally been called in and done really heroic service. What is here stated is the result of experience, and those who have followed the work of these simpler nurses are able to testify to their extreme value as an educational influence on the poor whom they serve, and who at present would not admit any others to live in their cottages.

It is impossible to close without lamenting the many omissions which, from lack of time and space, are no doubt perceptible in this brief survey. Nothing has been said of the many excellent colonial centers, and the faithful nursing-missionary work being done in the wild places of the earth by devoted women. Miss Marsden was the last before the public, a name of which every Englishwoman may be proud, for her perilous and heroic journey to succor the lepers in Eastern Siberia, an undertaking which is likely to prove of great benefit.

WORK DONE BY RELIGIOUS COMMUNITIES DEVOTED TO THE RELIEF OF THE SICK.

By Cardinal Gibbons, of Baltimore.

Among the numerous objects of commiseration that indigence and human infirmities daily place before us, none appeals so forcibly to philanthropy and heaven-inspired charity as the stricken victim of disease, whatever be his position in the social world. Hence, since the dawn of Christianity we find institutions for the relief of the afflicted.

Paganism knew nothing of compassion and charity. Ancient Rome, with all her boasted splendor, could find no room amid her palaces for the erection of asylums for the sick and maimed. But scarcely had the pure light of the Gospel beamed on this benighted "mistress of the world" when we find the first Christians devoting themselves to the relief of the plague-stricken and distressed. One of the unfailing attributes of religion seems to be the power of accomplishing great results silently and unostentatiously, and a spirit of self-sacrifice is the inheritance of her favored children; the fairest chapters in the history of our country warrant this assertion.

The Catholic Church, ever true to the teachings of her divine Founder, and the faithful imitator of His example, has never ceased to raise up devoted children whose lives are spent at the bedside of the sick and dying. Witness her religious communities, those thousands of men and women who, severing the strongest and tenderest ties of nature, consecrate themselves without reserve to the service of the sick and indigent. Who among us has not often met the Sisters of Charity, the Sisters of Mercy, the Sisters of St. Francis, the Sisters of St. Joseph, the Xaverian Brotherhood, and the Sœurs de Bon Secour?—these last, by nursing the sick in the homes of private families, are welcomed as angels of consolation for the much-needed relief they bring to the weary day-watcher. There is another community—the Little Sisters of the Poor; happy indeed is the city or town in which one of their blessed homes is reared. There are others, no less efficient in their work among the sick, but, being fewer in number, are not so well known as those above mentioned.

Self-sustaining institutions of these communities are to be found in nearly every State in the Union; our large cities cherish them as objects of just pride. We find them occupying the healthiest sites in the suburbs; again, they are erected in the crowded districts and near railroad junctions, where sickness and accidents are most frequent; we occasionally view their stately proportions reflected in the waters of our great lakes, and not unfrequently we see them near the beach where the invalid may have the benefit of the fresh sea-air.

Some of these institutions may be wholly or partly supported by the State, but even in such cases patients are devotedly cared for by the religious. After all, what would be the material aid furnished by the State were there no faithful hands to bestow immediate relief on the necessitous? But there was a time when the State did not provide thus for the sick and infirm. In this as in many other instances, religious communities were the pioneers; they had their humble infirmaries, asylums and hospitals for the sick, the homeless and the aged, long before the State thought of erecting imposing edifices to shelter the invalid. Their hands opened the virginal soil and cast into it the seed of practical charity, and we of to-day enjoy the fruit of their labor—health-restoring systems of hospitals and sanitariums throughout our land, magnificent living monuments of private charity.

And to the honor of religious communities be it said, that funds placed in their hands are conscientiously appropriated to the purpose for which they are given; no consideration of ambition or kindred is found here to bias or solicit favor, and the needy are the happy recipients of whatever fortune has bestowed on those whom religion has engaged in her service.

Where there are thousands equally deserving it would, perhaps, be invidious to select any one community, or any set of hospitals for commendation; still, while soliciting their kind indulgence for publicity herein given, I shall present a few statistics from hospitals under the care of the Sisters of Charity with which I am well acquainted. Need I say in passing, that in their homes of relief every species of human misery receives the personal attendance of these harbingers of peace and benediction? No exception is made to class or kind or religious denomination; the nameless sufferings of helpless infancy, the numberless diseases of youth and manhood, the last low moanings of the enfeebled octogenarian, receive alike their gentle ministrations; and their nightly watch is kept near the lone cell of him whose lamentations attest the ruin of the noble throne whereon reason once so proudly sat.

In the Charity Hospital, New Orleans, La., during the sixty-one years of its existence, no fewer than 468,837 patients have received from the Sisters that personal care and attention which their condition required; of this number, 399,852 recovered and were dismissed by the devoted physicians in charge.

The above figures include the persons attended and restored to health during the ravages of yellow fever, whose pestilential breath has so often swept over the southern portion of our country. During its visitations, neither fear of contagion nor of death itself could diminish the zeal of these devoted ministers of charity. When any of them fell victims to the plague, others immediately offered themselves to continue the work, despite the fate that seemed inevitable. What a roll of heroism might be displayed could we but scan the eternal records!

These same Sisters have labored for the past thirty years in the very heart of our national capital. In the Providence Hospital alone, more than 35,000 patients have been admitted; of this number, 24,493 were cared for gratuitously, receiving the same kind attention as that bestowed on others more favored by fortune.

In the Carney Hospital, South Boston, Mass., 18,888 patients were received from June, 1863, to January, 1893; 10,115 of these were charity patients.· An infant asylum was attached to this same institution from September, 1868, to 1874, during which period 1432 infants were admitted. An out-patient department was established in connection with this hospital in October, 1877; up to the present date 172,386 patients have received treatment.

Another establishment in Norfolk, belonging to the same community, received 25,201 patients from January, 1864, to April, 1893; 4507 of these were charity patients, and more than 9000 received in the wards medical attendance for a merely nominal sum.

In the Mullanphy Hospital, St. Louis, Mo., from January 1, 1876, to January 1, 1893, 18,576 sufferers were cared for; from December 1, 1889, to January 1, 1893, 7799 clinic patients were treated. In this, as in all the other establishments under the care of the Sisters, the surgical and medical departments have their special day and night nurses; twelve doctors belonging to the staff visit the departments daily, besides outside physicians who have private patients under the Sisters' care. An admirable feature in this hospital is a special ward for children not afflicted with contagious diseases, who are received free of charge; many of these little ones receive here for the first time in their lives nutritious food and intelligent care, to which they quickly respond and become bright, healthy and happy children.

Over all these the personal supervision of the Sisters is extended. It is needless to mention the assistance rendered to the sick and wounded during the late Civil War; the recollection of what was done in tent and ambulance is fresh in the minds of many, and from countless hearts the prayer of gratitude still ascends for the gentle but skilful nurses that brought them back to health and home.

There is to-day in the management of many of our Sisters' hospitals an important feature that cannot but commend itself, even to the most indifferent. It is the system of training as nurses intelligent young women who are desirous of adopting nursing as a profession. Under the guidance of the Sisters, from whom they learn the principles which underlie the intelligent treatment of the afflicted, they become skilful in the hospital wards, and acquire that gentleness and ease of manner, that devotion to duty so much appreciated by the physician and the patient.

The above gives but a limited idea of the work accomplished by our Catholic sisterhoods; for though much of their labor is seen and appreciated by the world, yet the greater part is known to God alone. When the desire of relieving the sufferings of humanity is prompted and ennobled by the love of God, it keeps alive that spirit of self-sacrifice and devotedness which we so much admire in those who consecrate their lives to the care of the sick.

No one will deny that there are many valuable books in the collection presented at the World's Columbian Exposition, but the volume of volumes would be that which would contain a full account of all that has been done by religious communities for the relief of the distressed of our favored land since its existence as the prosperous home of liberty.

THE TRAINING OF MALE AND FEMALE NURSES IN CATHOLIC ORDERS.

BY THE SANITÄTSRATH, DR. KÖLLEN,

Physician-in-chief to St. Hedwig's Hospital at Berlin.

The number of religious orders and similar congregations of the Catholic Church attending to sick-nursing in Germany is a very large one; in Prussia alone there are 49 different orders with 886 stations, and amongst these there are 5 male orders with 34 stations and 517 members, and 44 female orders with 852 stations and 7352 members.

As the Catholic Church predominates in most other German States over the Protestant, contrary to what obtains in Prussia, an idea may be formed of the great extent of nursing in the religious institutions of Germany, from these figures.

Amongst the most widely spread and active orders of Prussia, as also of the other German States, may be especially mentioned the Alexian Brothers, the Brothers of Mercy, the Franciscans, the Borromeans, the Poor Maids of Christ, the Sisters of Mercy, the Elisabethans, and the Gray Sisters.

The cause of this manifold form of religious orders for nursing must, however, not be sought in the various objects and regulations of these different orders, since these are on the whole the same and correspond to the common spirit that pervades these institutions. Although the activity of such orders presents such a varied appearance, the cause of this must be sought for in the depth of the religious life of the Catholic Church, a depth that permits of placing in the foreground in the various orders, now one and then another side of merciful activity. Most of the religious orders devote themselves to the nursing of the sick in hospitals; some confine themselves to district nursing, while others again do both; a few orders follow certain special lines of nursing, as the Alexian Brothers, for example, who devote themselves to the care of the insane.

Notwithstanding these differences, the training is everywhere inspired by the same objects in view and the same general rules, and the description which follows may hold good in general for all orders and congregations now existing in Germany, and the same in fact may be said to apply to all other European countries, allowing, of course, for some slight deviations resulting from the national character of the people and the state of civilization of the country.

The age of the applicant to one of the nursing orders must not exceed 30 years. Exceptions to this rule can only be made upon the special permission of the religious superiors. The applicant must furthermore furnish the superior of the order with a certificate from the civil magistrate of his home, as well as from his pastor, testifying to the good character of the family and his own faultless life. Should he have been a soldier, a statement must also be provided by the military authorities as to his conduct during the time of service. The applicant must be in good health and free from any bodily defect. His temperament must be cheerful, without tendency to melancholy and over-conscientious scruples, his bearing friendly. On the other hand, his admission depends upon the general impression gained of his entire mental development, as also of his character, and upon his being guided by the love of God and mankind, and upon his being filled by the desire to alleviate suffering by his general bearing as well as by his nursing.

As to his mental education, a sufficient knowledge of all elementary principles taught in schools is at least presupposed, and a degree of intelligence enabling him to understand the principles of mental life. The superiors of the orders, finally, must feel convinced that the applicant has previously tested himself thoroughly and earnestly, *i. e.* that he has remained faithful to his plans for at least one to two years, and that he has prepared himself, by means of good deeds and renunciations, for a profession demanding so much of self-sacrifice. Upon admission the candidate is handed over to the mother-institution, with which a larger hospital or insane asylum is connected, and here the first instruction is provided in monastic life and the nursing of the sick. To this end daily instructions are given of a theoretical as well as practical character. This is at first confined to all kinds of domestic work, such as washing, ironing, cooking, the cleaning and airing of rooms; then to the handling, lifting and carrying of patients, the cleansing of wounds, the disinfection of instruments and of the operating room, and the application of bandages, poultices, leeches, cupping, the adminstration of hypodermic injections, enemas, etc.

This instruction is furnished by members of the orders who have already obtained a sufficient degree of experience, and in the more important branches by the hospital physicians themselves.

In the course of this first instruction the superiors also obtain an idea of any special adaptability and inclination on the part of their pupils. Some manifest an especial talent for cooking, others for washing or needlework, and still others for various kinds of handicraft. Many wish to be occupied with true nursing, and amongst these some are especially adapted to the nursing of medical, others to surgical cases, and again others to children and the aged. Smaller, however, is the number of those who assist directly at operations, or those who pass the apothecary's examination and are able to take in hand the druggist's department of an hospital.

After such an education at the mother-institution, which extends over one to one and a half years, the candidate pledges himself for four, and in some religious orders for five years to the order. They are then sent away from the mother-institution as novices to daughter-institutions, *i. e.* to other hospitals or insane asylums belonging to the order, so as to perfect themselves by continuous daily practice.

Here their education continues in all branches, alternately in the medical, surgical and children's wards, as also in the more severe cases, the lighter and the chronic, or on the other hand again, according to special indications, in the kitchen or the drug-store, always, however, under the supervision of a superior and the various experienced officers.

During this time those who are especially talented in assisting at operations, or in the apothecary's department, for example, receive a special education under the guidance of the resident physicians or the apothecary respectively. For all, however, in addition to the technical training in sick-nursing, the most conscientious and faithful observance of the physician's orders, and especially a tender and loving treatment of the sick, at any personal sacrifice, are regarded as the great ends to be attained. After this period of training has been completed, and the novice has shown himself to be competent, he returns once more for a year to the mother-institution, in order to finish his education under the supervision of the superior-general, to obtain the finishing touches, so to speak, but especially to test himself once more before taking the final vow. Up to this time the novice has been at liberty to leave the order; if, however, he does not wish to do so after a final self-examination, and is deemed worthy by his superiors, he takes the eternal vow before the bishop and is formally admitted to the order. Here his novitiate is ended and he is now either retained in the mother-institution, or sent to some other house belonging to the order, where he is placed in a position corresponding to his ability, and where he is independent and is placed upon his own responsibility.

This is the course of training, with slight deviations, in all orders especially devoted to sick-nursing in Germany.

That such an education is a proper one is demonstrated by the results reached, especially within late years, in the nursing of the sick by Catholic orders.

Although the State and community have bestowed their attention and care upon sick-nursing more and more, it remains an indisputable fact that the hospitals of these orders not only maintain their position, but daily grow in importance, and in the esteem and confidence of all classes of the population.

The soil upon which these fruits have ripened, and from which the members of the orders, even after their training, draw strength and enthusiasm for their lives so full of pain and self-sacrifices, is the strict and uniform care of the spiritual life, and that complete devotion of one's entire existence to suffering humanity, from the love of God, based upon the evangelical rules of the Catholic creed.

[*Note.*—The original German article of Dr. Köllen has been lost and it is necessary to present a translation.—EDITORS.]

THE WORK OF DEACONESSES IN GERMANY.

FROM THE FLIEDNER INSTITUTE, KAISERWERTH, GERMANY.

The following resumé of the work of deaconesses in Germany has been written to accompany the book published in Kaiserwerth in 1886 as a memorial volume for the fiftieth anniversary of the founding of the Kaiserwerth institutions.

The beginnings of the work of deaconesses in modern times were small and unsightly like the mustard-seed. To-day their cause is bound up heart and soul with the Protestant church in Germany and deeply rooted in the life of our people. In the place of one mother-house at Kaiserwerth, begun fifty years ago with one deaconess, there are now sixty vast establishments with six thousand deaconesses in successful operation. The host of these volunteers against all kind of human need and misery are upon duty by day and night everywhere, from under the palms of Egypt unto the snow and ice of Lapland, from the sacred grounds of Zion and Lebanon unto the scene of the latest beginnings of Christian culture in the Far West of America. The man who gave the impulse to an efficient renewal of the ancient office of the women-helpers—a renewal adapted in its form to the wants of to-day—was Theodor Fliedner, a clergyman of the Protestant church. When in 1822, in his twenty-third year of age, he was appointed minister to the evangelical community of the small town of Kaiserwerth on the Rhine, the modest youth arrived in his parish on foot, in order to spare to his poor parishioners the cost of the usual formal welcome. Poverty was Fliedner's lot through all his life, and it was that of his parishioners; but their very destitution showed the way to him from which he brought back the stimulus to the great work of his life. When Fliedner had been for a few weeks in Kaiserwerth, a rich merchant, who had lent 500 thalers for the building of the evangelical church, became bankrupt, consequently the church had to be sold. Two other places were at the same time offered the young pastor, but he could not bear to witness the destruction of his parish. His faithfulness led him to travel about through the Rhine provinces, through Holland and England, to raise funds to save his church. He actually brought home the desired sum; but more than this, he had gained the knowledge of great charitable enterprises of other nations, especially that of care for the prisoners. Soon after his return he began laying to work in the same field. Journeys to this purpose caused his acquaintance with the Rhenish pastor Franz Klönne, who for a long time had urged on the public thought a revival of the ancient ministry of the deaconesses. Fliedner had actually found women-helpers officiating in the parishes of the Hollandish Mennonites. He resolved to found an asylum for discharged women-prisoners, and to apply to Christian womanhood for support of his work. In 1833 the first woman-prisoner, soon afterwards the first deaconess, arrived in Kaiserwerth. Only a very small summer-house, twelve feet square, in his own garden could as yet be obtained for the two. The book by J. Disselhof will tell you minutely how wonderfully the grain of mustard-seed became an overshadowing tree.

I here restrict myself to a short description of the present state of the cause, which cause, exclusively by Fliedner's never-relenting energy in persuading, working, collecting, leading, gained a vitality that will nevermore give way. In 1836 it was possible to buy a house, a very stately building then in the eyes of Fliedner. It is true that the price 2300 thalers could only be raised as a loan by the good pastor's indefatigable entreaties. But the sympathy with the work increased, and so did the establishment. The activity of the deaconesses from the care for prisoners soon extended to the nursing of any kind of the sick and the needy. Christian education of children as well as that of their teachers, the care for the insane and the Magdalens, became new branches of the work, which indeed tended to alleviate every sort of human misery, so far as woman's ministry might lend a helping hand. To-day we find in Kaiserwerth a great hospital, a fine church and a college, a home for old and invalid deaconesses, a workmen's house, an orphan asylum, an asylum for prisoners; we find kindergartens, a seminary, a library, preparatory schools for teachers and helpers, bathing-houses, and the cottages of the various officers in the vast establishment. Within a few years after its foundation the mother-house could open new stations all over the Rhine provinces. The number of these new places of work is to-day 107 in Rhineland, 36 in Westphalia. Filial houses were built in other provinces, and even in distant countries. It was granted to Fleidner to witness this wonderful development. His blessed life ended the 4th of October, 1864. He had been married twice, and each of his wives was a faithful helper in his work and a model to other deaconesses.

Let me now review in short the statutes for the order of the deaconesses. You will find ample and interesting information on the subject in the book by Disselhof. The thirty-fifth year is the utmost term for the admission of a "sister." She has to begin with a preparation of some years' studying and working in one of the headquarters. The preparation is fixed longer or shorter according to character, capacities and education of the individual. It comprises the practice of the most humble household work, as well as the higher instruction for all the above-mentioned disciplines. If at the end of an appointed time the novice is judged fit by the woman-superintendents of her house to be a deaconess, she is consecrated to the ministry in a religious ceremony. The relation to her family remains undisturbed, as well as her disposition and administration of her private fortune. At any time the sisters are in close connection with their mother-house, the government of which is in the hand of a lady superintendent (Frau-Oberin). The house appoints the position and mission of each of its members and takes care of them. They are at liberty to marry and to return to their parents if the latter want and require their nursing.

Until 1884 more than 60 houses of deaconesses, with nearly 6000 sisters and 1750 outside working places, had opened. I shall finally name the principal among the establishments.

The first of them was the Elizabeth Hospital in Berlin, founded under the protection of Queen Elizabeth of Prussia in 1837. The number of its deaconesses to-day is 101.

A hospital in Paris followed in 1841; it was re-established in 1867, once more in 1874, with to-day 15 sisters.

The hospital in Strassburg, 1842, has to-day 165 sisters; St. Loups in 1842, 54 sisters; Dresden, 1844, 218 sisters; Utrecht, 1844, 61 sisters; Berne, 1845, 210 sisters; Berlin, "Bethanien," 1847, 223 sisters; Stockholm, 1849, 136 sisters; Pittsburgh, now Rochester, U. S., in 1849, 18 sisters; Breslau, 1850, 175 sisters; Königsberg, 1850, 204 sisters; Stettin, 1850, 32 sisters; Ludwigslust, 1850, 140 sisters; Karlsruhe, 1851, 89 sisters; Riehen near Basel, 1852, 174 sisters; Neuendettelsau in Bavaria, 1854, 228 sisters; Stuttgart, 1854, 286 sisters; Augsburg, 1855, 63 sisters; Halle on the Saale, 1857, 70 sisters; Darmstadt, 1858, 135 sisters; Zürich, 1858, 80 sisters; St. Petersburg, 1859, 34 sisters; Speier, 1859, 70 sisters; Kraschnitz in Silesia, 1860, 74 sisters; Hannover, 1860, 189 sisters; Hamburg, "Bethesda," 1860, 27 sisters; London (in Hyde Park), 1861, 14 sisters; Danzig, 1862, 93 sisters; Kopenhagen, 1863, 115 sisters; Treysa, now in Kassel, 1864, 34 sisters; Haag in Holland, 1865, 35 sisters; Milan in Kurland, 1865, 14 sisters; Posen, 1865, 66 sisters; Budapest, 1866, 10 sisters; Frankenstein in Silesia, 1865, 121 sisters; Riga in Livland, 1866, 10 sisters; Berlin, "Lazarus Hospital," 1867, 43 sisters; London (Tottenham), 1867, 39 sisters; Reval in Esthland, 1867, 18 sisters; Helsingfors, Finland, 1867, 12 sisters; Altona, Holstein, 1867, 58 sisters; Bremen, 1868, 23 sisters; Christiania, 1868, 172 sisters; Wyburg, 1869, 5 sisters; Bielefeld, 1869, 352 sisters; New Torney near Stettin, 1869, 150 sisters; Braunschweig, 1870, 42 sisters; Frankfort-on-the-Main, 1870, 64 sisters; Flensburg, 1874, 76 sisters; Berlin, " Paul Gerhardt House," 1876, 55 sisters; Sarata in South Russia, 1867, 21 sisters; Nowawes near Potsdam, Gallneukirchen in Austria, " Salem " near Stettin, " Bethlehem " in Hamburg, Arnheim and Philadelphia, U. S.

THE VICTORIA HOUSE FOR THE CARE OF THE SICK AT BERLIN.

By Luise Fahrmann,

Superintendent of the Victoria House, Berlin, Germany.

The Victoria House in Berlin for the nursing of the sick owes its origin to her Majesty the Empress Frederick. Her Royal Highness desired to meet a two-fold need. First, she wished that the sick in their own homes, as well as those in hospitals, should have a share in the benefit of careful and humane nursing afforded by good, trained and educated women. Secondly, it was her Majesty's desire to open to young women of the educated ranks of life (but in poor circumstances and without occupation) an honorable, gratifying and blessed vocation, free from all restrictions of the Roman Catholic confessional.

Germany possesses, it is true, a great many evangelistic deaconesses and Roman Catholic sisters who do excellent work in the sphere of nursing, but on the other hand their number does not approach the demand, so that in a great many hospitals the nursing falls into the hands of uneducated and untrained male and female attendants, to whom the care of the sick is purely a means of livelihood. On the other hand, every woman is not willing to enter into a nunnery or a deaconesses' home, although willing and ready to assist her fellowmen in devoted surrender to a noble calling, and, in addition, to accomplish better and more satisfactory results in an organized and protected society than would be possible for one woman to achieve alone.

The Empress Frederick was anxious to gather just such women as the above into the society (to which she had given her name) and to train them into thorough nurses. In the year 1881 her Royal Highness introduced her plan to the Society of Domestic Hygiene, of which she was the patroness.

The beginning was a small one. They rented a house, which was dedicated and opened by her Majesty on the 4th of January. For the time being the superintendency was in the hands of a trained nurse of the Nightingale School in connection with St. Thomas Hospital, London, who was assisted by three nurses trained in German hospitals, and the aid of the Polytechnic Society of the Board of Health. Nevertheless, a wider development was only possible by means of connection with public hospitals, which opportunity soon presented itself. Therefore the Victoria House withdrew from the ranks of the Society of Domestic Hygiene, and three years afterwards, in the spring of 1886, it was organized as an independent society, and its labors proved so successful that at present, after ten years' independence, the Victoria House numbers 171 nurses, who are actively employed in 25 different districts. This number does not include all the other graduates who, after having received their training and fulfilled their term of service, hold other positions as teachers in the art of nursing.

The Victoria House is governed by a board of trustees, consisting of ladies and gentlemen, of which the presiding chairman is the State minister, Dr. Delbrück, who regulates the outside affairs of the institution. A committee of four ladies and two gentlemen attend to the current affairs of the home, the chairman being her Excellency Frau Von Helmholz. Those accepted are young women and widows of the educated class, between the ages of 20–35 years, with good character and sound health, without religious distinctions. Each candidate must produce a certificate of health, also a letter composed and written by herself, giving an account of her whole life; letters of recommendation from well-known persons, and, in default of this, a letter from her pastor, or a certificate of birth and baptism, and if possible, a candidate should apply personally. Applications of those whom the principal finds acceptable are handed in by her to the chairman of the committee, and only those accepted by these two persons are received into the Victoria House. There is no stated time for entering; this depends entirely upon the number of vacancies. After entering the Victoria House the probationer binds herself for three years (after receiving her training) to serve either in hospitals or in private houses, and to submit to all rules of the institution. As a guarantee of the above obligation, she deposits in the bank of this institution 300 marks, which are kept for her and returned at 4 per cent. interest at the expiration of her agreement. In case of non-fulfilment of the same, the money goes to the Pension Fund for Nurses. The training of the nurses is carried on in one or more hospitals, and requires one year; those less capable need longer time. Almost without exception the first six months are spent at the Universal Hospital, at Friedrichsheim, in Berlin, where an organized training school exists, and where the two chief physicians, Dr. Hahn and Dr. Färbringer, carry on the technical instruction which closes with a written examination. During the course of six months they are called pupil-nurses, after that sisters. The superintendent, who lives in the same house with the nurses, watches over them and trains them for their future calling. In the first six months they are reserved for hospital service and have a share in all the principal divisions of the work, being changed every three or four weeks to different posts. During the second half of the year they are considered as regular nurses, and have the opportunity given them of proving their fitness for bearing responsibility. The superintendent places them in different districts, where they have practice and training in the care of the sick under the supervision of head-nurses. At the end of the second six months, if they prove worthy, they assume the name and dress of Victoria nurses, and receive on the 21st of November, the Empress Frederick's birthday also Commemoration Day, a silver Victoria medal, which is often presented by her Majesty's own hand; this medal they have to return in event of their leaving the Victoria Society.

During the training the Victoria nurse receives her board, lodging, laundry, and uniform free. At the end of the first half of the year she receives 10 marks as pocket-money. The principal, with the chairman of the committee, is at liberty to dismiss at any time during the training any nurse who does not prove worthy of receiving the training. The pupil-nurse has a right to leave during the first three months, by giving two weeks' notice. If she avails herself of this opportunity, or is dismissed on account of bad behavior, she has to refund 50 marks per month as equivalent to her training. A rebate of 25 marks monthly is given if the cause of leaving is not the fault of the nurse. After the admission as nurse into the Victoria House, a certificate is given by the superintendent and committee, which entitles her to a uniform, board, lodging, laundry, and a salary of 300 marks a year, which increases 50 marks per year from the third year until it reaches 500 marks. In the case of those who show exceptional talent this salary is increased to 600 marks. With the exception of the above-named sum, the nurses are not allowed to accept any remuneration, and if any presents be given them they are to be handed over to the institution. At the end of three years' service the superintendent and chairman have power to dismiss any of the nurses, but this only occurs in the case of serious grievances, and only then when repeated warnings have been unheeded. In the event of urgent circumstances which make the withdrawal of a nurse from the institution compulsory, such cases receive prompt attention, and under these circumstances the board of trustees returns a nurse either in part or in whole the sum of money deposited by her. After the expiration of the three years a nurse can leave the Victoria House after giving notice three months ahead, and on the first day of the month. In case of sickness, the nurse receives free medical attention at the Victoria House, or at any other hospital where she is working. Every year of service (excepting the first year) each sister is given a month's vacation, and is allowed reduction on the different railroads when she goes to take her holiday trip. The salary is continued during sickness and vacation. Sometimes at the end of her contract she receives as an extra compensation an extended period of vacation from three to six months, but during this time her salary ceases.

Each nurse is required to save 50 marks yearly, to be put into the Fund for Aged and Infirm Nurses. This sum is deposited at the Prussian " Renten Versicherungsanstalt." If a nurse is still in the service of the Victoria House at the age of 60 she receives a pension. If she leaves the institution before that age she receives all money she has deposited, provided it has been in the Prussian Versicherungsanstalt five years, and after a year's notice is given she receives it back with compound interest. If a sister dies before the expiration of the above-given notice, the money falls into the hands of the aforementioned bank. In addition to these amounts paid by each nurse, the Victoria House contributes 30 marks yearly to the same savings bank, which increases the pension for aged nurses. Should a nurse withdraw from the Victoria House before her 60th year, then the contribution of the additional 30 marks yearly falls back to the Victoria House.

If a nurse becomes incapacitated before the age of 60 she is entitled to assistance from the Invalid's Fund of the Victoria House, which at present amounts to 56,713 marks. In each case the amount to be given is decided upon by the trustees. Besides these arrangements for disabled and aged nurses, there is another provision made for old age and accidents, although no nurse is entitled to its assistance until she is 70 years of age. Whereas the Victoria House has its own training school in which the nurses can receive their technical training, it entered, in 1884, into an agreement with the authorities of the city of Berlin, by which the Victoria sisters could receive their practical training at the city hospital of Friedrichsheim. By this arrangement the Victoria House promised two-thirds of their trained nurses for different city hospitals. In this way those who have received their first six months' training are eligible to serve in the city hospitals. The Victoria House receives a yearly income of 480 marks from the city of Berlin for each head-nurse in the city hospitals, and 360 marks for each sister, and these sums of money are divided among the sisters according to the agreement of the authorities of the Victoria House. Besides the 100 sisters who are now serving in the city hospitals, the Victoria House has a number of state and private institutions and associations to supply, partly to take charge of the sick and partly to direct and superintend. In the former case they have male and female attendants who assist, but do not belong to the Victoria House.

The compensation which is received at the Victoria House from these institutions amounts approximately to 500 marks yearly for each nurse, whether it be in the capacity of nurse or of superintendent. No difference is made in the salaries of the Victoria sisters whether they work as nurses or superintendents, for each one is expected to be placed in the position which she is best fitted for, and as such to do her work to the best of her ability. The income of the Victoria House up to 1892 consists of the earnings of the sisters, which amounted to 57,471 marks, besides presents and dues of members up to the present time, and the interest on 120,000 marks. This sum was a present from the Crown Prince and Princess of the German Empire to the Victoria House; this amount was presented to them in 1883 by the city of Berlin on the occasion of their silver wedding; they gave it for the building of a house for the Victoria sisters. It was not begun until 1892. The constant increase of the associations made the erection of a new building at last absolutely necessary. The city of Berlin appropriated 130,000 marks to the above sum and a building site, with the condition that the house should remain city property. The present home for the nurses is near the city hospital at Friedrichsheim, in which the superintendent and pupil-nurses have resided since 1884; they had also rented quarters in this neighborhood for private and sick nurses. In the new Victoria House, which will be located further out in the suburbs but near the hospital at Friedrichsheim, from the 1st October, 20 to 30 sisters will live here during the first six months of their training.

There are 36 rooms in this building for private and sick nurses, besides dining, sitting, reading and meeting rooms for all the sisters of the Victoria House. Here they meet at least twice a year, at the anniversary of the opening and at Christmas, and here they find a kind home and every care in time of sickness and in need of rest. All the Victoria sisters who are engaged in hospital work live and board there, and also the 61 sisters who are at present employed at the Friedrichsheim hospital who have hitherto lived at the hospital itself.

For each nurse the city of Berlin pays 1 mark .75 per day for each nurse, the same sum which it used to cost to board them. The sisters are responsible to the doctors in chief and to the assistant doctors in all their work in connection with the different institutions and associations. At the head of each district there is a head-nurse, who is assisted by subordinate sisters and pupil-nurses, for whom she is responsible for the conscientious fulfilment of their duties. In the larger hospitals one of the head-nurses acts as assistant to the superintendent; she is free in this capacity to give afternoons off duty to the sisters and pupil-nurses, and her advice is solicited in all difficulties. In circumstances too difficult for her to decide she applies to the superintendent for her decision; in any case she is required to consult the superintendent in all matters regarding the sisters of the institution. The duties of the nurses are equally arranged. The work is divided into day and night duty. The hours of duty in most of the hospitals are from 6 a. m. to 8 p. m.; the night duty from 8 p. m. to 9 a. m. If the night-duty nurses finish their work they may go off duty earlier. As a rule the night staff is changed every month, and for the sake of the nurses' health they are not required to go on night duty more than four times a year. Before going on duty at night they have supper all together. During the night they have a similar meal, which they take in the kitchen of the ward. They take a cup of coffee with the day-nurses, and at 10 o'clock they have breakfast, when they come off duty. From that time until 12 o'clock they generally spend out in the grounds of the hospital. They then sleep for 7 hours. Twice a week they are allowed to go out from 9 until 1 p. m. The day-nurses have one hour off duty daily, besides 9 hours free weekly. The pupil-nurses are required to be in the Victoria House by 10 p. m.

Whatever comes under the head of nursing is in the hands of the nurses, but all other work in the way of house-cleaning, etc., is done by men and women employed for that purpose. Orderlies are given the care of 20 to 40 male patients; they assist in keeping them in good order, in lifting and in carrying. This assistance is provided for the sisters by the different institutions and not by the Victoria House. In regard to the uniform, they all wear the same on duty. It consists of a light-blue wash dress, white apron and white cap. On Sundays they wear a dark-blue cashmere dress. On the street they wear a plain black mantle made in the latest style, and a small black inconspicuous bonnet faced with white ruching, and white ties. When the nurses are off duty they can wear what they please. They are allowed to attend concerts and theaters, but cannot go to public places alone, and must inform the superintendent or assistant of their intention of going.

There are no other restrictions, and it is expected that young women of their standing should conduct themselves as ladies. If they ever take advantage of these liberties they are expelled from the society. In the Victoria House no one is obliged to attend religious services. On Sunday every one has an opportunity of attending the Protestant services held in the building. They are allowed to attend services outside the hospital, provided this does not interfere with their duties, for we consider that our service to the sick is service to God. The majority of our sisters are Protestants. At present there are 171 sisters, out of which number 158 are Protestants, 9 Roman Catholics, and 4 belong to other denominations. So far there has never been any religious discord in the Victoria House.

ON NURSING IN SCOTLAND.

By Rachel Frances Lumsden,

Honorary Superintendent, Aberdeen Royal Infirmary.

The nursing of the sick in Scotland is a big subject, and I feel myself to be little qualified for the task which has been laid upon me. Let me begin by explaining that the word "infirmary" applies in Scotland to a large general hospital with a medical school attached to it, not, as in England, to one specially connected with a workhouse or union.

In Scotland our helpless paupers are nursed in the poorhouses.

The royal charter of the Edinburgh Royal Infirmary dates from 1736.

Before 1872 we shall not inquire how the nurses were trained, or how the sick were nursed, especially how they were cared for during the long dreary nights of pain and weariness, seeing that the poor night nurses, who were expected to watch and tend them, had to help the day nurses in scrubbing the wards and did not get to bed until late in the afternoon. Training there was none, in the light of present requirements, and the managers, realizing the necessity for improvement, sent to St. Thomas's Hospital in London, where Miss Nightingale's training school for nurses had been established, for a lady as superintendent, and twelve nurses, to initiate a new system and to reform the nursing in the infirmary. This reformation could not be accomplished at once, but required years of patient work. The old buildings were found unsuitable, so a new infirmary was built on a large and handsome scale, and finished in 1879, part of the old one being reserved for fever patients. The demand for nurses, and the number of nurses in the training school having increased, a new home for nurses has been lately opened.

It is built of red brick, two stories high, in the form of a quadrangle surrounding a red-tiled court. In the center of this court is a small fountain, and a bed of lovely tulips and hyacinths, which filled the air with sweetness in the April sunshine of the day on which I visited the home.

The new and the old home are connected by a pretty conservatory. The nurses who are in training for three years sleep in the new home, each having a bedroom; 121 can be accommodated. There is a large airy sick-room for five nurses, and two single rooms.

The nurses who are in training for only one year sleep in the old home, which is fitted up with cubicles. They are called pupils or probationers, and are sent from district homes or private nursing homes, and pay a fee of £10 per annum.

The nurses have a comfortably arranged reading-room, in which is a good lending library, with plenty of newspapers and periodicals. The recreation room in the new home is large and well proportioned, and its low roof, its windows at either end, and its two tiled fireplaces, give it a quaint, old-fashioned appearance. A more comfortable, luxurious, restful room could not be desired. I now quote from printed regulations.

"At present there are 35 nurses in training for the Royal Infirmary, and 28 pupils.

" The nurses are bound for three years. At the close of one year their training will usually be considered complete, and during the two following years they are required to take hospital, district, or private nursing, as may be offered to them by the lady superintendent.

"At the end of a year those who have passed satisfactorily through the course of instruction and training will be entered in the register as nurses.

" The course of instruction includes lectures on anatomy and physiology, on medical and surgical nursing, gynecological work, and fever nursing, also clinics in medical and surgical wards.

" Lessons are given in bandaging and instruments, and examinations are held after each course of lectures and teaching.

"Apart from the practical training in the wards, members of the medical and surgical staff of the infirmary give lectures to the probationers, while classes, to assist them in understanding these lectures, are held by some of the ladies in charge of the home and the wards. A series of lessons in sick cookery is also given by a teacher from the school of domestic economy."

Glasgow.

Glasgow, with its population of over half a million, has two large general hospitals or infirmaries.

The Royal Infirmary has 580 beds (100 less than the Edinburgh Royal), and the Western Infirmary 400; while a smaller one, the Victoria, with 150 beds, has lately been opened—making 1130 beds in Glasgow, against 680 in Edinburgh.

The Glasgow Royal Infirmary, established in 1791, more than 50 years later than those built in Edinburgh and Aberdeen, has lately undergone great changes, and no doubt improvements in the system of nursing.

"The matron has three assistants and 125 nurses divided into three grades: 30 staff nurses, 30 assistant nurses on day duty, 30 assistant nurses on night duty—these assistant nurses alternate every three months—30 probationers and 5 special nurses, making in all 125.

"The probationers rise at 4 a. m., and go off duty at 4.30 p. m., having to be in bed at 8 p. m.

"Before candidates are eligible they have to show a certificate of preliminary education, after which they have to go through a course of lectures and demonstrations in anatomy, physiology, hygiene, massage, care and knowledge of instruments, electricity, ward work and cookery, etc.

"These classes occupy three months, during which time the pupil provides board and lodging at her own expense, paying a fee of £5 5s. for the lectures."

The period of actual hospital training is two years, at the end of which time a final examination may be held, and a certificate of training given. There is a nurses' home.

At the Western Infirmary, a beautiful nurses' home has been finished lately, which is entered from the main building through a handsome conservatory. The infirmary stands on high open ground, and was built in 1874, but the plan of the building has drawbacks.

In Glasgow, amongst the various smaller special institutions, there is an extremely good maternity hospital, with 34 beds, where the training is excellent.

Aberdeen.

The Aberdeen Royal Infirmary dates from 1739. About that time, "the Magistrates being informed that there had been lately errected ane Infirmary in the City of Edinburgh, into which house all proper objects were received," sent "an ingenious man to see the Infirmary, and from it to make plans."

Not many years later, at the time of the rebellion in Scotland in 1745, Prince Charlie's wounded were placed in the Infirmary, and they were succeeded by the soldiers belonging to the Duke of Cumberland.

It is no wonder that after these troubled times, when the directors were again in office, we find them giving orders for an inventory of the furniture to be made:

"In doctor's room, two machines for broken legs.

Two chairs, one wanting an arm.

Nineteen single sheets, three of them needing mending; all for the patients and kitchen bed.

Three pans, but two of them useless.

A little pot, and middling pot, both very good.

A big pot, and a kettle pot, both very bad.

A little ladle and a cavie.*

Two stone little tullies for warming drink.

In east vault, a bathing tub and fixed bed"; and so on.

In these cells or vaults, paved with stone, the bedlamite patients were kept. A patient suffering from paralysis, and considered incurable, is ordered as the best treatment the doctor can think of for him: "The frequent use of cold water to be poured on his loins, rubbing with a dry cloth, and swallowing a spoonful of unbeaten mustard in the morning, and as much in the afternoon." Dr. John Gregorie, in 1751, writes to the managers on the subject of a bath for the infirmary, which had been under consideration for a year. He says, "Considering how useful, yea necessary, hot and cold bathing are in ye cure of many diseases, we cannot but earnestly wish to see this plan executed." The physicians determined to recommend the use of the bath to their patients in town and county, and evidently to defray the expense, "which was not to exceed two hundred guineas,"

* Hencoop.

students and apprentices coming to Aberdeen "are to pay one guinea to the Infirmary." At a general meeting the question of the bath was put to a vote, and on its being passed, "the Lord Provost is recommended when he goes up to Edinburgh to carry the plan and estimate of the bath with him, and to show it to proper judges." The number of patients increasing, five more beds are required, and they write "to Dalkeith for six bed-coverlets."

Herbs are grown in the "physick garden," and carefully stored for the use of the patients and for sale.

Later on, some twenty years ago, the night nurses, like those in Edinburgh, had hard work to do after they left the wards, having to help with the washing of the linen until 2 P. M. Coals were given out twice a week, and they had to carry the large heavy backets up to the wards.

Still later, in 1876, came ward assistants, which was a great improvement, but the nurses received little training.

In 1877 a further improvement in nursing spread to Aberdeen, when the Hospital for Sick Children began, but it was not until 1885 that the nursing in the Aberdeen Royal Infirmary was put upon a new system and a training school for nurses started. At that date the average number of patients was about the same as now, say 160 or 170. There were then only 25 nurses, and there was a scarlet fever ward, which has since been abolished, all fever cases being now sent to the City Hospital. The present nursing staff numbers over 50, including sisters, staff nurses, and probationers,* who are bound for three years, and whose training is not considered complete under that time. At the end of three years, after going through a final examination, they become staff nurses.

In addition to the practical training in the wards, nurses receive instruction from the medical and surgical staff, and examinations are held in anatomy and physiology, and also in the care and knowledge of instruments. Massage lessons are given to the staff nurses and nurses of two years' standing by a certified masseuse attached to the hospital, and only those who show a special aptitude of touch are continued in the class.

The annual holidays extend from three to four weeks; a long pass is given to each nurse once a week, and the usual length of night duty is three months.

The Jubilee Extension Scheme for improving the hospital, for

* 9 sisters, 8 staff nurses, 37 probationers.

which £30,000 has been subscribed, is still in process of execution, the administration and medical block having yet to be completed. The new surgical pavilion was opened in the end of 1892, by her Royal Highness the Princess Louise.

Dundee.

In Dundee, the Royal Infirmary, which was established in 1798, seven years after the one in Glasgow, is beautifully situated, overlooking the river Tay. The average number of patients is 163, much the same as in the Aberdeen Royal Infirmary. There is a special children's ward, and "the nursing staff numbers 32." Fever patients are sent to a special hospital.

Hospitals in Scotland for Sick Children.

Edinburgh.—The Edinburgh Hospital for Sick Children, established about thirty-five years ago, has hitherto occupied a somewhat cramped and inconvenient site, close to the Royal Infirmary. A new one is now in process of erection, in which the number of in-patients will be greatly increased. The present daily average is between 50 and 60. A dispensary is attached, and there is a large number of out-patients. No infectious cases are admitted.

Aberdeen.—Next in age comes the Aberdeen Hospital for Sick Children, which dates from 1877. In 1883 a large addition was built, together with a separate block for scarlet fever and measles cases. The daily average of in-patients is from 50 to 60. There is an out-door department, but no dispensary attached. The distinguishing feature of this hospital is its admission of scarlet fever, measles, and typhoid cases, and the consequently large staff of nurses, in proportion to the size of the hospital, which must be maintained. This staff is available for private nursing.

Glasgow.—The Glasgow Hospital for Sick Children has been in existence for ten years. The daily number of patients averages 65. There is a large and well-appointed dispensary. No infectious cases are admitted.

Dundee.—In Dundee, a ward for children is provided in the Royal Infirmary.

District Nursing in Scotland.

The establishment of Queen Victoria's Jubilee Institute, for nursing the sick poor in their own homes, has introduced a great and a greatly needed reform into the condition of the suffering poor. The Scottish branch, the headquarters of which are in Edinburgh, has already sent out numbers of nurses specially trained both in hospital and district work, to different towns in Scotland. The largest affiliated homes are in Glasgow, Dundee, and Paisley. One has been lately opened in Aberdeen, another in Inverness. Smaller branches are established all over Scotland.

Within the limits of this paper it is impossible to do more than refer briefly to the many smaller hospitals throughout Scotland, such as Paisley with 180 beds, Greenock, Kilmarnock, Dumfries, Ayr, Leith, Perth, Inverness, etc. The cottage hospitals and convalescent homes, which are yearly increasing in number, do a large amount of good.

Hospitals for Incurables.

I must not omit to mention that in Edinburgh, Glasgow, and Aberdeen we have hospitals for those patients who are beyond medical and surgical aid to cure, but whose sufferings can be lightened by the tender care of a good nurse.

LES ÉCOLES D'INFIRMIÈRES ANNEXÉES AUX HÔPITAUX CIVILS DE PARIS.

NOTE PAR LE PROFESSEUR LEON LE FORT,

Chirurgien de l'hôtel Dieu.

La création des écoles d'infirmières annexées aux hôpitaux de Paris se lie intimement à la question de l'expulsion des religieuses, ce que l'on a appele "la laïcisation des hôpitaux." Pour apprécier la valeur pratique de ces écoles, les résultats qu'elles voit données, il faut nécessairement donner un aperçu rapide de l'organisation des hôpitaux de Paris et des raisons qui ont amené leur laïcisation.

Les hôpitaux (consacrés au traitement des malades) et les hospices (où sont reçus les vieillards et infirmes) de Paris relèvent d'une même administration qu'on appelle : Administration centrale de l'assistance publique de Paris. Cette administration n'a pas seulement à s'occuper des malades, des infirmes et des vieillards, elle doit venir en aide aux pauvres, aux ouvriers sans travail, elle centralise

donc tout ce qui concerne le soulagement de la misère, les secours à
donner aux pauvres qu'ils soient jeunes ou vieux, bienportants ou
malades. Cette centralisation excessive comprend donc les hôpitaux, les hospices, les asiles, les maisons de secours, les bureaux de
bienfaisance et les secours à domicile pour les malades ayant un
domicile et pouvant se faire soigner dans leur famille.

A la tête de cette administration est un directeur (M. Peyron)
nommé par le ministre de l'intérieur. Il a à coté de lui un Conseil
de Surveillance composé de vingt membres.

Les ressources pécuniaires de cette administration consistent en
revenus provenant de dons et legs et du produit d'un impôt sur les
spectacles, concerts, etc., impôt appelé " le droit des pauvres," et
qui rapporte par an trois à quatre millions. Pendant longtemps
l'administration a pu vivre sur les propres revenus (c'est ce qui
existe encore pour la ville de Lyon) ; mais depuis plus de cinquante
ans, il n'en est plus de même.

L'augmentation de la population parisienne a eu pour résultat
l'augmentation du nombre des indigents, la création d'un certain
nombre d'hôpitaux. Pour suffire à ces dépenses, l'assistance publique a vendu des maisons, des terres, des rentes sur l'état, alienant
ainsi son capital. Ses revenus diminuant, en même temps que ses
dépenses augmentaient, il lui fallait demander à la ville de Paris,
representée par son conseil municipal, des sommes annuelles, de
plus en plus importantes.

La haute direction de l'assistance publique appartient au ministre
de l'intérieur et cette direction de droit fut jusqu'en 1870 une direction de fait. Le conseil municipal de Paris qui cherche à se rendre
indépendant a profité de l'influence que lui donnait le don pécuniaire qu'il fait chaque année à l'assistance publique, don qui dépasse
actuellement 20 millions par an. Loin de chercher à diminuer cette
subvention annuelle, il cherche au contraire à l'augmenter et voici
comment il y arrive. S'il faut créer un hôpital qui coute trois ou
quatre millions, il oblige l'assistance publique à se créer en alienant
une partie de son capital. Les revenus de l'assistance publique
diminuant de ce fait, le conseil municipal augmente d'autant son
allocation annuelle. Il en est résulté que le patrimonie des pauvres
a été dépensé et que c'est le conseil municipal qui est en quelque
sorte devenu le maître absolu de l'assistance publique. Nous ver-
rons tout à l'heure le résultat de cette situation. Je me borne à
examiner ce qui concerne les hôpitaux.

Chaque hôpital comprend un personnel qu'on peut diviser en quatre categories.

1º. Des agents de l'administration centrale qui sont : le directeur, l'econome, le pharmacien en chef et le personnel des bureaux. Tous sont des employés nommés et payés par l'assistance publique.

2º. Les médecins et chirurgiens des hôpitaux, nommés par voie de et dont la nomination est signée par le ministre de l'intérieur. Ces médecins et chirurgiens sont aidés par des élèves internes et par des élèves externes egalement nommés par le concours. (Il faut pour pouvoir être interne, avoir été d'abord externe.)

3º. Le personnel de surveillance des salles de malades, de la lingerie, de la cuisine. Ce personnel était, il y a quelques années uniquement constitué par les religieuses.

4º. Le personnel inférieur ou des infirmiers qui ont toujours été des laïques. Ce sont les infirmiers et infirmières qui font les lits, nettoient les malades, lavant les parquets, font en un mot tous les gros ouvrages. Quant aux pansements ils sont faits exclusivement par les élèves.

La laïcisation n'a eu pour effet que de chasser les sœurs des hôpitaux et de changer le personnel chargé de la surveillance des salles de malades et des divers services de l'hôpital.

A l'instigation d'un médecin, docteur Bourneville, un conseiller municipal, M. Talandier, proposa au conseil municipal de Paris des 1872 la création d'une école d'infirmières. Cette proposition ne fut pas accepté.

Le 10 Novembre 1877, le docteur Bourneville, qui avait été élu conseiller municipal, proposa lui-même cette mesure. Cette fois elle fut acceptée et le conseil municipal invita l'administration de l'assistance publique à créer deux écoles d'infirmières, l'une à l'hospice de Bicêtre, l'autre à celui de la Salpetrière.

Comme je l'ai dit tout à l'heure, les désirs du conseil municipal sont des ordres pour l'administration des hôpitaux, on s'occupa de suite de la création d'une école. Mais les infirmières sont en général des femmes sans éducation dont beaucoup ne savaient ni lire, ni écrire et la première école creé fut, ce que nous appelons en France, une école primaire où l'on se bornait à enseigner la lecture, l'écriture et le calcul. On chercha en même temps à leur donner quelques notions sur le rôle des infirmières. Dans ce but on traduisit en français une partie du *Manuel des infirmières anglaises* par Miss Veitch et cette traduction servit pour la lecture et pour les dictées.

Le veritable enseignement professionnel fut inauguré le 23 Juillet 1878. Cet enseignement comprenait 1° un cours d'administration fait par M. Lebas, directeur de la Salpetrière ; 2° un cours de pansements et de petite chirurgie fait par M. le Docteur Poirer ; 3° un cours d'anatomie fait par M. le Docteur Duret ; 4° un cours de physiologie fait par M. le Docteur Reynard.

Pendant l'année 1879 on joignit à cet enseignement théorique un enseignement pratique. On fit faire aux élèves infirmières des exercises de pansement et on leur apprit à recueillir le vaccin et à faire des vaccinations.

Jusque là l'enseignement n'était donné qu'à de simples infirmières chargées de faire le service des salles, mais n'ayant pas à s'élever jusqu'au service de surveillance et de direction encore confié aux religieuses. Lorsqu'en 1888 on eut laïcisé l'hôpital de la Pitié il fut nécessaire de donner un enseignement plus complet, plus élevé, afin de pouvoir recruter des femmes suffisamment instruites pour pouvoir remplacer les religieuses. C'est alors que fut creée l'école d'infirmières de la Pitié, école d'un ordre plus élève que celles de Bicêtre et de la Salpetrière.

L'école de la Pitié outre les cours d'anatomie, de physiologie et de petite chirurgie eut des cours d'hygiène, de petite pharmacie et un cours sur les soins à donner aux femmes en couches et aux enfants nouveau-nés. On admit à suivre ces cours non seulement les infirmières des hôpitaux, mais aussi des personnes n'ayant aucune attache avec les hôpitaux, mais desireuses de suivre les cours afin de s'instruire dans les soins à donner aux malades. En 1884 on alla plus loin et l'on obligea toutes les infirmières des hôpitaux de la Salpetrière, de Bicêtre et de la Pitié, hôpitaux où existaient des écoles à suivre les cours de ces écoles d'infirmières. On créa en même temps des diplômes qui n'étaient donnés qu'à la suite d'examens passés à la fin de l'année.

Ces diplômes sont assez libéralement donnés car jusqu'en 1891, il en avait été delivré 1118 et en 1891–92 il en fut donné 301, soit un total de 1419. Sur ces 1419 diplômes 688 sont attachés aux hôpitaux. Ils se separtissent ainsi :

Hommes.		Femmes.		Total.
Surveillants, . .	2	Surveillantes, . .	39	41
Sous surveillants,	16	Sous surveillantes,	134	150
Suppléants, . .	45	Suppléantes, . .	180	225
Infirmiers, . .	70	Infirmières, . .	202	272
	133		555	688

Comme on le voit le chiffer des infirmiers diplômés est fort minime et cependant dans les salles d'hommes le service est fait par des infirmiers et non par des infirmières. Le service de surveillance est confié à des femmes qui remplacent les religieuses. Je dirai tout à l'heure quel est le résultat pratique de la laïcisation et de la création des écoles d'infirmières.

Il serait trop long de vous transcrire le programme des cours, je me borne à vous l'envoyer. Il est extrait du compte rendu pour 1891-92.

Lorsqu'on éxamine ce programme il semble que ces leçons doivent s'adresser à des personnes dejà instruites. Il faut ici faire une distinction. Les surveillantes sont en général des personnes ayant dejà reçu de l'instruction et auxquelles ces cours peuvent profiter, mais quant aux infirmières qui savent à peine lire et écrire on ne voit pas à quoi des cours d'anatomie et de physiologie peuvent leur servir.

J'arrive maintenant aux résultats.

D'une manière général la laïcisation a été une déplorable mesure.

1° Dans l'esprit qu'il a inspirée, puisqu'elle n'a été faite qu'en vue de chasser la religion de l'hôpital. En même temps qu'on chassait les religieuses, on chassait les aumôniers.

2° Au point de vue pécuniaire. Chaque religieuse n'étant payée que 200 francs par an et comme toutes les religieuses d'un même hôpital mangeaient à la même table et couchaient en dortoir, les dépenses pour l'administration étaient minimes.

Les surveillantes qui les remplacent coutent 800 francs par an, plus indemnité de logement pour aux grand nombre soit en moyenne 16 à 1,800 francs par an.

Pour apprécier les resultats il faut distinguer les surveillantes et les infirmières.

L'esprit d'intolérance pour ou contre la religion a rendu injuste. Je déclare en ce qui me concerne que j'ai été très-satisfait des surveillantes que j'ai eues à Necker et à La Pitié et je ne les ai pas trouver inférieures aux religieuses. Pour elles, les écoles d'infirmières ont été une très-utile institution.

Si maintenant je passe aux infirmiers s'est tout autre chose. Les infirmiers sont payés de 28 à 30 francs par mois. Ils sont mediocrement nourris, couchent en dortoir et font un service possible. Pour ce prix on ne peut avoir que de détestables serviteurs. Pour compenser la faiblesse de leur salaire, ils se font payer par les pauvres malades pour leur rendre les plus légers services. Il est inutile de dire que les réglements défendent absolument cet abus.

Un domestique homme est payé à Paris de 80 à 120 francs par mois; on comprend que l'administration ne puisse avoir pour 30 francs par mois que des gens tarés aux trop paresseux pour faire un bon service chez un particulier. L'exemple suivant permet de juger la question bien que l'administration soit indulgente. A Bicêtre en une année d'après le compte-rendu de M. Bourneville lui-même on renvoya 87 infirmiers : 15 pour ivresse, 54 pour abandon de service, 16 pour insubordination, 2 pour actes d'immoralité.

En resumé si nous, chirurgiens des hôpitaux devons reconnaître que les écoles d'infirmières nous ont donné des surveillantes et des sous surveillantes très dignes du côte q'elles ont à remplir et qui remplacent les religieuses expulsées à cause de leur religion ; nous devons avouer aussi que rien ; en ce qui concerne les infirmiers, ne nous fait soupçonner qu'il éxiste pour eux une école. Ils sont aussi mauvais serviteurs que je les ai toujours connus dans les hôpitaux de Paris.

[Professor Le Fort died suddenly at his country residence, Oct. 19, 1893, at the age of 63. In 1861–62 he was sent by the government to examine the hospitals of England and of Germany, and his reports upon their organization and methods of management were and still are of much value and interest.

At one time he was in favor of the doing away with the nursing and administration of the French hospitals by religious orders, and of placing them under exclusively secular management, and when I wrote him asking for a brief statement of his views to present to the Congress, I was not aware that he had changed his opinions, as indicated in this paper. In a private note dated June 5, 1893, Professor Le Fort says that he may have been too sharp in the statement of his opinions, and from this and from my personal knowledge of his habit of forcibly giving his views I think it probable that his condemnation of the lay nurses and their training was more emphatic and unqualified than he would have made it upon second thoughts.—J. S. BILLINGS.]

WASHINGTON, Dec. 25, 1893.

LA SOURCE NORMAL EVANGELICAL SCHOOL FOR INDEPENDENT NURSES FOR THE SICK AT LAUSANNE, SWITZERLAND.

By Dr. Charles Krafft, *Director.*

I.—Principles of La Source.

Ambroise Paré, the great French surgeon of the 16th century, said, speaking of one of his patients: "I dress his wounds, God heals him." This simple and modest speech, as far removed from the mysticism which prays without acting as from the rashness which acts without praying; this beautiful motto of the christian physician—the care of the sick under the benediction, with the aid, of God—this is the fundamental principle of La Source.

To teach young women, married women, and widows, compassion and care for those who suffer; to teach them to seek in the Gospel the light and strength indispensable to whoever wishes to live and serve as a child of God—such is the aim of the school. A magnificent aim; placed so high as to seem beyond reach, but attainable through the grace of Him who never refuses His aid to those who believe in His goodness.

A number of institutions designed to train religious nurses place celibacy, renunciation of salary, the rule of obedience, and the wearing of a special garb, at the foundation of their structure.

La Source, obeying other inspirations, follows a different path. For her nurses she desires liberty in Christ, spontaneity, the development of their capabilities, modesty in the exercise of their calling, in outward appearance nothing to attract either the curiosity or the admiration of the public. She wishes for them respect for the laws of God, who made woman the companion of man, who permits no other leader for our souls than Himself, and who dignifies all remuneration by declaring that the laborer is worthy of his hire.

Upon her entrance into the school each pupil receives a short explanation of the principles to which the institution owes its origin, and which she is to follow and support. They are as follows:

Principles.

The school called La Source aims to train capable and pious nurses for the sick. It differs in the five following points from other institutions which pursue an analogous course:

1st. Its pupils conform to a common law only during their time of training.

2d. It does not bestow the title "sister" on its pupils.

3d. It does not require a special dress.

4th. It does not exact celibacy.

5th. The time of training finished, and the pupils having graduated as nurses, all money earned by them is received by them directly from their patients.

The school, placing at its foundation the five principles just enumerated, puts them in practice, that its example may show their justice.

Explanation.

1st. *Common Rule.*—During their training the pupils must submit, as they do in every school, to a common rule. But God, who gave each individual a conscience and a will, has, by the words of the Saviour, established for each one liberty of action.

Our school, the time of training ended, does not impose any rule whatever on its pupils. Their individual liberty is thus entirely preserved.

2d. *Sisters.*—La Source does not give the title of Sister to its pupils or graduate nurses, believing that they have no more right than other christian women who exercise a similar vocation, to bear this special title.

3d. *Costume.*—La Source does not require its pupils or graduates to wear a special dress. They, being prepared for their mission, follow it in the world as do other christians, protected by a husband, brothers, relations, friends, and by a strong religious education, and above all, by Him who directs and who guards each of His children.

4th. *Celibacy.*—La Source does not consider celibacy indispensable to the functions of an hospital nurse. Among married women there have been, and there are to-day, many noble careers in the service of the sick, many examples of devotion. In virtue of this fact, and of the higher law, the school admits to its teaching either married women, widows, or unmarried women.

5th. *Salary.*—God said " Thou shalt earn thy bread in the sweat of thy brow." The hospital nurse who, on principle, declines a salary places herself above this common law. The nurse or sister, deprived of capital or of revenue, finds herself, if she leaves the institution after some years of service, deprived of the legitimate resources which her work ought to have assured to her. Let us add that the gratuity of this work. is illusory, since the support of sisters is assured, during life, to those who remain affiliated with the order. Our school holds it honorable for women and for men alike to earn their daily bread. We see nothing in the law of God, either here or elsewhere, to be corrected. We render homage to those who, placed in a position of great wealth, consecrate it to the gratuitous care of the poor. But, if we see in this a privilege, we do not see in it a superiority. In our eyes, each nurse should remain free, either to accept remuneration or to refuse it.

II.—THE COUNCIL.

La Source is committed to the administration and to the care of a council, composed of twenty-five members.

The council forms an association which meets twice a year to deliberate on every question pertaining to the school. In the interval between these meetings, the council delegates its powers to a committee composed of three members.

III.—THE DIRECTOR.

The normal evangelical school of independent nurses for the sick was, from 1859 to 1891, a purely private institution. M. and Mme. de Gasparin confided the education of the pupils to a director, and this director was responsible to them only. MM. Muller, Panchaud, Reymond, filled successively this office for 32 years. The latter, M. A. Reymond, pastor, had directed the school for 28 consecutive years. Let me recall here that M. Reymond was always the ardent defender of the principles of La Source, that these fifty-six generations of pupils (two classes in a year) were the favorite work of his life, and that the nurses whom he trained remain sincerely attached to him both by bonds of gratitude and of respectful affection.

The school was changed in 1891. M. Reymond having retired from his arduous labor, the author of these lines, appointed by Mme. de Gasparin, became the director of La Source.

In this position he directs the progress of the school, lays down the course of study, appoints the practical work of the pupils, provides for their support, supervises the interior workings of the institution, is responsible for the preservation of all property, carries out the wishes of the council, etc., etc

The director chooses his own assistants and is responsible for them. The present director—a physician—has established a private clinic in the school building which is under his direct care. In this clinic the pupils obtain a large proportion of their practical work.

Dr. Krafft is assisted in part of his work by Mlle. Marie Le Coultre. She has the title of directress, and has the immediate charge of the establishment; she regulates the domestic arrangements of the school and clinic, assigns various tasks to the pupils, hears recitations, and gives special attention to their training in household affairs, besides being charged with a part of their moral teaching. The directress lives in the school building.

The director makes bi-annual reports to the council. He edits the journal of the school. (This journal is called "La Source," and appears every three months.)

IV.—THE LOCATION.

La Source, a beautiful villa surrounded by gardens, is situated in the near neighborhood of Lausanne. The air is pure. In front of the building stretch the shores and blue waters of Lake Leman, while beyond is unfolded the vast panorama of the Alps of Savoy and the Jura.

The property comprises a principal building with adjuncts, in all twenty buildings. Eleven of them are occupied by the offices of the director, the rooms of the directress and pupils, and nine by the clinic.

There is running water through all parts of the buildings, and there are bathing accommodations, operation rooms, isolated rooms for contagious diseases, etc.

In short, nothing is lacking which is necessary for the recovery and the comfort of the nurses and patients.

V.—INSTRUCTION.

The pupils of La Source are taught practically and theoretically. The theoretical course covers about 120 hours, distributed, an hour a day, over the five months of training.

The complete course is divided into five branches: hygiene, anatomy, physiology, pathology, therapeutics. These subjects are taken up in succession, each for one month. This course, given by the director, comprises obstetrics, to the extent necessary for the care of women in childbed. La Source does not furnish a complete course of midwifery.

Examinations.—After the five months' course of teaching, the pupils, both internes and externes, undergo an oral examination upon the five branches taught. The markings which they obtain, combined with the markings for practical work given by the director and the directress, determine the grade of their diploma—" very satisfactory," or "satisfactory," or "sufficient."

The practical instruction is obtained: 1. Among the sick poor of the town, who are for the most part placed under the care of the director, and are visited by the pupils ; 2. With the patients in the director's private clinic and polyclinic.

Head Nurse of the Clinic.

The best ones among the pupils may prolong their service. They then take the title and assume the duties of the chief of the clinic, exercising a direct supervision over the young pupils working in the town or in the clinic. They keep order, take care of the dressings, instruments, appliances used by the director in operations, and thus perfect themselves further in the practice of their art.

Each year, sixteen pupils, internes, without counting a smaller but variable number of externes, enter La Source and leave it, furnished with diplomas, or without.

La Source has always at least four internes, at most eight, receiving their training there.

VI.—Outline of a Day's Work.

The various occupations of the pupils are apportioned to them in series of three weeks.

One pupil appointed to the kitchen service learns there how to prepare special dishes for the sick. Another does household work. Two or three are busy in the clinic, whilst their companions visit the sick in the town, accompanied by the externes, at the wish of the latter.

The clinic, I may add, rarely admits externes to its service. Two large dormitories accommodate the internes. The head-nurse of the clinic occupies a special building.

At a quarter past six in the morning all are astir. The pupils make up their beds, arrange the rooms of the patients, and attend to different household details.

At 7.30 breakfast; at 7.50 the director reads family prayers, at which all assemble—a chapter from the Bible, a few verses of a hymn sung, a prayer. Such is the preparation for the duties of the day. From 8 to 9 theoretical instruction. The director, after having questioned the pupils upon the lessons given the day before (both theoretical and practical), and being assured that they have been understood, distributes the work for the day, designates the visits to be made in the town, and orders (and explains) the treatment for each patient.

The pupils take advantage of this opportunity to ask questions or to speak of any point which puzzles or embarrasses them. This conversation lasts perhaps quarter of an hour, then follows the lecture. The director then speaks slowly enough for the pupils, the most of whom have not much facility of composition, to take complete notes. He illustrates his remarks on the blackboard, by way of making the lectures more comprehensible.

At 9 o'clock, each pupil goes to her own particular work. Broom and brush in hand, the one assigned to the house sweeps stairs, corridors, dusts and brushes.

The kitchen-assistant goes with the cook to market, or prepares the midday meal. The nurses for the town patients go to those assigned to them. If the patients are attended by the director, he gives the nurse her orders; if they are attended by some other medical man, the nurse is responsible to him.

The head-nurse of the clinic and the three or four assistants appointed for this service work with the director and under his orders, until 11 or 12 o'clock, giving baths, applications of massage or of electricity, assisting at operations, etc.

From 12 to 12.30, dinner.

There is no fixed routine for the afternoon, save one hour devoted by the directress to the pupils' recitations and to familiar talk, when she endeavors to inculcate the moral and religious principles which will fortify them for the exigencies of their future vocation. This time having elapsed, the town nurses return to their patients, the others to the clinic, others write out their notes under the supervision and with the aid of the directress.

At 5 o'clock, a second visit made to the sick by the director gives him opportunity to notice the care given them by the pupils.

At 6.30, supper.

At 8 o'clock, prayers read by the director.

At 9.30, bed.

The nurses of the town take night duty in turn with the sick poor who are seriously ill or alone.

The pupils of the clinic also do night duty in turn while their companions take a rest, well earned by the work of the day, which is always full and often very fatiguing.

VII.—PUPILS, INTERNES AND EXTERNES.

The school is open not only to all applicants of the French tongue, but to every one, whatever her nationality, who is capable of speaking and writing French legibly. La Source admits indifferently, we repeat here, unmarried, married women, and widows. It receives externes and internes.

Internes.—Conditions: To belong to the Protestant church, to possess certificates of health and morals, and to have a steadfast intention of carrying on the work of a nurse.

The director admits, of the applicants, those who present the best testimonials and appear the most capable of worthily fulfilling their duties, and from among these he chooses the ones who, having the least means pecuniarily, need to support themselves while consecrating themselves to the service of the sick.

The lectures, board and lodging, light and fires, are provided. Laundry work and all the expenses of dress are paid by the pupils. The internes live in the buildings and take their meals there, under the supervision of the director, the directress, or Mme. Krafft, who takes the place of the latter during her absence.

Externes.—The externes are selected from the leisure class, among those who wish to employ some part of their time in the gratuitous care of the sick, or those who for any reason, such as difference of religion, delicate health, or special duties, are prevented from taking the whole course and fulfilling its duties.

There is the same instruction for the externes as for the internes. The former are, however, released from a part of the practical work. The teaching is not free to the externes. Each one pays 120 francs for the complete course of lectures. In special cases the director may, at his judgment, remit all or a part of the fixed price.

VIII.—PUPILS GRADUATED FROM LA SOURCE FROM 1859 TO 1892.

For want of the early records and correspondence, it is unfortunately not possible to furnish accurate statistics of the pupils who attended the school during the first four years of its existence. After this period we find the following records:

From 1863 to the end of September, 1892, 603 pupil nurses, 492 internes, 111 externes, graduated from La Source. Among these 519 were unmarried; 84 were married or widows. The number of regular pupils, taking the whole course of five months, has not varied greatly from the usual average, 16 a year. Sometimes the number rose to 18, rarely to 20.

The externes, who were not arranged for at the outset, did not form a part of the school during the first years. The school, at that time little known, did not gather without difficulty the ·16 applicants that she had undertaken to train. By the goodness of God, however, all difficulties disappeared and the school was enabled to carry out her programme.

During the first 22 years (up to 1870) only two externes applied at La Source. From 1870 to 1881 the same number was received annually. At the present time the applications each year are from 3 to 10, and we are now without any uncertainty on the score of recruits.

Nationality of the Pupils.

500 Swiss and 103 foreigners are distributed as follows:

Swiss.

Vaud,	271	Geneva,	18	Thurgovie,	6
Berne,	89	Zurich,	16	Appenzell,	4
Neuchatel,	53	Fribourg,	10	Grisons,	5
Basle,	4	Valois,	3	Soleure,	4
Argovie,	3	Glaris,	1		
Saint-Gall,	3	Luzerne,	1		

Foreigners.

France,	55	Denmark,	3	Italy,	1
Germany,	15	Belgium,	2	Austria,	1
Great Britain,	14	Russia,	7	Australia,	1
Holland,	4				

17 cantons of Switzerland have sent us pupils. 5 only, Uri, Schwytz, Unterwald, Zoug, Tessin, have no representative in the school.

To the canton of Vaud, on the other hand, belong more than half of the Swiss pupils. Ten foreign nations have done us the honor to profit by the varied resources that the school offers. Among these France occupies the first rank, having sent us 55 pupils out of 103 that we owe to other countries than our own.   The similarity of language partly explains this fact.

X.—WORK OF THE 603 PUPILS OF THE SCHOOL DURING AND AFTER THEIR TIME OF TRAINING.

We will not consider again the daily work of the pupils during the five months that they passed at La Source. A simple resumé of their visits and night duty will sufficiently illustrate.

From 1863 to 1892 (that is, in 29 years), 58,189 visits and 4932 nights of night duty with the sick in the town have been made by the pupils. These two totals give a mean of 2006 visits and 169 nights of night duty yearly. Let us add to this sum the large one of the visits made and the watching done in the ambulance service, particularly at Pontoise (Lausanne) during the Franco-Prussian war (1871).

After graduation, a considerable number of pupils were appointed to positions by the board. Others have found work for themselves in different countries, while some have given up their profession.

The pupils are classified under the following heads :

1st. Those working in hospitals, public or private infirmaries, missionary nurses—268.

2d. Those who are gratuitously working among the poor—92.

3d. Those who can no longer pursue their work, or who, for one reason and another, have never pursued it—59.

4th. Those whose address is unknown—131.

5th. Those whose deaths have been learned—53.

Our pupils may be found not only in Europe, but in Asia, in Africa, and in Australia. At home, the greatest number may be found by the borders of Leman, in Geneva, Vevey, and Montreux. Lausanne has few; the other Vaudois villages still fewer. However, they are to be found in most of the confederate cantons, especially Berne and Neuchatel.

In France,—Paris, Lyons, Marseilles, Bordeaux, Nice, Cannes, Aix, Alois, Saint-Hippolite, Montauban, and Annonay, employ our nurses.

In Italy they are working in Milan, Naples, Genoa, San Remo. Ten or twelve of them are working in the two Americas. Some are missionaries—two in China, two in Africa, etc.

Let us now repeat—for the question of principle has the first rank with us—our pupils having finished their course, are free,—free to work where they will, free to remain in communication with the management of the school, free to enter the category of those classified "address unknown."

We are satisfied to be able to give information concerning 472, or more than three-fourths of the whole number.

HISTORY OF AMERICAN TRAINING SCHOOLS.

By Miss Irene Sutliffe,

Directress New York Hospital Training School, Honorary Vice-chairman.

In the many directions in which American women have made rapid progress in the past quarter of a century, of none can they be more justly proud than of the Training Schools for Nurses.

It is both interesting and instructive to those engaged in the work to look back upon the condition of our large city hospitals before training schools were established, and upon the struggles of the pioneer schools. To quote from a description given by one whose efforts in organizing one of the most successful schools in this city (Chicago) are well known and appreciated: "We talked with many physicians, only a few of whom sympathized with us. We were met with such statements as this: 'Oh yes; but I know an old woman who has nursed for me for years, who beats any trained nurse.' In spite, however, of every opposition from institutions, physicians and politicians, we succeeded, after meetings, speeches, etc., in getting a few influential men to rally around us, and determined to make an effort to secure money for the experiment. This was done by personal solicitation from office to office. It was a most repulsive task for refined, dignified women to undertake, but there seemed to be no alternative, and not one flinched, but met it bravely and successfully." It is true that in many institutions the nursing was done by sisters of various religious orders, whose tenderness and sympathy were much appreciated, and whose gentle influence and holy lives must have made lasting impressions upon many; but the nursing skill was lacking, and in many cases the vows taken by those noble women greatly limited their sphere of usefulness as nurses.

It is to the women of America that we owe our pioneer schools, as well as so many other good works, and it is certainly very fitting that they should be the first to recognize the importance of so great a work for women, for in its scope of usefulness to humanity at large there is no work equal to it. These schools were so well organized that not only do many essential features remain unchanged up to the present day, but they have been followed up by other schools throughout the country.

It is impossible to get reliable statistics of the training schools of this country. As early as 1798 (thirty years before Elizabeth Fry gave instructions to nurses in Guy's Hospital, and thirty-six years before Pastor Fliedner founded at Kaiserwerth the Institute for Deaconesses, for the training of women to be nurses) Dr. Valentine Seaman gave a systematic course of instruction to the nurses of the New York Hospital. In the administration building of that hospital, underneath his portrait, is a letter of presentation, from which the following is quoted :

"In 1798 he organized in the New York Hospital the first regular Training School for Nurses, from which other schools have since been established, extending their blessings throughout the community."

From 1861 a system of regular instruction has been given at the Woman's Hospital, Philadelphia, followed by examinations and the awarding of certificates. The first recognized schools of which I can get information are the New England, in Boston, and the Woman's, in Philadelphia. These were organized in 1872. That they are not better known is probably due to the fact that they are connected with small hospitals, limited to women and children. In 1873 three schools were established : Bellevue in New York, the Massachusetts General in Boston, and the Connecticut in New Haven. These three schools have done continuously good work. Bellevue has trained more nurses than any other school (424). In 1875 the school on Blackwell's Island (New York City) was organized under the Department of Charities and Correction. The good this school has accomplished in Charity Hospital may be estimated by comparing one of the reports of 1874 with a recent one.

To quote : "In the fever ward (40 beds) the only nurse was a woman from the workhouse under a six months' sentence for drunkenness, who told the patients, without any sign of shame, the story of a most shameful life. There were no chairs with backs in the hospital ; round wooden benches were the only seats, and the only pillow one of chopped straw. In the fever ward the only bathing conveniences consisted of one tin basin, a piece of soap and a ragged bit of cloth passed from bed to bed." It was the opinion of the committee that a large part of the patients in this hospital were hungry every night; butter was used occasionally, and there had been no sugar for over two months, the supply being exhausted. Order and system now reign in these wards. The patients are cared for by earnest gentlewomen, with whom we cannot associate neglect and disorder.

In 1876 the New York Hospital School was organized, and in 1877 the Buffalo General School. From this time on scarcely a year has passed without new schools in various parts of the country, a large number being in the Eastern and Middle States, but spreading to the Pacific coast and the Gulf of Mexico. The Bureau of Education, in the report of 1892, gives only 36 schools in the United States, and it is exceedingly difficult to estimate the number with any degree of accuracy. I have succeeded in obtaining the names of 148 schools. In these there are estimated to be 3250 pupils, and from these schools 4850 nurses have been graduated.

The details of government in these schools vary greatly. In most of the older schools the government is not vested in the hospital authorities, but a separate incorporated society has entire control of the management. In others the school is under the same management as the hospital, and is, in fact, a department of it. While both methods have advantages, the latter seems to be growing in favor; first, perhaps, from a financial standpoint (many of the independent schools have no endowment, depending entirely upon contributions for support, and if these prove inadequate, which not infrequently happens, the partially trained nurses are sent out to private cases, the income from which service is used to supplement the deficiency); secondly, it would seem that if the hospital and school were united there would be less friction among the workers, as all would have a common interest, and the best work can be accomplished only when harmony and happiness prevail.

There is a unique school at Waltham, Massachusetts, which seems to show that, however valuable a hospital is to a school, it is not an absolute necessity. This school was organized in 1885, and the nurses are trained by the bedsides of poor patients in their own homes. Through this school a hospital has been started; the 46 graduates have an excellent reputation, and a number fill prominent positions.

District nursing is done by several schools; that is, nurses are sent out by the training school to care for the very poor who, on account of family claims and other reasons, are unable to go to the hospitals. This is an excellent charity, the nurses not only caring for the sick, but teaching the principles of cleanliness, ventilation and economy.

The Illinois School is the first, I think, to adopt the plan of providing nurses at greatly reduced rates to people unable to pay the regular charge for trained nurses. Through the generosity of a man whose name these nurses bear, this school sends thoroughly trained nurses for a small charge, ranging within the means of the applicant, who must give proof of inability to pay the regular charge. They are not sent to charity cases, as this branch is covered by the Visiting Nurses Association, but to those who are able to pay a moderate sum.

Many schools are under religious influence, mostly connected with church hospitals. Of these, St. Luke seems to be the favorite patron saint. In some of these schools the religious element enters into the training. I find in a number of schools regular religious instruction and special services at convenient times for the nurses. In some the nurses are trained for missionary work, as well as to be nurses. In the missionary school at Battle Creek, Michigan, the course is five years; both men and women are trained as missionary nurses and doctors. This school is large and the course of instruction very elaborate.

Although nursing is essentially a woman's work, still there are cases where for obvious reasons a man's services are required. To meet this demand a few schools for training men have been organized. The Mills School in New York was started in 1888 and its success has proved its necessity.

The Training School for Colored Women, at Hampton, Virginia, connected with the Dixie Hospital, has opened a new field of usefulness for educated colored women among their own people.

There are several clubs and associations for nurses, among which is the Guild of St. Barnabas for Nurses, copied, together with so much that is good and useful, from our English sisters. The object of this guild is "to assist its members in realizing the greatness of their calling and in maintaining a high standard of Christian life and work." There are branches in many of our large cities and its influence is extending. There are over 700 members in the United States.

Truly we may look back upon the work done in twenty years with some satisfaction. Our training schools compare favorably with those of other nations. The amount of good work they have done cannot be overestimated. The sick poor, as well as the rich, are cared for in the hospitals and at their homes, and each year the demands made upon the trained nurse enlarge. Asylums, schools, homes and other institutions seek nurses as matrons and superintendents, not alone for their knowledge of nursing, but in view of the fact that their training fits them for such positions. Schools are being established all over our country, and there is reason to think that before five years more have passed there will be few hospitals of any importance in the United States without schools for nurses.

Is there not some danger in this rapid growth in number? There is no danger of the supply exceeding the demand, for the demand increases much more rapidly than the supply. The danger is in deterioration. Not all schools are well organized; too often the only object is to secure the nursing of a few patients in the most economical manner. Many hospitals have no facilities for training nurses; most of the training consisting of lectures given in the evening, when the nurses are too tired to profit by them. This will not attract desirable women, who prefer the large, well organized schools. The result is young girls just out of the schoolroom are received, and often those whose education and intelligence are very inadequate.

We often hear of the spoiled nurse, and not with injustice. Many a nurse has left the protection of her Alma Mater with the highest aspirations and noblest aims, and all too soon these are forgotten and she thinks more of her own comfort than of the beauty of self-sacrifice, and of the amount received for her services rather than of her resolution to give the best that she has cheerfully and ungrudgingly to her work. Why is this? May it not be due to the fact that her life is hard and that she loses sight of the ideal, and not being able to resist the pressure of outside influences, she grasps at the material reward of her labor? Can nothing be done to prevent this? Would not a well regulated association of nurses do much towards correcting these evils? With a standard so high that only intelligent and honorable well-trained women will be recognized as trained nurses, and by an earnest endeavor to help and influence each other, much may be done to correct these dangers and elevate the Training Schools of America.

PROPER ORGANIZATION OF TRAINING SCHOOLS IN AMERICA.

BY MISS LOUISE DARCHE,

Superintendent of New York City Training School, Matron of City and Maternity Hospitals.

In this present age of charities and philanthropy, when the care of the sick, the insane, and the destitute occupies so prominently the thought and attention of a benevolently disposed public, the building of hospitals and the management of hospitals have become one of the leading questions of the day. The improved methods of caring for the sick, as introduced by the training-school system of nursing, are generally acknowledged, and I think rightly acknowledged, as one of the prime factors in bringing about the wide-spread and intelligent interest now so generally felt in hospital work.

With the higher intelligence and skill introduced by this method of nursing came the knowledge of higher possibilities of hospital development. Doctors were not slow to grasp the idea that a system and science in the treatment of the sick could now be introduced which before, owing to the low order of intelligence and the poor education of the old-time nurse, were impossible; that accurate reports, exact obedience, cleanliness and order came with the new nurse, and that inquiry and research into new fields could now be ventured upon, based on a knowledge gained from treatment faithfully carried out and as faithfully recorded.

This improvement in the nursing when brought about first received the notice and then the encouragement of the attending physicians and surgeons under whose observation the trial was first made. The change also soon made its impression upon the hospital authorities, when it was demonstrated that where noise and unseemly altercation had prevailed in the management of "unruly patients," peace and quiet now reigned, and the so-called unruly patient seemed to disappear and become a thing of the past simultaneously with the disappearance of the old-time way of nursing and the old-time nurse. The news of this improvement in the condition of the hospital wards and the care of the hospital patients, as a result of the introduction of the training-school system, in a very short time became generally known to the outside world. The friends of the patients told of it, visiting ladies and others interested in hospital work reported it, the physicians and surgeons constantly commented on the improved results as shown by hospital statistics, and made favorable mention of the new reforms brought about by this improved system of nursing. In this way and from its very beginning we see how the training-school system found favor on all sides, and it is not difficult to trace the vital influence and bearing which it has exerted in helping to make so popular, as it is to-day, the question of hospital management and hospital care of the sick.

In considering the subject of training-school management or organization in this country it will be well to try and understand the demand or great needs which first called this system into existence here ; second, to understand some of the difficulties which had to be surmounted and overcome at the very outset of the undertaking ; and third, to trace how, in overcoming these difficulties and obstacles, the fundamental principles which underlie all good training-school government were gradually and experimentally worked out and finally established. The first fundamental principle and starting point of all training-school organization is the fact that hospitals exist, that they contain patients, and that the patients require nursing.

When the ladies who inaugurated the first training-school in America formed into a committee for the purpose of starting a school for nurses, it was not because of the need of a school, as a school for nurses; nor was it for the purpose of creating a new field of labor for women, a profession; but simply and solely because of the great need of one of the great charity hospitals for better nursing. They had visited the hospital, they had seen the misery and disorder, and they decided that any hope of reform must depend upon introducing into the wards as nurses, women of an entirely different stamp from the nurses already there. But how to do this was a question which at first sight did not seem an easy one to solve. They readily appreciated the fact that no self-respecting woman would go into the hospital and nurse under the then existing condition of affairs—to sleep where the old-time nurse slept, to eat what the old-time nurse enjoyed, to work under the then hospital officials, and to be treated with as little respect and consideration as the nurse of that time expected to be treated and deserved to be treated.

The idea of a separate administration in the management of the nurses from that of the hospital administration presented itself as the only way out of this difficulty. The hospital authorities were visited, the matter laid before them, and a contract entered into which placed the responsibility and the management of the nursing of several wards in the hospital in the hands of what has proved to be the first board of managers of the first training school in America. As this board of managers was composed of women from the first families in the country, the moral support and backing necessary to the undertaking was at one stroke accomplished. The idea of a home for the nurses, separate and away from the hospital surroundings, was at once thought of and provided; a few venturesome women of the right fiber, some of them actuated by a misssionary spirit, consented to go into the work and engage as nurses; a superintendent was secured, and the enterprise started.

Thus were three distinct features of training-school organization mapped out, viz:

(1) Hospital needs were met in providing hospital patients with conscientious and intelligent women as nurses.

(2) The nursing had been placed under a separate management and head with a distinct aim and purpose.

(3) A home for the nurses had been provided.

It will not be a difficult matter to trace from this beginning how the training-school idea was gradually developed, and along the lines of the fundamental principles thus laid down. The separate management of the nursing department, first brought about because there seemed no other way of getting the proper control of the situation, has proved to be the corner-stone of all training-school organization. The contract entered into by the hospital authorities and the board of school managers at once indicated that the relationship between hospital management and nursing management could be established on a friendly, and at the same time on an independent footing; and it was soon proved that nursing under a distinct management and head could and *did* work harmoniously with the hospital management, and to the mutual benefit and advantage of both.

Starting with this basis to work upon, the board of managers of the school found an ever-widening field of usefulness opening up before them. Under the wise direction of their representative head, the superintendent, new methods of sick-nursing and of ward-management were introduced; the staff of nurses was increased to keep pace with the additional work entailed by the new methods; with the increasing popularity of the new movement more wards were placed under the school management, and more nurses were added.

As new nurses were admitted, the older and now more experienced naturally assumed the position of head-nurses and ward-instructors. The intermediate nurses were called seniors, with duties accordingly, and a system of graded responsibility, based on experience and merit, began to take shape. In addition to the practical instruction in the wards which went hand in hand with the accomplishment of the daily nursing, the superintendent started a system of class instruction, which was later supplemented by a course of lectures on the theoretical aspect of a nurse's work, given by the visiting physicians and surgeons of the hospital.

Thus the school idea in this scheme of nursing began to gain greater prominence as it was found that not only were the patients better cared for by reducing nursing to a system, but also, that in the system and through ·its operation, women were being daily trained as nurses; *that the work itself, accomplished by proper methods and under proper supervision, had an educative value,* this educative value becoming more apparent as the nurses advanced in their course of training and became more efficient in their work.

The school, which had thus far been developed as nearly as had seemed practicable on the plan for training nurses established by Florence Nightingale, at the St. Thomas Hospital, London, England, now began to assume proportions and a bearing distinctly American.

The school had been started on very democratic principles. The women who entered to train—whatever their previous position in life—were placed on the same level or plane, and none were engaged to do the higher or more special or nicer parts of the hospital nursing. They all began at the bottom, to work on and up to the more responsible duties as they showed capacity for advancement.

At first, of necessity, the undergraduates were obliged to act as head-nurses of the wards ; the importation of head-nurses or "sisters" from abroad being too expensive to be contemplated, and as yet there were no graduate nurses here. But by degrees, what was at first regarded as a misfortune came to be considered a part of the system, and it was found that by extending the course of training from one year to two, the services of the nurses after they had obtained the practical training of the first year could be retained and utilized as head-nurses. Had they graduated at the end of the first year and been at liberty to withdraw from the hospital, so great had become the demand already for their services outside, that no salary the hospital or school authorities could afford to offer would have been sufficient to retain them, even as head-nurses in the hospital, for a second year.

Aside from this view of the case, it soon became apparent that the second year of hospital service proved to be very valuable to the nurse herself, training her in self-reliance, perfecting her in technique, developing her judgment, and giving her that power to control others which is a very essential quality in the make-up of a nurse.

During the second year also, nurses at the first were very generally sent out to nurse in private families, and in this way to add to the funds of the school; but of late years this plan of utilizing the services of a nurse during her second year has been very generally discarded by our larger and better established training-schools.

In this way was inaugurated the "two years course of training" now so generally adopted and advertised in connection with our American training-schools.

At first sight it would appear that the course of training so-called had in this country been extended over a longer period of time than the training period of the nurse at the St. Thomas Hospital, London, England; but, on investigating the subject closely and on all sides, we find that this is not the case. To quote from the St. Thomas circular of information:

"The committee of the Nightingale Fund have made arrangements with the authorities of the St. Thomas Hospital for giving a year's training to women desirous of working as hospital nurses."

"The term of the probationer's* training is a complete year. It may, however, be extended by the committee for another quarter," etc.

"At close of year their training will usually be considered complete, and during the three years next succeeding the completion of their training they will be required to enter into service as hospital nurses in such situation as may from time to time be offered them by the committee."

"At the end of a year, those whom the committee find to have passed satisfactorily through the course of instruction and training will be entered on the register as certificated nurses, and will be recommended for employment accordingly."

"The committee have hitherto readily found employment for their certificated nurses in some public hospital or infirmary at salaries usually beginning at £20, with board, washing, etc. Engagements are not to be made except through the committee, and no engagement must be terminated without quarter's notice to the committee."

"The training establishment is maintained by the Nightingale Fund which was established, etc., etc. The nurses so trained are drafted into other public institutions, but it is not the object of the Fund to train for private nursing."

*Called pupil-nurses, or nurse-in-training, in this country.

"We do not give our nurses printed certificates, but simply enter the names of all certificated nurses in the register as such."

"Obligations signed by probationers after one month's trial: Having now become practically acquainted with the duties required of a hospital nurse, I am satisfied that I shall be able and willing, on the completion of my year's training, to enter into service for the space of three years at least in whatever situation the committee shall think suitable to my abilities, it being my intention from henceforth to devote myself to hospital employment; and further agree not to enter into any engagement without first having obtained the approval of the committee and not to leave any situation without giving due notice to the committee."

From the above it would appear that a woman wishing to train as nurse at the St. Thomas must, after passing satisfactorily a month of trial, sign a paper promising to give four years of service under the control and management of the Nightingale Fund Committee, the first year as probationer under training, the other three to act in the capacity of a hospital nurse. It would also appear that although at the end of the first year she is duly registered as a certificated nurse in the hospital books, she is not given her certificate, nor even after the fourth year does she receive it.

From these facts it would seem that a nurse is never graduated in the sense of being placed on her own responsibility, but must always remain under the supervising control and authority of the training committee. It is not surprising, then, that a departure from the original system should have been found necessary in this country, where the idea of pledging oneself to a corporation or society for a period of four years, not to say indefinitely, would have been regarded as almost impossible. The board of managers of the first training-school in America, therefore, very wisely decided upon a compromise between the one year thought necessary for training and the four years pledged by the St. Thomas system, and offered a two-years course. They also decided that at the end of the two years, the nurse having proved worthy, should receive the diploma or certificate of the school, with liberty to choose for herself her future line of action; and they further decided upon a yearly commencement, where the members of the graduating class each year might receive, with a parting address, the public and honorable recognition of the close of their services as nurses of the school.

Nor, again, is this departure from its original model to be wondered at, when we remember that the aim of the Nightingale Fund connected with the St. Thomas Hospital was, first, to train women as nurses, and then to draft them off to other hospitals and infirmaries, where, pledged to a central committee of control, they worked out the chief purpose of the fund in reorganizing and reforming the hospitals and infirmaries in which they were placed.

The purely philanthropic spirit of this "missionizing and reformative" plan has not only accomplished the wise purpose of its founder in revolutionizing the nursing in hospitals over all the English-speaking world, and that in an incredibly short space of time, but it has gone further and through secondary channels has provided skilled nursing in large measure for the sick wherever placed, whether rich or poor. It has also provided a useful, honorable, and self-supporting work for many women.

The Nightingale School must ever stand alone as unique in its scope and in its organization; the pioneer school of all schools—the conception of a noble woman whose generosity and philanthropic impulse set in motion a system of caring for the sick which has brought light and comfort into more dark places than perhaps any other movement of this century.

But to return to our subject: we now approach the third phase of training-school organization as seen from an American standpoint—and this is the School Registry, managed in the interests of its graduate nurses.

Our first board of lady managers having provided a reformed system of nursing in the wards of the great hospital, as they had set out to do, and having also in the process developed a nurse-training school for women, now decided to carry on their good work a little further and institute a plan of registration which would enable their graduate nurses to get employment readily, and under the auspices of the school, and would at the same time guarantee protection to those seeking the services of a nurse.

The plan adopted was a very simple one. The graduate nurse engaged a room in some part of the city to which she could resort when off duty, with the understanding that when available for duty she would report to the registry, and hold herself in readiness to answer any call that should be sent to her. The public generally, and physicians in particular, were notified that duly trained and qualified nurses could be secured through the school registry. A reasonable weekly fee was decided upon which the nurses were allowed to charge for their services while nursing in private families. A few sensible rules were formulated for the purpose of protecting the nurses from unjust or an undue amount of continuous duty, suggesting also their obligations to the registry, and to the families in which they should be engaged to nurse. A small yearly fee, sufficient to cover the expense of registry-calls, was instituted, to be paid by the nurse; the superintendent of the school was made responsible for the registry management, subject, as in the school management, to the approval of the managing committee; and the third phase of training-school organization was completed.

That this plan of registration succeeded is not surprising when we consider the forces thus set in motion. The newly graduated nurse, as she entered upon private duty under the supervision of her school, felt both stimulated and encouraged to prove herself worthy in this new field of labor. The school management feeling itself thus closely and directly represented to a critical public, naturally felt desirous of promoting a higher degree of excellence in the training and education of its student-nurse. The medical profession, finding a ready means of procuring trained nurses for private cases, patronized the registry, and the registry thus established continued to be appreciated and to flourish. Thus was the school in its threefold aspect completed, and stands to-day representative of training-school organization in America.

It is true, many and various deviations from this original design, to suit the exigencies of peculiar hospital management, have been made; but it is only when the fundamental principles first laid down by Miss Nightingale at the St. Thomas Hospital, England, and afterwards introduced here, are adhered to in all their essential entirety, that there will be harmonious and successful training-school development and organization.

The essential elements of proper training-school organization, then, may be briefly stated as:

(1). A hospital containing a fair proportion of medical, surgical, and obstetrical cases; the hospital constructed with ordinary conveniences for the care of patients.

(2). The understanding that the nursing is to be considered a distinct department in itself, whether managed under the hospital or a separate board of control.

(3). As head, a superintendent who will herself be a trained nurse and a woman of considerable executive ability.

(4). A home for nurses, removed from close proximity to the hospital wards, and so arranged that nurses when off duty may enjoy the ordinary comforts of home life.

(5). A definite course of lessons and lectures embracing all theoretical instruction necessary in the education of a nurse.

(6). A board of lecturers and examiners composed of visiting physicians and surgeons of the hospital, and who, with the superintendent, will conduct the final examinations and award diplomas.

(7). A school registry, to be managed in the interests of its graduate nurses.

One of the first points to determine in training-school organization is the relationship the school management shall maintain to the hospital management—whether the school will be under a separate board or committee, or whether it will be managed by the hospital board or committee. In the first case, a contract will be entered into which will make the school committee responsible to the hospital committee for the proper nursing of the hospital; in the second case, the head or superintendent appointed by the hospital board or committee to be over the nursing department, will be held responsible for the proper nursing of the hospital.

Good schools are conducted upon either plan, *the point being to have it distinctly understood that the nursing is considered a department in itself, and is to be organized and managed as such.*

This vital point having been settled and a superintendent appointed, several questions at once arise as to her jurisdiction: what shall her relationship towards the heads of the other departments of the hospital be? What the limit of her prerogatives? What her authority?

The importance of these questions demands the highest authority, and I cannot do better than quote Miss Nightingale on these points. In her paper on "Relation of Hospital Management to Efficient Nursing," she says:

"Vest the charge of financial matters and general supervision, and the whole administration of the infirmary, in the board or committee; *i. e.*, in the officer who is responsible to that board or committee. Vest the whole responsibility for nursing, internal management, for discipline and training of nurses, in the one female head of the nursing staff, whatever she may be called. The necessity of this is not matter of opinion, but of fact and experience."

"The training or nursing matron should be responsible to the governing authorities of the infirmary or hospital, or to any committee appointed by them for the purpose."

"There should be but one superintendent or training matron in the nursing department, and it follows as a matter of course that she should also be matron of the hospital. She may have a housekeeper subordinate to her, and, if the

training school be large, a deputy mistress (assistant superintendent) of probationers (pupil nurses)."

"She should be made responsible, too, for her results, and not for her
methods. Of course, if she does not exercise the authority entrusted to her
with judgment and discretion, it is then the legitimate province of the governing body to interfere and remove her."

"The matron or nursing superintendent must be held responsible for the
conduct, discipline, and duties of her nurses, for the discipline of her sick
wards, for the care and cleanliness of the sick, for the administration of diets
and medicine, for the care of linen and bedding, and probably for the patients'
clothing."

"The duties which each grade has to perform should be laid down by
regulation, and all that the medical department or the governing body of the
hospital has a right to require is that the regulation duties shall be faithfully
performed."

"Any remissness or neglect of duty, as a breach of discipline, can only be
dealt with to any good purpose by report to the matron (superintendent of
nurses) of the infirmary."

"No good ever comes of the constituted authorities placing themselves in
the office which they have sanctioned her occupying. No good ever comes of
any one interfering between the head of the nursing department and her
nurses. It is fatal to discipline."

"It is necessary to dwell strongly on this point, because there has been not
unfrequently a disposition shown to make the nursing establishment responsible, on the side of discipline, to the medical officer or to the governor of the
hospital. Any attempt to introduce such a system would be merely to try anew
and fail anew in an attempt which has frequently been made. In disciplining
matters, a woman can only understand a woman."

"Simplicity of rules, placing the nurses in all matters regarding treatment
of the sick absolutely under orders of medical men, and in all disciplining
matters absolutely under the female superintendent, to whom the medical
officer shall report all cases of neglect, is very important. At the outset there
must be a clear and recorded definition of these classes of jurisdiction."

From the above it is evident that Miss Nightingale considers it of
the first importance that the question of the duties, responsibilities,
and limit of authority of the head of the nursing department or
school should be unmistakably understood and defined from the
very beginning, and she has left no doubt in our minds as to what
she considers this responsibility and authority should be.

Given a hospital, a home for nurses, and a competent head for the
school, authorized to work on the lines laid down by Miss Nightingale, the development of any individual school is but a matter of
time and of detail management. A definite understanding and statement should be made regarding the number of hours of daily work

which will be expected of a nurse; the time which will be allowed daily for rest and study ; the course of lessons and lectures which will be given, the facilities for practical training, and the outlook or prospects of future usefulness open to graduates of the school.

The subjects taught in training schools are usually anatomy and physiology, materia medica, and methods of nursing, for a first year's course ; and diseases, surgery, obstetrics, hygiene, sanitation, etc., for a second year's course. Usually a class receives a weekly lesson, with a course of from 30 to 40 lectures, for 18 or 20 months out of the two years ; but to what extent or in what proportion, each school determines for itself. In America many of the large schools have gradually worked up to a standard of excellence, which the smaller and less important training schools look upon as the standard of training-school education ; but we of the larger schools are not satisfied, and know that a general standard of excellence must be arrived at before trained nursing can take that stand among the professions which it is entitled to take, but which it will never take until its training methods are more *universally* exact, and its course of instruction in every school more definitely and strictly laid down.

It is much to be desired that some plan might be devised by means of which a closer intercourse between training schools might be brought about. We need to co-operate in the interests of the profession, to promote what is good and to eliminate what is bad. Much has been accomplished, but much remains to be accomplished ; and we must bear in mind that any successful development in the future will lie in unitedly establishing and unitedly keeping the standard of our work at its highest possible point. From its nature nursing is peculiarly a woman's work ; a woman originated the training-school system in England, women started it in this country, women have brought it to its present stage of development, and it is to women we must look for its future advancement.

DISCUSSION.

MISS LEVINS, of Chicago.—There is only one point I want to make in regard to the last speaker's address, and that was her final point, that it is desirable to have more uniformity of action among nurses at large. As she spoke I was reminded of the remark of Mr. Burdett, yesterday, that we should follow the privilege of personal service, and there can be no successful alumnæ association or national association or international association until each one comes to feel a personal pride and interest and pleasure in furthering the interest of her own organization and of her workers as a class. So in our Chicago alumnæ or in your private alumnæ, and in the efforts being made to establish a national association, and ultimately, as your chairman has suggested, an international association that will never be planted upon a successful basis unless the feeling expressed by the gentleman yesterday is taken into individual consideration, that there is a privilege in personal service in each one trying to attend the meetings and doing all she can to further the interests of the associations, either the alumnæ, national or international.

MISS MCKECHNIE, of Louisville, Kentucky.—I would like to ask Miss Darche in connection with one point of her paper about the registry : if the training school has anything to do with arranging the prices of nurses when they go out from the school.

MISS DARCHE.—I understand where there is a school registry managed by the superintendent of the training school, that there are set rules and set charges. It is generally more for obstetric and contagious cases than ordinary cases. Each school has generally adopted, I believe, the standard set by the first school, of from $20 to $25 a week, according to the case. In the smaller towns where it is not so expensive to live, they very easily can work for $15 a week, and they will receive as much benefit as those who charge more in the cities.

MISS WALD, of New York.—Why should a training school or hospital have the right of deciding what a nurse shall charge? She should have the privilege of setting her own price. It is as much professional work as that of the physician.

MISS DARCHE.—I will answer that question. As I understand the school registry, it is perfectly optional with the graduating nurse to belong to that registry or not. If she belongs to it she must conform to the rules of the registry. If she wishes to be independent and get her cases independent of the registry, she may charge what she pleases.

MISS ALSTON, of New York.—I was going to say that I think the graduates of the training school really find a great protection to have these prices set. Their prices are often contested, and if they have a paper on which it is stated what they can charge, then all they have to do is to present this paper to the family and they will know that they have the sanction of the board, and nothing more can be said.

MRS. NIXON, of Chicago.—It is a common remark in Chicago amongst society people, that "none but a pauper or millionaire can enjoy the luxury of a nurse," and I was very much surprised to hear from the first paper that the Creerar organization was the first institution to meet the needs of the largest of our population, that is, people receiving small salaries; and I would like to repeat the suggestion made by the president of the Illinois Training School to the graduating class last week, that each graduate should agree to take one case a year under the system of the Creerar fund, which will give a nurse from $3 to $10 a week, and render her services to people whose salaries will not admit of paying more. I think that would be a fine thing for the nurses of every city represented here. There are nurses, I know, who give their services at a very low figure in a private way, but if some organization of that kind could be formed I think it would meet a great want in this country.

MISS WALD.—I should like to ask how that could be regulated. One case might last a week and the next three months.

MRS. NIXON.—I understand they take a case for so long, and if it runs over they divide up with another. It was simply a suggestion made by our president. I don't know whether the nurses would be willing to subscribe to it or not.

MISS SHIELD, of Indiana.—I would like to ask Miss Darche if the nurses are allowed to charge less than the directory fees.

MISS DARCHE.—I think the idea generally is, if you want to give your time for less, to give a whole week or a few days for nothing, but don't lower the price of the registry.

MISS ROGERS, of Washington.—It seems to me this fixed method is a little unfair to the older nurses, if they can only demand what a nurse doing her first private work can demand. It looks to me like a very unfair adjustment of things if a nurse, after ten years' experience, is only as valuable as one doing her first week.

MISS SUTLIFFE, of New York.—I think the nurses ought to charge what they think their services are worth, provided they make that known before they register.

THE CHAIRMAN.—I suppose you mean they would not charge less?

MISS SUTLIFFE.—They ought not to charge less than the regular charge.

MISS DARCHE.—Some registries are conducted on the plan of a range of prices, from $25 up to $30. A nurse can say that she will not go out for less than $25 a week or $30 a week, but she has to take chances of getting employment from those people. The other way is the way I spoke of in my paper where they have a regular schedule of prices, and the older nurses find after a while that they don't need the aid of the registry at all, they get cases independent of them, and they can charge what they wish. It is for the protection and care of the younger ones. Generally, a nurse prefers to be associated.

THE CHAIRMAN.—There was a statement in the paper of Miss Sutliffe which I think is not correct, that the Creerar fund was the first to send out nurses at moderate prices to families with moderate means. I have not corrected it before because I could not remember the name of the fund in New York. It started some five years ago and was called the Dubois fund, but I am not positive that it is in existence now, but I think it is. If any one can tell us about it it will rectify the error.

MISS LETT, of Chicago.—I think in some schools the graduate nurses give their superintendents the privilege of assigning them for two weeks to poor patients. I have had it so for two years. This year I had two weeks given to me whenever I liked to use it to devote to people that cannot afford to pay. I think that spirit ought to be encouraged in every training school.

MISS McKECHNIE, of Kentucky.—The Dubois fund was in operation last year.

THE CHAIRMAN.—Then it is probably in operation yet, and the Creerar fund is the second.

TRAINED NURSES AS SUPERINTENDENTS OF HOSPITALS.

By MISS E. P. DAVIS,

Superintendent of the University of Pennsylvania Hospital, Honorary Vice-Chairman.

A woman who has taken the training required to fit her to graduate from any of our large, well organized, well conducted training schools for nurses, must, it can easily be seen, have many advantages and therefore be better prepared, other things being equal, to be the superintendent of a hospital than the man or woman who has little or no hospital experience.

True, the training of a nurse has not in the past in any way been looking towards being superintendent of an hospital as the ultimatum; nevertheless, the general training in institution nursing, discipline and routine which she has received tends to develop exactly the qualities requisite for such a position.

In looking about for a person to fill the position under consideration there are several qualifications which it seems peculiarly desirable that a candidate should possess.

He or she should be a person of liberal education, large executive ability and adaptability, firmly grounded in principles of justice and morality; one who can work side by side with an equal without friction, or direct subordinates without antagonizing them.

A probationer is accepted as a nurse if she, during her month or two months, as the case may be, of probation, gives evidence of possessing the majority of the above-mentioned qualities in a more or less marked degree. If then she is selected to fill the office of superintendent we may feel assured that she is a woman of some education, as only such are accepted in first-class training schools. It does not remain to be proven that she is a person of responsibility; that has already been demonstrated by the ability with which she discharged her duties and the manner in which she carefully avoided encroaching upon the prerogative of others when placed in positions of trust.

The officers of the training school have come to rely as much on her justice and veracity as on her tact and judgment. She has always been depended upon to carry out an order unquestioningly, if issued by the proper authority. When she comes to be superintendent she will not be less loyal to the management of the hospital than she was to the school, and will expect and insist upon a like intelligent fidelity from her fellow-officers and subordinates.

She has been instructed in the theory of ward and hospital cleanliness. Still better, she has been obliged to minutely and laboriously practice it. Acting on the principle that nothing is clean if it can be made cleaner, she has day after day systematically and carefully gone through the same routine of thoroughly cleansing patients and hospital paraphernalia alike. She is taught that it is not enough that things look clean: to be aseptic they must *be* clean. From having thus had a personal acquaintance with its details she will be able to judge of the quantity and quality of the work performed.

She has held positions where it was her duty to instruct, to criticize and to inspect. As the head of the hospital, the ability to perform all of these functions will constantly be called into operation in a much broader and more varied degree.

She has some knowledge of the quantity of material to be used in hospitals in contradistinction to other institutions, such as the number of sheets, towels, etc., allowed to each bed. She knows about hospital equipments, such as bedsteads, mattresses, etc., which are considered the best theoretically and which are the best practically; she knows about instruments, their care and cost; about surgical appliances and dressings, their preparation and preservation, etc.

She knows if a hospital is well furnished with necessary things, and if such supplies are too lavishly used; and she knows how to devise means to check such expenditures without detriment to the good service rendered.

She has been taught to be ready for emergencies of all kinds, to be self-possessed, never to lose her presence of mind under any circumstances, to act coolly and promptly in the most trying situations, so that there may be no unnecessary discomfort and no lives endangered by short-sightedness in preparing for the unexpected, or lack of dexterity in cases that require promptness and decision in execution.

The care of the sick is the central point in a hospital round which all things else revolve. The time and talent of every one connected with the institution is expended for the benefit of the patients; it goes without saying that the knowledge of the personal care of the sick will be her strong point—the patients will certainly lose nothing by having a trained nurse as a hospital superintendent.

She has been trained to be systematic, and has also become impressed with the desirability of reducing all departments of her charge to the same condition. In that respect she will meet with the hearty co-operation of her assistant, who will also be a trained nurse, thereby materially lessening the friction that sometimes exists between an untrained superintendent and a trained assistant.

If for any reason a person directly in charge of the nursing (directress of nurses, superintendent or assistant superintendent of nurses, or whatever she may styled) is unexpectedly obliged to leave, or becomes so ill that her place will have to be filled, the nursing need in no way become demoralized; the superintendent, if she be a trained nurse, can have the direct oversight of the work and carry it on quite successfully until the place be satisfactorily filled.

She comes to her work single-minded, she does not make the hospital a stepping-stone to some other ambition, she has not the care of a family to divide her time and thought, and thereby materially lessens the expense of the hospital in providing them suitable apartments, maintenance and service.

I see but one disadvantage to a hospital having a trained nurse for a superintendent, and in some instances that may not exist,—the total lack of business training. Very few women who enter a training school have the faintest idea of business methods, and the training develops that quality least of all. She has to compete with men who for years have been engaged in some occupation or profession where their business ability has been more or less called into exercise, and she also has to compete with women whose business ability is almost, if not altogether, their only qualification.

It has become a recognized fact that trained nurses have made successful hospital superintendents without any business training, but only the person herself knows the amount of brain and nerve force she has been obliged to expend in order to acquaint herself with the details of the accounts and office-work generally. All her other qualifications would have counted for nothing if she could not have mastered this one serious impediment, and her efforts, instead of being crowned with success, would have proven a dismal failure.

With so many advantages to begin with, I cannot see any reason why she should not go on broadening and extending her sphere of usefulness and knowledge in this direction.

Seeing that trained nurses are taking their places as superintendents, it behooves us who are in the work to look to it that they are properly fitted for it. I think you will agree with me that the time has come either to add the necessary business course to the present curriculum of the school, to have an extended term devoted to this course, or a postgraduate course, eligible only to those showing a special inclination or aptitude for the work.

Let her not be handicapped longer by want of preparation, but be fully equipped to do justice to the school from which she graduates, to herself as a woman, and to the people who employ her.

I venture to hope that when the time comes that the trained nurse has also become the trained superintendent, that we can recommend her to that position with the same confidence that we now do a trained nurse to a nurse's position; that no hospital management will offer or expect her to accept a salary less than they would offer to an untrained person, but be prepared to acknowledge the benefits of the training in the same proportionate way that a trained nurse receives compensation over an untrained one.

DISCUSSION.

MISS ROGERS, of Washington.—I don't know as I can offer any discussion, but I would be glad to emphasize the point upon special preparation for the superintendency of a hospital. So many small hospitals combine the superintendent of nurses and the superintendent of the hospital; they cannot afford two separate officers, and they combine these officers, and it is found more and more that the trained nurse who takes the position of superintendent of nursing also becomes the head and front of the hospital, and nine times out of ten has no experience except that of a head-nurse in a large hospital. This does not teach her to take care of the business management of the hospital, to attend to the surgeons, to look after the laundries, and to take care of the accounts, and it does not give her the tact required to please these various people. The smaller the hospital, as a rule, the larger the management. I have known a hospital with 80 beds and 100 managers, and you will find perhaps, after a year or two of such work, that you are totally unfitted for your proper duties, because you have exhausted your nerves and brains and stomach trying to train yourselves to be everything to every manager. You have also to put their ideas on one side, when they do not agree with yours, without making bad feeling. I think if the training schools of the larger hospitals could give an extra course of three or six months as assistant superintendent, to the nurse, it would give her a general oversight over the whole thing, and she would please the public in general much more. I think there would be fewer vacancies caused by death if we had a little more of that sort of training.

MISS DENNIS, of Syracuse.—As president of a small hospital, I wish to say to Miss Rogers that all she has stated is true. I am so fortunate, and have been for some years, as to have a superintendent that covers all these points and more satisfactorily, and I wish to second Miss Rogers' point on the necessity of a short business training for nurses in small hospitals. We have thirty beds and twenty-four managers, so the beds have a little advantage of the management.

MISS DARCHE.—It is a pity we cannot arrange some plan of training managers and directors on their side. I think they would realize the situation a little bit.

THE ORIGIN AND PRESENT WORK OF QUEEN VICTORIA'S JUBILEE INSTITUTE FOR NURSES.

By Miss Amy Hughes,

Superintendent, Metropolitan and National Nursing Association, London, Eng.,
Honorary Chairman.

In coming before you as a representative of "Queen Victoria's Jubilee Institute for Nurses," it may not be amiss if in the first place I give a short sketch of district work, what it is and what it entails, before referring to the special objects for which the "Queen's Institute" was founded.

I. District nursing is the technical name for the work of nursing the sick poor in their own homes.

There is no doubt that this strikes many minds at first as an unnecessary form for philanthropy to take, if not an absolutely unwise one.

To those who know something of the slums and alleys of large cities and the small crowded cottages of the country, it would appear that the only means of restoring health or lessening discomfort to the inhabitants who are stricken with disease, would be to remove them without delay to places where fresh air, cleanliness and proper food are awaiting them.

A quotation from an admirable work on the care of the sick at home and in hospital, by the well-known Dr. Billroth, forcibly expresses these opinions, which may be shared by many now present:

" It is evident that the essential conditions of rational and successful sick-nursing, . . . such as good air, light, warmth, bedding, good food, etc., are altogether wanting in the homes of the poor. Of what use are the gratuitous supply and regular giving of medicines, if every necessary is wanting even for ordinary healthy living? It is not that the nurse shrinks from enduring the privations and injurious influences existing in the cottages and hovels, but it is the impossibility of being useful under such circumstances, that renders home nursing unattainable for the poor. One can comfort them in their cottages, and give them food and medicine gratuitously, but to nurse and treat them there with any prospect of success cannot be done."

In answer to this and other equally strong arguments, four important considerations may be urged in reply.

1. There are innumerable forms of chronic disease which are unsuitable for treatment in general hospitals, but which may be as well attended in their own homes by skilled workers. These cases include cancer in its many phases, paralysis, chronic rheumatism, and bronchitis, ulcers, phthisis in its last stages, and many obstetric cases. By bringing trained nursing to these sufferers, it prevents the overcrowding of the public hospitals and infirmaries, leaving vacancies for cases that can be cured, without condemning the rejected ones to suffer without any alleviation of their misery.

Again, cases frequently occur where medical aid has been called in so late that any attempt to remove the patient to more favorable surroundings would probably cause a fatal ending to the illness. Here the only chance is to call in skilled assistance, and in spite of all disadvantages to place the patient in as good condition as experience and training will suggest, and it is wonderful what can thus be done.

2. The visiting of these unwholesome quarters by trained workers brings sanitation into the worst hovels, as the nurse is bound to inculcate some knowledge, however elementary, of cleanliness and ventilation. Besides, she is able to bring unsanitary conditions under the notice of the proper authorities, and thus nuisances are removed which would become hotbeds of infection if not thus reported.

3. Many homes are kept together, and untold misery prevented by the head of the family being able to remain as a moral support to the rest. Many instances might be quoted where the presence of the father or mother, even though very ill, has been the means of keeping order and regularity in a home, while without this the whole establishment would have been broken up. The moral advantages, especially where there are young children, can hardly be overestimated.

4. This form of nursing the poor stands comparison most favorably with the nursing in hospitals, as regards its cost. In proportion to its results, it is much less expensive.

It spite of all objections, therefore, the necessity for home nursing has long been recognized, and its practicability demonstrated thoroughly.

It was first definitely formulated in Liverpool in 1859, a trained nurse being sent to work in a small district.

The experiment proved so successful, such good results being obtained, not only in alleviating suffering, but in the moral good effected, that its promoter, Mr. W. Rathbone, M. P., was encouraged to extend the work, and within four years the whole of Liverpool was divided into 18 districts, each supplied by a trained nurse. This success gave an impulse to the work all over the country, and parochial nurses were started in many towns.

II. I pass on now to the work of district nursing in its immediate connection with the "Queen's Institute."

In 1868 the East London Nursing Society was started by the Hon. Mrs. Stuart Wortley, Mr. R. Ingram, and others. This provides trained nurses, who each live in the district she nurses, several of them being under the charge of a trained matron. This society is now in affiliation with the Institute.

In 1874 the Metropolitan and National Nursing Association was brought into existence, with a view of raising the whole standard of district work to higher level. This movement was initiated by the Council of the Order of St. John of Jerusalem, and set on foot by Lady Strangford, Mr. Ingram, Sir H. W. Acland, Sir Rutherford Alcock, Mr. Rathbone, Mr. Bonham Carter, and others interested in the work. The Duke of Westminster also gave his support, and has been a friend to district nursing ever since.

It was resolved to adopt the principle that the nurses should live together in homes under a trained district superintendent, and Miss Florence Lees, now Mrs. Dacre Craven, was the first superintendent of the central home. It was also decided to select nurses from the class of gentlewomen, with a view to bringing women of higher education and refinement to grapple with the special difficulties of the work, and the experiment has proved eminently successful.

From this center several homes were rapidly started, until in 1887 there were nine established in London on these principles, and some in the country.

In 1887 was founded "Queen Victoria's Jubilee Institute for Nurses," which has gathered up into one grand system all the previously existing forms of district nursing. Its origin and work are most admirably described by the president, the Rev. A. L. B. Peile, Master of St. Katharine's Royal Hospital.

This hospital was founded in 1148 by Queen Matilda, wife of Stephen, and received various royal charters in the reigns of other sovereigns. In the charter of Queen Philippa, wife of Edward III, it was particularly charged upon the sisters, as belonging to their office, that they should nurse the sick in time of illness, and otherwise minister to their necessities. It seemed, therefore, most suitable in founding an institute for training nurses for the sick poor in their own homes, that St. Katharine's, associated of old with such work in the past, should be the headquarters of a larger effort in the same direction for the future.

I cannot do better than quote the Master's account of its origin:

" It is the outcome of the offering of the women of England which was made by them to her most gracious Majesty Queen Victoria on the completion of the fifty years of her most illustrious reign. After her Majesty had associated that gift with the late Prince Consort by erecting a statue to his memory in Windsor Park, and had accepted a personal gift at the special desire of the donors, there remained a considerable balance of £70,000, which her Majesty desired to devote to some special object of public usefulness. With that fine instinct of queenly love, and tenderness and sympathy for others, her Majesty determined to devote this large sum in trust for the purpose of training nurses to minister in times of sickness to the poor in their own homes ; and for this purpose appointed as trustees of the fund the Duke of Westminster, Sir James Paget and Sir Rutherford Alcock. It was her wish that the poor should have the advantages of skilled and thoroughly trained nurses in the time of sickness equally with their richer neighbors—with this great exception, that while those who can afford to do so pay for the nurses' services, the poor may freely have the best that can be had, absolutely without any cost to themselves."

In order to carry out this trust in the best possible way, a provisional committee was appointed to set the work in motion, and then the Institute was incorporated by royal charter. The council consists of 24 members, to be elected by the Queen every three years ; the president alone, as Master of St. Katharine's, being permanent, in virtue of his office.

It was decided to utilize all the valuable experience gained by the working of the various existing systems, and therefore the council drew up a form of conditions of affiliation, which was circulated to the committees of the different associations, so that they might judge whether they felt it desirable to seek affiliation with the Queen's Institute. The result of this has been that in the report of the council for 1892 it is stated there are now 52 affiliated associations in England, 36 in Scotland, 6 in Ireland, and 7 in Wales.

The central home of the Metropolitan and National Nursing Association was selected as the central training home for the Institute in England. Scotland, Wales and Ireland have also central homes in their respective capitals for training their own nurses. The various committees of the Queen's Institute deal with different branches of the work. To the "Affiliation Committee," for instance, come all applications from existing associations who desire to affiliate, or from places who wish to start nursing work under the auspices of the Queen's Institute. By so doing, associations obtain the help and support of the Institute, they are supplied with fully trained Queen's nurses, and have the great advantage of the inspector's visits, by which a uniform standard of training and work is maintained all over the kingdom.

Affiliation in no way interferes with the arrangements of local committees, which make their own rules and arrangements, provided always the conditions of affiliation are maintained.

One of the most essential is that the work must be absolutely unsectarian, both as to the training of nurses and the nursing of the poor. If this were not insisted upon, the nurse might be looked upon as a proselytizer, and her work regarded as a cover for other objects. Nurses of all denominations are accepted, and the council always endeavor to suit the nurse to the post to which she is to be sent.

It is also required that nurses in town should live in a Home, and not in separate lodgings, under a superintendent, and that all the nurses employed be fully trained. The value and importance of the inspector's office can hardly be overestimated.

When an association desires affiliation, or an appeal for starting work is received, all information possible is obtained by means of printed forms, and if satisfactory, the inspector makes a personal visit, and her report guides the decision of the committee. In thus accepting or starting an association, it is required that the expense of the work must be undertaken by those who wish to establish it.

The inspector gives full information regarding the expenses that must be incurred, the lines upon which the work is carried out, and, in fact, makes the whole plan of the Institute intelligible to those who wish to join it.

And when an association is thus started, the subsequent value of the inspector's visits is inestimable. Being herself a trained nurse, her advice and help are a boon to the nurses themselves and those interested in the work. There is no interference with local arrangements; all that is done is to see that the conditions of affiliation are carried out, and that the nursing itself is well and thoroughly done. Every home and nurse belonging to the Institute in the United Kingdom is thus systematically visited, and this has done more to establish and consolidate the work than almost anything else.

And not only in towns is the work going on, but in the country villages and hamlets. The Rural Nursing Association had already come into existence to meet the difficulty of providing skilled nursing for scattered country folk, and it is now affiliated and known as the Rural Branch of Queen Victoria's Jubilee Institute. It has its own committee and superintendent of nurses, but works under the Institute entirely.

It provides nurses for towns not exceeding a population of 9000, and for all country districts.

In Scotland the work is carried on by a Scotch Council. There is a central training home for nurses in Edinburgh, besides homes in Glasgow, Dundee, and other centers.

The Scottish branch works as does every affiliated association. The work of the nurses is subject to inspection from the Institute, and the full affiliation of each local association is dependent upon the report of the inspector.

Quarterly reports are made to the council of the Institute from the Scottish council, besides the report given by the inspector.

In Ireland the work was much more difficult to initiate, but though slow, its progress has been steady. In Dublin there are two training homes, one at St. Patrick's, for Protestant nurses, and one in Mary Street, for Roman Catholics, both under the care of one superintendent, specially appointed by the Institute.

Three branches have been started, and the work is progressing as quickly as the supply of nurses and increase of funds will permit.

In Wales the central home is at Cardiff, where nurses, especially Welsh-speaking ones, are trained for the work. It is steadily proceeding, though not yet so widely spread as it will be when the object for which the Institute was set on foot is more widely recognized.

III. Having thus briefly sketched the outlines of the rise and progress of district nursing, from the one nurse in Liverpool in 1859 to the grand system spreading rapidly over every part of Great Britain and Ireland at the present time, I must add a few words regarding the nurses themselves, their training and their work.

The council of the Queen's Institute requires that every candidate for the post of Queen's nurse must have had at least one year's consecutive experience in one of the approved general hospitals, which are large enough to furnish full experience in nursing every kind of case, and where theoretical instruction is also given to the probationers. This is followed by six months' experience in district work, including the care of women and infants after childbirth, under the constant supervision of the superintendent of one of the recognized training homes. This is the minimum of training required, but the majority of the nurses have received from two to four years' hospital experience, including fever duty and obstetrical training, and many in addition hold the diploma of the London Obstetrical Society, qualifying them to practice as midwives, or are certificated monthly nurses. The Institute is prepared to give midwifery training to any candidate willing to practice that branch of nursing, which is frequently essential in country posts.

Before accepting any application for a probationer, full inquiries are made regarding the past history and personal character of the candidate, as well as her nursing qualifications. Every candidate is passed by the inspector before being sent to the training home. The first month is considered as a trial of the probationer's fitness for the work, and if at the end of this time she appears suitable, and the superintendent is able to send a satisfactory report to the inspector, the nurse signs an agreement to remain in the employment of the Institute for two years from the end of the district training, in consideration of the expenses incurred for her during that period. A report of every detail of her work is sent each month by the superintendent to the inspector, who herself sees the nurse's work. During these six months the nurse is known as a Queen's probationer, and has the advantage of attending three courses of lectures on hygiene, fevers and obstetric nursing given by well-known authorities. If the training ends satisfactorily, the nurse is appointed to a suitable post, and is recommended as deserving to be placed on the roll of Queen's nurses. She receives a brassard worked with the Queen's cypher, and the bronze medal of the Institute.

These details are thus given fully to show how thoroughly the Institute endeavors to investigate and ascertain the suitability of nurses employed under it.

The advantages of requiring the nurses to live together under a superintendent in districts which need several workers are many and tangible ones.

The common life promotes zeal and *esprit de corps;* the work is more methodically arranged by one head ; waste of time and strength being prevented by having the superintendent on the spot if any difficulty arises.   The nurses are relieved from any housekeeping anxieties, thus enabling them to rest in mind and body when off duty, and the general tone and standard of work are better maintained.

The general plan of the work is as follows: The superintendent puts herself personally, or through the honorable secretary, into communication with the parish doctors and other medical men practising among the poor, the poor-law authorities, the clergy, district visitors, sisterhoods, bible readers, mission women, the Charity Organization Society, the Society for the Relief of Distress, and other persons or societies working amongst the poor. Applications for nursing services, when received at the Home, are visited as soon as possible. If it is a proper " nursing case," the patient, and if necessary the rooms, are put into nursing order.

When the case has been sent by a doctor, his orders are carried out, and in all cases the nurse receives his instructions in writing, on forms supplied specially for the purpose.

No case is retained on the books which is not under a qualified medical practitioner.

Every nurse visits her patients once daily, acute cases twice, or much oftener if necessary, Sundays and week-days alike, making a regular round, and recording notes of each case for the doctor in attendance.   The time the nurse stays and the attention she gives to each patient depend on the nature of the particular case.

The relatives and friends of the patient can often be taught to keep the room in a proper condition to ensure good ventilation, etc.   In cases where no one is at hand, the nurse will do the work herself.

Nurses are not allowed to give money or relief of any kind except under special circumstances, with the approval of the superintendent.

No nurse ceases to visit the patients assigned to her until they are taken off the books by the superintendent.

That it is desirable to secure the services of educated and refined women has been proved by experience.

The responsibilities of a district nurse are infinitely greater than those of one working in a hospital with the doctors to turn to in any emergency, therefore the more highly trained and intelligent nurse is better fitted to exercise this responsibility.   The same higher education and greater refinement exercise a beneficial influence over the patients and their friends. It needs genuine tact, innate courtesy, to deal successfully with the ignorance and prejudices of the poor. A successful district nurse must be able to command their respect and win their love if she is to carry out the reforms so needed in their homes, and if she is to exert any real and permanent influence for good over them.

I have thus briefly endeavored to lay before you the general plan of the working of the Queen's Institute. It is yet in the early stages of its growth, but during the few years since the Queen's Jubilee, when it was called into existence, it has been able to make a considerable advance in its efforts to train nurses to work among the sick poor in their own homes. It is not saying too much to express the opinion that a very decided impetus has been given to this work through its agency, and that the position it holds as being under the direct influence of the Queen has made it the center of this form of nursing, and has called forth a great deal of local effort in every part of the kingdom in setting on foot nursing associations where they had not previously existed, and in uniting and organizing many which were working independently and without a uniform standard.

DISTRICT NURSING.

By Miss C. E. M. Somerville,

Lawrence General Hospital, Lawrence, Mass.

District nursing is now recognized as a distinct branch of the great nursing profession. The last quarter of the century was well advanced when America caught the reflection of England's light, and the era of trained nursing for the poor began in this country. At this date in the last decade, let us see how far the rays have penetrated in one direction, and ask if we are not justified in hoping that the new century will find us in the full blaze of sunlight, and that the darkness, disease and foul air of our tenements will have been dispelled and purified through the systematic efforts of organized trained nursing.

As far as I have been able to learn, the first society to employ the services of a hospital-trained nurse for the care of the sick poor in their homes was the Woman's Branch of the New York City Mission and Tract Society. Its report of 1877 says : " A new power for good has been introduced this year—the missionary nurse. Prepared in the training school, she is thoroughly competent to do all that is necessary in cases of extreme illness, and has been an unspeakable comfort to many who have had no one to minister to them."

Something more than seven years ago the systematic nursing of the poor in Boston found a first footing under the auspices of the Woman's Education Association. Its fundamental aim was to teach the people some of the principles and simple arts of nursing, and the name given to the branch was " The Instructive District Nursing." Direct access to the sick was reached through and in conjunction with the Boston Dispensary. In two years it grew strong enough to become an independent charity, and was incorporated as the " Instructive District Nursing Association "; and beginning with one nurse, this Association can now say that not one unresponded call for nursing help need be given anywhere within the city of Boston. Its methods are these :

The board of managers, consisting at present of nineteen ladies, has the entire management of the business of the Association. This board can at any time have the assistance of the advisory board.

The Association works, for the most part, in connection with the Boston Dispensary.

All nurses must be graduates of a regular hospital training school. One nurse is assigned to each of the ten dispensary districts, and meets the dispensary physician of her district each week-day ; from him she receives the list of cases to which he has been called, and she usually visits the sick with him ; sometimes she makes the round of visits alone after obtaining his written or verbal instructions.

Nurses are expected to work eight hours each week-day, but only in exceptional cases on Sundays, holidays, or nights. The nurses receive $40 per month during three months' probation, and then $45 per month; after two years' service the salary is $50 per month. In addition, each nurse is allowed $5 per month for car fares, and $2 per month for charwoman and the necessary washing for patients ; also one month's vacation without loss of pay, a substitute at $40 per month being provided.

There are two managers for each district, to whom the district nurse reports at a stated time each week at the office of the Association. All the nurses meet the president of the Association at the office once each month for general consultation and for discussion of some given subject or paper. The president also receives each month from each nurse a written report describing in detail the cases she has attended, and especially the instruction which she has given. Articles needed in the sick-room are kept at four places in the city, and are loaned under the direction of the nurses, who are responsible for their return to the supply committee. The Association furnishes, upon request of any physician of standing, extra nurses for special cases, in emergencies, or for night duty. The office of the Association, 64 Park Building, 2 Park Square, is open each week-day from 9 a. m. to 2 p. m., and is in charge of a salaried agent, who keeps the records of the nurses' visits and assists the managers in various ways.

By the request of the managers the following account of an average day's work was prepared for the annual meeting by the senior member of the staff of nurses now engaged in service:

The Experience of a Single Day.

I am very often asked, " What do you mean by district nursing? Where do you get your patients, and what do you do for them?"

I answer that the Instructive District Nursing Association employs nurses to take care of any patients who send to the Boston Dispensary for one of the out-patient doctors.

I find the easiest way to give an idea of what is done is to describe some of the cases; or, better still, outline a day's work.

For instance, a few days ago, starting at 8 a. m., I go first to see the patient who is more dangerously sick than any of the others— a little girl with bronchial pneumonia and whooping-cough. I find her mother has kept the room warm and well aired, and carefully carried out the directions given about her medicine, stimulant, and nourishment. As her temperature is high, I give her a sponge bath. I then rub her chest with camphorated oil, and put on a cotton jacket I had made for her.

Then I go to see a little boy just recovering from pneumonia, who is weak and very stiff. I give him a good rubbing, and show his mother how to make a custard and beef-tea for him.

Then to see our oldest case, who says she is a hundred. She has had the grippe, has been quite sick, but is now improving. She is not in pain; so I wash her face and hands, rub her back with alcohol, make an eggnog, and leave her calling down numberless blessings on me.

The next case is a two-year-old girl who has bronchitis. I have been at this house before, and am glad to find the sick child in bed and a hot flannel on her chest. I give her medicine and milk, which she refused to take from her grandmother. I notice the four-weeks-old baby is being fed from a cup of tea, as there is no milk in the house. I promise to ask the doctor for a diet order, and show the grandmother how to prepare the baby's food properly. I next see a woman who has erysipelas. I show her daughter how to make and apply the wash ordered by the doctor, and how to make some beef-tea.

Then I go to the dispensary to get some supplies, and to the loan closet to get some sheets and pillow-cases for a needy patient. I meet the physician at 12 o'clock and report the cases I have seen this morning and the preceding afternoon; ask for the diet order, get the new orders, and go with the doctor to see a man who has an abscess which needs to be lanced. When this is done I wash the arm, make a poultice, and put on a sling.

After my luncheon I begin the afternoon round by going to see a woman who has a bruised and crushed ankle. This patient ought to be in the hospital, but does not want to leave her young baby and five children. I dress the wound, put on a splint, and caution her to use it as little as possible.

Then to see two chronic cases—one a woman with an ulcer on her leg. I show her how to dress this. As she cannot leave her room and is fond of reading, I lend her some of the books given by one of the managers for this purpose. The other patient is a young girl with phthisis, whose mother is glad of any suggestions for Maggie's pleasure or comfort.

The next call is to a family where the seven children have a painful skin disease. I showed their mother how to wash them and to apply the ordered ointment. Any amount of old linen is needed here. One of the children had brought home a stray dog that was afterward found to be covered with sores. The children had all played with the dog, and this was the result—truly a case of mistaken kindness.

The next house I visit is one of the most dismal in the district. Sounds of quarreling come from every room. The halls and stairs are dark and dirty. The patient's room is up three flights, and contains only a stove, table, and old sofa-bed. He is a boy with acute rheumatism. They have not yet sent for the medicine which the doctor ordered the day before. I get the mother to go for this while I do up the patient's knees in cotton-wool and bandage. This boy's sister was also a patient; her neck and face were burned. As I dressed this for her she explained that in a friendly scuffle she fell across the stove. She neglected doing anything for it until afraid that her neck was growing crooked. I have twice since found this young woman so intoxicated that she could not be roused sufficiently to have her neck dressed; so I fear this is one of the few hopeless cases.

The next visit is to a German woman, who is in bed, with her face and head, particularly about her eyes, badly burned. She had been heating a can of milk with the stopper in, and it exploded in her face. One of her neighbors told her to put ink on it. She did so, and the result was startling, to say the least. It takes much time and patience to get this properly dressed, as the woman is weak and nervous and understands very little English. She has five small children, and her husband is doing the best he can for her. I stay and show him how to make some gruel for the patient and to prepare the milk for the baby.

I next go across the street to a nine-year-old girl who has had both feet frostbitten. I wash these and poultice as the doctor directed. Four of her schoolmates are here, and watch these doings with great interest.

Then I go to the little girl I saw first in the morning, take her temperature and pulse, and make her comfortable for the night.

The last visit is to a woman who has gastritis. She cannot retain nourishment, and has much pain. A neighbor who had been a patient some time before came in, made the bed, put the room in order, and offered to make a poultice. She did this very nicely while I peptonized some milk which the patient was able to take.

Almost every day I find some former patient carrying out many of the simple directions that have been given during some former sickness. While this may be taken as a fair day's work, there are many cases requiring hours of care, as, for example, where a child is very sick and the mother also sick, or in emergencies—as hemorrhages, confinements, or operations.

Very often I am asked why I like district better than private nursing; to which I answer that the great variety of cases met with in district work is a valuable experience, while the outdoor exercise, the freedom from care at night and on Sunday, are also among the pleasant features of the work. For although we frequently make Sunday visits to very sick patients, they are not required by either the managers or physician.

There seem to be three classes to deal with in our work—a few who are too old to change their ways, a few who are indifferent through intemperate habits, and a large number who are grateful for the help and instructions given. I may say that I have been civilly received in all cases, even enthusiastically at times, according to the nationality of the patient.

Terms.

1. For those in comfortable circumstances a visiting nurse can be furnished, and the charge must, in such cases, fully cover the expense to the society, fifty cents or one dollar a visit, according to the time required.

2. From those able to give no more, the car fare is expected, being generally ten cents a visit.

3. A *visiting* nurse is furnished without charge to those who are quite unable to pay for her service.

4. Visiting nurses will remain with a patient for the first 24 hours after a major surgical operation, and will visit after that daily as required. Should a patient need continuous care, an outside nurse must be engaged and paid for by the patient.

5. The hours of the nurses are from 8 o'clock in the morning until 8 at night. After that time they cannot respond to calls.

6. The nurses will visit in the morning those cases which have been reported the previous day, while those coming to the office before 12 o'clock will receive attention that afternoon.

7. The nurses are for the use of the public, and it is desired that physicians and others interested in the sick shall send for them. The service should be paid for whenever possible, as the society is supported entirely by voluntary contributions.

8. In addition to the trained visiting nurses the society also has a few *pupil* nurses that can sometimes remain with a patient for a moderate compensation by the week.

NOTE.—At the office of the Visiting Nurse Society nurses are registered who can be engaged by the week at a moderate expense.

Almost simultaneously with Boston, Philadelphia founded her Visiting Nurse Society, whose object is to give to the poor and those of moderate means the best home nursing possible under existing circumstances. The service is free to the very poor; other patients pay according to their means.

The Visiting Nurse Association of Chicago was organized in 1889. " This Association is formed for the benefit and assistance of those otherwise unable to secure skilled attendance in time of illness; to promote cleanliness, and to teach proper care of the sick, and to establish and maintain one or more hospitals for the sick, or a home or homes for the accommodation of nurses." That it is an assured success we glean from the statement that whereas in 1890 the number of patients was 1407, in 1892 it was 2478, an increase of over 1000 patients. This number entailed the making of 17,346 visits.

" Nine nurses are now employed, one of them being a head-nurse. From the very poor no pay is expected. Occasionally a patient is able to give something to the Association. No nurse is paid by the patients. The nurses are at the call of any one needing them, the Association being independent. The nurses distribute old clothing, food, beef-teas, condensed milk, milk tickets, malt, cod-liver oil, etc. They attend every kind of case, fevers, maternity, surgical, except the well-known contagious diseases, small-pox, scarlet fever, and diphtheria; to those a special nurse is sent."

Boston, Philadelphia and Chicago have the largest unsectarian district or visiting nurse associations in America. New York, Brooklyn, Buffalo, Baltimore, Kansas City and Newport (Rhode Island) support smaller societies, and carry out their work on plans similar to those already described. Hampton, Virginia, includes district nursing in its training school for nurses. The object of this school is to train colored nurses for missionary, hospital or private nursing. Since October, 1892, about 45 cases have been cared for by the district nurses, and about 150 visits paid.

The custom of assigning the pupils of the school to district nursing, for an allotted time, prevails in some hospitals.

The Methodist Episcopal Church, with its indefatigable zeal, has planted a Deaconess' Home in almost every city of the Union. Their first object is to inculcate religion; and the deaconesses devote themselves to the care of the sick in the poorest parts of the city. They have regular papers printed monthly, preparatory schools and hospitals in connection with their work.

Such is a bird's-eye-view of district nursing in the United States—a cursory glance certainly, but we see in it the planting of a great charity, and the promise of a glorious achievement.

On whom does the success of this charity largely depend? My sister nurses, a duty lies before us which only we can fulfil. There are battles in the warfare against dirt and disease which can be effectually fought only by the trained hands, prompted by christian hearts and guided by disciplined characters of the women of the nursing profession. Our co-operation with the Board of Health would result in the banishment of the sweating system. We could stir public opinion till householders would be obliged to make their tenements habitable. And before such weapons as scrubbing-brushes and brooms cholera must beat a hasty retreat. This mighty foe cannot be grappled with single-handed. If the many small societies throughout this broad land were to agree to become one national association, varying the general methods of that organization only in such details as would best suit individual cities, what might we not accomplish! This is not an untried scheme. Let the doubting ones and faint-hearted look for one moment at our fair sister, the Red Cross Society, and take courage. I am told that the nurses of the Chicago society go forth with the white cross on their arm—a fitting emblem of the purity and self-sacrifice of their mission.

We have accompanied the nurse in her rounds of one day, in order to acquaint ourselves with her duties, and have seen what she accomplished. What about the nurse herself? Do we picture her simply as one who has what is called "a knack with sick people," and "a desire to do good"? Two indispensable qualities they certainly are; but the truth presses itself upon us more and more that to successfully wrestle with disease we must be master of the art, and to teach a subject we must understand it. The two years' course of training and discipline of hospital life is not too long an apprenticeship for the would-be district nurse. And here let me emphasize the great importance of refinement, cultivation and self-devotion, in addition to thorough hospital training, as essential qualifications of a district nurse. Even more than in private nursing is it necessary that the district nurse shall be a woman of high character, and with strong religious feeling, so that she may consecrate herself to her work in true missionary spirit. It is a work which should be represented by every rank in life.

Suffering and helplessness appeal to every true woman's heart, and the stories repeated of her response to them never lose their charm. Thirty years ago women of high social standing heard the cry from the battlefield, and stepped from their luxurious homes into bare hospital wards, without a thought of doing anything worthy of record ; and stories of their action fall on our ears like musical echoes. Surely humanity calls as loudly for help now as then ! The victims of disease are more numerous and the battlefields cover a broader area than those of the civil war. The Princess Christian, in an article, says, " Public sick nursing is a work which will make the 19th century remembered as the one in which women found their vocation, and followed it even to the sacrifice of their lives." And a London paper expresses itself in these words : " Amidst all the wrangles concerning what is woman's true mission, to what trade, craft, or profession may she belong, what art she may practice, to what position she may aspire, or on what board she may sit, one point has never been called in question—her heaven born gift and right of being a nurse."

This profession of ours is a great heart in whose center Christ must be the power to send the life-blood through the channels of the world.

ON DISTRICT NURSING.

By Mrs. Dacre Craven, *née* Florence S. Lees.

District nursing, or the care of the sick poor in their own homes, by educated women who had received some training for that purpose, has existed among Christian nations from the earliest ages.

Religious women formed themselves into communities for this purpose, and the daughters of the rich and noble in every Christian land were sent to these communities to be educated in the care of the sick and wounded, as well as in the preparation of the simple dressings and remedies used at those times.

In England the Hospital of St. Katharine, originally founded in 1148 by Queen Matilda, wife of Stephen,* was chartered by Philippa, Queen of Edward III, and the care of the sick poor in the neighborhood of the hospital was imposed as one of their duties upon the members of the community, who were women of noble birth dedicated to the service of God.

The first paid secular nurses for the poor in England were sent out by Anglican sisterhoods, and in London by the Order of St.

* With the intention of securing repose for the souls of two of her children.

John, at that time connected with King's College Hospital ; but it was not until Mr. William Rathbone, the then member for Liverpool, founded the district nursing institute in connection with the infirmary there, that district nurses were recognized as having a distinct work of their own. The nurses were taken from the lower grade of women. It was the pioneer of work of a similar kind throughout the country, founded upon the same principles.

But it was not until the Order of St. John of Jerusalem, in 1874, inaugurated the National Nursing Association, to provide more fully trained nurses for the poor, that a sub-committee of inquiry was appointed (to which, with the late Lady Stangford, I acted as honorary secretary) to ascertain how far existing institutions throughout England fulfilled the requirements of nursing the sick poor in their own homes, and of teaching and introducing among them rules of health, cleanliness, order and ventilation.

The result of that inquiry showed that where the visiting nurse had to give relief as well as to nurse, it ended by her being an almoner and doing no real nursing service for the patients she visited, with the exception of a few surgical cases, and at some of these the nurses actually prescribed the treatment and boasted of curing wounds which no doctor had ever seen. But this was not nursing. It was therefore decided to found the Metropolitan and National Nursing Association, in 1875, for providing trained nurses for the sick poor, of which the present Duke of Westminster became chairman, and a very important resolution was adopted,* upon my recommendation, namely, to recruit the nurses entirely from the class known as gentlewomen.

There were several grounds for this decision suggested by me, and these were chiefly that, in nursing the poor in their own homes, nurses were placed in positions of greater responsibility in carrying out the doctor's orders than in hospitals ; that women of education would be more capable of exercising such responsibility; that the vocation would attract a large number of ladies anxious for some independent employment, and that a corps of nurses recruited altogether among ladies would have a greater influence over the patients, and by their higher social position would tend to raise the whole body of professional nurses in the consideration of the public.

All this has been fully justified by experience. Yet, when I first

* See page 49, *On the History and Progress of District Nursing*, by William Rathbone, M. P.

suggested it, and indeed made it a condition of my accepting the post offered to me of acting as superintendent-general to the new Association, it was strongly opposed by all the members of the then committee, with the one exception of the Duke of Westminster. Even Miss Nightingale said to me, "I don't believe you will find it answer, but *try* it—try it for a year."

And it *has* been tried and *has succeeded*, although in Liverpool and other places the nurses are still taken from women of a lower grade; yet the high standard established and maintained by the Metropolitan and National Nursing Association has exercised an influence over the whole country, and one might also add, over Europe.

The nurses were educated on the following plan. The candidates were selected by the superintendent, and on completion of the hospital training, which every nurse had to pass through, they had to spend six months in a special course of district training, in the Central Home, under the superintendent, who accompanied each nurse to every new "case" and taught her how to extemporize needful appliances and to place the room in nursing order. She also taught the nurses, what they could not learn in hospital, the care of the mother and infant after its birth, or what may be termed maternity practice, and how to teach the mothers what to do and what not to do; and where "cases" of scarlet fever could be obtained, she taught her finally how to nurse and disinfect in contagious disease. During the six months training in district work the nurses received more advanced lectures than were obtainable in hospitals where lectures had to be adapted to women of a lower grade and education.

These lectures were on anatomy, physiology (the latter including some lectures on the diseases of women), and hygiene, including the peptonizing of foods. Nurses had to read up for these lectures, and at the end of each course undergo an examination by the lecturers. They were then placed on the roll of trained district nurses of the Association.

In a letter from Miss Nightingale to the secretary of the Association in April, 1876, she said: "As to your success—what is not your success? To raise the homes of your patients so that they never fall back again to dirt and disorder: such is your nurse's influence.

"To pull through life and death cases—cases which it would be an honor to pull through with all the appurtenances of hospitals, or of the richest in the land, and this without any sick-room appurtenances at all.

" To keep whole families out of pauperism by preventing the home from being broken up and nursing the breadwinner back to health.

" To drag the noble art of nursing out of the sink of relief-doles.

" To show rich and poor what nursing is and what it is not. To carry out practically the principles of preventing disease by stopping its causes, and the causes of infections which spread disease.

" Last, but not least, to show a common life able to sustain the workers in this saving, but hardest work, under a working head who will personally keep the training and nursing at its highest point. Is not this a great success ? District nursing, so solitary, so without the cheer and the stimulus of a big corps of fellow-workers in the bustle of a public hospital, but also without many of its cares and strains, requires what it has with you, the constant supervision and inspiration of a genius of nursing and a common home. May it spread with such a standard over the whole of London and the whole of the land."

As I was superintendent of the Central Home at that time, and the "genius of nursing " referred to, I trust I may be forgiven for stating somewhat in detail what I consider district nurses should be, and their special work.

District nurses should feel themselves beyond and before all things the servants of the sick poor. They instruct, but practically and by example.

District nursing means the care of the sick poor in their own homes, where there are no proper appliances, and where the nurse can rarely see the doctor—in some cases not at all. She must know how to put the room of each patient into such good sanitary conditions that the patient may have a fair chance of recovery, and how to extemporize hospital appliances where these are required.

She must be so well trained in nursing duties as not only to know how to observe and report correctly on every case under her charge, but to allow no change to pass unnoticed, and to be able to apply provisionally suitable treatment until the medical man shall have arrived.

She must know how to purify the foul air of the room without making a draught; to make it clean, and insure cleanliness being observed ; to dust without making a dust; to ice drinks without ice ;

to filter water without a filter ; to make outside blinds out of inner ones, and indeed the great art of keeping a room cool, or of raising its temperature as may be required, out of such materials as can be found in the homes of the poor.

She must know how to make beef-tea, etc., and light puddings and drinks, and how to bake without an oven.

She must be content to be servant and teacher by turns, and must have the tact and sympathy required to command the patients' entire confidence and that of their friends.

All nursing service must be performed with her own hands, but she must teach the patient's friends how to keep the room in nursing order, how to change the linen of helpless patients, and how to give nourishment, etc.

But it requires special training to know how to sponge a patient between blankets without uncovering him ; and to make and apply poultices or dressings without the risk of chill or pain.

A district nurse must have a real love for the poor, and a real desire to lessen the misery she may see among them, and such tact as well as skill that she will do what is best for her patients, even against their will. No district nurse should ever give alms or relief of any kind, beyond the highest of all, that of nursing service.

Food is required more for convalescents than in cases of acute disease, and giving it leads to the so-called nurse becoming a simple almoner, and having a larger number of patients than it would be possible for any woman to nurse, or even to visit daily.

A nurse's business is *to nurse*, but she has also to teach the poor those sanitary laws which are household words with the well-to-do, and how they can beautify or improve their surroundings with the things they possess.

The room of a patient, once put in sanitary order, is kept so, but the nurse has daily to wash her patient between blankets, to make the bed without removal of patient, and perform all other nursing duties required. If there is a relative able to assist, the nurse teaches her how to do it, but she does not leave it for her to do until the patient is out of danger.

The nurse daily dusts the room, arranges for its proper ventilation and temperature, washes all utensils, dirty glasses, etc., and when necessary disinfects utensils and drains; sweeps up the fireplace, fetches fresh water and fills the kettle, and, if there is no one else to do it, prepares and makes what nourishment is required for her patient.

We never allowed any room where we nursed to remain in a dirty or disorderly condition, our rule being that " nurses shall be responsible for the personal cleanliness of each patient under their charge, and for the care and cleanliness of the room."

" Each nurse shall on every visit see that the room, furniture, and utensils of each patient are clean, or clean them herself."

Sometimes it has been said that it was a waste of a trained nurse's time and strength to do what was termed charwoman's work, but they forget that where there is serious illness, it requires special training to put a room into nursing order and to keep it so, without noise and without dirt.

I have always found gentlewomen of good birth and breeding more ready than women less delicately reared to perform the most trying and repulsive services for the sick poor, which could add in any way to their comfort or well-being.

Through the nurses, sanitary defects in the homes of the poor have been brought to the notice of the officer of health. Dust-bins have been emptied and disinfected ; drainage disinfected and water supply examined, and cisterns cleaned.

And this has been done through the nurse performing the so called " menial service " for her patients, for as she emptied slops, carried down dust, or fetched water, she had opportunities for observing the sanitary condition of things in the tenement or crowded lodging-house, which she could not have obtained in any other way.

And yet if as a nurse I am capable of judging nursing work, I can fairly say that the *nursing* services rendered by these ladies have been the highest attainable. In cases of scarlet fever, small-pox or other contagious disease, a nurse is set apart (each in turn) for fever duty *only*, and is not allowed to come in contact with the other nurses, until she has herself been disinfected, and changed her dress, etc. I had had the good fortune to nurse small-pox in Paris, at the time of the great epidemic there, and I was therefore able to personally instruct the district nurses in nursing a disease which is not admitted in England to our general hospitals.

The district nurses do not, as a rule, except during their training, attend maternity cases, unless there are complications rendering skilled obstetric nursing necessary for the recovery of the patient, in which case they only attend such other cases as the doctor may approve.

Yet I think it is impossible to overestimate the good that has been done by nursing these poor women into convalescence and teaching them the care necessary for themselves as well as the newly-born infant, and how to wash and dress the latter and to feed it. A doctor lately observed that wherever one of the district nurses went to a maternity case he knew there would be no trouble about the infant's *eyes* or its feeding.

I cannot conclude without referring to the good work of these nurses in their care of the dying and the dead.

Some years ago it was suggested to me by a medical man that it would be well to instruct district nurses on the best positions in which to place the dying, according to their ailment (there were no written directions with regard to this until my " Guide to District Nurses " was published in 1889), so that they might breathe to the last without unnecessary effort or pain ; but to the Sœurs Augustines of the old Hôtel Dieu at Paris I owe my best lessons in the last offices for the dead, offices so reverently performed that a district nurse once observed to me, " It takes away all the horrors of death ! I hope a district nurse will do for me, when my time comes, what they do for their poor patients."

To district nurses, then, belong the highest privileges a nurse can claim—to nurse the sick back to health ; to cheer and brighten the homes of the poor ; to comfort the fatherless and widow ; to ease the dying, and to perform the last nursing duties required by the dead. But it is not so easy to summarize the sympathy and love which render the visit of the nurse the brightest spot in the day, not only to the patient, but to the patient's friends.

When people speak of the hardships of a district nurse's life they forget that it is a life in which love and human sympathy have so large a share that patients cease to be mere " cases," and may be rather termed the friends and children of these " servants of the poor."

I cannot better conclude than by stating that in Great Britain our Queen has so fully realized the good effected by the district nurses that she has devoted the Women's Jubilee Fund to providing trained nurses for the sick poor, as her representatives among them, so that district nurses in this country are now known as " Queen's nurses," but still their proudest title must ever be that they are also the devoted servants of the sick poor.

DISCUSSION ON DISTRICT NURSING.

MRS. DUDLEY.—I wish to ask a question. The system outlined by Miss Hughes, in her paper on English nursing among the poor, is so different from ours that I would like to ask Miss Hughes, with the chairman's permission, about the time allowed to each case in England.

MISS HUGHES.—The time given to each case varies according to what is really required to be done. It depends upon whether you have to wash the patient and make the bed and prepare the food or not. We generally say, as a matter of routine, in teaching a nurse, to allow half an hour for a man and three-quarters of an hour for a woman, because of her hair. It averages from half an hour to an hour. The chronic cases that require less care we devote about half an hour to.

MRS. DUDLEY.—You have no rule, then? no specified time?

MISS HUGHES.—No, not at all. We have no set rule.

MRS. DUDLEY.—These papers have been very interesting, and of course district nursing in Chicago is so comparatively new, compared with Philadelphia or Boston, that I should like very much, with the chairman's permission, to have Miss Bruebaker, of Philadelphia, if she is here this afternoon, take part in the discussion and tell us somewhat about the Philadelphia work.

THE CHAIRMAN.—Miss Bruebaker does not appear to be present.

MRS. DUDLEY.—Then I would like to ask our own head-nurse in Chicago, Miss Wakem, to speak in behalf of our association. Miss Somerville's paper has so thoroughly covered the work done here in Chicago and Boston that there is not very much to be said about ourselves specially. We differ somewhat from Philadelphia in the fact that so far we have given our work, although we have expected, of course, and we have asked patients, if they could, to return something to the society, if it were only ten cents for the car-fare, but that has not been generally done. Most of the work has been given freely without any return whatever. But in Philadelphia, as I understand from the reports there, and also from what the president has written me, the system is quite different. There they aim to make it self-supporting, or as near that as possible; they aim to have their patients pay something, so as to take away any possibility of pauperizing; and I am very sorry Miss Bruebaker, who is the representative of that society, is not here to tell us how far that has prevailed and whether she feels it is a good plan or not.

MISS McDONNELL.—May I ask how your society is supported?

MRS. DUDLEY.—Our society is supported by voluntary contributions. We have had various gifts from societies and churches, and from foot-ball games and a charity ball, but mainly from subscriptions. Several of our nurses now are supported by ladies here. If any of you have seen our reports you will notice that we call our nurses by the name of the donor of the fund supporting the nurse, and we hope in the future this will grow and that our nurses will be supported in that manner, so that the directors and officers of the association may not need to ask for funds. At present I think we have four nurses supported in that way.

MISS WAKEM.—We have seven. One is permanently endowed, and six nurses are supported for the present year.

MRS. DUDLEY.—It is possible, of course, that the support will be continued. One gentleman has given $15,0co, the income from which will support a nurse permanently. Of course, we should like to see that system carried out further. It would very much aid the work and make it much more agreeable and pleasant for everybody concerned.

MISS WAKEM.—One of our nurses is supported entirely by a band of the King's Daughters, and has been for two years. The other five nurses have been supported by individual ladies, and we hope in the future the churches will support some. One or two churches have offered, if they can get over the non-sectarian limit, to do so. I would like to ask Miss Somerville one question. How is it possible for a nurse in a day of eight hours to make 21 visits? Your paper said 21 visits and that it was an average day's work.

MISS SOMERVILLE.—She frequently makes that many.

MISS WAKEM.—We have found it impossible to make more than eight or nine, and that is by working as late as half-past eight in the evening.

MISS SOMERVILLE.—We don't go from one end of the town to the other, you remember. The dispensary service of Boston is divided off into districts, and a doctor is assigned for each district, and a nurse is assigned to that district also, so that her distances are not a very difficult matter.

MISS WAKEM.—We are divided into districts, you know, all over the city, but we have found that our distances are so very great, and also the street-cars do not run sufficiently to allow us to do that number. One of our nurses who works in a very crowded part of the city has made 21 visits, but her district is much smaller, and she may have as many as five patients in one house.

MISS SOMERVILLE.—We sometimes have four in one street. Many dressings, you understand, will not take more than 15 minutes. I used to spend about that time unless I had a patient to bathe.

MISS WAKEM.—In that report of yours there are six full baths and a great many things that take a long time, and you spoke of it as an average day's work. That is why I asked.

MISS SOMERVILLE.—I think 16 or 17 visits would be about the average number. This was given to show the kind of work done rather than to show the number of visits. That was why she took that special day's work.

THE CHAIRMAN.—I am obliged to close this discussion, but it is not to be closed finally, as the president of the Chicago Visiting District Nurses' Association, Mrs. Dudley, proposes to hold a meeting in room 23, from two to three o'clock, Friday afternoon, to which you are all invited.

MR. HENRY C. BURDETT, of England.—I would like to ask how much it costs to pay the district nurses of Chicago, and also whether the street-cars take the nurses free.

MRS. DUDLEY.—It has cost us this last year a little over $8000, from December, 1891, to December, 1892.

MR. BURDETT.—If I wanted to endow a nurse, what would I have to give per annum?

MRS. DUDLEY.—$900 is what we allow in round numbers for a nurse. Did you ask about street-car fare?

MR. BURDETT.—Yes, do they give it to you free?

MRS. DUDLEY.—No, we have to pay our car-fare, and it is a very large item of expense.

MR. BURDETT.—Then Chicago is the only city that does not give car-fare free. I hope after this meeting they will give it to you free. If I wanted to endow a nurse in London it would be about eighty pounds per annum. That gives you an idea of the cost.

NURSES' HOMES.

By Miss K. L. Lett.

[It is with deep sorrow that we record the death of Katharine Lilla Lett, at St. Luke's Hospital, Chicago, November 4, 1893. Miss Lett had many friends among nurses, who sorrowfully realize how hard it is to do without her. As an able and enthusiastic worker in nursing and for nurses her place cannot soon be filled. She entered Bellevue in 1884, and from that time until within a few weeks of her death her work as a nurse was constant and varied, qualifying her well for the responsible duties as Superintendent of St. Luke's School for Nurses in Chicago, which position she held for the past five years. Her executive ability and judgment were excellent, and her opinions on nursing affairs always received the attentive consideration of her co-workers. She was faithful in her attendance at the Nurses' International Congress last June, and an active and enthusiastic member. Although at the time in delicate health and with much extra work to attend to, she prepared and read the following paper and took part in a number of discussions. In her rooms at St. Luke's the first committee meeting was held for the purpose of organizing " The American Society of Superintendents of Training Schools for Nurses," of which she became a charter member, and she looked forward with keen interest to attending their first meeting in New York in January, 1894.

She was a Canadian by birth and education and a most devout churchwoman, ever forgetful of herself in her love for her work and religion.

Her illness was brief, as she wished it to be, and our comfort is in knowing that she was quite happy in being to the last in her beloved hospital and in touch with her work.—I. A. HAMPTON.]

Not long ago some one remarked to me, rather discouragingly, that the above was not a subject of much scope.

I hope to prove that this is a mistake, or at least to show how important it is that nurses should be properly housed.

I shall dwell chiefly upon the home of the pupil-nurse, as it is of more consequence than the home of the nurse pursuing her vocation after she has graduated.

The situation of the home, to begin with, ought to be suitable. By that I mean that it should be convenient to the hospital with which the nurses are connected, and at the same time not placed, as the authorities of a large eastern hospital proposed when discussing the location of a home for their nurses, close to the morgue, dissecting house and other less cheerful buildings. Fortunately for the nurses, the proposition was not carried into effect, as the superintendent of the training school rather objected.

It is well when there is a covered way from the home to the hospital, but it is not a necessity. Nurses being obliged to cross a street or to walk a block is no great disadvantage, and when such is the custom, indispositions are not any more frequent or more serious than when the nurses live in the hospital.

The home need not be luxurious, but it ought to be comfortable. Hygienic principles should be uppermost, and no economy should be practised in regard to sanitary appliances. Baths should be found in proportion to the number of persons (one for every fifteen is a fair requirement), and no restrictions should be enforced in the matter of the free use of hot and cold water. To describe in full all measures necessary to insure good hygiene would be tiresome. One thing, however, which is frequently overlooked must be mentioned, namely, the importance of each nurse having a room of her own. In most homes some of the nurses can enjoy this privilege, but there are few, if any, where all the rooms are so arranged, and there are homes where there are not only two nurses in one room, but two in one bed. It is better for a nurse to have a small room alone than to share a larger one with a second person. It is wise to have the home well equipped in other respects, and entirely separate in all its domestic arrangements from the hospital. For instance, a good home should have its own laundry. Nurses suffer and have suffered from the destruction, loss and poor washing to which their clothes have been subjected when sent to the hospital laundry, which as a rule is wretched.

Of no small importance is the culinary department and the dining-room ; to have them well arranged, well managed and well appointed is an absolute necessity, therefore I speak emphatically because, sometimes, the governing bodies do not realize that this is so.

In addition a reception room, a class room and lecture room, servants' quarters, pantries, closets, etc., are also indispensable requirements in order to make the home complete.

To some it may seem that this description is rather an extravagant one, but remember that the home is not merely for board and lodging, it is a factor in the education of the nurses.

In the well-ordered home many lessons in neatness may be given, and it is seldom that these lessons are unnecessary. It also helps to keep the nurses happy, and happy people will always do good work. Finally, it is conducive to health on account of being detached. It is almost impossible to prevent the hospital air from permeating apartments not detached, or to prevent the nurses, in spite of iron-clad rules to the contrary, from returning to the wards when "off duty."

A number of general hospitals in this country have homes for their nurses which are almost perfect in their appointments. In England and abroad the accommodation for a long time was very poor, but now it is otherwise.

The time has gone by for nurses to sleep in rooms off the wards, and to have their meals in or adjacent to them. In the hospitals for insane, however, there is comparatively little improvement even where there is supposed to be a training school. Spacious apartments and separate houses are provided for the officers, but that is all; where the nurses and attendants are to live does not seem to occur to the builders of these huge institutions. It is exhausting to mind and body caring for the insane, and for those who do so to be obliged to sleep off the wards, even if the patients near by are quiet at night, is not at all the same as living in a separate house or even in a remote part of the building. No set of nurses receive so little consideration as those who care for the insane; their accommodations are poor, their food coarse, badly prepared and badly served.

At the same time it is not difficult to understand why this is so. The nurses in these hospitals are indirectly under political domination, while the nurses in general hospitals, so far as their maintenance and presence in the institution are concerned, are independent of all such government; and the nurses of the insane live anywhere and have no homes. Perhaps it may be urged that these women are not of as good a class as those we find in general hospitals and therefore do not require such good homes. In a manner this is true, nevertheless there ought to be a number of good class women in these hospitals who do require and have been accustomed to good homes.

No class ought to sleep off wards, because better care will be given and more interest taken in this unfortunate class of patients by the nurses, if the nurses, when off duty, leave not only the wards but the hospital and go to their own special home. The absence of these homes and separate apartments is what frequently prevents good class women from working in State hospitals, and there, if anywhere, the intelligent self-possessed woman, with good executive ability, is indeed needed. People finely organized simply cannot sleep in rooms adjoining a refractory ward, when possibly they have been in all day; the strain would be too great. Besides, nurses whose rooms are adjacent to-the wards may yield to the temptation to retire to them when on duty, regardless of the consequence to the patient or patients requiring constant vigilance. What then can be done in order to secure homes for nurses in asylums for the insane? Nothing, except to wait for the State authorities to realize some of the above-mentioned facts.

The homes of other nurses are generally erected by charitable and munificent people, or sometimes they are given as memorials. Instead of calling them as we do not infrequently, I think it would be an improvement to give them a name appropriate to the circumstances under which they were built, and to avoid the use of the term "training school," which is harsh and unsuggestive, as has been remarked by a colleague, of anything educational, and which, as has been stated, they ought to be. Moreover, it is a misleading name, because the popular idea of training makes us think of boys in a reformatory, as was lately demonstrated by a party of ladies, after having been taken through an hospital and nurses' apartments, in both of which they seemed interested, asking, most ingenuously, " but where is the training school?"

The nursing institute is unknown in this country, and as the system is not at all likely to be introduced, as it is not in accord with the characteristics of our schools, I shall not enlarge upon it.

Good homes, however, are needed for our graduates. Establishing such homes has been discussed from time to time, but difficulties seemingly insurmountable always arise, so the idea has never become a reality, and the graduates go on living as they have always done, in boarding-houses more or less uncomfortable and certainly very forlorn.

In all large cities the number of nurses is now quite large. As the warm weather each year comes round, I cannot help wishing that there were more people like the gentleman who gave as a memorial to his wife, the Edith Home to the Bellevue nurses. It is a pleasant cottage on Bell Island, near New York, where tired nurses can rest and forget for a season all about the hospital and everything else that may have grown irksome to them.

Much more could be said about nurses' homes, but my time is limited. One thing is certain, however, that there is nothing more elevating, sweeter or refining than a good home influence, and there is no class of people who need the comforts of home more than nurses.

DISCUSSION.

MISS HUGHES.—I might say that the hospital in which I was trained is built in two wings, and the graduate nurses live in a building situated between these wings. It is quite away from the ward, in a detached building. In another hospital in London, the staff of nurses are not so fortunate as to live in a home of their own, but their quarters are in the top of the building, and they leave the wards entirely. In another large hospital, St. Bartholomew's, the nurses' home is distinct. A few of them, I believe, still live in the hospital, but the others are five or ten minutes' walk from it. In St. Thomas Hospital there is a nurses' home. Their dining-room is distinct, and their sleeping apartments, though under the roof of the hospital, are quite separate.

THE CHAIRMAN.—Miss Sutliffe, Superintendent of the New York Training School for Nurses, in connection with the New York Hospital, will please say something about the latest improvement in homes for nurses.

MISS SUTLIFFE.—In the first place, we have on the top of our building a garden-house which is covered by an awning, where the nurses can rest in the evening, by themselves, and they do it thoroughly. Each nurse has a room by herself, and each two nurses has a sitting-room. There are five flats, which are occupied by 60 nurses connected with the school. They also have a large reception room and library. There is no covered passageway from the hospital to the school, it being deemed desirable that the nurses should have this opportunity of getting the air. It is perhaps 30 or 40 feet from the hospital. The dining-room is not in the building.

MR. H. C. BURDETT.—In no country in the world are nurses' homes equal to the nurses' homes in Scotland. At the Western Infirmary at Glasgow there are dining-rooms and sitting-rooms and class-rooms for the nurses, and every nurse has a separate bedroom to herself. There are also bath-rooms, and everything is as comfortable as it is possible to make it. I think the class-room is a new departure in the right direction. There are also attached to that institution certain outdoor nurses, who, by an excellent arrangement, have a separate entrance from the street, and they cannot enter their rooms until their clothes have been changed. At the Edinburgh Royal Infirmary they have erected a home designed by the best architects in Scotland, and interiorly it is decorated in a different manner for each room. It includes class-rooms as well as the other rooms. I noticed in New York the other day, in the New York Hospital, they have taken a new departure which I think has much to recommend it. In that home every two nurses have a separate sitting-room—that is, two bedrooms open into a sitting room. They are comfortable and attractive. Miss Lett has said that in this country there is no proper provision for the attendant upon the insane. I think that requires a little modification, because the system which Dr. Cowles has evolved is certainly a most excellent one. It is due to him and to Americans to know what he has done with reference to the training of attendants on the insane. If you want to know how the attendants on the insane are treated in England you should go to the Burywood Asylum. You will find there an excellent arrangement, with a separate home, and class-rooms, and thorough training for both male and female attendants. The difficulty, however, is that nobody has come forward to enter and be trained under that system, except those nurses who are required for the immediate necessities of the institution.

I quite agree with Miss Lett that those nurses who are in outside institutions, working among the public, should have proper accommodations. We have now in London certain spinsteries, they are called—that is, blocks which are devoted entirely to lady workers, where they have their own separate apartments; and I would like to see every city in the United States have its own spinstery. The nurse is the link between the institution and the public, and it is most important that she should be provided with every requisite and encouraged to maintain her self-respect. All of us can take courage and thank God that progress in the last ten years has been so enormous in the amelioration of the condition of the nurse, and in the next ten years I hope the nurses will be put in their proper position and their calling recognized, and that they will be placed in a position to do all the work devolving upon them efficiently and with dispatch.

MISS LETT.—I said there was comparatively little provision for attendants upon the insane. I have had some experience in an insane asylum. There were some nurses living even in the refractory wards. In a hospital in New York City I found a few trained nurses with very poor accommodations. All the regular attendants were living in rooms off the wards. Whether they were refractory wards or not it is the same throughout, and from what I know of other asylums I find it is pretty much the same throughout the country. The hours were long, and I had a great deal of sympathy for the nurses.

MR. BURDETT.—Dr. Cowles has been trying to get an insane asylum built for some years. So far as his means allowed he has produced great results and has made proper provision for all the nurses.

I agree with you that the asylums in this country and our own have much to learn, with reference to their treatment of nurses ; but as Dr. Cowles has started the movement, I want it brought out here that an attempt had been made in the right direction.

DR. HURD.—I will say for Miss Lett's information that I was at the Buffalo State Hospital (for the insane) in the State of New York, a few days ago and had the pleasure of inspecting a nurses' home, with accommodations for 30 nurses, which is in process of erection, to be completed and occupied within the next six weeks. The location of the building is unfortunate, but the building itself is admirably arranged, with class-rooms, recreation rooms, and individual bedrooms.

MISS L. L. DOCK.—While I think Mr. Burdett's suggestion on the subject of spinsteries is attractive, I doubt if our nurses would consent to the idea of having homes provided for them, as it were by wholesale, by kindly-disposed people, because they always like to make their own little homes, together or singly, and even prefer to have them less comfortable and have their lives more isolated.

MR. BURDETT.—I only proposed to have buildings erected where the nurses would have proper accommodations. There is no charity about it at all. I have had, during the last month, letters from 25 nurses, in all parts of the United States, saying they feel that they ought to have better accommodations. This word " charity " is very often misapplied. In our country, and even in this country, there is not a man, no matter how high his degree, who can say that he has got to his present position without having touched what some persons, I think a little too hastily, are apt to call charity. Your great universities are the result of large sums of money given by liberal people, and we go to them and send our children there, and we don't consider ourselves in any sense participants in charity. You must allow yourselves to be helped as every other class of people has been helped, by those people who have more money than they know what to do with.

A DELEGATE.—I would like to ask if one had to choose between having the nurses directly in the house, or having a nurses' home at a comfortable distance, say 3 or 4 blocks away, which would be preferable. I understand the idea is that the nurses' home is adjoining the hospital, but not in it.

THE CHAIRMAN.—I notice that in Miss Lett's paper there are different kinds of nurses' homes mentioned. It is all very well when you have a wealthy man who gives a memorial to his wife or daughter, and puts $50,000, $100,000, or $150,000 into a home, or when some corporation that has an ample amount of funds builds a nurses' training-school with all manner of comforts and improvements.

Another thing is to prepare for the actual necessities, without luxury, in providing for a training school for nurses. It is about time that some concrete recommendation on this subject should begin to come from the more experienced nurses themselves. Heretofore, those of us who have had to plan hospitals have done the best we could. We have called in architects to help us, but there is very little help to be obtained from architects in hospital construction, because they put the money on the outside, where you don't want it ; and I think it is time that we should have plans for nurses' homes prepared by superintendents who know what is wanted. In many cases the supply of money will be limited and things will have to be done in the cheapest way, and you can't rely on the fact that the appropriation which you may have this year will be the one you will have next.

To answer the question that was asked by the last speaker. In my judgment it makes little difference whether the nurses' home is 40 feet or a square and a half away from the hospital. The difference in the walk amounts to very little in our cities. When it rains or snows your waterproof and rubber shoes will protect you. I would rather have an open space and a good building a square and a half away than to have an incomplete building 30 or 40 feet away, where the lecture-room and the sitting-room and other rooms were left out because there was not space for them.

MISSION TRAINING SCHOOLS AND NURSING.

By Miss Linda Richards,

Superintendent of the Women's and Children's Hospital, Roxbury, Mass.

In our own country and in England training schools have become so much a part of all well regulated hospitals that no one expects to find even the smallest of our hospitals without its own training school; and very excellent schools do we often find in some of these small hospitals. This is a matter to which much time and thought—yes, and money—have been given. But in doing so much for our own schools, have we forgotten that there are other lands which can date back to our own? Do we realize that while doing for our own land we have been indirectly working for heathen lands? Will it be of interest to be told a few facts concerning it? Can we to-day in our own hospitals, so nearly perfect, realize how totally unlike our beautiful hospitals and our own training schools those in other lands must of necessity be? Can we realize how much patient toil and real sacrifice the organizing of one of these schools costs to the person who does the work of the pioneer in the matter? And more than all this, can we realize how necessary to the organizing and carrying on of such a work a thoroughly trained nurse who is ready to meet any emergency is? It may be that some facts concerning all this will be of interest to those who care for this work at all. It may be that some will care to know that this nursing reform, so recently confined to our eastern cities, has traveled across the continent; that it has flown across the wide Pacific and taken root in Japan, that country we as Americans are so fond of; that in that country, filled to overflowing with restless, changeable, progressive little people, training schools fashioned after our own have sprung up like mushrooms, and that to-day there are in Japan several well-organized training schools, and that they have all been organized since 1885, when a graduate nurse of one of our oldest training schools was sent out by a mission board to organize a training school for nurses, for the purpose of making one more channel by which Christian teaching might be taken into the homes of the Japanese.

Let us go with this nurse as we find her on a cold winter's day nearing the shores of "beautiful Japan." Very beautiful it indeed is, and so it seemed to our friend as in the moonlight she stood upon the deck of the steamer as she sailed into port. Very grand and beautiful was the wonderful "Fuji-Yama," the pride of Japan, as it stood out in the bright moonlight, covered with snow from base to summit —a thing of grand beauty never to be forgotten. She was happy at the thought of soon being upon land again. But with the joy came the feeling of great loneliness to this woman who stood looking at the far-away beautiful mountains, the near shore, and the scores of strange-looking little rowboats which rushed to the sides of the steamer as soon as the anchor was dropped. The whole scene was very new and so very strange; the language of these boatmen so meaningless, and she must, if she ever becomes useful, learn this language. As she stood there by herself she wondered if she had not made a mistake in going to this country for the purpose for which she had gone. But it was too late now for looking backward; she must look into the future. She had gone from a sense of duty; she would trust that she had been led aright. But these thoughts were soon driven away as men came on board the steamer to change the baggage to a steamer going south. Our nurse must go farther; this was not to be her home. She was soon in one of those queer-looking little rowboats, and in a few moments was standing on the shores of Japan. A little drive in one of the little two-wheeled carriages which one finds all over Japan, took her to the house of a missionary, who kindly gave her all the desired information concerning the remainder of her journey. She again set off, and was soon on the comfortable steamer bound for Kobe. Here she was to land and take the train for the beautiful historical city of Kyoto, of which we hear so much; for in this beautiful city, surrounded by mountains whose sides are adorned by temples, her work was to be. Very uneventful was the journey save from the ever-increasing strangeness of it all, and in due time she had reached her destination. We find no interest in following her through the first weeks of her stay. Her time and energies were given to the study of the language. Very difficult indeed was the task. But to be of use she must know something of the language, and soon we find her in a city in the southern part of Japan where there were very few of her own countrymen, devoting herself to the study, and soon the words had a meaning for her and also a familiar sound. Then with the heat of summer came the cholera, which every summer visits some part of Japan, and in the city where we find our nurse it rages. She offers to go into a hospital to take care of the sick ; one of the missionaries, well versed in the language, offering to go as interpreter. The offer was refused with thanks, and she sat by her open window studying the language, every now and again looking up to see a new case of cholera taken to the hospital, probably to die. Very useless did she feel, we may be sure. For six weeks during the extreme heat did she live there with cholera raging ; still not a feeling of fear troubled her. She did make some progress in acquiring the language.

During the summer five women had been found who wished to enter the training school. The women had to be sought out; they did not seek for admission, as nurses do in America and England. An old mission-house had been set apart for hospital work, and in it the work commenced. There were ten rooms in the house; two were large rooms, five were medium-sized rooms, and three were very small. There were also two little rooms outside which were used for nurses and the one servant. In these rooms six patients were made comfortable. Five nurses were accommodated. Two missionaries also lived in the same house, the largest room of which was used as a dispensary, and on the back piazza a little room was built of rough boards, which bore the dignified name of " pharmacy." You surely will hardly believe me when I tell you that no one complained of want of room, and that good work was done in that very inconvenient place. The hospital appliances were, as far as possible, those produced in Japan, and strange indeed did some of them seem to our nurse, who had worked in model hospitals in America and England. But she had some lessons to learn, and she was often surprised to see how much could be done in a land where so little could be found to work with. But the nurses must be instructed to use the products of their own country ; so foreign conveniences were very little used. The nurses at first were nearly useless. They knew very little of work, and nothing of taking care of the sick. Object-lessons were daily and hourly to be given, and both teacher and pupils were forced to learn patience. Lessons from text-books were given daily, but very simple were the books first used. Let us go with them to a class recitation and study. We will find them sitting around a small, low table. All are sitting upon their heels on the floor, all are writing with little brushes. The lesson has been put by the teacher into the very simplest of language for the interpreter, that she in turn may put it into very simple Japanese for them to write in their books, to learn to recite on the morrow, when they will, after reciting, write another lesson for the following day. These women, we must remember, have had very few educational advantages, and the teacher must commence her instructions in a very simple manner. But they learn quite rapidly, and at the end of six months of constant teaching the nurse feels that she did not make a mistake in going to Japan.

Let us see what manner of women are these little nurses—very short indeed, none of them more than five feet in height—very cheerful and even-tempered, very patient and exceedingly polite; always willing to do anything. Never punctual; this they must be taught. Not thorough in work; this they have never learned. On what terms have they entered the school? They receive no pay, and they board themselves or their friends board them while they are in training. It will naturally follow that not many hours of labor can be expected of them daily. Then, too, each day they must have one class-recitation and two lectures. Still, five nurses and the teacher could take care of six patients the first year. At the end of the first year the hospital had been enlarged so that 24 patients could be accommodated. A nurses' home had been built. What would American nurses think of such a home? The Japanese nurses thought it nice. A small house had been built for the two missionaries. Seven new nurses entered the school; so there were twelve nurses, and by that time the senior nurses had become very valuable indeed. At the end of two years from the time of opening the school the first class graduated. Two of the graduates were retained in the school, two married at once, and one died. The third class numbered eleven; the fourth class numbered thirteen. The school is now six years old—yes, nearly seven years old. About fifty nurses have graduated from it, and a few months ago not a graduate nurse was available for any call the school might have. A few of the graduates have married, and the others, with two or three exceptions, are in government hospitals in different cities in Japan. They are universally respected and are sought for by hospitals far and near, showing that their training has made them valuable.

What of the training schools in the Japanese hospitals? Some of them are most excellent, and they can give a nurse a more varied experience than a small mission hospital will ever be able to give. But our American training schools have done a grand work for Japan in sending nurses to them. In China and Corea the time has not come for training schools, though the Chinese women would make most excellent nurses. Trained nurses are sent to China by nearly every mission which has missionaries in China, and the good they do no one can estimate. In India missionary nurses have done and are doing a grand work. But we need not leave our own country to see good work done by trained nurses who have taken up mission work. In the district nursing which now we find in many cities, our trained nurses are doing a most excellent mission work—the mission of cleanliness taken into houses which have not known the meaning of such a word until instructed by the faithful nurse. Who shall say that this is not mission nursing? The mission work done to the poor and destitute who enter our hospitals is often overlooked. But it is a grand mission work of kindness and help to these poor sick and suffering ones, which our training-school nurses are constantly doing as they are receiving their training. In the city mission work in New York City there are several trained nurses who are doing most efficient work. A double mission work is the work of the trained nurse. Let us bid her " God speed."

NECESSITY OF AN AMERICAN NURSES' ASSOCIATION.

By Edith A. Draper,

Superintendent of Illinois Training School, Chicago.

It has been with considerable hesitancy that I have undertaken to present to your notice a most important work which lies before us. I have listened with so much pleasure to the papers which have gone before, all relating to work accomplished, and descriptive of the rapid strides with which our profession has advanced; yet we have so much to achieve, and the future holds out so much for us, if we meet it in the right way, and I know that to every thinking woman amongst us the needs for a national organization are becoming more and more strongly realized, until now our success for the future depends upon our unity.

I am afraid I cannot do the subject justice, but am glad to introduce it, hoping I may be fortunate enough to revive the interest shown once before, or at least promote the movement by leading to its discussion. We have had a notable example set us, and should be willing to follow the lead of our cousins across the water, in the advancement of this undisputed woman's work and nursing. Setting aside any spirit of rivalry, and admitting frankly that we are younger and less experienced, but that we have intelligence enough to recognize a good thing when we see it, and ambition *ad libitum* to strenuously endeavor to be the possessors of that good thing.

We have, as a profession, just emerged from infancy and attained our majority, it being twenty-one years since first an English woman introduced the system of training nurses in this country. A passing tribute to Sister Helen, the first superintendent of Bellevue, would not come amiss now, and could she see to what proportions her seedling has grown she would, I am convinced, feel amply repaid for her endeavors.

The plan so ably sketched some time ago, in our nursing periodical, through some misfortune has not matured. Whether the time was not propitious, or a competent leader not forthcoming, or because energy and enthusiasm were lacking, or whatever the reason, to the majority of toilers for the sick in this broad land even the name of such an organization is utterly unknown.

We have gathered here from East and West, from far and near, actuated by the desire to take part in the World's Exhibition, this union of nations in one vast representation. It would be fitting to commemorate the time by adding our mite to the history of the Exhibition, and becoming an united organization, a body of women trained to be of unquestioned benefit to mankind and not lacking in love and sympathy for each other.

If I may urge the cause which appears to me so important an one for us, I would add that if we are ever to be ready for action surely now is the time. " There is a tide in the affairs of men which, taken at the flood, leads on to fortune." Surely the tide is high for us now and it were a thousand pities to allow so grand an opportunity to slip by. We represent a number of schools, our English friends are here to give us their experience and advice, the medical fraternity are ready to offer their support, and the way seems clear; our combined efforts will surely be crowned with success.

The difficulties to be encountered, one must truthfully admit, will be mainly of our own manufacture. What we need is energy of purpose, enthusiasm, a spirit of philanthropy more developed, and ambition to lift our profession to a height to which the eyes of the nation shall look up and not down. Nothing is more conducive to the ruination of a project than lukewarmness and a conservatism which does not look beyond individual benefits.   These are our main hindrances, but not insurmountable ones, for though acknowledging these faults, we are aware of counterbalancing virtues and know that the day will come when America will be justly proud of this association of her countrywomen.

By a national association we mean a society with legal recognition, that every nurse who is a member of the same will be guaranteed for by the association and entitled to its benefits; and that we will be a recognized profession just as doctors are.

The objects to be attained would be schemes for professional and financial assistance, and, perhaps I should have put first, arrangements for conferences and lectures, that by meeting as frequently as possible we might gain a better knowledge of each other, which would result most undoubtedly in mutual appreciation, and consequently aid in the advancement of other schemes.

We have been accused, and with some justice, of envy, malice and all uncharitableness toward each other; schools of one system antagonistic to schools of another, and nurses of the larger cities and hospitals looking with contempt upon nurses trained in the smaller places.   Upon this petty, narrow-minded state a quietus might be placed by the system of registering (for a standard of equality would be exacted), so that all members of the association would be considered equally competent as far as their technical knowledge went. To protect the public, the medical profession and ourselves, no better means have been suggested than this.

People may be spared, if they so desire, the imposition of the ignorant woman, who, not fit for anything else, is good enough for a nurse; from the so-called "natural nurse," who believes herself endowed from above with the necessary knowledge to undertake any case, no matter how critical, without wasting time on a preliminary training; from the rejected probationer, who endangers life with the infinitesimal scraps of information she has gleaned in a short stay in the hospital; and, lastly, from the woman who, expelled from her school for cause, pursues unchecked this means of livelihood.

To the many excellent women who have nursed successfully for years, without thorough training, it may seem an arbitrary measure that they should be excluded from the association; but if we are aiming at beneficial results to the many, the inconvenience to the few we may regret but cannot avoid.

I imagine we would all concur readily in deciding that the standard for membership be high; a certified diploma, at least two years training in a hospital, endorsements of work well done and testimonials of character above reproach, should be required.

As a means of discipline this association would prove a power. We might imitate the Society of Loyal Orangewomen, whose regulations state that a member will be fined or expelled who does not "behave as becometh an Orangewoman." An even more laudable undertaking would be the scheme for benefiting nurses in a financial way.

Notwithstanding the objections which have been raised on the score of patronage and the repugnance of the self-respecting toward anything savoring of charity, the assurance of material aid when overtaken by sickness, of a sufficiency to keep the wolf from the door when growing old and unable to discharge the arduous duties of a nurse any longer, would bring consolation and relief to many a weary worker.

In this country, though fairly well paid, nurses are not able to save to any great extent; whether the calls upon their slender means are too great, or possibly through sickness or their own improvidence, the fact cannot be controverted that pecuniary aid is not infrequently needed by members of our profession, and I imagine would be received without any loss of self-respect.

The Alumnæ Associations furnish help by drawing upon members, and such help is not considered degrading : why should a larger and more far-reaching fund be so regarded ?

If we can help others by lending our aid to this undertaking we must put aside all feelings which may tend to obstruct its advance. The endowment of beds for nurses in hospitals would meet with the approval of any nurse who has been ill in a boarding-house, and those of us who have not experienced this nightmare should, selfishly speaking, be most anxious to give our aid, as fortune may not always deal so kindly with us, and the vicissitudes which have overtaken others may in time overtake us.

Another and equally important aim would be the promotion of conferences and lectures as often as practicable. Those thoroughly interested in the work would find a way to attend occasional meetings, and each State association might send one or more representatives, so that in business matters all might have a voice ; and through the medium of a publication, those unable to attend might keep up their interest. To advance we must unite! Otherwise, factions will arise and stagnation result. We know that nurses who have graduated ten or twelve years ago feel that they are not keeping pace with the advancement of medicine and science; that the recent graduate is oftentimes preferred before them, though in experience she may be a child. What better help can we give these nurses than the promotion of lectures, theoretical and practical, the encouragement of publications pertaining to our needs, and the free interchange of all the newest and best ideas?

Somewhere I have read that this plan is not feasible, and that we are sundered too far, geographically. We have immense territory to scatter over, it is true, but the difficulty does not seem to me insurmountable—rather an incentive to action.

I suppose the railways might be induced to give us excursion rates, annually. We are as deserving of consideration from them as the Christian Endeavor or any other society; and in the interim, lectures furnished by the Association and examinations held, something on the order of University Extension courses, would in each town or State be of inestimable value to those ambitious to be among the foremost in our calling. The opportunity to travel when annual meetings were held would be hailed with delight by every intelligent nurse and the appointment as delegate be regarded as an honor.

I have only touched lightly upon the many advantages to be obtained, and have not attempted any plan of organization. The subject is of vital interest to us all, and if I have succeeded in promoting its discussion my object has been attained.

THE BENEFITS OF ALUMNÆ ASSOCIATIONS.

By Isabel McIsaac,

Assistant Superintendent Illinois Training School, Chicago, Ill.

In presenting this short paper on the benefits of alumnæ associations, I must plead an ignorance of any further knowledge and experience than have been acquired by an eighteen months' connection with our own society. I do not wish to set it before you as an example, but rather for criticism and suggestion. Alumnæ societies have been started by several schools, but it is yet early to decide which plan is most successful. We are indebted to the New Haven school for many suggestions.

In our constitution we pledge ourselves first to " support by our personal efforts and interest the organization to be known as the Alumnæ Association of the Illinois Training School for Nurses." The first article announces our objects, which are :

The union of graduates for mutual help and protection.

To advance the standing and best interests of trained nurses, to co-operate in sustaining the rules of the directory, and to place the profession of nursing upon the highest plane attainable.

To further the interests of the Illinois Training School by giving it our hearty support to make it the foremost among such institutions.

To promote social intercourse and good fellowship among the graduates, to extend aid to those in trouble, and to establish a fund for the benefit of any sick among our members."

If the high sentiments expressed in this first article be carried out, how wide the field and how infinite the benefit! To quote further:

" Graduates of the Illinois Training School in good standing are eligible for membership, but any person upon the payment of $10 may become an honorary member, and upon the payment of $50 a beneficiary of the association, the amount thus obtained to be used towards the permanent endowment of a room in the Presbyterian Hospital. The initiation fee is $5, payable to the treasurer upon admission. The annual fee is $3, payable at the annual meeting. These fees to constitute the sick benefit fund. In case of necessity the executive committee can make an assessment to defray the burial expenses of any member."

In eighteen months we have paid out about $275, and have $519.70 in our endowment fund and $301 in the sick benefit.

" The officers to consist of a president, vice-president, secretary and assistant, and treasurer, elected by ballot at the annual meeting, and to hold office one year. The president to preside at all meetings, and the officers of the association to constitute the executive committee. A visiting committee, consisting of one member from each class appointed by the president, to visit sick members, ascertain their needs and see that they are properly cared for. It shall be the duty of the executive committee to investigate charges brought against any member, and if they find such member guilty of conduct unbecoming a nurse, they shall present the facts to the society for action, but no member shall be recommended for expulsion until she has had notice and opportunity for a full hearing before the executive committee."

" The amount allowed a member from the sick benefit fund to equal the cost of a private room at the Presbyterian Hospital, or if unable to enter the hospital, a sum not to exceed $10 per week for a period of six weeks. In case of necessity the executive committee may increase the amount and extend the time. Applications for sick benefits to be made to the secretary and by her to the executive committee."

This is an outline of our purposes. It needs no argument to convince us that "in union lies strength," and " in knowledge, power." We have for ourselves a most honorable calling, one which compels respect of all mankind. We are just beginning to realize how much higher we may go.

The system of training will soon be enlarged in every way. The successful nurse will be she who keeps abreast of the times. How better can it be done than by the maintenance of alumnæ associations?

The difficulties are our indifference and lack of enthusiasm. The routine life of a nurse tends to narrowness, and that to selfishness. The irregular habits interfere with study and recreation, and it requires enthusiasm, and a realizing sense of the immense improvement to be derived from concentrated efforts, to lift us out of a meager intelligence and commercial spirit. If every school establishes alumnæ associations the obstacles to a national organization will rapidly disappear, and if only members in good standing, active members—not merely those who pay their fees but never come near the meetings—are eligible for membership in the national league, each will be a stimulus to the other. Then let the national organization establish a code of ethics which shall govern all auxiliary bodies. It can define the conditions constituting "good and regular " standing in the auxiliary associations, thus establishing a high grade of excellence for membership ; it can provide rules and procedures for discipline. The practical working of a national league will bring to the front the best material for the heads of schools.

We have the example of the honorable bodies of the medical profession. Our societies should be based upon simple business principles, but let us guard against the idea of their being only a medium for financial aid, and still further should we avoid any idea savoring of charity in the ordering of sick benefit funds. It is mutual help, not charity. The furtherance of post-graduate study should be encouraged in every way. During the winter our society had the benefit of several lectures from eminent medical men, notably upon cholera and yellow-fever epidemics, other contagious diseases, and the nursing of abdominal surgery ; these were given most cheerfully by busy doctors and were much appreciated. We need better literature and more of it on nursing. If we demanded it by our better intelligence it would be forthcoming. The really good books on nursing could be counted upon one's fingers. During the past six months two volumes by nurses and for nurses have emanated from the Johns Hopkins School which throw strong light upon dark places ; we needed them. Let us show our appreciation. We have but one journal, which all schools should feel it a duty to support in every possible way. The heads of all schools should bring these associations to the notice of undergraduates long before they leave the school.

We have fought for firm footing. We can by united effort lift ourselves to honorable permanency. " United we stand, divided we fall."

DISCUSSION.

MISS ALSTON.—I think that the subject of an association for American nurses is something in which we are all particularly interested, and I think that both of the papers which have been read cover the ground entirely. First of all, we must have an alumnæ association for every school. Our own school has one which is still very much in its infancy. We have a sinking fund of $400. We expect to have our association in full running order by fall, when our graduates return from their vacation and we can call a general meeting.

It has been my idea—perhaps it is a wrong one, but I have thought that the benefit to sick nurses should come from their own association; that is, from the alumnæ association. That the national association should be to arouse us more to the necessity of keeping up the standard of nurses to what it should be. I think nurses are too much inclined to get in a rut and become very selfish, and I think we all as individuals feel how easy it is to say things are going on fairly well and be inactive. It seems to me there is no better time in which to take some steps toward starting a national association, for I am sure we would all derive a great deal of help from it.

MISS DARCHE.—I am a graduate of the Bellevue Hospital Training School and also a member of the alumnæ association, but I have not the printed rules with me. I know there is a large fund of four or six thousand dollars that has been contributed, and I know there is in the hospital a suite of four rooms for sick nurses given by ladies interested in the school, and also a fund for sick nurses, and the alumnæ association is supposed to look after the care of the graduates when they are sick.

MISS BETTS, of Brooklyn.—I would like to ask if it is not general for each hospital to look after its own graduates when they are ill? It has always been done in my school, treating them as private patients and free of charge, and I supposed it was general, but I don't know.

MISS MCISAAC.—I think that is done wherever it is practicable.

MISS MCKECHNIE.—May I ask if the room is only for the alumnæ association of your training school, or if it is not for all members?

MISS MCISAAC.—Yes, but in our case the training-school management and the hospital management are separate, and we cannot ask the hospital to provide free of charge a room for nurses who belong to our school. That was our idea in entering on founding our own alumnæ association.

MISS READ, of Baltimore.—I think each hospital or alumnæ association would prefer that its members should be cared for by its own association rather than by its hospital.

THE CHAIRMAN.—I hope that in the course of time we will be able to evolve Alumnæ associations, American Nurse associations and a Superintendents' convention, but to accomplish all this thoroughly will require time and careful thought. Haste is to be avoided, and our meeting here in Chicago is the first step in the right direction. Superintendents being the heads of schools have a great deal of influence, not only among their pupil nurses, but graduate nurses, and until we can get superintendents united regarding the fundamental principles of the work, we cannot expect the nurses to work and to unite and to be as successful as they must be later on when we hold ideas in common. The next thing we can take steps towards accomplishing is to organize a superintendents' society and also alumnæ associations in connection with every good school in the country. The alumnæ associations should be as nearly alike as possible. Of course some of the details must be different according to the special demands of each school or hospital, but their requirements and aims should be practically the same. I do not think superintendents should take too active a part in such associations; they should be organized and sustained by the graduates of the schools. Until these alumnæ associations are in good working order it will be impossible to organize a national association, because in that we must have schools and hospitals and nurses represented, and we can only have the schools represented through the board of managers and superintendents, and the nurses can only be represented through their alumnæ, so the organization of the alumnæ associations and superintendents' society is necessary before we can have any qualified members for the larger national association, for only those graduates who are recognized members of their own school alumnæ association should be considered eligible for membership in the national association, their vouchers being their own alumnæ.

Before the congress adjourns it is desirable that we should hold a superintendents' meeting with the view to forming a superintendents' society.

THE ROYAL NATIONAL PENSION FUND FOR NURSES.

By L. M. Gordon,

Matron St. Thomas Hospital, London.

My paper on the Royal National Pension Fund shall be short, but I hope your consideration of the important subject of nurses' pensions will be long and practical. For the sake of definiteness the argument may be divided into two parts: (1) the nurses; (2) the fund. Nurses are scientific persons, more or less. They know the value of this scientific axiom, "If you would deal with a thing as you ought, you must first see it as it is." Now if nurses wish to deal with their own classes as they ought, they must see themselves exactly as they are. I am a nurse. In order to see my class as it really is I have thought it wise to use, not only my own eyes, but the eyes of a sister woman as well, and, more important still, the eyes of a brother man. The following brief description of nurses is made on the inspection and report of three pairs of eyes: two pairs belonging to women, and one pair to a man. Nurses are, of course, considered here from the special point of view of the provision of pensions for old age.

I.— *The Nurses.*

My sister woman declares of nurses that, as a class, they are healthy young women and happy. They are happy because they are fully employed and intelligently controlled and governed. But because they are healthy and happy they do not think of the future. Is that a true view of the case? You will probably consider that it is. But supposing it to be true, does it argue any very great blameworthiness on the part of nurses? Are nurses very foolish and very wicked because they do not, whilst still in the bloom of youth, look forward into the dim vista of old age, and begin straightway to lay by money for that nebulous and uncertain future? I think not! They must, on an impartial consideration, be acquitted of the charge of decided folly, and still more of the charge of wickedness. On the contrary, there is a certain merit in living by the day, in being happy in our work, and in reposing a general and intelligent trust in the Providence which wisely rules the world.

But though nurses are not to be actually blamed for not initiating a pension fund for themselves, it certainly would be prudent on their part to take full advantage of such a fund when it is initiated. Nay, more, it is probable that they will blame themselves, and that very severely, if, having had the opportunity of making provision for old age by the simple method of joining an established institution, they find themselves in old age friendless, helpless and destitute.

"Nurses are lacking in enterprise," says their sister nurse and critic. They are often anxious and unhappy about the future. But though they are both anxious and unhappy, they would rather sit down and fold their hands in despair than boldly face the inevitable and make a way to competence by their own intelligence and determination. Now, is this a true charge to bring against nurses? If it be, then the lookout for women generally is of the most melancholy kind; for nurses are at the very head of their sex in intelligence, capacity and training. But if the most competent of women cannot face and provide for their own future by their own efforts, what are the vast numbers of the unintelligent and the incompetent to do? It looks as if the sex as a whole had made up its mind that it is and must forever remain inferior to and dependent upon man.

Women, and more particularly American women, will hardly accept this as their final and inevitable destiny. Nevertheless, the history of the past three or four years would seem to confirm the proposition that American nurses are really deficient in enterprise. A beginning was made with the establishment of a national pension fund for nurses in America, an American national fund, and a very hopeful beginning. Now one would have thought that the energetic and self-reliant matrons, sisters and nurses of the American hospitals, and, still more, those independent women who sail out into the open sea of the nursing world on their own account, would have hailed such a beginning with enthusiasm and established the fund as a going concern out of hand. But where is the American National Pension Fund to-day ? Where are the traces even of its foundations, which but two short years ago were so well and hopefully laid ? Well may my nursing friend and sister say that "nurses as a class are lacking in enterprise."

A "tendency to weak grumbling" is said to be characteristic of nurses. It is also said that their grumbling leads to nothing. Of course no *man* would say this of women ; it is women who say it of one another. But really, if women are going in the future to be their own guides, their own masters, and their own breadwinners, they must learn to carry their discontent beyond the stage of mere ineffectual grumbling.

"There is *occasionally* a wise woman who looks ahead," says our candid feminine critic. Very cautious praise this ! The wise woman, according to Miss ———, is only an "occasional" person, a *rara avis*, a kind of creature to be critically inspected by naturalists and classified apart with a strictly limited number of the same order. But even when such a woman is found she can by no means proceed to the goal of a provision for old age by a mere wish. How can a woman in America, or even in England apart from the R. N. P. F., set about making adequate provision for old age ? She has no knowledge of investment, and extremely little to invest. In England she is practically shut up to the postoffice or the building society. Now the postoffice gives the poorest possible pension which money can purchase. As for building societies, many of them seem to have been designed to play the part of spiders for the easier destruction of helpless and unsuspecting flies. The very name "building society" now excites terror in the Englishwoman's mind.

From all this we are led to the certain conclusions that nurses are not provident in youth, but that they ought to be; that there are no facilities in America which specially develop thrift in nurses, but that there ought to be; and that of England the very same things might be said, had it not been for the existence of the Royal National Pension Fund. The fund, by its existence, has created a new faculty in the minds of the nurses of England, the faculty for persistent thrift. By the possession and use of this faculty British nurses have placed themselves in the vanguard of those brave and honorable women who essay to fight the battles of the world for themselves, and, unaided, to conquer in the strife.

II.— *The Pension Fund.*

Let us come now, in the second place, to close quarters with the Royal National Pension Fund itself. We will briefly consider its history first, and then its present position. The pension fund had its origin in the sufferings of nurses. The blood of the martyrs has ever been the seed of the Church. It has been the same with the pension fund. Had there been no Nurse Steers to contract fatal illnesses in the course of their duty, to be disabled by such illnesses, to be neglected because disabled, and to die helpless in the poorhouse, there would have been no Pension Fund. Nurse Steer did not spend two of her last years as a pauper among paupers and then die in middle life and fill a pauper's grave for nothing. Her sufferings and her sad fate gave rise to the idea of the Pension Fund.

It was fortunate—was it not providential?—that this idea of a pension fund originated in the mind of one of the most practical, competent and resolute men of his time? Mr. Henry C. Burdett is the founder of the pension fund. Without him would there have been any such fund before the world to-day?

Mr. Burdett set his mind upon starting the fund with £50,000 sterling—that is, with about a quarter of a million dollars. The first person to take up this idea of £50,000 resolutely and practically was an American, not an Englishman. The chief official of the pension fund to-day, the chairman of its board of managers, is an American, not an Englishman. The first of these two noble Americans was Mr. Junius S. Morgan. The second is Mr. Morgan's son-in-law, Mr. Walter H. Burns. Is it a mere coincidence that this pension fund for British nurses owes so much to Americans? Is it not rather a providential call to other Americans to arise and establish a similar fund for their own country?

The £50,000 was raised in due time, and I always love to publish the names of those who furnished that magnificent sum for such a purpose. The four donors were Lord Rothschild, Mr. Junius S. Morgan, Mr. H. Hucks Gibbs and Mr. E. A. Hambro. All these persons ought to be and will be canonized in the nurses' calendar of practical saints throughout the world. Their gifts enabled an experiment to be made which has been so conspicuously successful that it may be said to have completely revolutionized the condition and prospects of nursing in all civilized countries. This fund having been so well and successfully established in England, we may be quite sure that trained nurses in all other civilized countries will give themselves no permanent repose of mind until a provision of equal simplicity, security and adequacy is made for them.

The public mind ought to be impressed with one fact in connection with the history of the pension fund, and that is that the highest persons in the British State took it up and gave it an impetus which made it at once conspicuously and permanently successful. The Prince and Princess of Wales, in two years, by their judicious and even enthusiastic help, won a position for the pension fund in the estimation of the public and the nursing world which it might not otherwise have attained in twenty years. That was a signal service, and a service to be gratefully remembered. But it was also an example for great and exalted personages in other countries. Why should not the President of the United States, and the distinguished lady who shares that high position with him, place themselves at the head of a movement of American nurses, and establish on this side of the Atlantic a pension fund greater, richer, more extensive and more adequate than even the pioneer fund in the mother-country. Perhaps this may yet be done!

The example of the Royal National Pension Fund must, one would think, be very contagious. Its success has been so steady, so rapid, and so complete in every detail that other countries will surely wish to emulate the island in the western sea. (Perhaps being in America one ought rather to say the island in the eastern sea?) By the courtesy of the manager of the fund I am enabled to lay before you some facts and figures of the most gratifying and convincing character.

Perhaps I should have indicated before that the pension fund really consists of two parts: an annuity branch, and a sick-pay branch. At any rate I beg now that you will have this fact in your

minds. The first and principal object of the pension fund is, as the
name implies, the provision of retiring pensions for nurses when they
are beginning to get too old for work. Let me indicate to you by
half a dozen figures the rapid growth of this annuity branch of the
fund. In 1889 the invested annuity funds amounted to a little over
£51,000; in 1890 they had risen to over £73,000; in 1891 to over
£96,000; in 1892 to over £123,000; and during the four and a half
months of the present year the amount has gone up to over
£134,000. That is to say, with interest at 4 per cent, the pension
fund has already available for distribution in pensions an income of
£5400 a year, or between 25 and 30,000 dollars of annual income.

This striking record of success is emphasized by a consideration
of the increasing number of nurses who have joined the fund for pensions year by year. At the end of 1889 the number of nurses stood
at 1039; twelve months later it had risen to 1475; the following year
to 2099; and in December, 1892, it had reached 2585. At the present
moment the actual number of nurses who have joined the fund for
pensions is 2792.

The sick-pay branch of the pension fund was felt to be somewhat
of an experiment, but it has proved to be successful and useful
beyond all expectation. I will not give you in detail the figures for
this department, but the following will indicate with clearness its
rapid progress and its marked service to nurses. In 1889 there were
only 198 sick-pay policies issued; in 1892 there were 604. In 1889
only 10 nurses received sick pay; in 1892 there were 89 nurses who
claimed this benefit. In 1889, £49 were disbursed in sick pay; 1892,
£ 392, or nearly ten times as much, was distributed.

The annuity and sick-pay branches constitute the two chief departments of the pension fund. But it is to be remembered that the
Junius S. Morgan Benevolent Fund has proved to a considerable
number of distressed, disabled and sometimes destitute nurses a
veritable salvation from despair. This fund has only been in operation for about two years. In 1891 it distributed £45 19s 4d to 15
nurses; and in 1892 the disbursements amounted to £238 1s 2d and
31 nurses were benefited.

Those three departments of pensions, sick pay and benevolent
help to the disabled, constitute the tripod on which the Royal
National Pension Fund stands. But in addition it acts in the capacity
of a savings bank for nurses, and receives temporary deposits and
pays interest on them. Moreover, it is also an insurance society and

a general place of refuge, as well as a paternal adviser to all who associate with it as members.

Two of the points mentioned or implied ought to be specially emphasized; the first is that by the exertions of Mr. Burdett and the splendid generosity of the four merchants already named the fund possesses an endowment of £50,000. The second is that the business is carried out on mutual principles. There are no shareholders and no paid directors. Whatever profit is made by the investment of the nurses' premiums and of the £50,000 endowment is divided equally among all the nurses in proportion to the amount of their pensions.

Thus I have given you, in briefest outline, the story of an institution which, as I have said, is destined to revolutionize the economic conditions and prospects of the whole nursing world. The purpose of my paper would be frustrated if I did not add one pregnant word of practical application. The word to America, to the President and to leading citizens and their wives is this: You see what great and blessed things have been done in England for a most meritorious and ill-paid class: " Go ye and do likewise " for the nurses of your great continent. Nay, may we not say and say truly, that as Great Britain has made generous provision for her nurses in old age, and has thus transformed nursing from an anxious to a happy calling, so all other civilized and Christian countries should forthwith set about making such a wise, right and most necessary provision for every one of their deserving nurses?

OBSTETRIC NURSING.

By Miss Georgina Pope,

Superintendent Columbia Hospital, Washington, D. C.

When I first went to Bellevue Hospital and understood what care had to be bestowed upon the ill of mankind to mitigate suffering, to check disease, to prevent the spread of infection, and indeed to save life, I wondered how any patient once entering its wards could have gone out alive under the system of nursing in vogue before the training school was established. Going back these many years, the care of these unfortunates was entrusted not only to those of their number who were not bedridden, but even to the criminals who, being sent to the workhouse for long or short sentences, were transferred to the hospital to care for the sick and dying of its overcrowded wards, while the nursing in the outside world was conducted by grannies and maiden aunts who were thought unfitted for anything else. It is unnecessary to dwell further upon the character of the nurses and quality of the nursing in this recently benighted age.

When Florence Nightingale, in 1854, with a corps of 92 volunteer nurses went to the Crimea, the seeds of the present efficiency of nursing were sown. Nor were these seeds slow in germination and growth. Miss Nightingale has lived to see nursing taken out of the hands of the most degraded of humanity and raised to a profession in which even the daughters of nobility deem it not beneath them to serve.

In the time of the Pharaohs of Egypt and of the Hebrews, obstetrics seems to have been wholly in the hands of midwives. That the science did not advance is evident from the fact that women were not only considered unfit for education, but that this most unfortunate art was left to the most ignorant. Primitive obstetrics was guided, we might say, by instinct. The savage mother when about to be confined left the village of her tribe, and digging a shallow hole in the ground by the side of some stream, combined the cleanliness of fresh earth with the bath in the river, immediately after the completion of her labor.

At the time of Hippocrates, 400 B. C., obstetrics, still in the hands of midwives, had not advanced as rapidly as medicine and surgery, the priest being called in to a difficult case more often than the surgeon. Efforts in this age seem to have been towards saving the mother regardless of the fate of the child. After 1550 A. D. more attention was given to the preservation of the life of the child. Just after this time instruments began to be used in midwifery, their invention giving an impulse to the further development of the obstetric art.

Now that the surgeon had begun to take up the study of obstetrics the progress is somewhat greater, but not so rapid as after about 1801, when obstetrics seemed to break away from surgery, and we find schools opened to midwives and students for its special study. This was the turning-point for midwifery, and as a separate science it soon grew to such importance as to rival surgery, which had been, we might say, its mother. Men no longer looked on it as work for old women, but something to be studied carefully. To the exact anatomical description given previously by Smellie were added the physiological investigations of later workers. This work, so comparatively new, progressed with a rapidity scarcely equaled by that of any other branch of the medical profession. Anæsthesia was employed, and the operations, before almost impossible, were made plain and easy, and the woman, from having been forced to suffer pain the like of which seems scarcely to have an equal, "remembereth her travail no more," not only because "a man is born into the world," but because God has blest man with an agent that renders her suffering nearly nothing. But still the maternities were visited with a scourge nearly as disastrous in its effects as smallpox. It was not until the true nature of puerperal infection was discovered that midwifery could truly be called a science; and it is here that obstetric nursing comes in play as the most important part of all this science. It is through the nurse that the skillful accoucheur expects to combat the frightful disease, and I intend to show in this paper how she can become of no less importance than the physician himself in guarding the health and preserving the lives of the mothers and the children, adding to the average of years of human life, and more than all, in preventing the suffering of the mother.

When a patient comes under observation it should be the endeavor of the nurse to place her in circumstances best fitted for her condition ; and as nervous symptoms are predominant, absolute quiet and freedom from excitement, with careful attention to all the secretions, with at least a bi-weekly bath, and a well regulated diet, are of prime importance. I do not think too much attention can be paid to the first-named prerequisite, because the mind of the pregnant woman is very susceptible to disturbing impressions, and the influence of a good nurse at such a time is immeasurable:

The lying-in ward or room should be well ventilated and as free from unnecessary furniture as possible. Especially in this work absolute cleanliness is demanded. The preparation of the bed depends upon whether it is in a hospital or private house. In the former, where we have delivery rooms with tables, delivery pads, and the patient is dressed and bandaged before being taken to her bed, the process is much more simple—a clean tick filled with fresh straw is provided for each patient, over that a sheet tucked in neatly and pinned at each corner, then across the middle of the bed should be put a rubber sheet a yard and a half square, over that a draw sheet and

both of these firmly pinned to the mattress, one pillow for the first
day or two, and the top sheet and spread of the ordinary bed. In a
private house, the delivery bed entails much more work. A single
bed with a hair mattress is best, placed in the room so as to be accessible on either side, then a sheet over that, a rubber sheet a yard and
a half square, and draw sheet, both of which should be firmly pinned
to the mattress, this with a pillow is the permanent bed, then over
that place another rubber and draw sheet and a Kelly pad (which I
would here suggest should be in the possession of every obstetrical
nurse), a piece of oilcloth on the right side of the bed to protect the
carpet, and a pail for the pad to drain into, a top sheet and blanket.
After the third stage of labor the pad is gently withdrawn, the
patient washed and dressed on the temporary bed, after which it is
also removed, leaving a clean and comfortable bed as the permanent one. A wood wool or jute pad of a foot and a half square
covered with cheese-cloth, placed under the buttocks, is desirable for
the first twenty-four hours; it is soft and comfortable to the patient,
absorbs readily, and can be changed much more easily than the
sheet.

For every case of labor there should be at hand plenty of hot and
cold water and ice, with two large basins, for a possible resuscitation
of the infant—several sheets, plenty of towels, a binder and a small
blanket to receive the baby. On the obstetrical table should always
be found a hypodermic syringe, with ergotine, fluid extract ergot,
persulphate of iron, chloroform, a graduated glass, solutions of
bichloride and of carbolic acid, carbolized vaseline, cotton-seed oil,
saturated solution boracic acid and wipes for the baby's eyes, several
pieces of string nine inches long to tie the cord, safety pins, pins,
sutures, needles, needle-holder, scissors, catheter, sponges, cotton,
and the post-partum dressings. A great deal of care is necessary in
the selection and preparation of these dressings, that nothing septic
may be brought in contact with the patient.

At the beginning of the first stage of labor the patient should be
given a warm bath, an enema of soap-suds and a vaginal douche of
bichloride $\frac{1}{3000}$ or carbolic $\frac{1}{60}$; see that the bladder is empty, if necessary passing the catheter. Her nightgown should be folded up under
the arms, and she may wear stockings and a plain white skirt, opened
all the way down the back; this latter need not necessarily be in the
doctor's way, and affords a covering to the patient which cannot be
thrown off in the restlessness of her pains. After the waters have

broken, and from time to time during the progress of labor, the vulva and thighs should be washed off with a solution of bichloride $\frac{1}{3000}$. When the pains begin to be regular and hard with short intervals, if the doctor has not arrived it would be well for the nurse to examine the patient, first washing her hands with liberal use of a nail-brush, and then soaking them in some antiseptic solution, then lubricating the fingers of the examining hand with carbolized vaseline. If the os is dilated to the size of a 25-cent piece, and the pains regular and hard, the doctor should be sent for at once, the nurse in the meanwhile encouraging and cheering the patient, and getting everything he may need close at hand, so that there may be no running out of the room after he gets there. A nurse should always try and anticipate a doctor's wants. If the case be normal he will not need assistance until the second stage is over. As soon as the head is born she may wash out the baby's eyes (with a saturated solution of boric acid), also the mouth, freeing it from any mucus. After the child is born most physicians wait until the pulsation in the cord ceases before tying, so as to give the child the benefit of the extra blood in the placenta. If it does not cry or breathe well, she may give it a sharp slap over the buttocks, or sprinkle a little cold water on the chest; if it cries lustily she may wrap it in a small blanket, oil it over with vaseline or cotton-seed oil, and put it in the cradle, laying it on its right side and looking at it now and then to see that it is still breathing.

It is generally twenty minutes before the after-birth is expelled. During this time the physician, or nurse at his direction, makes firm pressure on the uterus through the abdominal wall, continuing this until after the delivery of the placenta, when, if well contracted, it will feel firm and hard, of about the size of a cricket-ball. She should have a small basin close at hand to receive the placenta, which the physician will usually wish to examine to see if it has all come away and to make some measurements.

After even a normal birth most physicians will order a vaginal douche of bichloride $\frac{1}{3000}$ or carbolic $\frac{1}{60}$, temperature 110° F. The external parts are washed off with some of the same solution and dusted with iodoform, a piece of bichloride padding 9 inches long and 4 inches wide is laid next the vulva, and then the post-partum pad, made of oakum or jute, the ends of which are pinned posteriorly and anteriorly to the binder. A straight binder is, I think, the nicer, from 14 to 16 inches in width, pinned down the front with small pins and firmly fitted to the figure on either side with safety-pins. A post-partum should be dressed every four hours for the first 24 hours, after that every eight hours until the ninth day, after that the antiseptic dressing may be dispensed with, the patient still wearing the oakum or jute pad until the lochia ceases.

This describes a normal birth, but there may be complications which will require rapid and skilled services on the part of the nurse. If before the physician comes the patient should develop symptoms of eclampsia or mania, he should be sent for in all haste ; in the meantime, for eclampsia she should endeavor to keep the tongue from being bitten or the patient otherwise injuring herself, and if possible, to have prepared a large bath of hot water, which the doctor may use in the treatment of the case. In the mania her efforts should be to calm and control the patient.

Then we may have a forceps case. For this there is generally an assistant doctor and extra nurse; if not, there will be needed two low chairs or stools, the same height as the bed; the patient is placed across the bed, a foot on each chair, and the buttocks brought close to the edge. Added to the usual preparations will be a large basin of carbolic $\frac{1}{40}$, into which are submerged the forceps; before handing to the doctor she will oil the blades with carbolized oil and hand one blade at a time, after this a towel, as the handles become very slippery from the oil and discharges. She can then support the knees and be ready to aid the doctor in any emergency that may arise.

In a case of lacerated perineum the patient will be placed on the bed as for a forceps case, and the instruments as carefully prepared, and the surgeon will require scissors, uterine dressing forceps, needles, sutures, cotton or sponges in an antiseptic solution. After this operation, greatest care, if possible, is needed to prevent infection and to insure healing. It may be required to pass the catheter at intervals to prevent the urine dripping over the wound.

Perhaps there is no time when a nurse can be of more assistance to a doctor than when the patient has a post-partum hemorrhage : to give him promptly each thing he may call for without becoming excited and awkward is very essential.

Sometimes the baby requires resuscitation; for this several methods are used, the most common one the hot and ice-cold alternate dip; two large basins, one with ice and cold water, the other with hot water, temperature 115°–120°, the baby is dipped first into one and then the other; often this means will succeed. Again the doctor will try other ways. He may need a catheter to pass down the trachea, through which he will blow air into the lungs, clearing away any mucus that may be there; again he may try Schultze's or Sylvester's methods of artificial respiration, for each of which the nurse must be prepared to assist, not forgetting to watch the mother also, that all is well with her.

During the labor, if the patient should ask for a glass of milk, give it to her, and indeed if she desires it she may have some at frequent intervals after the completion of her labor; do not starve your patient, be guided in the diet by the physician, some allow a liberal diet while others restrict it. In Columbia Hospital we give a light diet for the first five days; for the first two days feeding them every three hours, giving them milk, oatmeal gruel, cracked wheat cereal, chicken soup, tea and toast, and crackers and milk; on the third and fourth days, in addition to any of these, soft-boiled eggs and a small piece of steak or mutton chops, and on and after the fifth day she has a regular diet excepting fresh vegetables.

The care of the breasts should begin before labor, preventing pressure from clothing, and if the nipples are extremely tender bathing them with a solution of alcohol and alum. The baby may be put to the breast as soon as the mother wakes from her first sleep; he will probably get no milk, but it will excite contraction of the uterus. There is in the breasts at this time a substance called colostrum; this the baby gets, and it is said to cause an evacuation of the bowels. This should suffice for nourishment for the baby until the milk comes; do not give him catnip-tea, Winslow's Soothing Syrup, or any other of the popular nostrums suggested by kind (?) friends. After the flow of milk is established the baby should be put to the breast every two hours during the day, and at night after nursing at 11 p. m., not again until 5 a. m. This insures good rest for the mother and better digestion and habits for the child. If the nipples become cracked, besides greater care being taken to keep them perfectly clean, they may be painted in the fissure with a solution of nitrate of silver, or painted over with a mixture of sub-nitrate of bismuth and castor oil, or whatever way the physician may order. If the nitrate of silver is used, great care must be taken to wash it off well before putting the baby again to the breast. You cannot devote too much attention to the nipples, for much depends upon the nurse whether they become inflamed and suppurate.

After the mother is cared for and left to sleep, the nurse prepares to wash the baby. Before beginning she should have everything needed close beside her, a small bath, or large basin of water 100° F., a little white castile soap; a piece of sheet-lint makes a nice soft washcloth, or in hospitals a piece of jute, which can be used once and thrown away. The nurse should wear a rubber apron and over that a small blanket; place the baby across her knees and wash first its face and then all over carefully; if it has been oiled well after birth it will aid much in removing the vernix caseosa, then it can be put in the bath, and after being dried thoroughly with a soft towel (old linen makes the nicest baby towels) especial care should be taken to see that it is well dried in all the creases, a little lycopodium or fuller's earth may be used, but careful drying is much more essential. Next the care of the cord. It may be dusted over with a little iodoform and boric acid, $\frac{1}{3}$, and wrapped with a small piece of borated cotton; this need not be changed unless there is fresh bleeding or it becomes wet from any cause. Never use oil or vaseline; it delays the cord dropping off and causes an odor. The fewer clothes and bands about a baby the better. In our hospital we have discarded the latter altogether; in private houses most mothers will insist upon a band; if so, be careful that it is too loose to do harm. A little flannel shirt, high neck and long sleeves, two small diapers rather than one large one, the one folded into a square and put just over the genitals, and the other pinned on the outside in the ordinary manner, one flannel skirt with a band sewed or pinned on with small safety-pins, and a single little slip is all the baby needs. After its toilet is completed, as soon as its mother wakes it may be put to the breast, then into its cradle, beginning even at this early age to train it to regular habits. The baby should be nursed every two hours during the day, as said before, except at night. Great care should be taken to wash its mouth after each nursing. The nurse should pay special attention to know that the baby's bowels move and that it urinates, especially during the first twenty-four hours.

In case of death of the mother, or if from any cause she cannot nurse her baby, after a healthy wet nurse, the best substitute is cow's milk, adding lime-water, $\frac{1}{3}$, and a little sugar; if, after giving this a good trial, it does not suit the baby, some good patent foods may be tried. If possible, keep the baby, at any rate for the first few weeks, from being handled round and danced by admiring relatives. Animal nature sets us an example in the care of its young, and yet no animal is born in a more undeveloped state than the human baby. Quiet sleep and regular feeding go far to make a good baby and healthy child.

In conclusion I must not forget to say something about that dread scourge, septicaemia. Cleanliness is the sheet-anchor for its prevention, and I mean by cleanliness surgical cleanliness; the time was when anything was considered good enough for the bed and dressings of a lying-in patient. The preparation in regard to asepsis, the handling of the patient, and the examinations should be made with as much care as for a laparotomy. The nurse usually has nearly all of this part under her control, and even though the physicians may seem somewhat hurried, she can do a great deal of suggesting with her basins of hot water, soap, nail-brushes and plenty of clean towels. I predict that when nursing shall have reached the height to which it is destined, childbed-fever will be a thing of the past, and only interesting as a matter of history.

MIDWIFERY AS A PROFESSION FOR WOMEN.

BY ZEPHERINA P. SMITH, *née* VEITCH,

President of the Midwives Institute, London.

Midwifery as a profession for women is a somewhat vexed question. Many people hold that it is unsuited for them. Again, others say it is particularly their province. Again, opinions differ as to how far women should go in practice, whether they should be limited to natural labor only, or whether they should qualify for the full practice, even to undertaking instrumental cases. It is impossible to discuss the question thoroughly, in a paper which must deal briefly with its subject, therefore we must face the fact that it has been calculated that in the British Isles alone the number of women who give assistance in childbirth is probably about 9000. Therefore, whatever opinions may be concerning the expediency of women as midwives, the question before us is, if 9000 women are practicing, should they be educated to fulfill their duties with safety to mother and child, or should they be allowed to obtain their knowledge as best they can?—which must mean experience gained at great risk to their patients. There can be but one answer to such a question, in any serious mind. A very large proportion of these women have had no training, nor education of any kind, beyond the experience they have gained in the number of cases they may have attended. So far back as 1813, the Society of Apothecaries made an attempt to get Parliament to pass enactments for the examination and control of midwives, but they failed to get any legislation on the subject, as all who have since tried have also failed. In 1872, the Obstetrical Society of London, recognizing the serious mischief done by these untaught, ignorant women who called themselves midwives, endeavored to improve matters by offering to give certificates to any women who could pass an examination to their satisfaction, showing that they had been thoroughly taught how to conduct a case of natural labor with safety to mother and child, and the Society appointed a body of examiners for this purpose. At first few women presented themselves for examination; in the first year only 6 passed in the two examinations which were held. But partly in consequence of a very superior class of women taking up the profession, and no doubt the general improvement in nurses during the past twenty years, no less than 75 women received their certificates from the Obstetrical Society in the examination held in January, 1893.

Some ten years ago, a few women who realized the very unsatisfactory condition of midwives both as regarded their training and social position, formed a society—The Matron's Aid Society—having for its object the better training of midwives, and the improvement of their position generally, with the ultimate object of endeavoring to get a bill passed for the registration of all women who called themselves midwives and acted as such. This society has grown into the present "Midwives Institute," which in 1889 was incorporated by act of Parliament. It carries on the work of the former society, and has further added to its usefulness by a registry for members, a good medical lending library, and club room, and medical lectures, by which means those members who are preparing themselves for the Obstetrical Society's examination can obtain most valuable help in their studies.

It is through the efforts of this society that at last the bill for registration of midwives was before the House last session, and that a select committee was appointed to examine into the question. At the present time any woman in Great Britain can place "Midwife" upon her doorplate, and undertake the duties this word implies, without being answerable to any person or persons for her training, and so long as she has no fatal case she can practice without interference. It is scarcely possible to form anything like a correct idea of the mischief done by these women, as too often lifelong injury is done, even when life itself is not destroyed. Legislation ought to be brought to bear upon the subject, and no woman should be allowed to style herself midwife who cannot show that she has received an education fitting her to practice.

So far we have considered the question of midwifery as a profession for women, and whatever may be the individual feeling concerning this question, all will agree that if women do act as midwives they certainly ought to be thoroughly instructed in their duties. The public generally have a very indefinite idea of what a midwife is, and a very deep-rooted objection to the word, which in itself is a very inoffensive word, meaning with-woman, or in Latin with-mother. For the very great dislike to the word we must look to the disgrace brought upon it by the malpractices of the women who professed to be midwives. Before entering upon the question of the due instruction of these women, let me clearly state what is meant by the word midwife, viz. a woman who undertakes to act as a doctor in cases of labor. A midwife must not be confounded with a certificated nurse; the latter is in no way trained to act as a doctor, only as a nurse who thoroughly understands her duties to a lying-in woman and her child. A midwife, according to the Obstetrical Society's diploma, is only certified to be able to attend cases of natural labor, which may roughly be classed as those cases which proceed to a close without interference or complications. Her education enables her at once to decide, when called to a patient, whether the case is one which she can safely manage herself, or whether it will be necessary to seek further medical skill; and this is most important, for in all cases of midwifery the loss of time may result in the death of the patient, while timely aid would turn what might be a serious case into one without danger to mother or child.

Here follows the question of training and education. This is a very difficult question to settle in the present state of things concerning midwives. I can therefore only give my opinion of what I consider should be the education for women who intend to practice midwifery. If the bill passes the House, some definite rules will be laid down, and schools appointed for regular education and examination of all acting as midwives. From my own personal experience,

I am convinced that every woman who undertakes these serious duties should in the first place obtain a good training as a nurse to the sick—say at least a year's work in a general hospital ; then I fully concur in Dr. Smith Napier's opinion: " Speaking broadly, I would suggest: (1) Six months' training in a good lying-in hospital, or three months' training in such an institution with nine months' additional pupilage under a recognized practitioner of midwifery. (2) The personal conduction of at least twenty confinements. (3) A searching examination conducted by a competent, duly constituted board." But this education would only fit a woman to undertake what I have roughly described as natural labor. Should she desire to go further in the practice of midwifery—which I in nowise advocate, at least for the generality of women—she would have to give more time to study, and she would have to attend some school where she could learn the use of instruments, etc. In my opinion, any woman desiring to practice in this way ought to qualify as a woman doctor, otherwise I do not see how she is to do full justice to those who employ her. There can be no doubt that the more thoroughly a woman is trained and educated for her work, the better will she do it to the advantage of her patient, and the more knowledge she has, the less likely will she be to delay sending for medical skill when she finds the case requires it. She may attain a very considerable proficiency in her calling, and make a highly honorable position for herself, without attempting to reach so far as qualifying for a doctor, for which only a small proportion of women are in any way fitted. In the necessarily small space of a paper such as this is, it is impossible to do more than touch upon the salient points of my subject, and therefore I have been obliged to condense what I have said, and to leave out details into which I should have liked to enter, as my personal interest in the question of midwives is very great, but I hope I may have said enough to lead others to examine into the question for themselves.

NURSING OF THE INSANE.

By Miss M. E. May,

State Hospital, Rochester, N. Y.

The civil and social status of the insane, and the manner in which they were to be treated, were determined for long ages by religious and philosophic hypotheses.

The earliest records of cases of insanity are given in the Old Testament. Saul (1063 B. C.), possessed by an evil spirit, was comforted by the music of David's harp, and became well again.

Nebuchadnezzar, King of Babylon, "was driven from men, and did eat grass as oxen" (Dan. iv. 33), and at the end of six years (569-563 B. C.) he recovered and was re-established upon his throne.

"In ancient Egypt, cases of mental derangement were sent to the temples to be cured by the priests, and they were regarded as afflicted by the gods or possessed by demons. Similar views of divine inspiration or of diabolical possession prevailed generally until the time of Hippocrates (460 B. C.)."* The "Father of Medicine" taught that the brain was the organ of the mind, and that it was subject to physical laws and diseases like other organs, and that insanity followed abnormal conditions of the brain. He described disorders of the mind that essentially correspond with mania, melancholia and dementia, and divined the important bearings of heredity, and dwelt on the value of a study of temperaments in the treatment of cases. These teachings became the accepted medical doctrine, and were enlarged upon by others for some centuries. Galen (130 A. D.) distinguished between insanity and the delirium of fever.

"These comparatively enlightened views of the nature of insanity were unfortunately destined not to endure. With the downfall of the Roman Empire and with the decline of civilization, gross ignorance and superstition with regard to the insane again prevailed, and their lot became more wretched, if possible, than at any previous time."* Thousands of the insane were executed as witches, and comparatively few among them found protection and humane treatment in cloisters. This pitiful state of the insane continued throughout the middle ages, except in Oriental lands where superstitious theories as to their inspiration served the purpose of averting harsh

---

* *Reference Handbook of the Medical Sciences.*

measures, and it was not until long after the Reformation, and the revival of letters and of science, that there was any very essential change for the better in their condition. Although special buildings were erected for the reception of the insane in Italy in the latter part of the fourteenth century, and in Spain in the beginning of the fifteenth, and although subsequently in various countries efforts were made for their safekeeping, it may still be asserted that the care extended to them was simply custodial, even until the latter part of the eighteenth century.

In the latter part of the eighteenth century and the beginning of the nineteenth, Pinel in France (1745–1826) and William Tuke in England (1732–1822), did much for the improvement of the condition of the insane in these countries, by removing the excessive mechanical restraint then considered necessary, and by introducing more humane treatment into the institutions in which they were interested.

In our own country, Dorothea Lynde Dix, in the first half of the nineteenth century, began her great life-work in behalf of the insane ; her efforts to improve the condition of the insane never ceasing until her death in 1887. To her zeal and energy the present plan of caring for the insane in America was largely due.

At the beginning of the nineteenth century there were only four insane asylums in the whole United States, and only one of these had been entirely built by a State government. " They were, in the order of the dates of their foundation, those of Philadelphia, Pa., 1752 ; of Williamsburgh, Va. (the first State Asylum), 1773 ; of New York, 1791 ; of Baltimore, Md., 1797."

In 1813 the attention of certain Philadelphia Friends was drawn to the work of William Tuke in England ; they began to collect money, and three years later an asylum was opened, in which the insane might see that they were "regarded as men and brethren."

The original purpose of this asylum was the care of members of the Society of Friends, but in a few years after its opening all sectarian restrictions were removed, and now only a small proportion of the patients are in membership with the Friends.

In 1817 the McLean Asylum for the Insane, now the McLean Hospital, was established in Somerville, Mass., and from that time many other asylums were built ; a higher standard of care was aimed at, the old idea of custodial care being all that was necessary had died out, and the new plan of studying each case and prescribing a course of treatment for it took its place. In this course of treatment, employment for the insane is an important factor.

There are in all hospitals for the insane in America a medical superintendent, assisted by one or more physicians, and a steward; in many hospitals there is a woman physician. In New York State the law requires that a woman physician shall be on the medical staff of each State hospital.

In arranging the daily life of patients in a hospital for the insane, the medical superintendent plans that they shall be grouped into families, according to the amount of self-control they are able individually to exercise. This method of classification results in a psychological school for the training of the patients in the exercise of self-control. Each family or ward contributes from its members to a large number of industrial classes, and its daily life is arranged in such a manner that each member is urged to take part in some educational or industrial occupation. The hospital is furnished so as to make it seem as home-like as possible to the patients, and the hours of the day are arranged so that their work, their meals, and their rest shall accord closely with comfortable home-life.

The patients help with the ward work, in the laundry, kitchens, sewing-room, shoe-shop, tailor-shop, carpenter-shop, engine-house, garden, farm, and in many other industries. Then there are indoor and outdoor games provided, entertainments of different kinds, a library, daily papers on the wards, the daily walk or drive when the weather permits, each of these being used as a means of treatment.

Schools for the instruction of patients are being generally established; trained teachers are employed, and object-teaching is particularly prominent. Reading, writing, arithmetic, grammar, geography and many other subjects are taught. In some of these schools there are classes in drawing, painting, modeling in clay, and wood-carving. Many hospitals have gymnasiums in which patients are instructed in physical training.

By the last half of the present century a reform had taken place in the treatment of the insane by the medical profession; then it was necessary that there should be nurses who could intelligently carry out the orders of the physicians. A course of training for nurses of the insane was thought of.

In 1854, the year of the beginning of Florence Nightingale's work in the Crimea, Dr. Browne began a course of lectures to attendants, at Crichton Institution in England; this was the "first attempt to educate the attendants upon the insane." This lasted only a short time. Many physicians were interested in "true nursing reform," and the influence of the general hospitals was strongly felt in Europe and America ; but the first attempts to start training schools in asylums failed, and in 1879 there was not in any asylum in the world an organized school for the training of attendants. To Massachusetts belongs the honor of having first successfully carried into effect the plan of an asylum training school. The trustees and superintendent of McLean Hospital determined in 1879 to establish a school for the training of attendants in that asylum, and in three years the school was inaugurated. " It was planned that the school should be not simply for the instruction of attendants upon the insane, but also to fit young men and women, as in general hospitals, to undertake general nursing." The training of women nurses in this school has gone on without intermission since 1882. The formal training of men was begun four years later. An arrangement was made in 1886 with the Boston Training School at the Massachusetts General Hospital, by which any female graduate of the McLean Hospital Training School who wished to have additional practical experience and instruction in general nursing, had the privilege, under the usual conditions, of entering that school and receiving its diploma after completing satisfactorily the studies of its senior year.

The instruction in McLean Hospital Training School includes the general care of the sick, the managing of helpless patients in bed, in moving and changing bed and body linen, making of beds, giving baths, keeping patients warm or cool, preventing and dressing bed sores, bandaging, applying fomentations, poultices and minor dressings, the preparing and serving of food, the administering of enemata, and the use of the catheter; attendance upon patients requiring diversion and companionship, the observation of mental symptoms, delusions, hallucinations, delirium and stupor, and the care of violent, excited and suicidal patients. The nurses are also given instruction in the best practical methods of supplying fresh air, warming and ventilating sick-rooms in a proper manner, and are taught to take proper care of rooms and wards, in keeping all utensils perfectly clean and disinfected; to observe the sick accurately in regard to the state of the secretions, pulse, breathing, skin, temperature, sleep, appetite, effect of diet, of stimulants and medicine ; the giving of massage and the managing of convalescents.

In October, 1883, Dr. Andrews began a course of instruction to the women attendants at the Buffalo State Hospital for the Insane.

Two years later a course of instruction for men attendants was begun, and a number of graduates go out from this training school each year. During the past ten years many hospitals have begun to train their attendants. These hospitals report that the advantages derived from the attendants being trained become more apparent each year. The course of training usually extends over a period of two years. Many graduates remain in the service of the institution and receive an increase of wages in recognition of their having successfully completed the course of study. Some leave the institution to do private nursing ; others are employed in other institutions at higher wages than they could command if they were not graduates of a training school, while some of the men have taken up the study of medicine. The experience in surgical nursing is not great, but there are always some capital operations which give the attendants the opportunity of learning how to prepare themselves and a patient for an operation, how to prepare the room and assist at the operation. The standard of training required differs in different hospitals. There has been some discussion amongst superintendents in America about having a uniform standard of training, but as yet no plan has been acted apon.

When graduates remain in the institution they are given charge of a ward, or industrial department, with as many assistant attendants as the work of their department requires ; these they instruct in the work of the department. Each ward has a graduate, a senior attendant (who takes charge of the ward in the absence of the head attendant), and one or more junior attendants.

As to the benefits to the insane and the hospital resulting from the systematic training of nurses, Dr. Edward Cowles, in his report of the McLean Hospital Training School for 1889, in speaking of the character of the service rendered by these nurses, says : " It is difficult to present this adequately. It is given to the experienced superintendent alone to appreciate such a thing as this. He knows what it is under such responsibilities to *feel* what his household is doing, and the spirit with which it is being done. The paramount consideration, however, is the relation of the nurse to the patient. From this side there are constantly coming, in a multitude of ways, from patients and their friends, spontaneous expressions of the most significant kind, testifying to a gratifying appreciation of the uniform kindness and helpfulness of the nurses to the sick. In the very nature of the case there must sometimes be control and restriction of the patients, and inevitably misconception and complaint on their part. But when such patients grow fond of their nurses, and the testimony of convalescents is uniformly to their credit, the evidence is unquestionable."

Dr. Cowles goes on to say: " The proof is satisfactory to me that it is the knowledge given to the nurse by careful instruction which brings satisfaction to her from the exercise of the ability to intelligently direct her sympathies. With such stimulation, she knows what is needed, and when and why to give her sympathy; she knows the wrong of not giving it. On the side of the physician, the advantage of the new order of things might be stated strongly. To have nurses in every ward who can make an intelligent analysis of mental symptoms and detect many of the important particulars in which disorder exists, is not only to have instruments in one's hands for the precise application of remedial influences of moral treatment of a kind before unavailable, but it enlarges the physician's own knowledge of morbid conditions. The asylum thus becomes an hospital in truth, and both the humane and scientific spirit are invited to dwell and flourish in it."

DISCUSSION.

A DELEGATE.—I would like to ask Miss May if it is not rather confusing to call an asylum an hospital, and an attendant a nurse? Doesn't it mix up the ideas of the different work ?

MISS MAY.—I think perhaps it does, but in New York State it has become a law that all the State hospitals for the insane shall be called hospitals. I never call an attendant a nurse, myself, but Dr. Cowles, in his report, I think almost invariably does.

CHAIRMAN.—I think the tendency in insane asylums is to call them hospitals instead of asylums. I have heard various superintendents object to the name "asylum," and I think they are trying as far as possible to call them hospitals.

THE HISTORY OF WORKHOUSE REFORM.

By Miss Louisa Twining.

It is not an easy task to write the history of a movement that has been carried on in various ways and with varying success during a period of forty years, but as I am asked to give some account of what has been accomplished, I will endeavor to do so, believing that I am perhaps the only one remaining of the first small body of " reformers " in the cause of workhouse management.

In 1850 a pamphlet on this subject was written by two ladies, Mrs. May and Mrs. Archer, and it was the first publication that turned my attention to it. The pamphlet was called "A Plan for Rendering the Union Poorhouses National Houses of Mercy "; and I may add that the same plea is now again being urged by the Countess of Meath and myself.

But there was an even earlier effort than this which must not be forgotten. One hundred years before, a now well-nigh forgotten philanthropist, Jonas Hanway, born in 1712, was led to consider the sad state of the infant parish poor. He even traveled through Europe (no easy matter in those days) to ascertain what was done in other countries, and on his return published the results of his investigations. The workhouse of St. Clement Danes in the Strand is particularly named in relation to this matter, and I may mention the coincidence that it was in this very Strand Union that my investigations and visits were first carried on. In 1761, Hanway, after ten years of toil and unceasing work, obtained an act for regulating the treatment of parish children. It forbade their being kept in the workhouses; all were to be sent into the country to be nursed until six years old; and there is no doubt that thousands of lives were thus preserved. In 1855 a volume of " Practical Lectures to Ladies " was published, containing one by the Rev. J. S. Brewer, on "Workhouse Visiting," which showed that consideration for the poor inmates was beginning to be felt.

In 1853, through interest in a respectable old woman whom I had long visited in her little room (which she was obliged to give up for the workhouse, her eyesight failing her for needlework), I was led to follow her into her dreaded retreat; and from that day, now forty years ago, my interest in and desire to help the inmates may be dated, and has never since ceased. Their utter loneliness, their prison-like separation from the outer world, was the first thing that struck me; for I learnt that no one was allowed to enter, except the friends and relations on certain fixed days, and there were, of course, many poor, lonely creatures who had neither relation nor friend. There were at least five hundred inmates in that one workhouse, of every class and description, and of all ages; no separation of classes being then made. I obtained permission to visit when I liked, but my endeavors to extend this privilege to other ladies, when referred to the Board of Guardians, consisting of local tradesmen, were unsuccessful. The Central (then the Poor Law) Board having been consulted, it was decided that there could be no giving way to such an innovation as was proposed, which threatened to overthrow "the discipline of the workhouse" and perhaps create a revolution! A subsequent application from myself was "reluctantly declined" as "forming an inconvenient precedent"; a phrase we are all familiar with in connection with suggested reforms. I may here quote from a little book of my "Recollections," published in 1880: "The plan was thus stopped for a time, but not relinquished; and the individual visits were continued, by which much knowledge was acquired of the internal arrangements of the workhouse, and of the many cruel and unknown miseries which were inflicted on the inmates. For what could the best of matrons effect for good or comfort when she was the sole woman in authority over that vast household, with literally no helper or assistant but pauper women?"

In the following year, 1854, another effort was made, and a personal interview was granted by the President and Secretary of the Poor Law Board, when a kind promise was given that, if the plan were carried on quietly, no objection would be made. So by degrees, some friends being enlisted in the work and others becoming interested in it, the visiting system gradually extended. There was one visitor for every ward for many years (until, indeed, the removal of the old workhouse) both on week-days and Sundays; with tea-parties at Christmas, in which the whole staff of visitors, ladies and gentlemen, joined.

In 1857 I was induced to send a letter to the "Guardian," a weekly high-class Church newspaper, with some remarks and suggestions concerning "Homes for the Aged Poor," and this was the beginning of a long-continued correspondence. These letters were republished in 1857 as a pamphlet, called "Metropolitan Workhouses and their Inmates"; one other having already appeared in 1855, with the title, "A Few Words about the Inmates of our Workhouses."

In 1858, Mrs. G. W. Sheppard, of Frome, wrote a pamphlet, "Sunshine in the Workhouse," and in the following year, "Christmas Eve in a Workhouse"; both of which helped to bring the forgotten inmates, who were indeed "out of mind" as well as "out of sight," to the notice of the outer world.

In 1857, a young nobleman, Lord Raynham, was led to consider the subject, in consequence of the disclosures that had been made public. He brought forward a motion in the House of Commons that a select committee should be appointed to inquire into the condition and administration of metropolitan workhouses; referring to the state of St. Pancras Workhouse (one of the largest in London), where an investigation had just been made, resulting in a verdict of "horrible" from one of the first of London physicians. But though the motion was well supported, after an "official" reply from the president of the Poor Law Board, it was lost. For years after this apparent failure, the very committee then asked for was appointed; and exactly ten years later, in 1867, the result appeared in the bill introduced by Mr. Gathorne Hardy (now Lord Cranbrook) and subsequently passed. By this grand effort the metropolitan infirmaries for the sick were entirely separated from the workhouses and placed under the management of other officers. In 1858 I wrote a long article in the "Church of England Monthly Review" on "Workhouses and Women's Work," afterwards published as a pamphlet, which was widely reviewed by the daily press. Other movements were going on. In 1855 the matter of training nurses was brought before the Epidemiological Society of London by an eminent physician, Dr. Edward Sieveking, who proposed that the able-bodied women in workhouses should thus be made useful; and in 1858 a circular of the Poor Law Board sanctioned the plan, which, I may say here, was never found practicable, owing to the generally degraded character and antecedents of this class. In connection with this part of our subject, I may add the satisfactory information that the idea thus started has taken, since 1879, a practical and entirely successful form in the formation of the "Workhouse Infirmary Nursing Association," which has now one hundred and thirty nurses at work throughout the country, many of them trained by the funds of the association; the demand for the nurses being beyond the number that can be supplied.

In 1857 a great step was made by a proposal to form a central society for the promotion of workhouse visiting. This suggestion was brought forward at the first meeting of the "Social Science Association," which met at Birmingham ; when I contributed a paper in the department of social economy on the "Condition of Workhouses"—the first, I believe, that had ever come before the public. The plan was afterwards developed in London, under the presidency of the Hon. Wm. Cowper (afterwards Lord Mount-Temple), and a large and influential committee of men and women was formed, I being the honorary secretary. Its rules and objects were : 1. The care of children, and their after-care as well (a plan now largely developed). 2. For the sick and afflicted. 3. For the ignorant and depraved, their instruction, and the encouragement of useful occupation. Thus the seeds were sown for many subsequent developments ; one of which, in connection with the last-named object, is the "Brabazon" scheme for providing work and suitable occupation for both men and women who are unable to assist in the regular work for the house. This scheme is now being increasingly adopted in many workhouses in London and the country, its origin being due to Lady Meath, who has the satisfaction of seeing her scheme now carried out in America as well as at home.

In the year 1859 another departure was made by the publication of a periodical called the *Journal of the Workhouse Visiting Society*, which at first appeared every two months, and then quarterly. Much useful information was thus distributed, and the plan was continued till 1865, when it was felt it had done its useful work of enlightenment and it ceased. In this periodical may be found the suggestion of nearly every movement now being carried out. The first meeting of the society was held in 1859, "the first occasion on which the claims of the workhouse inmates on the sympathy of the public have been advocated," as was said at the time. Two bishops and many influential clergymen and laymen spoke, to advocate the cause. A committee of visitors was formed for one of the city workhouses, under the auspices of the Lady Mayoress, and in 1860 one was appointed also for St. Pancras Workhouse.

In 1862 a bill was carried through Parliament—chiefly owing to the exertions of the Hon. Mrs. Way, who had already established a school for pauper girls in Surrey—establishing the legality of payments by the guardians to homes certified by the central board. The rescue of children and girls from the contamination of pauper intercourse was the first object to engage the attention of visitors ;

with the result that a home was opened in London for girls, who returned to the workhouse after being sent to service. This was done in 1861, under an influential committee, of which the Baroness Burdett-Coutts was one, while she generously furnished the house and paid the rent during three years. The management devolved upon me, and for many years I lived almost entirely at the home, into which thirty girls could be taken. I may mention here that this home was carried on till 1878, when the house was taken for the remaining years of the lease by a committee of ladies who were beginning to carry out the plans of Mrs. Nassau Senior, appointed in 1875 as the first woman inspector under the Poor Law Board, for the schools. This was the starting-point of the now widely extended Metropolitan Association for Befriending Young Servants, number-ing thousands, under the care of a large staff of visitors, and with homes also. Many hundreds of girls may be said to have been saved from ruin during the twenty years work of this association.

In 1860 a commission was appointed to consider the state of education in England, and as pauper schools were included, I was asked to give evidence about them. The two chief points I dwelt upon as evils were, the want of industrial training for girls, and the herding of them together in masses. Both evils have been largely done away with since by means of boarding-out children (begun in 1870, and suggested in our Journal in 1864), and by cottage homes, started by voluntary effort, and certified by the Local Government Board. An association to promote this last plan was begun in 1891.*

In 1860 attention was drawn to the condition of incurables in work-houses by Miss Frances Power Cobbe, who had visited the workhouse at Bristol and had become acquainted with the sadly defective care of them. She wrote a paper called "A Plea for Destitute Incur-ables," which was read at a Social Science Congress at Glasgow, and afterwards brought before the central board. A petition was framed, signed by ninety of the leading physicians and surgeons of the Lon-don hospitals, asking permission to give voluntary aid to such sufferers (of whom there was supposed to be 80,000 in the workhouses) by means of trained nurses; comforts and appliances suitable to their sad condition being supplied from a central fund. Seven Boards of Guardians consented to try the plan, and it was carried on for two years; but after that time, objection was urged that it was

* At the present time Miss Mason is acting as Inspector, under the Local Government Board, of all children boarded out.

illegal and contrary to the intentions of the Poor Law. In 1865 a deputation of the Workhouse Visiting Society waited upon the president of the Poor Law Board (Mr. Villiers) with a statement and petition as to the general condition of the sick in workhouse infirmaries. Two meetings, attended by twenty-one members of Parliament and medical men, were held at Mrs. Gladstone's house to arrange this matter. This effort cannot be said to have been a failure, considering the great results that have followed from its endeavors and example. The petition is remarkable for embodying all subsequent reforms, but it is too long to be given here. The admission of additional medical men and students into Poor Law institutions was then urged, and is still earnestly desired. Of the gentlemen who formed that deputation, only two are now living. Impressed by the needs of sick paupers, it was decided to take a house adjoining the Girl's Industrial Home, for the reception of incurable women chiefly, and in the first instance from workhouses, their cost (as in the workhouse) being paid by the guardians, as in the case of the girls. This plan was successfully carried on for twenty-eight years, but owing to the improvements in the London infirmaries, their inmates ceased, after a time, to be received.

An inquiry was also instituted as to the number of *paid* nurses employed in workhouses: in most of which it was found there were only paupers to attend the sick.

In 1861 another Parliamentary Commission was appointed, at which much valuable evidence was given. Other committees followed in 1888 and 1891. Among the earlier efforts must be named a letter to the *Times*, written by me in 1858 on workhouse nurses. Then followed in 1866 the " Lancet Commission," carried out by the editors of that paper, for an investigation into all matters connected with the sick in workhouses. It was well said that this and many other endeavors to expose very grave evils were but following up the efforts of private persons; public opinion and the press supplying a force that compelled official action, " the foremost banners being borne by private individuals."

In 1867 Mr. Villiers acknowledged to a deputation that "a case had been made out," and although he left office before a bill could be prepared, one was carried through by his successor, Mr. Gathorne Hardy. The separation of the various classes of workhouse inmates was one of the chief features of this bill; and though it is not even now entirely carried out, children and the sick were removed from the "workhouse," so called, as well as lunatics, the imbecile, and all infectious cases. Of these latter classes the Metropolitan Asylums Board, a body formed from the guardians of the various unions represented, has taken charge. Its labors are on a truly gigantic scale.

The first grand reform in the management of the sick was begun at Liverpool, when, in 1865, Agnes Jones, a devoted lady and highly trained nurse, was appointed, in the enormous workhouse of 1200 inmates, as superintendent of the infirmary. A second such appointment was made at the Sick Asylum, Highgate, when Miss Hill, one of the Nightingale nurses of St. Thomas Hospital, went there in 1880. These were the first instances of educated and trained women taking such posts.

During the last few years women acting as guardians of the poor have aided the work of reform in no small degree, and by an increase in their number, year by year, we look forward to still further progress in the right direction. The first of these ladies was elected in the parish of Kensington in the year 1875, and now about one hundred and thirty women are acting as guardians of the poor in England, Wales, and Scotland.

I have now completed my sketch, but the full extent of all that has been accomplished can only be known to those who were eye-witnesses of a state of things now happily passed away.

In conclusion, may I be allowed to point out the moral of this history, which may be commended to all who are engaged in any similar work and undertaking. It is comprised in three words—Patience, Perseverance, and Faith.

THE INSTRUCTION OF THE SISTERS OF THE RED CROSS.

By Dr. M. Goering,

Physician-in-chief of the League of the Red Cross, Bremen, Germany.

Permit me to express sincere thanks for the recent invitation to take part in the work of the International Congress of Charities, Correction and Philanthropy, in Chicago, in which I see not only an honorable recognition of my personal work, but also of the success of the present society for the education of trained nurses, the interests of whose training schools have been confided to me since their foundation. It therefore appears proper that the regulations of our society or league be submitted for your kind inspection. My work upon the instruction of trained nurses, as well as their guidance through their professional career, has found practical illustrations in them. I have endeavored to give a comprehensive demonstration of them in two accompanying treatises.* The one is a dissertation on the subject, " The Training of the Sisters of the Red Cross," which I delivered on October 17, 1882, in a conference of delegates of the Red Cross held in Bremen. The other forms the preface to a text-book for nurses which I wrote, after fifteen years teaching, in 1891. From both writings I should like to select as the chief exponents of my views the following points and place them before you for discussion :

1. A natural capacity for nursing is possessed by the female sex, provided an individual liking for the work exists.

2. The main difficulties encountered by nurses are not to be found in mere manual duties, but in meeting the demands upon character and inner life.

3. The vocation of nursing is not only a life for, but with the sick.

4. The training of a nurse must take into consideration the whole character or personality of the pupil or sister. She must be sustained and encouraged in conscientious self-culture, by the influence of teachers selected for this purpose, by working with other trained nurses, by the continual supervision of the superintendent, and by the minute directions given her in conversations with the attending physicians regarding her own individual work.

5. The results of such training give the best ground for judging of the qualifications of the pupil-sister.

6. The acquisition of the most perfect self-control (usually as necessary for patient as for nurse) must be considered as the principal aim in training.

7. A method of instruction which is wholly individualizing is as

* Dr. Goering's paper is accompanied by the following works : 1. Statuten für den Verein zur Ausbildung von Krankenpflegerinnen zu Bremen. Bremen, 1891.—2. Die Berufsausbildung der Schwestern vom rothen Kreuz. Correferat erstattet für die Delegirten-Conferenz der Pflegevereine unter dem rothen Kreuz (Bremen, 17 October, 1882), von Dr. M. Goering, etc. Bremen, 1882.— 3. Lehrbuch für Krankenpflegerinnen von Dr. Goering, dirig. Arzt, etc. Bremen, 1891.—[EDITORS.]

necessary for the trained nurse as the strictly generalizing method is essential for the sister of some other Order.

8. To adapt the character of the nurse to the peculiar demands of nursing requires a longer time. Training courses of a few weeks or months are not enough. The period of training should be at least one year, provided this be spent continuously in one of the training schools or sisterhoods.

9. Experience shows that nursing is not a real life-work, or but very rarely so, when the nurse remains dependent upon herself.

10. The trained nurse needs the connection with the mother house ôr school, which will offer her a firm support and encouragement, and become as well a continued source of culture and improvement.

11. Sister leagues should care for the professional nurse in active duty in the same manner as other organizations do for sisters of religious orders.

12. In addition to a professional education, the work of training demands imperatively a thorough and far-reaching technical knowledge on the part of the teacher, sister or instructress. She should enter upon regular duty and learn nursing from its very rudiments, performing every duty and service within the circle of nursing.

13. A third problem which this training has to solve is the theoretical teaching of the pupil-nurse. The knowledge gained by it must give an intelligent insight into the principles of practical work. Its general tendency must be to free the mind of the nurse on the one hand from the many notions about medical science not only false but harmful, which are prevalent among the laity, and on the other hand to bring her reasoning powers nearer to those of the physicians.

14. The conception of theoretical knowledge which is necessary and serviceable must be determined on the one hand by the social standing and education of the head-nurse ("Lehr-schwester"), and on the other by the nature of the service which is contemplated. In comparison with service in hospitals, private or parish nursing makes higher demands both upon the whole personality and upon the entire store of technical and theoretical knowledge.

15. An over-estimate of the value of theoretical knowledge on the part of the nurse should be foreseen and prevented throughout her general training and education.

16. The control of this training, including its educational side, must be absolute and centered in one head or principal. It rests

with weightiest responsibility upon the doctor and his indispensable helpmate, the superintendent, whose special and general qualifications determine the success of the school.

17. The favorable development of trained nursing will ever depend upon the devotion with which the physician gives himself to the entire education of the nurses, and the fact that he does not allow it to be narrowed down simply to theoretical and technical knowledge.

18. Nursing alone offers women a vocation comparable with the professions of men, but only when followed without sad or morbid motives, and to the exclusion of all other minor, outside considerations.

19. In professional nursing the laborer is worthy of his hire. The value of the services of the person is measured here also by thoroughness in the profession, not by any special ability or individual ability in the same.

For twenty years trained nursing has been chief of my interests. To some degree, in a comparative study of its varieties, my sympathies incline to professional nursing.

At one time I hoped to take part personally in the transactions of the Congress in Chicago, but owing to many duties here, the fulfillment of the plan is denied me.

[Owing to an accident, Dr. Goering's original communication was lost, and it has been impossible to compare the above imperfect translation with the original.]

NURSING IN HOMES, PRIVATE HOSPITALS AND SANITARIUMS.

By Mrs. S. M. Baker,

Medical Matron of the Surgical Department of the Battle Creek Sanitarium.

After a quarter of a century's experience, Florence Nightingale said she had found that the happiest people, those fondest of their occupation, and the most thankful for life, were those engaged in sick-nursing. Though our experience has been a shorter one, and though it has not been among wounded heroes, but in the hospital and in the home, among all grades of society, we can heartily re-echo her words.

As nurses, we all understand the regulations and routine of hospital work. Not all of us perhaps have had the privilege of going into the home and taking from the hands of nervous and anxious friends, whose very anxiety has led them into all kinds of imprudence, a sick one whose lamp of life is just ready to go out for want of skilled care.

Perhaps a word from us may be a help to such, if a few be here, and may be of some encouragement to those chiefly engaged in private nursing, whose courage may sometimes flag when lacking the stimulus of companionship in their work.

There is no need to speak of the sacredness of the nurse's calling: how, when she enters a home, the dearest and most sacred things in the family are entrusted to her care, the life of the dear one, and perhaps her spiritual guidance. Much of the family life comes under the observation of the nurse, and even the skeleton in the closet is often revealed to her, sometimes unwittingly, and again with a half hope that one who is so helpful in other things may help here also. There is no need to suggest that her influence, if she be devoted, self-sacrificing and intelligent, may reach out to every department in the home, and most valuable are the lessons that it may be her privilege to teach in the saving of time and strength, in the laying up of those riches beyond price,—health in the body, knowledge in the mind, and Christ in the heart.

Emerson's words to the careful housewife contain a thought that applies as well to the nurse. " I pray you, most excellent wife, cumber not yourself and me to get a curiously rich dinner for this man and woman who have just alighted at our gate . . . but rather let that stranger see, if he will, in your looks, accents and behavior, your thought and will, that which he cannot buy at any price in any city." It is within the knowledge and province of the nurse to give something more than she is hired to give—something that money cannot buy—to help those with whom she comes in contact professionally to a higher plane of living, because she comes nearer to their inner life.

The prevailing ignorance among the masses of people simply on the preparation of healthful food is astonishing. To answer the purpose of nutrition, food must be of the right material and properly prepared. But there are house-mothers who, even in this advanced day of reforms, will take to the sick, rich pie, cakes, creams, and dainties prepared in the most indigestible manner, with wines and condiments, and abundance of sweets—food which throws the digestive organs into disturbance and has no strength-giving power. Even those who have learned that such food is injurious to the sick will still carry them tea, coffee, wine, meat-broths, and hot buttered toast, jellies, etc., expecting them to gain strength on what is only stimulating or indigestible.

"Science in the Kitchen" tells us that the purpose of food at all times is to supply materials for repairing the waste which is constantly going on in the vital economy. Hence the importance of knowing the comparative values of foods. In the care of the sick, with whom the waste is greater and the vital forces less active, it is needful to know not only what food is most nutritious, but also what will bring the least tax upon the weakened digestive powers. Soft, warm breads of any kind, fresh, lightly toasted bread included, are indigestible, for simple reasons: first, their softness allows them to be swallowed without proper mastication, and the starch which should have been changed to glucose in the mouth goes into the stomach in lumps which cannot be easily acted upon by the digestive juices. To make it still more indigestible, it is penetrated through and through by the fat of the butter, and fat we know is an effectual barrier to the action of the gastric juice.

The nurse will find it necessary to show the anxious wife or mother why fresh warm bread is pernicious, and why the toast should be browned through, instead of on the surface only. She must explain that tea and coffee are only stimulants; that milk is to be eaten as a food rather than taken as a drink; that condiments are irritating, and bring about the condition "necessary for the acquirement of a taste for intoxicating liquors"; that it has been estimated that "the evils of bad cookery and ill-selected food exceed those of strong drink"; that much cold food or drink in the stomach lessens the temperature, and consequently the power of digestion; that mastication is the only part of digestion over which we have direct control, and is habitually slighted, and the food thus passed into the stomach wants the preparatory step in digestion. So it must be explained that prepared crackers, beaten biscuit, breakfast rolls, zweibach or bread twenty-four hours old, are wholesome food, while hot soda biscuit, or fresh raised bread, or fresh half-toasted bread is not so.

For our very feeble patient, whose powers of digestion are weak,

the food must be more concentrated, nutritious, and easily assimilated. Delicious gruels, made from the grains; milk, either pure or
made into junket; eggs prepared in a variety of simple and attractive ways; cream and fruit toasts made from zweibach; refreshing
beverages, made of baked milk, almond milk, barley lemonade, egg
lemonade, apple beverage; and nature's own delicacies, the fruits,
can be attractively arranged, pleasing to the eye and palate. This
comes not only under the oversight and work of the nurse, but also
under her teaching.

If the food question comes under the influence of the nurse, even
more do the treatments for the relief of the patient. The rational
medicine of the present day is requiring less of drugs and more of
natural remedies. The wife or mother to whose relief the trained
nurse comes when sickness enters the home, does not know, perhaps, the stimulating or relaxing and soothing effects of the simple
remedies, heat and water. How few really know when tired themselves, or when a child is tired or nervous, that a hot bath, followed
by a cool pour, is relaxing to tired muscles and soothing to irritated
nerves; that heat to the spine will reduce temperature, local inflammation and hemorrhage, and in case of excessive nervousness or
excitement, that the most soothing effects come from alternate heat
and cold to the spine, along which the nerve-centers lie.

How few, outside of the trained profession, understand that of the
different forms of hydropathic treatment, one will produce a tonic
effect, another a sedative, another a moderate eliminative, another
a full eliminative effect; that one will diminish pelvic congestion,
another will reduce cerebral congestion, and so on through the list
of ailments and remedial measures. The relief from pain which a
hot sitz-bath and foot-bath will give, the invigorating effect of a cool
shallow bath, the soothing influence of the hot spray, or alternate
hot and cold sponging of the spine, the comfort of a blanket-pack or
home-arranged Turkish bath in conditions requiring their use, or of
the cool wet-sheet pack in fevers, the indescribable exhilaration of
a salt glow are something known only to those who have witnessed
their magic working.

In the struggle with the disease which the nurse has aided the
physician in combating by means of some one or two of these lines
of treatment, the value of which the intelligent physician is coming
more and more to appreciate, she has instilled the idea of the
rational use of dietetics and of the simple and universal remedy,

water, into the minds and hearts of the family, and now that the crisis is past, she has come to the waiting time, often the weary waiting for the return of strength. Can the nurse do more than to see that the diet, treatment, fresh air and sunshine are made to do their part in bringing the longed-for strength? The long unused muscles of the patient are weak and almost useless, and she must find her strength in the use of them. She must have exercise to quicken the sluggish circulation, to stimulate the nutrition and carry off the waste. Even while still in bed, she can be led through a gradually increasing scale of exercises. Beginning with hand and arm flexing and foot and leg flexing, after a few days she can attempt head rotating or arm raising. Perhaps she is too feeble to raise the arm more than a little or a few times the first day, the next a little higher, till the arms can be extended directly upward. Then turning from side to side, or other exercise as she can bear, being careful always not to overdo. As she is able to sit up in a chair, trunk bending, twisting, or rotating may be added to the other movements; then the breathing exercises after meals; the quick and the slow and deep inhalations and exhalations, broadening the chest, developing the lungs, purifying and enriching the blood, and sending the glow of returning health to the cheek. These movements are all supplementary to the massage, with its active and passive movements; and the patient is on her feet in quicker time and with more strength than she would have had without the exercise.

The criticism has sometimes been made that hospital training schools for nurses did not accomplish all that is desirable in the preparation of nurses for work in caring for the sick in private homes. Hospital work is somewhat routine in character, and necessarily runs in more or less definitely fixed grooves which are determined by the general class of work to which a hospital is devoted, or by the predilections of superintendents or of the house or consulting physicians. In hospital work, also, everything is done under the eye and, to a very large degree, under the immediate direction of the physician. The work in a public hospital is necessarily simplified as far as possible in consequence of the large number of cases which must be cared for by each individual nurse; and the facilities of public hospitals do not always afford so great a variety of remedial agencies, especially those of a hygienic or non-medical character, as might be provided if the business managers were at liberty to draw upon an unlimited fund for the support of their work. The facilities of dietetic, electro-therapeutic, hydropathic, kinesipathic and other hygienic measures of treatment furnished by ordinary public hospitals are, to say the least, very meager ; and consequently, nurses trained in such hospitals do not always have an opportunity for acquiring thorough familiarity with these remedial means. This deficiency is certainly very largely compensated for by the superior opportunities offered by the experience and training in the treatment of emergency cases of various sorts. Notwithstanding, the hospital trained nurse, when she leaves the supervision of her instructors and starts out upon an independent career as a trained nurse, often finds herself longing for a more thoroughly furnished armamentarium in her battle with disease and suffering in district and private nursing. A well-equipped sanitarium, provided with ample facilities for the administration of every form of hydropathic measures ; for the use of electricity in every form ; for the utilization of massage, Swedish movements, Swedish gymnastics, and the various forms of physical culture ; mechanical appliances for active and passive exercise; diet kitchens and surgical wards with every facility for aseptic surgery, and for the application of all rational hygienic as well as medicinal and mechanical agencies in the treatment of medical and surgical cases, is certainly an ideal place for the training of the nurse for working in the private home, in district nursing, and, in fact, wherever her lot may be cast. The course of training in such a school necessarily includes not only the subjects usually taught in hospital training schools, but theoretical and practical instruction in the therapeutics of water, electricity, massage, manual and mechanical Swedish movement, medical dietetics, scientific cookery, and a thorough course in exercise and physical culture. My experience has been that nurses appreciate the last-named feature as much as any other portion of such a course of training. The personal advantages which the nurse derives from the possession of strength, enduring muscles, perfect digestion, capacious lungs, strong waist, a back that never aches, an elastic step, a dignified and energetic bearing, are beyond estimate.

The training in physical culture, massage, and Swedish movements gives the nurse full command of all the advantages to be derived from measures of treatment which operate through the muscular system in the treatment and cure of disease, and which enables her to accomplish in many cases for her patient what cannot be accomplished by drugs or by any other means.

The resources afforded by electricity, especially the galvanic and faradic currents, are not at the full command of a nurse unless she has had months of daily experience in its use, and has learned well its potency and modes of application to the great variety of morbid conditions to which it is adapted. She must know more than this, she must have learned so well the secret of the battery by which the current is produced, whether faradic or galvanic, that in case the instrument fails to work (which it is quite likely to do when it is needed most) she can give it the magical touch which will unlock its potent forces; or, if need be, she may construct out of the raw material a battery capable of accomplishing useful results.

Sanitariums afford a specially favorable field for the study and application of medical dietetics. The absence of a regulation diet makes it possible to adapt the bill of fare to the needs of each individual patient, with a degree of accuracy which cannot be attempted under less favorable conditions. Facilities for analysis of stomach fluids and other secretions afford a basis for the exact study of the dietetic needs of patients, which affords the nurse educational advantages of no small value.

But perhaps the most practical advantages of all derived by the nurse from training in a well-equipped and scientifically organized sanitarium are derived from the daily and hourly experience in the use of hydropathic measures of every description. Water is a simple remedy which is universal, and is a most convenient means of utilizing those most potent of therapeutic measures, heat and cold, which act upon the central nervous system and through it upon the whole body, in a manner little less than marvelous. The nurse who is able to take the results of such a course of training into the home, into her work as a district nurse, or to a foreign field as a missionary nurse, is equipped for work of the highest usefulness, and feels a confidence in meeting every form of human malady not to be derived from any less thoroughgoing system of training.

In the sanitarium, private hospital and home, the nurse has the further advantage of an opportunity for the more exact treatment and study of her cases than in ordinary public hospital work, in consequence of the smaller number of patients usually placed under the care of each individual nurse. In well-organized private sanitariums patients who require nursing usually receive the whole attention of a single nurse, and sometimes of two nurses, one for the day, the other for the night. The application of so large a variety of measures of treatment gives the nurse abundance of work to do, even in caring for a single patient, and one which might not be considered of the most critical class, as for example the case of a rest cure patient, of which the following is a sample programme: 7 a. m., light rubbing and toilet. 8 a. m., first breakfast. 9 a. m., gentle massage of the stomach for fifteen minutes, then patient is allowed to rest three-quarters of an hour, while the nurse makes arrangement for morning treatment. 10 a. m., hot application to spine, cool saline sponge-bath, followed by vigorous massage or general faradization. 12 m., second breakfast. 1 to 3 p. m., rest in room, insolation in wheel-chair, hammock or cot on the porch or in the grove. 3 p. m., dinner. 4.30 p. m., light gymnastics or mechanical Swedish movements. 7 p. m., lunch. 9 p. m., sponging or rubbing of spine and preparation for the night. The treatment is varied from day to day according to each individual case or to suit certain conditions.

In carrying out such a programme the nurse will certainly find no time for idleness, and besides the treatment enumerated there is a vast number of little things to be done for the patient, such as reading, writing letters, keeping visitors away, doing little errands, and above all else, "making sunshine" for the patient.

In the care of surgical cases fresh from the operating room there is, of course, much more to be done. The following example is an exact copy of the hourly notes made by the day and night nurses in charge of a patient during the first twenty-four hours after an operation for the removal of diseased tubes and ovaries. The case was a critical one. Tubes distended with pus and adhesions numerous and dense. Operation completed at 5 p. m., patient placed in bed surrounded with hot bottles. Pulse to be taken every 15 minutes, temperature every two hours; drainage tube to be examined every three hours. 8 p. m., nausea, ice-bag to throat, fomentation to spine, temperature taken. 9 p. m., fomentation to stomach, position changed. 10 p. m., vaginal douche, ice-bag refilled for application to throat, temperature taken. 12. Faradization to stomach and spine temperature. 1 a. m., ice-bag over dressing; patient slept about 15 minutes. 2 a. m., enema to remove gas from bowels, temperature. 3 a. m., drainage tube examined and fluid withdrawn. 4 a. m., patient slept a few minutes, temperature. 5 a. m., patient vomiting, application to stomach and throat renewed. 6 a. m., fluid withdrawn from drainage tube, fomentation to stomach, ice-bag to throat. 7 a. m., hot vaginal douche, patient slept an hour. 9 a. m., faradization to stomach and spine. 10 a. m., hot bags to back and ice to throat, temperature. 11 a. m., fomentation to stomach. 12 m., hot vaginal douche, fluid withdrawn from tube, temperature. 1 p. m., ice-bag to throat, hot bag to stomach, patient slept an hour. 2 p. m., cool compress to head, temperature. 3 p. m., hot bag to spine. 4 p. m., faradization to spine, hot foot-bath, temperature. 5 p. m., fomentation to stomach, cool compress to head. Of course, in the care of such a case there are innumerable attentions necessary, such as turning of patient, changing head, rubbing limbs, and a great variety of other attentions which require the constant and faithful service of a nurse.

The results of such assiduous attention on the part of a well-trained nurse ought to be better than those ordinarily attained, especially in the treatment of acute and surgical cases ; and that the results are superior is abundantly attested by the records of private hospitals and sanitariums where such care is given. In one hospital, with the work of which I am familiar, and in the wards of which many serious surgical cases, including an average of two or more abdominal cases occur weekly, stitch abscess rarely ever occurs even after the most tedious operations, peritonitis is almost absolutely unknown, and erysipelatous inflammation of wounds is never seen. In my own wards I have seen 150 ovariotomies for removal of diseased ovaries or appendages, with an equal number of successive recoveries and without a single case of peritonitis. The operations were, without doubt, skilfully performed, but the operator makes no claim to greater skill than some other operators whose record of recoveries is by no means so great, and does not hesitate to attribute the extraordinary success to the thorough preparation of the patient, including aseptic dietary and careful nursing after the operation.

All the methods used at a sanitarium or private hospital are not adapted to the home, but a very large share of the hydropathic, electric and dietetic measures employed in the sanitarium, together with the resources of massage, physical culture, Swedish movements, Swedish gymnastics, can be utilized in the great proportion of cases requiring nursing at home.

Nursing in homes and private hospitals or sanitariums affords the intelligent nurse an admirable opportunity to do an educational work for her patient, of the greatest importance as a means both of cure and of prevention of future suffering and disease. In taking charge of a case, a nurse may limit her work absolutely to the care of the sick, and on leaving, may feel that she has done her duty. She will carry with her the abundant gratitude of the patient and her family; but her province can extend farther. If her heart is sincerely in her work, and her training thorough, her influence will not stop with teaching the science of dietetics, or ventilation, or disinfection, exercise, the use of heat and water; but her quick penetration will often find in a home the members of the family living by false standards, either through ignorance or carelessness. One of the most painful and appalling errors to a wide-awake nurse who understands the principles underlying healthful dress is the prevailing ignorance on that subject, and the discomfort and misery following in its train. The inequality of warmth over different parts of the body, the weight suspended from the hips, the tight bands and stays about the waist, the sweeping skirts, the high-heeled shoes, are destructive to the comfort and health, and consequently to the happiness of thousands of families.

At the Battle Creek Sanitarium training school we are taught that this error must be corrected by example as well as precept, and we dress with equal warmth from neck to ankles, constricting bands and stays are entirely discarded, and lungs and limbs are alike free in their action.

Dress-reform strikes unpleasantly those who do not understand just what is to be gained by it, and it is the nurse's privilege to teach why the old way will bring discomfort and irritability, even if worse evils are escaped. We heard at the Woman's Congress that ninety-five diseases and disorders come from bad dressing. The nurse will find it an argument in overcoming the prejudice against this most stubbornly opposed of reforms, that the stigma is being lifted, first by the leading ladies of the land agitating it until it is being better understood, and second because the masses have discovered to their surprise that beauty and reform in dress can walk hand in hand, and that the bloomer costume is by no means a requirement of reform.

When the nurse has converted her patient to the principles of healthful dressing, and has shown her how to adapt her style of dress to it, she has put her in a position, quoting again from an address at the Woman's Congress, where her life may "be greatly richer when not handicapped by dress."

Is this all a nurse can do? Perhaps the life of the patient has been heretofore only for selfish pleasures and ambitions. It may be she has never felt before that "it is not all of life to live." As the nurse ministers to her from day to day, she looks to her for words of counsel and light on a subject which to the sufferer is dark and misty. This is the most golden opportunity of all the nurse's work, and in the dark moments when the friends of the sufferer turn to her for courage and comfort, what comfort can she give if she cannot bring them to the feet of the Great Physician?

Often it is the unrest and the disappointments of life, or its hurry and rush, that have brought the physical suffering that we are called to alleviate, and the nurse who can show the sufferer how to find the higher strength with which to meet life will have given to her patient a help as much more potent than physical ministrations alone as the spiritual life is higher than the physical. Indeed, as the two are so closely and indissolubly linked, the ministering to the mind diseased is often an important factor in the recovery of the patient. It is much to alleviate physical suffering; it is a satisfying work to minister to the comfort of others, to save life, as is often our privilege; but as the life beyond is infinitely greater than this life, so is our satisfaction and our reward infinitely greater if we can help those to whom we minister to appreciate that life and the relations of this one to it. The grateful thanks of the patient whom we have nursed back to health are very pleasant, but sweeter still is the assurance that the life thus restored has taken on a new meaning and has been consecrated to a higher service than before.

Not always can we see that done in the homes of our patients which we would be glad to see done; but if we work "as unto Him," seeking to leave, as results of our effort, healthier bodies, purer homes, sweeter lives and nobler aspirations as we go from home to home, we can safely leave the results with the Great Physician under whom we serve.

LONDON HOSPITAL NURSES' HOME.

By Eva C. E. Lückes,

Matron London Hospital.

When the London Hospital authorities decided in 1880 to reorganize their nursing department and establish a training school for nurses, the want of suitable and sufficient accommodation for the increased numbers required was the most serious obstacle to be overcome. This experience is common to nearly all institutions in similar circumstances. The accommodation which sufficed for the class of nurses formerly employed was deficient both in quality and quantity and wholly inadequate to more modern requirements.

A comfortable "Home for Nurses," adapted to their needs in every respect, is the first essential for every hospital in connection with which a training school for nurses is to be established. The committee of the London Hospital fully realized this, and were indefatigable in their endeavors to procure the necessary funds for this important purpose, with the result that in 1886 the present large building was fit for habitation, and in May, 1887, was in good working order, in readiness for the formal opening by their Royal Highnesses the Prince and Princess of Wales.

In this short paper I only propose to state briefly the principles we endeavored to carry out for the comfort and well-being of our nurses and probationers. We determined that each worker should be provided with a separate bedroom, and that all the cubicles in the old buildings should be ultimately abolished and transformed into separate rooms in due course. This plan was adopted, and has proved a source of great comfort to the nurses and a useful means of improving the general discipline throughout. Each nurse is responsible to the "Home Sister" for the neatness of her own room. She is required to make her bed, and observe such minor regulations as are needed for the maintenance of order throughout the building, but servants are provided to do all the necessary cleaning. We endeavor to arrange that it shall be somebody's business to provide for the needs of the nurses, and that they, being cared for themselves, shall be ready to devote themselves with all the more energy to the care of the patients.

There are about 22 of these small bedrooms on each floor, with adequate bath-room accommodation for this number. At the entrance of the Nurses' Home there is an "Inquiry Office," where letters are delivered, parcels received, and visitors to the nurses promptly attended to and given the necessary directions. There is a large dining-hall reserved exclusively for meals, and adjoining, a second dining-room allotted to the use of the sisters at certain hours, and otherwise used as an extra sitting-room in which nurses may receive their friends if their own large sitting-room is occupied by other members of the nursing staff. Next to the dining-hall is a serving-room in which the food is received by means of a lift coming direct from the

Nurses' Home kitchen. The Nurses' Home kitchen, the servants' quarters, and all the servants employed in that building are distinctly separate from the hospital.

In addition to the sitting-room referred to there is a large, airy sick-room where nurses and probationers are cared for when they are not well. This is literally reserved for "Home" nursing, as when any of them are suffering from serious illness they are at once removed to small rooms, reserved for this purpose, leading out of some of the wards. There is a large box-room at the top of the building reserved exclusively for the nurses' use. The Nurses' Home also contains several bedrooms and sitting-rooms for the use of some of the sisters who fill responsible posts either in the Nurses' Home or the hospital, and careful arrangements are made for adequate supervision throughout.

We have no separate chapel, and no separate lecture-hall for the nurses, as these are admirably provided for in the hospital. We have also been obliged to have a room in the hospital fitted up with the necessary appliances for practical instructions to the probationers in sick-room cookery. Had space permitted we should have preferred this to be arranged in the Nurses' Home, in the vicinity of the sick-room sister, if convenient, but in any case it is best to have a room adapted for this purpose apart from the ordinary Nurses' Home kitchen. Our Nurses' Home only contains 102 of the small, separate bedrooms described, but sleeping accommodation on the same principle has been provided in various parts of the establishment for our nursing staff of 250 persons.

Our sisters (28 in number) are each provided with their own sitting-rooms, but the dining and sitting-rooms in the Nurses' Home are sufficient in size for all our nursing staff, whether they are sleeping in the Nurses' Home or in other parts of the building allotted to their use. I need scarcely say that if it were a matter of choice— apart from considerations of space and of expense—we should prefer to locate all our nurses under the same roof, but the old accommodation has been so well adapted to the requirements of to-day that we cannot honestly complain of any practical inconvenience.

I fear this brief sketch of the existing conditions of the London Hospital Nurses' Home can only be interesting to a few, but it may serve to illustrate the kind of domestic arrangements deemed desirable for nurses in this country. It is evident that if we can manage to carry out these principles on so large a scale, smaller institutions should be able to achieve the same result with less difficulty, and, doubtless, in many cases they succeed in doing so. I forbear to enlarge upon the importance from every point of view of securing a happy and comfortable "Home for Nurses," for I think the time has arrived when all that can be said in favor of this view will be freely conceded.

ASSOCIATION FOR THE TRAINING OF ATTENDANTS.

By Mrs. D. H. Kinney,

Teacher of Dept. of Mass. E. and H. Ass. for the Training of Attendants.

The work concerning which I have the honor of addressing you is the instruction of women in the care of chronic invalids, feeble elderly persons and little children. The credit of originating such a work is due to Mrs. Charles N. Judson, President of the Brooklyn Young Women's Christian Association, New York. Miss Katharine M. Adams, of the Red Cross Society, has been the able and devoted teacher from the outset.

In May, 1892, the Massachusetts Emergency and Hygiene Association undertook the same kind of work, through the influence of Miss Abby C. Howes, a member of the executive committee of the Massachusetts association, and a friend of Miss Adams, from whom she had heard of the success of the Brooklyn work. Miss Howes was appointed chairman of a special committee for consideration of plans relating to the instruction of the "attendants," and through her energy and wisdom, and that of her committee, their purposes have been rarely successful.

And yet this new department was but the natural outgrowth of previous work of the Emergency Association. Starting as an independent organization nine years ago (after a short existence as a committee of the Woman's Education Association), that it might extend its sphere of usefulness, it first arranged for the systematic instruction of police and firemen in what to do in cases of emergencies. By the action of the Police and the Civil Service Commissioners, attendance upon these lectures was made obligatory, and the promotion of the men to a certain degree was made dependent upon passing the examination.

The ladies also desired playgrounds in the city school-yards during the summer vacation, and during the last two years also assumed charge of the first open-air gymnasium for women in the world, which is part of the park system of Boston. 200,000 children were under its care last season, in these various open spaces.

Simultaneously with this work the Association gave courses of lectures to voluntary associations of young men, and courses on hygiene and home-nursing to young women. The former were given by doctors only, the latter by a corps of ladies, specially prepared for the work, some even going to the Lying-in Hospital to be taught the best way to wash a baby. Everything pertaining to the care and feeding of little children was specially emphasized in these talks. Therefore when Miss Howes proposed the Brooklyn plan of instruction, the Association was all ready, through its previous record and its distinct looking forward to a similar plan towards which it had been slowly working, to embrace her enthusiasm and to make systematic efforts for its realization.

As the plan took definite shape, the more and more evident it became that there was no phase or aspect of it which did not at once commend itself to all thoughtful and philanthropic minds. Properly carried on, it held within itself the possibilities of benefit to the community at large, and to the individuals who took it up as their vocation. The physicians who were consulted signified at once their approval and promised their support. One eminent in his profession exclaimed : " I could place a dozen such women as you propose to prepare, in situations, if they were ready to take them." And ever since the first class received their certificates he has given practical evidence of his sincerity. As soon as the superintendents of the representative hospitals and training schools understood that the work was not to be allowed to interfere or encroach in any way upon that of the trained nurses they extended most cordial sympathy, and publicly acknowledged that there was a wide field open for such a class of workers.

There was great difficulty in choosing a name which should forever render impossible any confusion in the mind of the public or in the mind of the worker herself, concerning her position or her duties with those of the trained nurse. Finally it was decided to call such workers "attendants," the name by which they are now generally known.

The office of these women in their relations to the household into which they might go was epitomized in the pertinent idea, "To save work, never to increase it," and this has been the center about which all their instruction has been grouped. The Association did not attempt to enlarge upon this underlying principle further than to say that the women were to be willing to take their meals wherever it was most convenient to the family whom they served. For the first year they were pledged to bring to the Association a report from their employers, endorsed by the physician—had one been in attendance—and under no conditions to accept more than $7 per week and their living for their services.

The Association, through the courtesy of the Boston Medical Library Association, was able to offer its pupils the great advantages of registering at the Bureau for Trained Nurses, where a special department was opened for them. This permission to register gave a sure foundation to the instruction, and served both as a guarantee of its worth and of the certainty of obtaining places. The women, as it were, passed into the charge of the bureau, which properly reserved the right to drop the name of any attendant for any reason which it might deem sufficient.

The work thus planned by the Association was as follows:

I. By a course of lessons and practical instruction to prepare women to care for convalescents, chronic invalids, feeble elderly persons and little children.

II. To require all who took the course of instruction to pass the examinations, which should be conducted by a physician.

III. To duly certificate such as had passed, and to see that their names were entered as attendants at the registry.

IV. To limit the price for the first year, with the distinct understanding that it was *never in future* to be as much as that asked by trained nurses.

V. To impress upon the public and the women that they were in no sense *nurses;* that there was in the community a great and crying need for intelligent help for tired mothers; for gentle watchfulness over those who, having borne the burden and heat of the day, were walking with tottering steps in lengthening shadows, and for encouraging assistance to those who were slowly coming back from illness into the world of active life and work.

The work of instructing the classes was put into the hands of a graduate of the Massachusetts General Hospital, chosen for her especial qualifications as teacher, who in addition to teaching was expected as well to be able to lecture to classes of ladies who might wish to learn for the benefit of their families something of the "gospel of hygienic righteousness." Under the wise supervision of the special committee, a schedule was prepared for the instruction of the attendants. There were no text-books used, but each wrote out from the dictation of the teacher what she was expected to learn.

The classes have been conducted like any recitation, the work of the previous day being gone over, and as much given in advance as the pupils were able to take. Enough elementary physiology has been taught by the aid of a manikin to give the women a clear idea of the working of the lungs, heart and digestive organs. In connection with the lessons in respiration, the importance and best means of ventilation were taught; with digestion, the way of preparing and serving food, not a few of the women having later taken courses in invalid cookery; with the study of the intestinal canal, the regulation of the bowels, enemata and kindred preparations; care of the skin, with baths; prevention of bed-sores, the preparation and care of poultices, fomentations, blisters, plasters; care of the hair, eye, ear, throat, mouth. Though not allowed to take acute cases, they have had special instruction given on the care of the dead. Pupils have been taught to change the bed and body clothing of a bedridden patient, and what their special duties and responsibilities are in the case of the aged. The course has included the feeding, bathing and habits of children, pupils being taught what may be done for croup, convulsions and other emergencies till medical help can be reached.

Special emphasis throughout the course is being constantly laid upon the fact that the attendants are never to assume, in any way, responsibilities which do not belong to them, and never to give any medicine of any kind whatever without orders. Such conditions as might, in the course of their duties to convalescents, old people or children, require the attention of a physician have been carefully pointed out to them. They have been taught to read a clinical thermometer and to count a pulse.

The Association agreed that it was wise not to accept any candidates under 20 years of age, nor any who could not read and write intelligently. The fee for 30 lessons was placed at the very low price of $3, in order that the expense might not stand in the way of any who wished to take up the work. The number of applications for admission to classes was so large that it was found necessary to exclude from the regular $3 classes all who did not intend to use the knowledge gained as a means of self-support.

The work was actually commenced on November 1, 1892, by the issuing of a circular. By the middle of the same month three classes were already at work—one of twelve pupils having daily lessons, one of fifteen in the School of Domestic Science with two weekly lessons, another of ten meeting two evenings in the week at the Young Women's Christian Association. This was composed entirely of girls who were working in various capacities during the day, in shops and households. Later a class of ten ladies received the same instruction, giving three mornings each week to it. This course was supplemented by four lectures on the duties of a nurse in contagious and infectious diseases. For this teaching they paid the Association at the rate of 50 cents per lesson or $17 for 34 lessons. A more interested and enthusiastic class it would be difficult to imagine. Eight out of the ten took a thorough written examination. One paper was marked 100 per cent "cum laude."

On the completion of the course the first daily class sent a most gratifying note to the Association, acknowledging their indebtedness for the opportunity afforded them. When they finished a second daily class was ready to begin, who in turn were followed by a third, making in all 34 attendants registered in Boston.

On February 6 a class of 20 was started in Worcester. To this class came one young woman whose railroad fares cost her $96. There was another who spent $15 in traveling expenses, and another who came from Providence to Worcester twice every week. On one occasion a woman left to attend the class at 2 p. m. in a driving snow-storm at 8 a. m., and had not gone the ten miles between Worcester and her home by five o'clock that same afternoon, and yet it was she who said to the superintendent of the Young Women's Christian Association, "Even if I do not get any certificate I shall feel well paid by what I have learned for all the trouble to which I have been put."

The classes have been examined individually and orally by the president of the Association and one other physician of the lecture committee. Those who have passed satisfactorily have been given certificates, only two having failed. The large majority have been constantly employed since registering. The reports from their employers have been without exception most satisfactory and gratifying.

There have been during the season 7 regular classes, numbering 66 pupils, and one special class of 10 ladies. 34 women registered in Boston, 16 in Worcester.

The teacher has given during the winter 32 lectures to ladies, in various cities: Boston 9, Milton 4, Worcester 9, Somerville 2, Cambridge 4, Norwich 2, Framingham 2.

The Association has not been disappointed in the financial aspects of the work; even at the small charge made for the lessons, two-thirds of the expenses were covered by the receipts. Next fall the tuition fee will, however, be doubled, for, as a wise woman remarked not long since, " It seems as if a woman ought to be willing to pay as much for her preparation for a life-work as she would give for having a dress made."

The work is growing rapidly. Summer classes are held in Syracuse, Auburn, N. Y., while towns in Maine have asked for lectures, and Boston, Worcester, Fall River and other places in Massachusetts have arranged for winter classes. With all the success there has been a most wholesome seasoning of mistakes and difficulties, and there are problems in connection with it yet to be solved, the solution of which will make the enterprise a still wider-reaching power for good in our land; and who shall dare to set the limit of what it may yet be and do?

IV

DISPENSARIES.

DISPENSARIES HISTORICALLY AND LOCALLY CONSIDERED.

By Charles C. Savage,

President of the Demilt Dispensary and Trustee of the Roosevelt Hospital.

The best method of providing medical attendance for the sick poor, without debasing them, has long been the problem of philanthropists and social economists. Theories are constructed that seem perfectly adapted to the end desired, but, brought to the test of practical application, they prove defective or insufficient. The problem remains unsolved, because national habits, modes of living, density of population, variety of dwellings, migratory traits, etc., demand differing systems. Each community should devise a flexible plan, based on economic laws, enabling it to do the most good and the least harm. Cities outgrow methods with the increase and changing habits of the population, and the devices for housing the working people. I believe in conserving the good, but it is not wise to be so anchored to the past as to be unable to move with the scientific progress of the present, when it offers a better way.

It is essential for the welfare and safety of any large community that medical and sanitary safeguards be provided for the dependent and wage-earning classes, either through municipal or private charity. This obligation cannot be neglected without incurring a fatal penalty.

This leads to the question, how can the mentally and physically strong and healthy, best aid the mentally and physically weak, and especially the sick among them, with the least danger of paralyzing self-respect,—the backbone of character? Dependence on getting something for nothing is pauperizing, whether the party be a resident of a palace or a tenement. Useful labor is the divine remedy for this danger. The duty of the state or municipality to care for the chronic physically dependent ought not to be doubted by any social thinker. It is an imposition on private charity to ask its aid for this variety of poor. When legal provision is made for incurable dependents, I believe it is true humanity to let them suffer until they accept it. Private charity should expend its energy, and can most effectively assist those who are in temporary need. But this crutch should be withdrawn the moment the necessity for it has passed; otherwise dependence on, and bestowing of private charity, become a crime. It weakens efforts for self-support, instead of being a help over a hard place. It may enervate where it should invigorate. The true design of charity is to remove the occasion for it, and thus assist the recipient to help himself. I do not forget that there will be exceptions to this rule. They should, however, have a personal, beneficent motive to commend its violation. I have enunciated these introductory thoughts as germane to my special topic.

The primary intent in organizing a dispensary is briefly defined in the charter of the Demilt Dispensary : " The particular business and objects shall be providing and furnishing medical and surgical aid and medicines to such persons as may be in need thereof, and unable by reason of poverty to procure the same."

The beginning of institutions with the functions of dispensaries and hospitals is clouded in uncertainty. We have traditional accounts of mythological incantations, religious rites and physicians' prescriptions used for ills of the flesh. As sickness has existed throughout time, it was needful to devise methods of treating all manner of diseases. The Hebrew Bible gives direction for the healing " of whatsoever sickness there be." There are records of ways employed in Egypt as early as the eleventh century B. C. In Greece, four hundred years B. C., there were state physicians who invoked Apollo and other gods to help them. They appointed slave doctors to look after the ailments of the poor. There is weak authority for inferring that hospitals were connected with the temple of Æsculapius. Persia, India and China had their priests and prescribers to medicate the sick.

Hippocrates, who lived 460–357 B. C., is called " the Father of Medicine." He belonged to a line of physicians. He bound himself by oath that " he would all his life visit the sick and give them advice *gratis*." Here we find the germ of out-patient relief for the poor. May I not, therefore, add to his recognized title, also *the Father of Dispensaries?*

The evidence of the erection of buildings, of the nature of our charitable institutions, for the reception and treatment of the sick, before the Christian era, is more traditional than historical. In the early Christian centuries an *infirmaria* was attached to the monasteries, where the monks ministered to the sick who sought their shelter.

The oldest hospital I have noted was built at Cæsarea, about 375 A. D. Another was founded in Rome in 380. The Maison Dieu in Paris (now known as the Hotel Dieu Hospital), near 600 A. D. Apologies for hospitals were established by the Crusaders during the Middle Ages. Medical knowledge was crude. The hospitals of this period have been called a " curse to civilization," but civilization itself was then little more than the barbarism of humanity. It is not right to judge the methods of that age by the modern standard, but rather give credit to the attempts to alleviate suffering. The first hospital built in England was in 1080. St. Bartholomew's, in London, was begun in 1123, and refounded on a secular basis by royal charter, in 1544, under the charge of physicians.* It was the first building in any way worthy of the name of hospital. The service was so imperfect as to be little more than a pretense to relieve its inmates. There was a great increase of hospitals in Great Britain in the eighteenth century of a somewhat improved standard; but they were still low in merit as medical institutions, and vastly overcrowded, rendering them at times pest-breeders instead of life-preservers. This state of affairs originated a plan of treating patients who could not be received into the hospitals. They were called out-patients.

The outcome of this pressure of patients was the opening of the first medical dispensary, as a distinct institution, in 1770. It was

* This hospital, at its foundation, had an independent constitution and a separate estate, though under the control of the Priory. It was stated in the first charter that it was a hospital distinctly for the sick, for maternity, and the orphans of such mothers as died in it. The hospital and its revenues came into the possession of Henry VIII in 1537. He granted the charter of 1544 reorganizing it, and in 1547 a new charter, in which he restored to the foundation the larger portion of its former revenues. In this charter the king states as the motive for his act : " Considering the miserable estate of the poor, aged, sick, low, and impotent people, as well men as women, lying and going about begging in the common streets of the said City of London, and the suburbs of the same, to the great paine and sorrowe of the same poore, aged, sick, and impotent people, and to the great infection, hurt and annoyance of His Grace's loving subjects, which of necessity must daily goe and pass by the same poore, sick, low and impotent people, being infected with divers great and horrible sicknesses and diseases." At this time the hospital had 100 beds, with one physician and three surgeons. In 1892 it contained 746 beds.

allied to St. Bartholomew's Hospital, and entitled "the Royal General Dispensary." Its charter says, "for the relief of the sick poor, without regard to place of abode." The humane and economic results of this out-patient plan were so manifest, that between the years 1774 and 1789 nine other dispensaries were established in various parts of London. They are still in existence, and many others have been added, until London is well supplied with general and specific medical institutions. This seed for the relief of suffering humanity yielded such good fruit that it was planted in all the principal towns of Great Britain and carried to the Continent of Europe. There they are mainly the adjuncts of hospitals with governmental support. As early as 1805 dispensaries were the subject of Parliamentary investigation and regulation, for the purpose of correcting abuses. Subsequently medical provision for the poor was made compulsory in rural districts. The medical service is more defective than in this country.* The patients are too generally considered and valued as clinic material.

This brief outline of the origin of dispensaries has been given as prefatory history to their transplanting to the United States. The governments and habits of the people abroad are so unlike ours that only the fundamental ideas of foreign dispensaries can be utilized here. If it were thought desirable to imitate them closely the attempt would prove a failure.

Philadelphia has the honor of establishing the first dispensary in America, in April, 1786. It was incorporated in 1796 as the "Philadelphia Dispensary." The charter defines its design in these quaint words: "The principal object of this institution is to afford relief to the poor in those cases where removal to a public hospital would, for any approved reason, be ineligible." The chief originators of this

---

* A report published in London says: "At least one-fourth of the population of London receives gratuitous medical treatment. This is necessarily of a very imperfect kind. Besides the delay and hardship often endured in obtaining admission by means of subscribers' letters, three hours is the average time the patients have to wait in crowded infectious rooms, while the actual time often extends to seven hours, and, after all, they only get the smallest dividend of attention from the overworked medical man, who knows nothing of their individual constitution and habits. For home treatment no provision whatever is made, and deaths frequently occur from the absence of any (gratuitous) means of securing prompt medical attendance." There are days when the doctor prescribes for over fifty casualty patients an hour. Severe cases he can refer to another physician.

practical regard for the sick poor appear to have been Friends. They issued an appeal or " plan "* "to the ladies and gentlemen of Philadelphia" to attend "a meeting at the City Tavern," with a subscrip-

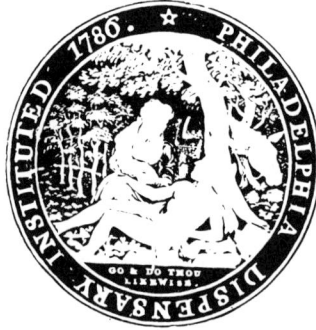

tion paper attached. The price of membership was one guinea, and that, or its equivalent in dollars, is still the terms. There were 187

---

* The reasons for this movement are so interestingly and forcibly stated that I copy them in full here : *"Plan* of the Philadelphia Dispensary for the Medical Relief of the Poor. To the Ladies and Gentlemen of Philadelphia.

"In all large cities there are many poor persons afflicted by diseases, whose former circumstances and habits of independence will not permit them to expose themselves as patients in a public hospital. There are also many diseases and accidents, of so acute and dangerous a nature, that the removal of patients afflicted by them is attended with many obvious inconveniences, and there are some diseases of such a nature that the air of an hospital, crowded with patients, is injurious to them. A number of gentlemen having taken these things into consideration, have proposed to establish a *Public Dispensary* in the city of Philadelphia for the Medical relief of the Poor. The particular advantages of this will be as follows :—

"1st. The sick may be attended and relieved in their houses, without the pain and inconveniences of being separated from their families.

" 2d. The sick may be relieved at a much less expense to the public than in an hospital, where provisions, bedding, fire-wood and nurses are required for their accommodation, and

" 3d. The sick may be relieved in a manner perfectly consistent with those noble feelings of the human heart, which are inseparable from virtuous poverty, and in a manner also strictly agreeable to the refined precepts of Christianity, which inculcate secrecy in acts of charity and benevolence." This is followed with rules for the government, the call for subscriptions and names of twelve gentlemen who will act as Managers until the members select others. Two of them are clergymen, but none appear to be physicians.

contributors before the opening. Among the first are Benjamin Franklin, Robert Morris and Charles Biddle. The seal adopted was a picture of the good Samaritan in the act of helping, with the emphatic motto, " Go, & do thou likewise."

The New York City Medical Society, in 1790, appointed a committee " to digest and publish a plan of a dispensary for the medical relief of the sick poor of the city, and to make an offer of the professional services of the members of the society to carry it into effect." This movement resulted, in 1791, in the organization of the second dispensary in the United States, to be known as "the New York Dispensary," with fourteen members of the Medical Society for its professional staff.

The third dispensary organized was in Boston, in 1796, under the patronage of the Chamber of Commerce, with the title of " The Boston Dispensary for the relief of the sick poor."

The Baltimore General Dispensary was established in 1801, under the auspices of leading clergymen and citizens. So marked were the benign results that it was chartered by the State in 1807. It received the first charter granted to a charitable institution. The preamble gives as a reason, that it " has been extensively beneficial in its effects in relieving the poor from sickness, and preserving the health of the city," " and the General Assembly are desirous to encourage and give permanence to an institution of such public utility."

It would be of interest to continue these historical data and give the date and name of the first dispensary organized in the chief cities of North America. Also to describe the methods devised to determine who are the sick poor entitled to gratuitous treatment, and how they are reached and attended in various localities. Each city has its local conditions, which necessarily have a modifying influence. The value of such data would be suggestive rather than comparative.

The method of admittance in London is by tickets issued on the recommendation of subscribers or physicians attached to the dispensary. It is open to serious abuses, and has too much red tape for this country to tolerate. The least possible machinery facilitates admittance to the sick and the detection of imposture. *Any one* can receive free treatment, no questions asked, in the out-patient department of the hospitals in Germany, France, and Austria. The Boston dispensary has a number of sub-stations. The increase of population must interfere with this original plan. Cincinnati, through its Board of Health, has a large corps of physicians who attend the "worthy and deserving poor." How they draw the line on this definition I do not know. They must meet sickness that should be abated, without regard to moral traits. Even a pauper afflicted should be cared for somehow, if not for humanity's sake, yet for the well-being of the community. But I must not linger, however attractive the study.

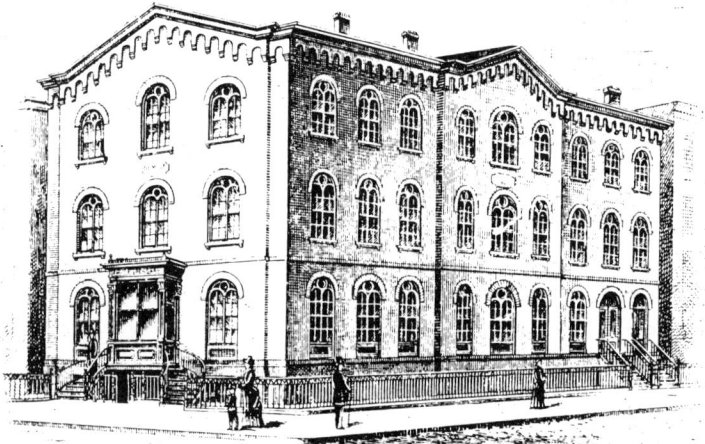

DEMILT DISPENSARY.

The dispensaries in New York City may be divided into three classes. They shade into each other, frequently doing work in common, or to the same patient, yet they are organized on different models, for varying purposes.

First. The original or general dispensaries, whose prime motive is the providing of medical and surgical treatment, with the prescribed remedies for the sick poor. They do this purely as a matter of sympathy or humanity for the sufferer unable to care for self. They restore such to health and ability to labor as speedily as possible, or alleviate the distress of the dying. They diminish the dangers of poverty, pauperism and crime. They are available as a sanitary protection and restraint from the spread of contagious or infectious disease throughout the community. They expose pest-breeders and violations of sanitary laws. They aim to do this and more at the least cost to beneficence or taxation.

The physicians attached to dispensaries, being in close touch with the poor as they are massed in the tenement houses or visit the dispensaries for help, are the first to know of the outbreak or increasing prevalence of an infectious disease. They are now required to report the same to the Board of Health, for removal and suppression by legally authorized action. The general dispensaries have a definite territory in which they administer medical relief. A building is erected at a central point in the district, to be within reach of the tenement-house population. Any one sick can apply, without formality, for professional treatment. At the building he will be attended by a specialist.* Formerly the advice of the physician was restricted to patients residing in the dispensary territory. Little notice is now taken of where the applicant lives. Experience has proved that reliance cannot be placed on the true residence being given, when the applicant desires to conceal it. This deception is adopted by chronic sick revolvers or tramps, who delight in visiting each dispensary, in hope their disease may be cured. The house or the prescribing physician, if he suspects the applicant is able to pay for advice, makes inquiry sufficient to decide, and treatment is rendered or refused on this decision. The line, however, is not rigidly drawn ; the patient is given the benefit of a doubt. There is very little counterfeiting of sickness, the general belief being that the physician can detect fraud.

No physician is allowed to charge a fee to a dispensary patient. The attending physicians are expected to donate their services, but some of the down-town dispensaries have found an advantage in paying a small salary.

To each of the general dispensaries are attached visiting physicians, who attend the sick in their homes when unable to come to the building. These physicians are paid a salary by the dispensary. They confine their visits to a special district. Application is made at the building, at any hour it is open, for their services, without con-

* The usual divisions are, General Medicine, General Surgery, Heart and Lungs, Throat, Eye and Ear, Skin, Special Diseases of Women, of Children, Nervous Diseases, Oral Surgery, and Vaccination. The Demilt Dispensary has also an evening class for women, with any disease, whose employment prevents their presence during the day. This class is under the care of female physicians exclusively.

ditions. The patient is visited within the day, and revisited so long as the sickness requires. Thus dispensary districts cover the whole city. No indigent person need suffer unattended by a physician. A professional nurse is a valuable assistant. She co-operates with the physician by instructing the household how to care for the sick, and by enforcing order and cleanliness.

The dispensaries do not undertake maternity cases, as they interfere with the prompt visitation of other patients. A large majority of the poor save in advance, and have a pride in paying the physician something for this service. Gratuitous arrangements can be made by the indigent. There are several maternity hospitals, and some of them will send, in special cases, a physician to the home. In 1890 the Midwifery Dispensary was opened. In 1892 it attended 2071 patients at their residences, nearly all foreign-born. The women, previous to confinement, register and are examined at the dispensary, except in emergency. It affords professional opportunity to a large number of undergraduates and graduates, under the supervision of expert physicians.

There are nine general dispensaries, organized as the increase of population necessitated the covering of extended territory, viz.: The New York, in 1791 ; the Northern, 1827 ; the Eastern (renamed the Good Samaritan), 1832 ; the Demilt, 1851; the Northwestern, 1852; the Northeastern, 1862 ; the Manhattan, 1862; the Harlem, 1868. To these should be added the German on the eastern side of the city, 1857, though it is deficient in visiting physicians.

Second. Within the last twenty-five years the principal hospitals have added an out-patient or dispensary department. They do not attend patients at their homes, but they perform a large gratuitous service in an annex to the hospital. It is not certain that the motive for their existence is so much humanity as to provide clinic opportunities for physicians connected with them, and patients for the hospitals. Their methods are similar to those adopted in the general dispensaries. They do not appear to diminish the number of patients depending on the general dispensaries. A large supply is found, if not created, by their existence, even though the hospitals are usually located outside of the so-called poor districts.

Third. Dispensaries for the treatment of special medical or surgical diseases. These have multiplied in recent years in number and variety parallel with the rapid increase of specialists in the profession. If their necessity is determined by the number of the sick who patronize them, there is cause for their existence. All of the general dispensaries have a system of classifying patients for treatment. Yet it is admitted that these special institutions give their patients the professional skill and the aid of the best equipment,—equal to that which can be obtained by the wealthy. This is to the advantage of the poor, but it is to the disadvantage of the poor physicians. It is in this class of dispensaries the clinic knowledge and professional experience are obtained which give specialists their pre-eminence in hospital and private practice. The first organized of these special dispensaries was the New York Eye and Ear Infirmary, in 1820. Some of them now have, by reason of required surgical operations, hospital wards.

Fourth. To these three divisions must be added another, to complete our statement of the medical resources of the poor in New York. The Homeopaths provide dispensaries, hospitals and special institutions. I do not find they have any systematic arrangements to treat the poor in their homes. Their buildings are located in the city above its center, and out of the midst of the poorer population. Some of them have a large number of patients.

New York City has sixty-three dispensaries and infirmaries in the four classes described, where the sick can obtain free treatment. They are governed by a board of managers or trustees, who raise funds for their maintenance, and appoint the medical staff. In addition, there are churches, missions, secret and trade societies, and private or unofficial associations giving like assistance to those in whom they have a personal interest. There is no lack of remedial agencies for all who can present themselves for treatment at an institution. If neglect exists, it is deficient provision for the very sick and dying, living in cheap apartments, who cannot be removed to a hospital for domestic reasons. These have a more positive claim on philanthropy than on the unrequited private physician.*

* I have limited this review to private institutions, depending on voluntary aid, bequests and pay-patients for income. It is impossible to ascertain how many persons came under treatment in the public hospitals and dispensaries under the charge of the City "Commissioners of Public Charities and Correction," and supported by taxation. The inmates are frequently transferred from one building to another, discharged, and return after short intervals. In 1892, 30,422 persons were assigned by permits to the City hospitals; to which should be added the sick already inmates of other departments for the City dependents and the criminal institutions. Bellevue Dispensary and its two branches report 89,738 outdoor patients. The deaths in New York in 1892 were 44,329, of whom 18,684 were children under five years of age.

In London there are over fifty Provident Dispensaries, and they are also established in the principal cities of England. The members pay a small sum monthly, which entitles them to the services of a physician in sickness. These dispensaries have been organized to supersede what is known as the "Club Doctor System" which provides medical assistance for male members only. The Provident dispensaries are designed to be co-operative, self-supporting, and thus exclude the charitable element of dispensaries. The physicians receive an equitable proportion of the dues paid by the members, instead of a salary, direct from the organization. Each family has the right to choose its own family doctor from the staff of the dispensary, and the physician is expected to become acquainted with the sanitary condition of the dwelling, the normal idiocrasy of each member of the household, and promptly respond to a call for his services. In midwifery the doctor is paid extra by the person attended. The theory is that these voluntary associations encourage thrift and foresight among the poor for the hour of need. I have had no personal observation of the merits and demerits of such organizations. They are praised and condemned by those who have investigated them. The opponents assert that if permissible in Great Britain, they should not be encouraged in the United States. An analogy to them is found in the Prudential Life Insurance, which is a great success in New York and vicinity. By the weekly payment of from five to fifty cents, a specified sum is guaranteed for the burial of the insured. As the poor are over-solicitous for a "decent burial," they will practice self-denial to make prompt payments and secure a respectable home for their remains.

The question, should dispensaries continue to furnish medicines free to all their patients, was frequently discussed by dispensary managers. The custom was sanctioned by the early founders. Was it right to make a radical departure and demand pay? In 1878 a conference of delegates from the general dispensaries met for consultation on the subject. The result of their deliberations was the adoption of a resolution, that "It is expedient a charge should be made by all the dispensaries to those applying for aid, when the applicant is able to make such payment." It was believed that a large proportion of those receiving the benefits of the dispensaries, who were unable to pay the usual fee of a physician in private practice, or the price for filling a prescription in a drug-store, could and were willing to pay the average cost of the medicine to the dispensary. A uniform charge of ten cents for each prescription filled was deemed an equitable price. Patients were to be supplied free who, by reason of poverty, were unable to pay this small sum, so that none in physical distress should be turned away unserved.* This charge has been more successful than was anticipated, both in upholding the self-respect of patients and its financial assistance to the dispensaries. Its tendency is to cause the patients to assume that the help of a dispensary is a right rather than a favor. But we do not expect gratitude as a reward for doing good. The result of the present system is that about 85 per cent of those coming to the dispensary and 70 per cent of such as are visited at their homes are able to meet this nominal charge without much inconvenience.† Vaccination is free to all, and compulsory of school children, for sanitary reasons.

The population of New York City in 1891 was 1,680,796. Of this number, 1,225,411 persons lived in 37,358 tenement houses containing three or more families. 276,565 of these persons were heads of families. Probably nine-tenths of them were foreign-born, or one remove therefrom. They depend mainly on their daily labor or charity for daily needs. In more colloquial words, "they live from hand to mouth." The rent of their rooms ranges from three to fifteen dollars a month. During the past forty years the most prosperous families and skilled mechanics have abandoned the lower and east and west sides of the city, as the poorer classes have encroached on these sections. A noticeable feature of this division of the population is the grouping of nationalities in certain boundaries. The Italians are in close proximity. The Germans have their favorite portion. The Irish have several spots about which they locate. The Hebrews, especially the Russian and Polish, are so clannish as to nearly dispossess other nationalities in certain wards. Even the Chinese are clustered in their streets, and the negroes are found near each other. The dispensaries covering such portions of the city

---

* Lately I noticed a well-dressed woman applying for the free stamp on her prescription paper. An inquiry proved that she was a widow, with five small children dependent on her labor for maintenance. One was sick, and she could not pay even ten cents without seriously missing it. Her request was granted without hesitation. This was no exception to the fact that good clothes are not sure evidence of ability to pay.

† Two of the dispensaries now vary the plan by collecting the ten cents on admission, from those able to pay. One has never charged for medicines, but probably will hereafter.

find it requisite to provide physicians who can talk in the language of the foreign cities in the midst of our city.*

A few statistics showing some of the work of the general dispensaries are here reported:

NAME.	Patients at Dispensary.	Patients at home.	Total new patients.	Consultations.	Prescriptions.	Sent to hospitals.
New York	42,912	3,570	46,482	123,025	115,162	906
Good Samaritan (Eastern).	89,116	6,117	95,233	148,018	107,808	581
Northern	11,516	3,582	15,098	..	22,524	205
Demilt	25,254	4,857	30,111	71,300	59,704	142
Northwestern	25,920	4,043	29,963	..	74,866	94
Northeastern	18,299	3,395	21,694	..	59,141	37
Harlem	2,357	286	2,643	6,795	64,154	17
Manhattan.	..	..	3,857	4,136	3,437	..
German,	..	..	28,232	71,584	45,846	..

Of the patients of the New York Dispensary, 13,587 were Italians, the Good Samaritan had 43,574 Russians, Northwestern 8,255 Irish, Demilt 7,366 Irish, the German 17,000 German-speaking. The children of foreign-born parents are not included in the foregoing figures. The Good Samaritan reports the nationality of the parents of children under ten years of age. Thus, Russian adults 43,579, children 31,933; Austro-Hungarian 6,843, children 2,017; Germans 3,071, children 912; Roumania 2,589, children 689; Ireland 1,231, children 224; United States (more than one remove from foreign-born) 36,898, children 2,247.

I copy the foregoing figures as independent statements to show some of the statistics furnished by the dispensaries. They are worthless for comparison because of the different methods of reporting. The cost per patient, regardless of number of consultations and prescriptions received, appears to vary between thirteen and forty-one cents, viz: 13, 21, 26, 38, 41 cents. Statistics of London dispensaries show an average cost of 47 cents a patient.

The lack of a uniform system of registering and presenting the statistics of the New York dispensaries is regretted. Unsuccessful efforts have been made on several occasions to arrange a single plan.

* The foreign-born population of New York has had marked modifications by successive tides of immigration. First came the Irish, then the German, followed by Scandinavians, though these are apt to make it only a temporary abiding-place. Now Italians and Russian and Polish Jews are settling here in vast numbers.

It is unsafe to trust the figures given in the published reports, even if correct by themselves, for comparison or induction. The number who receive gratuitous medical advice from the various medical charities, some time during the year, has been estimated as high as 500,000. More conservative calculations range between 300,000 and 350,000, or one in four of the tenement-house population.* I believe this is an overestimate, if we eliminate all the duplications.†

* London, with a population of 4,221,452, treated in a year 1,158,026 out-patients, or 274 per 1000 of its total inhabitants. In 1891 there were treated in St. Bartholomew's Hospital (including those of the Royal General Dispensary) 155,348 out-patients ; St. Thomas's, 18,779 out-patients and 72,576 minor casualties ; Guy's, 34,759 out-patients and 22,150 casualties ; London, 112,092 out-patients, which includes 66,376 casualties ; University, 42,225 out-patients. In India the records of 1889-90 show that there were 1,642 hospitals and dispensaries, which treated 265,000 hospital and 11,978,000 out-patients.

I am indebted to "The Hospital," London, for the following statistics of dispensary assistance in twelve of the principal cities of Great Britain :

	Population.	Out-patients.	Proportion per 1000.
Dublin,	353,082	162,164	459
Liverpool,	517,116	198,378	383
Edinburgh,	261,970	95,535	365
Birmingham,	429,906	144,559	336
Manchester,	506,469	146,298	288
London,	4,221,452	1,158,026	274
Glasgow,	567,143	85,839	151
Norwich,	101,316	10,577	104
Cardiff,	130,283	11,058	85
Halifax,	83,109	4,198	50
Portsmouth,	160,128	6,863	42
Oldham,	132,000	3,711	28

To understand the full significance of these figures it must be remembered that a very large proportion (Mr. Burdett estimates 50 per cent.) must be added to them in each town of those in receipt of free medical aid from the poor law infirmaries and free dispensaries.

† Since this paper was completed, an article on City Dispensaries has been published in the *Evening Post*. The views of the writer in regard to them are parallel with mine on the main points, except as to the number of persons treated. He gives detailed figures, yielding the gross sum of 628,486, from which he deducts as duplicates 176,057, leaving the net number of 452,429 distinct individuals receiving dispensary aid the last year. This means that one in three of the poor population are sick each year and depend on dispensaries. I think it too large an estimate. Patients from the surrounding cities are an element in the count which cannot be determined, as they usually give a false city address.

It is usual to register an applicant or a new patient on his first presentation, and he is given a numbered card for treatment. He can return on this card for consultation until discharged or he discharges himself. Afterwards in the year he may re-apply for the same or some other disease. He is again registered as a new patient. It is not an uncommon event for the same patient to consult different dispensaries. In each he is recorded as a new patient.*

Thus it will happen that the aggregate of new patients treated and reported is no evidence that that number of different individuals have received the assistance of the dispensaries. This difficulty is much easier stated than remedied. The dependent and unskilled wage-earning population is too shifting to follow for identification. And they do not hesitate to give false names and addresses if they think it advisable. To illustrate, a dispensary had 221 cases investigated with the following result: Able to pay 42, not able to pay 92, insufficient information 7, wrong address 80. The latter may be design, or misunderstood, or out-of-town residents. It is probable the most of these were not under treatment when the report of the case was returned. Investigation by other dispensaries shows similar results.†

The social problem involved in this investigation I will not consider.

The voluntary and involuntary gratuitous services of the medical profession to public humane institutions and private individuals are undoubtedly in excess of the gifts of an equal number of lay citizens. For this generous use of their skill and time they are worthy of the highest commendation, and it is unstintedly bestowed by managers and trustees who witness its vast extent. Figures will picture to the mind where words fail to express it. The benevolence of the patrons

---

* I know an institution in which a patient may be recorded twelve times in the year, and so be reported as twelve different patients.

† In the most attractive dispensary of the city, possessing an elegant building, a complete equipment and high-grade physicians, the patients are largely of a class one might judge able to compensate a physician. The Charity Organization investigated 1,500 cases selected out of 35,000 applicants. The answer was that about one-quarter were able to pay, another quarter had given a wrong address (possibly from an aversion to its being known that they had applied for dispensary aid or because they resided out of the city), and the remaining half were recommended as worthy of medical charity by reason of poverty. For another dispensary the same Society made investigation of 212 cases and returned answer that 55 were able to pay, 58 were not found at the address given, 18 information not conclusive, and 81 unable to pay. These referred cases were deemed questionable out of nearly 30,000 patients.

of the Demilt Dispensary has provided in the last forty years for its current expenses close to $300,000. In that time the medical profession has contributed 2,625,000 consultations. These should not be valued at less than one dollar each. Some of these physicians were receiving from five to twenty-five dollars for similar consultations in private practice. The experience gained in the dispensaries is so useful that physicians compete for an appointment, and cheerfully render the required service. It is a reflex benefit to them in their pay practice, and this is somewhat a compensation. The managers, as a rule, leave to the medical staff the responsibility of deciding who shall receive free relief, so that no injustice shall be done to the profession or imposition encouraged.

No questions pertaining to medical charities have been more frequently and inconclusively discussed than—does gratuitous relief have a demoralizing result on recipients, and does it wrongfully interfere with the rights and emoluments of practitioners? These questions have received the profoundest study of investigators in social science, and the medical profession, without reaching a final conclusion. Superficial thinkers are divided between yes and no. These vital complex problems still remain unsolved. It would be presumptuous for me to decide what is the truth.

Recently there has been discussion in medical journals and daily newspapers on the alleged abuses of dispensary aid. It is admitted "that dispensaries do an immense amount of good by relieving the suffering of the most deserving among the poorer classes of the community." But it is charged that "they do also an immense amount of harm, both by fostering habits of improvidence among their beneficiaries (who may be at first driven to them by necessity, but subsequently go to them from choice), and also by the indiscriminate way in which these institutions receive applications for their bounty."

Another physician asserts that the chief cause of abuse is "the keen rivalry and competition of the various medical schools and educational institutions, and the multiplication of dispensaries," and he adds: "Many of these are organized by well-disposed people, whose sympathies are excited by some tale of physical suffering and are ignorant of the ample provisions already provided. Little do they realize the harm they are doing by encouraging imposture and mendicancy." This writer omits to state that this multiplication of institutions has been caused through the active efforts of physicians desirous of appointments in them for clinic purposes and positions, who take advantage of the ignorance of the benevolent and appeal to their sympathy. He suggests a remedy by organizing a society with power to investigate, and by "co-operation prevent many of the existing abuses." This suggestion is impracticable of execution. I fear, if organized, it would make a spasmodic effort and die. Physicians would be earnest opponents of a genuine remedial plan, as its first work would be the consolidation or closing of some medical charities. Must we carefully scrutinize every generous, friendly act lest it demoralize the recipient? Are Christmas, Easter, wedding and funeral gifts wrong because they are open to abuses? Should not a society be organized to investigate and regulate such gratuities, that they may not "encourage imposture and mendicancy"?

A layman answers some of these charges, viewed from another standpoint. I incorporate his argument in mine. Are these charges true? Let us look at them in the cold light of practical utility. The first business of a community is to keep itself in a condition of the most effective economic or productive usefulness, at the least possible outlay either to the community or its individuals. To this end the dispensaries perform a capital service. Does it lead to mendicancy when the masses listen to free music in our parks, because perchance more favored folks pay three dollars for an opera entertainment? Does our free-school system lead to improvidence and debasement? It is believed that it will be protective of health to extend our free or cheap bath system. Will that, too, entail improvidence and pauperism? Is it demoralizing to read books loaned from a free library, supported by charitable gifts, when the reader has the means to buy them? Or does demoralization follow, not because the recipient has ability to pay for what he gets, but from premeditative reliance on aids and the designed remission of personal efforts? In other words, the degrading influence follows from the intended misuse of provided charity.

Obviously it is no easy matter to establish a standard of "worthiness." It is difficult to go behind appearances. Last year one dispensary treated over ninety thousand people. What sort of investigation could be made of this mass of shifting humanity, largely composed of foreigners who cannot speak the English language? Shall they be left unserved in their suffering, and in danger of its acute increase until investigated? If appearances are to guide, the rough-looking mechanic, in his working clothes, who earns not less than fifteen dollars a week, would pass unquestioned; but the clerk, whose position requires that he present a decent appearance, though eking out a mere existence for himself and family on a dollar a day, would be challenged as an "impostor." The first and best preventive of pauperism or dependency is health and strength to labor. The economic foundation, in the last analysis, is also the moral foundation. The "poor man's doctor" is too often either inexperienced or incompetent or worse, a scheming quack from whom the poor should be protected. To neither does the community owe a living or "protection." Through the dispensaries, with their carefully selected physicians, the poor classes have the benefit of the best service. This is true economy for the saving of health and wealth. It is this knowledge that nerves the more fastidious among the poor to submit themselves to the ordeal of the free clinic. Their one paramount thought is relief and cure.

The subject broadens before us. Within recent years the grade of dispensary work has greatly improved. The most skilled practitioners are seeking its advantages, and giving of their ability in return. These betterments naturally attract a more worthy class of people. The dispensary is no longer the source of dread that it was in former times. Are the friends and sustainers of dispensaries going in the wrong direction? It is a good time to discuss and decide before more are added. The question must be settled on broad lines of intention. It cannot be settled on the narrow lines of discrimination against individuals. The task is too great. In a shifting population like New York, it is nearly superhuman. Fallible man has not the ability to draw the line with exactness between those who should and those who should not receive gratuitous treatment. Because of this inability, shall the dispensaries be closed to those who apply for their aid, and the helpless invalids left to the tender mercies of municipal officials, at an enormous increase of cost and suffering, or wait in their distress until investigated?

Whatever faults and abuses may exist in dispensaries and hospitals, I think reasoning philanthropists and economists agree, as stated in my beginning, that they are an absolute necessity in any dense community. The proof of this is their existence in all the principal cities where modern civilization has a foothold. The emergency of sickness among the poor must be met by suitable means for its relief, regardless of their financial ability. Humanity in time of suffering cannot stop to coldly deliberate on what will be the after effects on the patient of its interposition. There are hours of extremity and danger when assistance must be extended without regard to moral consequences. The safety and health of the populace as a whole is a higher law than individual welfare, and must be protected, possibly to the demoralizing of the individual. The obligation, therefore, is on the citizens to provide sanitary remedies and refuges, either through taxation or private beneficence. I do not think the poor are actually pauperized by this kind of charity, as is too often done by promiscuous almsgiving. The poor do not reason about how to obtain free medical help as they do how to procure a living without labor. They rather accept the dispensary as their "family physician," thoughtless of degrading risk. May not the absence of pre-planned motive be a protection to self-respect? I am quite sure, from more than forty years' observation, that dispensary charity is the most helpful and least hurtful of the numberless ways to assist the poor, without breaking down their self-respect, and lessening efforts for self-support. There should be no place for a charity which eventuates in undermining self-respect and weakening self-reliance.

Another question has been agitated in the past. How should the board of managers of a dispensary be constructed? Shall the members be confined to laymen or shall physicians and laymen be elected?—the latter to manage the financial resources, and the former to select and make rules for the medical staff. Each side has its advocates, and both plans are employed. Very much depends on the character and energy of the men chosen, and their willingness to devote ample time and thought to the legislation and administration. Neither physician nor layman has a monopoly of these requisites. Whatever method is adopted, neither should retain in the board gentlemen who fail to actively participate in the management. Such should be eliminated, and vitality sustained by an infusion of live members. I do not believe in ornamental managers whose merit rests on social position or wealth. The natural tendency of all voluntary enterprises is to deteriorate without constant vigilance. Gradually the employees combine in themselves the legislative and executive control, and the managers become only nominally the source of authority. A lay board presents advantages in considering legislation and the appointment of those who are to form the executive staff. The bond of professional etiquette and friendship that attaches to a physician, somewhat hampers his freedom and makes him subject to the charge of partiality, however conscientious in the selection.

The Demilt and some other dispensaries never have had a physician in the board. No disrespect to the profession is intended. It is designed to assure an unbiased integrity in appointment on professional merit alone, and better supervision of the service. Also to avoid favoritism to the graduates of any special medical college.* The chief purpose of our work is to benefit suffering humanity and incidentally to recompense the attending physicians by the experience obtained. This latter advantage, we believe, should be impartially offered to all the profession on competitive terms, with the certitude that proficiency and experience will win the appointment. The one law governing the committee on the medical staff is to select those best qualified for the special duties, without fear or favor.

Some of the medical profession do not class the clinic advantages of dispensaries at their practical worth. Probably ten times as many physicians are cultured by them as have opportunity for hospital investigations. Dispensaries are not primary schools for the instruction of students, but post-graduate educators in advanced and original studies and preparation for instruction in hospitals and medical schools, or for higher skill in private practice, with its larger compensation as a reward. As one proof of this, I refer to the names of those who have had the opportunity to enlarge their culture and make it a stepping-stone to eminence in the medical world by devoting years to dispensary practice. To many it has proved the foundation of later accepted authority in the science of medicine and surgery. Dispensaries are with us to stay for good or evil. I think, therefore, the ignoring or belittling of them in the deliberations of county, state and national associations in the past is to be deplored. I trust hereafter the members of such organizations will think so, too, and that they will give a portion of their thought and action to the best methods of elevating the grade where it is defective, co-operating with trustees to dislodge any abuses, and thus improving and extending the usefulness of dispensaries to both patients and physicians. This can never be done while they are disparaged, or held as inferior auxiliaries in medical progress.

In conclusion, if this exposition of dispensaries shall stimulate thought in regard thereto and healthy criticism; if it shall lead to improved methods in management and service; if it shall be helpful

---

* The Philadelphia Dispensary has this rule : "nor shall the physician on any occasion permit his office to be made subservient to the use of any school, clique, institution or person, whatever."

in carrying out their original intent to promptly aid the sick who are unable to pay for treatment; if it shall enlighten any in regard to their value as sanitary protectors from the spread of contagious and pestilential disease; if it shall stimulate managers to be vigilant in suppressing abuses either by patients or physicians, it will not be in vain that attention has been directed to this great department of charity and humanity.

The work of dispensaries and hospitals has no finality. There is an hour when sickness overtakes each individual. No station in life is exempt. Each day has its catalogue of accidents, disease and death. This unavoidable penalty of life involves a never-ending demand for the skill, the time and the sympathy of those who are called to the ministry of healing as physicians. It appeals with equal force to the generosity of philanthropists in behalf of those who, by reason of poverty, are unable to procure needful medical aids to health, or relief from needless suffering on their way to the grave.

V.

FIRST AID TO THE INJURED.

UEBER BLUTLOSE OPERATIONEN.

Von Dr. Friedrich von Esmarch,

Kiel, Germany.

Es sind jetzt zwanzig Jahre verflossen, seitdem ich das Glück hatte, ein Verfahren zu erfinden, welches es möglich macht, bei allen Operationen an den Extremitäten, nicht bloss bei Amputationen, den Blutverlust zu vermeiden, den störenden Zufluss des Blutes während der Operation fernzuhalten und so an Lebenden wie an der Leiche zu operiren.

Die Erfindung war die Frucht zwanzigjähriger Bemühungen, bei blutigen Operationen den Blutverlust auf das geringste Maass zu beschränken. Sie breitete sich in kurzer Zeit über die ganze Erde aus, fand viele begeisterte Lobredner, aber auch manche Gegner und Prioritätsbestreiter.

Von vielen Seiten wurde geltend gemacht, dass schon lange vor mir dieser oder jener Chirurg bei Amputationen die abzuschneidenden Glieder vorher eingewickelt und hochgehalten habe, dass auch die Anwendung des Kautschuks zum Umschnüren nicht neu sei und so weiter.

Ich musste das zugeben, konnte auch nachweisen, dass ich selbst schon seit zwanzig Jahren die Einwicklung des emporgehaltenen Gliedes vor Amputationen geübt, ohne zu wissen, dass schon Brünninghausen dies Verfahren angewendet und im Jahre 1818 empfohlen hatte.

Ich konnte aber auch jenen Prioritätsansprüchen gegenüber es betonen, dass das Wesentliche meiner Erfindung nicht das Verfahren sei, durch welches ich bei Amputationen den Blutverlust verhindere oder einschränke, sondern der ganz neue Gedanke, dass der Chirurg bei jeder Operation, wo es möglich ist, den Blutverlust vermeiden solle und dazu gab ich das von mir bereits erprobte Verfahren an.

Sehr bald wurden auch die Mängel und Nachtheile, welche das Verfahren haben sollte, hervorgehoben, Warnungen und Verbesserungsvorschläge daran geknüpft, ja von manchen Chirurgen wurde es ganz verworfen und empfohlen, zu den alten Methoden, namentlich zum alten Tourniquet oder zur Digitalcompression der Gefässstämme zurückzukehren.

Die Hauptvorwürfe, welche man dem Verfahren gemacht hat und noch macht, sind: die oft eintretenden Nachblutungen; die Lähmung der durch den Schnürschlauch gedrückten Nerven; das Absterben von Hautlappen oder Wundrändern; die Gefahr, dass septische Stoffe oder Elemente bösartiger Neubildungen oder Thromben durch die Einwicklung in den Kreislauf getrieben werden könnten.

Ich habe mich redlich bemüht, das zuerst geschilderte Verfahren weiter auszubilden zu verbessern und zu vereinfachen, auch von Zeit zu Zeit darüber Mittheilungen gemacht, in denen ich hervorhob, dass die Nachtheile, welche man der Anwendung der künstlichen Blutleere zum Vorwurf macht, sämmtlich nicht von der Methode, sondern von einer verkehrten Anwendung derselben, namentlich von einer zu gewaltsamen Umschnürung mit dem zuerst von mir angegebenen Gummischlauch, abhängen.

Aber trotzdem schleppen sich diese Vorwürfe gegen die künstliche Blutleere von einem Handbuche ins andere, von einer Auflage zur anderen fort und zeigen, dass die Verfasser immer noch nicht sich bemüht haben, die Verbesserungen des Verfahrens kennen zu lernen. Ich halte es deshalb nicht für unnütz, noch einmal die Art und Weise zu schildern, in welcher in den letzten fünfzehn Jahren die künstliche Blutleere in meiner Klinik geübt wird, und bemerke dazu, dass wir niemals die oben angeführten Nachtheile beobachtet haben.

Das Verfahren besteht bekanntlich im Wesentlichen aus zwei Theilen; es bezweckt: 1. Das Heraustreiben des Blutes durch die Venen aus den Gefässen des zu operirenden Körpertheils; 2. die Verhinderung des arteriellen Blutzuflusses während der Operation.

Für den ersten Zweck verwende ich vor Allem die elastische Umwicklung des Gliedes von unten nach oben und wo diese gefährlich erscheint (wenn entzündliche oder eitrige Heerde, Thromben in den Venen oder bösartige Neubildungen in dem Gliede vorhanden sind) die senkrechte Erhebung des Gliedes, bis dasselbe deutlich blass geworden ist.

Zur Umwicklung gebrauche ich, nach wie vor, dünne Binden von reinem braunem Kautschuk, welche natürlich vorher zu sterilisiren sind. Aber auch durch leinene oder baumwollene Binden, welche trocken angelegt und dann nass gemacht werden, lässt sich derselbe Zweck erreichen. Die Binde wird bis zu der Stelle hinauf geführt, wo der Schnürgurt angelegt werden soll und hier zunächst durch Unterschieben des Bindenkopfes unter die letzte Tour befestigt. Dann folgt 2. die Anlegung des Schnürgurts zur Verhinderung des arteriellen Blutzuflusses. Dazu verwende ich nur noch in ganz seltenen Fällen, bei Exarticulationen im Hüft- und Schultergelenk und bei Amputationen dicht unter denselben, den zuerst von mir gebrauchten Kautschukschlauch, wo ich aber in neuester Zeit die von Bardeleben empfohlene vorherige Unterbindung der Hauptgefässstämme (der Arteria und Vena iliaca communis und der Art- und Vena subclavia) vorziehe. Auch bei Operationen am Penis und Scrotum verwende ich ganz dünne Kautschukschläuche.

Seit vielen Jahren schon gebrauche ich in allen anderen Fällen einen aus gewebtem Kautschukstoff bestehenden Gurt, der 5 cm. breit, 140 cm. lang und stark genug ist, um auch bei sehr muskulösen Männern die Arteria femoralis so zusammenzupressen, dass kein arterielles Blut mehr in das abgeschnürte Glied gelangen kann (Esmarch's Aderpresse, Schnürgurt). Für de Anlegung dieser Aderpresse gelten folgende Regeln :

1. Am besten legt man den Gurt an den Stellen an, wo reichlich Weichtheile den Knochen bedecken, weil die Arterien durch die zusammengeschnürten Muskeln zusammengedrückt werden sollen. In der Regel wird von mir die Mitte des Oberarms und die Mitte des Oberschenkels dazu benutzt. Nicht zweckmässig ist es, Körperstellen zu wählen, wo viele Knochen und Sehnen und wenig Muskeln vorhanden sind, zum Beispiel die Gegend dicht oberhalb des Ellbogengelenks, des Kniegelenks oder die Gegend der Knöchel.

2. Je weiter oberhalb der Operationsstelle der Gurt angelegt werden kann, desto besser, theils der Infektionsgefahr wegen (die übrigens durch vorherige Sterilisation des Gurtes und durch Umwickeln des angelegten Gurtes mit einer sterilisirten Binde zu verhüten ist), theils weil erst nach Anlegung des oft weit hinauf reichenden Compressionsverbandes, ev. einer Schiene, der Gurt wieder abgenommen werden soll.

3. Die Touren des Gurtes müssen unter stärkster Dehnung und

so angelegt werden, dass sie sich alle einander decken. Der Anfang der Binde wird gleich durch den Druck der ersten Tour befestigt.

4. Das Ende des Gurtes befestigte ich anfangs durch eine Sicherheitsnadel (baby's pin). Dann verwendete ich den von Nicaise angegebenen Verschluss mit Ringen und Haken, aber schon seit mehr als zehn Jahren gebrauche ich ausschliesslich eine einfache verschiebbare Klemmschnalle mit Haken.

5. Da dieser Schnürgurt infolge der eingewebten Seiden- oder Baumwollenfäden nur eine begrenzte Dehnbarkeit besitzt, so lässt sich damit eine übermässige Einschnürung garnicht ausführen. Ich habe auch niemals weder eine Drucklähmung, noch eine Gangrän der Hautränder und -Lappen in Folge der künstlichen Blutleere eintreten sehen, wie sie, meiner Ansicht nach, nur durch übermässige Dehnung von dicken Kautschukschläuchen hervorgebracht werden kann. Auch bemühe ich mich, in meiner Klinik meine Schüler in der Anwendung der künstlichen Blutleere zu unterrichten, indem ich sie oft unter meiner Aufsicht und Leitung den Gurt anlegen lasse.

6. Wenn das zu operirende Glied ödematös geschwollen ist, dann kann es vorkommen, dass der Schnürgurt seine Wirkung versagt, weil er das Serum aus den Maschen des Gewebes herauspresst und die Wirkung des Druckes dann nachlässt. In solchem Falle wird das vorher blasse Glied langsam wieder roth und das Operationsfeld von Blut überschwemmt. Nimmt man den Gurt ab, so sieht man, dass derselbe eine tiefe Furche in die Weichtheile gedrückt hat. Man muss dann die Wunde rasch mit Schwämmen comprimiren, das Glied hoch heben und den Gurt aufs Neue in die gedrückte Furche anlegen und warten, bis die Blutung vollkommen steht.

7. Der Schnürgurt wird in der Regel erst abgenommen, wenn die ganze Operation beendet und der Verband angelegt ist. Dann wird das Glied senkrecht in die Höhe gerichtet und nun der Gurt rasch abgewickelt (nicht langsam!). Der Patient wird mit erhobenem Gliede ins Bett gebracht und so gelagert, dass das Glied (oder der Stumpf) noch eine halbe Stunde nach oben gerichtet bleibt; dann wird auch dieses horizontal gelagert.

8. Handelt es sich um die Entfernung eines Gliedes durch Amputation oder Exarticulation, dann werden nach vollkommen blutloser Ausführung der Operation selbst alle sichtbaren Gefässe zuerst mit Schieberpincetten gefasst und dann sorgfältig mit Catgut unterbunden. Die Gefässmündungen sind auf den blutlosen Schnittflächen

leicht zu erkennen und man braucht dazu keineswegs die früher von mir empfohlenen Durchschnittsmodelle nach Prof. Pansch zur Hand zu haben.

9. Nachdem dann die ganze Wunde durch tiefe und oberflächliche Nähte sorgfältig vereinigt, ein aseptischer Druckverband mit Mooskissen und Gazebinden und darüber eine dünne Kautschukbinde mit mässigem Druck angelegt ist, wird der Schnürgurt abgenommen, wie oben geschildert.

10. Bei Resectionen, Nekrotomieen, Extirpationen und anderen grösseren Operationen werden nur die grösseren Gefässe unterbunden, welche man während der Operation als solche erkennt, was bei der Blutleere nicht schwer ist. Dann wird die Wunde entweder durch die Naht vereinigt oder tamponirt und darnach der Druckverband angelegt, der in der Regel mehrere Wochen liegen bleibt.

11. Daraus geht hervor, dass wir mit der so gefürchteten in Folge der augenblicklichen Gefässlähmung eintretenden Blutung garnichts zu thun haben, und da wir fast niemals eine auch nur nennenswerthe Nachblutung beobachten, so darf ich behaupten, dass in meiner Klinik in der That alle Operationen an den Extremitäten ohne Blutverlust vollzogen werden.

Der von mir angegebene Schnürgurt ist bereits in vielen Armeen statt des alten Tourniquets eingeführt worden. Da aber die Kautschukstoffe bei langem Aufbewahren in Arsenalen und namentlich in sehr heissen und sehr kalten Klimaten bald verderben, so habe ich für diese Zwecke einen ähnlichen Gurt aus Messingspiralfedern mit Lederüberzug herstellen lassen, welcher viele Jahre lang aufbewahrt werden kann, ohne zu verderben.

In derselben Weise lässt sich der von mir angegebene Hosenträger verwenden, welcher aus einem 150 cm. langen und 4 cm. breiten Gurt besteht. Er muss aber aus gutem, hinreichend elastischem Kautschukgewebe gefertigt sein, wie ihn Franz Clouth in Köln für den Deutschen Samariter Verein liefert.

Ich habe diesen Hosenträger erfunden zum Zwecke der ersten Hülfe bei Verletzungen grosser Gefässe. Die Anwendung desselben wird in unseren Samariterschulen gelehrt und es sind bereits zahlreiche Fälle zur Kunde des Deutschen Samariter Vereins gekommen, in denen durch diese Hosenträger das entfliehende Leben Schwerverletzter erhalten wurde.

Die Frage, wie lange ein gut angelegter Schnürgurt liegen bleiben kann, ohne wesentlichen Schaden zu verursachen, ist noch eine offene.

Ich selbst habe bei grossen mühsamen Operationen die arterielle Zufuhr bis zu 2½ Stunden ferngehalten, ohne irgend einen Nachtheil davon zu beobachten. Ich bin aber davon überzeugt, dass man die Zeit viel länger hinausschieben kann. Dafür sprechen folgende Thatsachen:

Cohnheim konnte bei Warmblütern die Blutcirculation auf 6–8 Stunden vollständig unterbrechen, ohne dass üble Folgen eintraten.

Riedel berichtete über einen Fall aus der Göttinger Klinik, in welchem wegen einer Zerschmetterung des Armes durch ein Eisenbahnrad eine elastische Binde 6 Stunden lang gelegen ohne Nachtheil. Denn die Verletzung wurde unter conservativer Behandlung geheilt.

F. Fischer berichtet aus Lücke's Klinik in Strassburg (D. Z. f. Chir. 1885, 22, III., S. 245), über eine Schnittwunde am Vorderarm mit arterieller Blutung, wobei die elastische Schnürbinde 17 Stunden gelegen hatte, ohne dass der Arm brandig geworden. Die Wunde wurde mit vollkommener Brauchbarkeit der Hand geheilt.

Im Jahre 1882 berichteten mir zwei hochangesehene praktische Aerzte in Emden, über zwei Fälle von schweren Maschinenverletzungen des Armes, welche sich am Abend ereignet und wo die Blutung durch elastische Umschnürung gestillt war. Die Verletzten kamen erst um Mitternacht ins Krankenhaus und wegen mangelnder Assistenz konnte erst am anderen Morgen um 10 Uhr die Amputation vorgenommen werden. Beide Fälle heilten ohne besondere Störungen, obwohl der Schnürgurt mindestens 12 Stunden gelegen hatte.

Ich schliesse aus diesen Beobachtungen, dass man in solchen bedrohlichen Fällen die arterielle Zufuhr ohne besonderen Nachtheil mindestens 12 Stunden lang unterbrechen darf.

Von besonderem Werthe für die erste Hülfe von Laien (Samaritern) ist die elastische Umschnürung desshalb, weil für die Anwendung derselben keine anatomische Kenntniss nothwendig ist. Es braucht dabei nicht, wie beim alten Tourniquet, eine Pelotte auf den Stamm der Arterie gelegt zu werden, sondern die Umschnürung ist wirksam an jeder Stelle, wo Weichtheile genügend vorhanden sind. Auch kann sich der umschnürende Gurt oder Strang auf dem Transport weder verschieben, noch seine Wirksamkeit einbüssen, wenn nur das Ende so gut befestigt wird, dass es sich nicht lösen kann.

RED CROSS AND FIRST-AID SOCIETIES.

By Mr. John Furley,

London.

It requires no assurance on my part that it is a very high honor to have been invited to contribute a paper to this International Congress held in connection with your great universal exhibition. The subject proposed to me is that of "Red Cross and First Aid Societies," a comprehensive work, towards the development of which the best years of my life have been devoted.

But when first the invitation was given, I naturally hesitated before consenting to address an American audience on such a matter. My thoughts at once reverted to that period when this continent was the scene of a struggle to which the history of the world offers no parallel, either in its immediate effects or in those glorious results which have established a Union which, for the sake of civilization and humanity, it is to be hoped may never again be disturbed.

An almost insuperable difficulty presented itself when I looked at the title of this paper; the subject is so extensive, and its history is so crowded with interesting details, that it would not be possible to do more than trace a slight sketch of the origin of Red Cross and first-aid societies in the limit of time allowed. My task, therefore, has consisted less in searching for material than in selecting from the mass of facts which I had at hand.

The convention of Geneva which was drawn up in 1864, and has since received the adhesion of 36 governments, was the outcome of the sad and terrible experience of centuries of war, and Red Cross societies were the natural sequel to this international treaty. It is generally, but erroneously, supposed that the convention of Geneva had in view the formation of a Red Cross organization, and that the numerous societies which have since been established under its flag are regulated by some occult international tribunal. Undoubtedly the international committee, composed of five or six Swiss gentlemen sitting at Geneva, has contributed largely to the solidarity of the Red Cross movement, but it cannot be too widely known that each Red Cross Society has a separate and national existence, although its objects are international; each has its own constitution and rules, and these are quite independent of foreign control.

Nor can there be any doubt that sympathy with suffering, and the excitement engendered by the prospect of war, may always be relied on at critical times to fill up the ranks of any army hospital corps with recruits of more or less efficiency. We have seen this in the past. But a few years ago the standard of qualification for nurses and ambulancers was very much below what it is in the present day. Something more is now required of volunteers than a willingness to serve, and considering the multitude from which a selection may be made, there is no reason why the highest efficiency should not be maintained. War, notwithstanding our boasted civilization, still exercises a magnetic effect on a large proportion of the population. On its outbreak hundreds of men and women are influenced by the thought that humanity claims their presence as near as possible to the battlefield, and, if circumstances prevent this, their humane instincts impel them to do their utmost from a distance to relieve the sufferings of the victims. This feeling has been a useful factor for many years in the social life of nations, and not only have civil and military hospitals thereby been gainers, but the influence of first-aid instruction, nursing classes, improved hospital management, and sanitation generally, has more or less permeated the populations of the world.

This great change is indisputably the result of the institution of Red Cross societies which almost immediately followed the adoption of the convention of Geneva by the great powers of Europe. People who were anxious to assist in alleviating the sufferings of the victims of war soon discovered that their ability to do so was in no degree commensurate with their inclination. Reflection convinced them that a serious apprenticehip was necessary if they were to be of use instead of hindrance, and this led them to seek for practical knowledge by giving attention to home needs and to the vast requirements of civil life in the always open field of human suffering. Thus has been brought about a change which is probably one of the most remarkable and important of modern times,—preparation for the ambulance necessities of war has been found to be the best school for providing hospital requirements in time of peace.

Two articles of the convention of Geneva sufficiently indicate its objects. Firstly, "ambulances and military hospitals shall be acknowledged to be neuter, and, as such, shall be protected and respected by belligerents as long as any sick and wounded may be therein." And, secondly, "a distinctive and uniform flag shall be adopted for hospitals and ambulances. . . . An arm-badge shall also be allowed for individuals neutralized, but the delivery thereof shall be left to military authority. The flag and the arm-badge shall bear a Red Cross on a white ground." Thus it will be seen that the intention of the framers of the convention was confined to war-time, and the Red Cross is a badge which has only a military significance. It is true that the use of this badge has been very much abused. It is indiscriminately adopted by those who have no title to it in time of peace, and some of those who now display it will sustain a rude shock should they attempt in any future war to use it without proper military authority.

A want of knowledge on this subject has led to so much error that no apology is necessary for again insisting that those who bear the Red Cross as a badge should be legally empowered to do so; and this can only be under military sanction, otherwise during a campaign it would become utterly worthless and, indeed, a menace to discipline.

Without disparaging the efforts which were made in bygone times to mitigate the horrors of war, it must be admitted that no systematic and concentrated effort was made in this direction until the present century. Nursing, and the relief of suffering, have ever been recognized as the special province of women, and we are, therefore, not surprised by the fact that in all the more serious attempts to grapple with the problem women have taken a conspicuous share. Consider, for instance, the work which was organized in 1813 by the Frauenverein of Frankfort, a society of women which subsequently, during 50 years of peace, was maintained in activity by ministering to the necessities of the sick and suffering, and was thus able to reassume its military rôle within fifteen days after the outbreak of a war in which the German fatherland was involved. Need we be reminded of the initiative taken, in 1854, during the Crimean war by Miss Florence Nightingale, with the sanction of the British Government, and of the impetus thus given to the extension of woman's sphere of usefulness in that particular department which is pre-eminently her own? The names of many other women who have played a heroic part in this vast field of humanity also arise. And of these women, some of the humblest are not the least distinguished by brave devotion to self-imposed duty. And others there are of exalted rank to whom the world is especially indebted for the assistance they have afforded by precept and example.

It will never be forgotten what the Empress Augusta of Germany
accomplished, not only for the Red Cross societies under her own
immediate patronage, but also for kindred societies in other countries. It is no exaggeration to say that for a long period she did
more towards the development of what, for brevity, may be termed
Red Cross work, than any other individual. And now that she is
gone her guiding influence is followed by her granddaughter, the
present Empress of Germany, and by her daughter, the Grand
Duchess of Baden. The Empress of Russia is another lady who,
from her high position, has stepped down to work in the ranks with
those who are struggling to contend with the terrible results of war,
as well as with the results of pestilence and famine from which her
adopted country has suffered so severely. Nor can we pass over
what Queen Victoria has done in the encouragement of those of her
own sex who are laboring as nurses both in peace and war; and in
this her gracious Majesty has had the active assistance of all her
daughters. Such examples, and I might name others, are of the
highest value, and I am confident this is acknowledged by the self-
reliant and practical women of the United States.

Red Cross societies are intended to act, and have been accepted,
as supplementary to the medical department of armies in the field,
and as such their representatives are entitled to that neutrality which
was sanctioned by the convention of Geneva, so long as they strictly
conform to military authority. The active sphere of each of these
societies during peace must depend, more or less, on national characteristics : they cannot be moulded on one pattern. But the moment
a war breaks out, any society desiring to perform its part must adopt
the position defined for it by the belligerent powers, and, if unwilling
to do so, it had better altogether abstain from interference.

Hitherto the assistance given by these societies has been somewhat irregular, but during the last few years the principal military
powers of Europe, notably France and Germany, have so organized
and incorporated hospital volunteer aid that their example may be
safely followed, subject to such modification as may be rendered
necessary by difference of race and institutions.

It has been generally recognized on the continent of Europe that,
in time of peace, each national Red Cross society should be engaged
in strengthening and developing relations with the military authorities under whom they will have to act in time of war; in organizing
the *personnel* in such a manner as will best enable it to co-operate

with the army medical staff and hospital corps, and in studying and adapting ambulance material to all the conditions of locality and climate under which it may be employed.

These are the first principles which should guide the central committee of a National Red Cross Society and all its branches. But, naturally, the civilians who are engaged in this work have their thoughts more directed to the wants of peace than the requirements of war. And here it is we find the real strength of such an institution, because its members, whilst attending to the daily necessities of those who are suffering from the accidents and epidemics of civil life, are, in a great measure, qualifying themselves for the demands which may be made upon them in the event of war. Thousands of men and women who never contemplate the possibility of leaving home to take part in war, willingly co-operate in giving first-aid to those who are injured in the occupations of civil life, and amongst these a strong nucleus can readily be found who may be relied on for active help in war at home or abroad.

The United States of America are happily more free than European nations from the constant anticipation of war, and I know how practical is the ambulance system on this side of the Atlantic. But I leave to others better qualified than myself to describe this.

I may, however, mention the work of the St. John Ambulance Association in my own country, which was established, in 1877, with the object of giving instruction to people of all classes in the best means of rendering first-aid to the injured. The growth of this society has been almost phenomenal; probably no institution ever gained a more rapid popularity. Its aims were at first limited to work in time of peace, but should a war occur in which England may be engaged, there is no doubt that the British National Aid Society (the name adopted by the British Red Cross Society) will find in the St. John Ambulance Association some of its most effective recruits.

In Germany the Samariter-verein, founded in 1882, has followed very closely on the lines of the St. John Ambulance Association.

In France l'Association des dames Françaises, and l'Union des femmes de France have been quite recently placed by a decree of the government on the same footing as the Société de secours aux blessés militaires, the French Red Cross Society.

In other countries, notably in Austria and Russia, orders of knighthood and other societies are engaged in similar work. And, indeed, everywhere in the civilized world may be found thousands of men and women who, whilst actively engaged in relieving the sufferings of the sick and injured during peace, are qualifying themselves for service under military control and discipline in time of war.

But no true idea can be obtained of the close connection which must necessarily exist between Red Cross organizations, having always in view the probability of war, and first-aid societies established to meet the needs of peace, if the subject of ambulance material be omitted from consideration. For several years the training of hospital *personnel* and improvements in ambulance material have made simultaneous progress; and military members of the medical profession are the first to admit that they have gained much advantage from the practical experience obtained through the efforts of civilians. In peaceful times there are few governments which will venture to spend much money on the non-combatant portion of armies, and the consequence is that, with one or two exceptions, should war suddenly break out, these armies would be found very deficient in the means of coping with the results of great battles, without the assistance of the civilian supplement, on which they can now rely.

Personal experience enables me to speak confidently in this matter. In some European States the links which connect the civil and military ambulance organizations are of the most intimate character —notably in France and Germany. In my own country there is no such union, although the most friendly sympathy exists. But I am bold enough to predict that the first indication of a great war would accomplish a fusion similar to that which has been encouraged and effected by the other great military powers.

Large stores of weapons, ammunition and accoutrements are indispensable to an army, and no fear of waste or deterioration, or the fact that the progress of science may render the patterns of one year obsolete in the next, can deter a government from the great expenditure of money which is the bugbear of political economists. But fortunately, civilians in their struggle to alleviate the sufferings of those who fall on the battlefield of daily life are not hampered in the same manner. They can devise and continue to invent new ambulance material, with the assurance that any merits will be appreciated and at once utilized. Contrast the present position of the United States of America, and, indeed, of all the states of Europe, with regard to hospital and ambulance appliances with that of 25 years ago. Whether for civil or military purposes the progress has been equally marked and beneficial. And this is due to the efforts of civilians acting in a large degree under the friendly advice and approval of military surgeons, who fully recognize the advantage of such co-operation in case of war. We note this in every item that is used for ambulance purposes, from bandages to stretchers and wagons.

It is perhaps natural that in a paper like this personal experience should occasionally crop out, and I am sure I shall not be accused of egotism if, in order to show that my statements do not rest only on theory, I mention two simple facts which, better than anything else, will illustrate my meaning. A considerable number of ambulance carriages have been built on patterns supplied by me and under my personal supervision, nearly all of which have been designed for civil hospitals, collieries and factories. Now the ordinary stretcher in use in the British army is about 7 feet 8 inches in length, and it has therefore been necessary to build military ambulance carriages of a suitable size. But for civil use the stretcher handles can be telescoped, and the carriages can, therefore, be made less in length, and consequently less unwieldy. I have never lost sight of the desirability of uniting to the fullest extent possible the *personnel* and *matériel* employed in civil and military ambulances. With this view, every accident-carriage which has been designed and built under my responsibility during the last few years has been so constructed that it can be used for the stretchers with telescopic handles, whilst by a simple arrangement, which does not add an inch to the body of the carriage, it will also take the full-length military regulation stretchers. By this means Great Britain now possesses ambulance carriages in daily use for civil purposes which can at any time be employed for home military use.

This is one example of the double service to which ambulance material can be put. I will now briefly refer to the dual employment as it affects the *personnel*.

For some years the St. John Ambulance Association has encouraged the formation of ambulance corps for civil purposes amongst those who hold its certificates of efficiency, and the endeavor has been attended with the most satisfactory results. Recently another step in advance has been made, for in some instances these corps have adopted a certain degree of military training. I need cite only one example;—in a colliery district a few months ago, 180 officers

and men were inspected, with the sanction of the Secretary of State
for War, by the Director-General of the Army Medical Department,
and they proved themselves well qualified to act as a valuable supplement for home service to the Army Medical Service Corps. I
may further remark that this corps, with the addition of another
body of miners from the same district, and under the same command,
comprising a total number of 413 officers and men, had the honor of
being inspected by H. M. Queen Victoria at Windsor Castle on the
6th of last May.

These two illustrations indicate, better than any other facts that
could be mentioned, the mutual relation which can exist between
Red Cross and first-aid societies on the one side, and the official
sanitary service of an army on the other. I am not sanguine enough
to think that in these days when business and pleasure, and even
philanthropy, are conducted at a pace which is exhausting without
being complete, relations will be as well organized as they should be.
It must be left for another war to bring home to the official mind the
advantages to be derived from such a union. Meanwhile, the work
is not wasted, as is testified by the effects of the labors of the large
numbers of men and women who are daily doing-their best to lessen
the preventible suffering arising from accidents in civil life. It would
be impossible to exaggerate the benefits to humanity which have
resulted from the efforts in all countries to which I have referred.

Time will not allow me to enter into details, and therefore I have
only briefly sketched the general outlines of the beneficent work
which has already been accomplished, and which is being daily
extended. Others, perhaps, will take up and elaborate this subject,
and will tell you how this is being done, and they can inform you
how the work in each country has been adapted to local requirements and national characteristics. It is not only that people of all
classes have found an opportunity close to their own doors and in
the midst of their daily avocations to do something in a practical
manner towards the alleviation of the sorrow and suffering which are
caused by sickness and accident, but they are qualifying themselves
to minimize those terrible effects of war which Red Cross societies
were in their origin designed to mitigate.

FIRST AID TO THE INJURED FROM THE ARMY STANDPOINT.

BY MAJOR CHARLES SMART, Surgeon, U. S. A.

Provision for first aid to the injured has been the subject of earnest study by medical officers of our army for several years back. The War of the Rebellion gave the army medical department a large experience, which has not been altogether lost by lapse of years; for although most of those who were personally engaged on the great battlefields have dropped from the ranks of active workers, many of them have placed their views on record, or impressed them on younger officers who have served with them as subordinates.

In the way of efficient arrangements for the administration of first aid in our military service there have been two obstacles which greatly delayed our progress. Ordinarily the paramount duty of a military bureau in times of peace is to keep itself in training for the emergencies of future war; but the quarter of a century of peace and prosperity enjoyed by our country since the close of the civil war has been so beset with Indian hostilities that the medical department has had little opportunity of keeping itself in proper training. This seeming paradox is due to the fact that the conditions of field service against the Indian tribes differ so radically from those of civilized warfare. Under the latter there is always some place of relative safety towards the rear or base of supplies, where the wounded may be gathered and become the object of systematized care, no matter what may be the issue of the contest. Under the former, on the contrary, there is no such place. There is no rear for the men of a cavalry troop assailed by Indians, many days' march from the nearest military post; there is no protection for the wounded, save what is afforded by the nature of the ground held by their comrades, and every available man must fight until the savage enemy becomes disheartened and withdraws, or is driven off by fresh arrivals on the scene of action. Systematic methods for aid to the wounded have had little opportunity for development under such conditions. Witness the fate of General Custer and the men of the Seventh Cavalry at the Little Big Horn river. Assistant Surgeon Lord and his hospital men merely accompanied the soldiers to their death.

The difficulty of providing first aid to such expeditionary columns operating in a country impassable for wheeled vehicles, by a system which on enlargement would meet the necessities of civilized warfare, was one of the obstacles which delayed the progress of the medical department of the army in this direction until the past few years. The other obstacle was the failure of that vague power known in military parlance as *superior authority*, to provide suitable men for hospital purposes. Medical officers generally got what they wanted during our great war, on account of the extent and importance of their field of practice. Thus, when a medical director called for certain men for hospital duty, he usually obtained the good men he asked for. After the war the whole military establishment fell back almost to its ante-bellum status, and when the medical officer of a military post asked the commanding officer of that post, probably the captain of the only company stationed there, for certain men for hospital work, it by no means followed that he got the men he asked for. The commanding officer disliked to lose good soldiers from the ranks, but readily spared any man who was broken down, valueless from innate stupidity, or worse than worthless from dissipation. The men whom he could get, not the men whom he wanted, were those that the medical officer had to prepare for the duties of giving first aid to the injured; and afterwards, when by dint of care and assiduous personal attention to their physical and moral well-being he had repaired the broken constitution, awakened the intelligence, uprooted the evil habits and endowed these men with possibilities of future worth, they were probably transferred to the ranks, and the hospital provided with substitutes as worthless as those that had originally been sent. After laboring in vain to build a hospital system with such bricks, the most enthusiastic medical officer generally subsided into a state of resignation, or gave vent to his suppressed energies by formulating for the benefit of the Surgeon-General what seemed an Utopian dream of a hospital corps, every member of which was sober, trustworthy and intelligent, and fully conversant with every duty that the exigencies of the service might call upon him to perform. Not, indeed, that the Surgeon-General was ignorant of all this, but that superior authority was slow to move the wheels of progress out of the old-time ruts.

However, in 1887, Congress was led to appreciate and remove one of these great difficulties in the way of first aid to the injured soldier, by authorizing the organization of the Hospital Corps, its members to be selected, educated, drilled and disciplined by the medical officers themselves; whereupon these officers began earnestly to build up

the organization, and to so systematize its work that the same principles would regulate its action in times of peace as in times of stupendous war. This work is now well in progress, but with its methods
the present paper has no concern, as it is limited to the executive
details of first aid. To understand these details, however, a slight
reference to certain of the administrative methods is needful.

General aptitude or intelligence, with some primary or elementary
education, is a *sine quâ non* to enlistment in the hospital corps. On
this selected soil the medical officer has to raise all the technical
knowledge of disease and injury that is necessary to enable the individual to do good and not harm, when his responsibilities come upon
him and he is face to face with some appalling accident with no intelligence but his own to guide the hand that is to succor. All men,
citizens or soldiers, who are to render first aid must have more or
less of this knowledge, because the clearer their perceptions of what
is to be done, the greater will be their self-possession and ability to
act. People generally lose their heads in the presence of accident
and suffering. The man who knows something of what has to be
done preserves his presence of mind. If he has been familiarized by
drill in the management of emergencies with the idea of his own
responsibility, he retains his presence of mind and ability to do good,
although knowing little of the conditions or special treatment of the
particular case. The advantages of drill in first aid are obvious;
but its importance to the hospital corps soldier is vastly greater than
to the citizen Samaritan. Drill and correlated discipline have to
support him in his duties to the injured under the appalling knowledge that he is himself liable to be struck down at any moment. He
must retain his presence of mind not only when confronted with
death and injury to others, but when every rifle-shot and bullet-hum
suggests the imminence of personal danger. Great courage or thorough discipline, or an adequate combination of the two, is required
under such conditions for the performance of duties calling for the
exercise of knowledge, tact, delicacy, and a humane consideration for
the sufferings of others.

Behold, then, the men on whom the injured of the army have to
rely, men to whom no Christian would deny the honor of wearing
the cross of Christ as the badge of their military service. The points
next in order are, What do they do, and how do they do it?

First aid to the injured in war has not the same extent of significance to the soldier as to the citizen. To the latter it means all that

is done on behalf of the wounded until they are *en route* from the
privations, exposures and dangers of the battlefield to the shelter,
care and comforts of permanent hospitals. In fact, it comprises the
whole battlefield service of the army medical department,—the
gathering of the fallen by the litter-bearers, their transportation by
ambulance wagons to the field hospitals, and their preparation there
for transmission from the lines of the army for their homeward journey,
by way of the post or station which is the base of military operations.
To the soldier, however, first aid is that which finds him where he
fell on the skirmish line or line of battle, which puts a canteen to his
lips to revive him, stops the flowing blood, straightens the fractured
limb, giving him cheering words meanwhile, and carries him to the
friendly side of the house a little way off, or behind the breastworks
or over the brow of the hill, where he will be safe from stray bullets
and have the doctor help to make him comfortable before transfer-
ring him to an ambulance for transportation to the field hospital.
When first aid has done these things it has done all that the soldier
expects, all that he wants ; for when he reaches the canvas tents of
the hospital, where the skilled operative surgeons of each brigade
are at work, and where all the resources of the medical department
are drawn upon for the comfort of the wounded, he takes his bowl of
beef tea and disposes of himself to rest, satisfied that whatever may
hereafter be done on his behalf is not in the nature of first aid, but in
that of regular hospital treatment for his wounds. The soldier's view
is the correct one, and is the analogue of the citizen's view of first aid
in all cases excepting only that of the battlefield.

When the command with which a medical officer and a detachment
of the hospital corps are on duty is in the line of battle, and in momen-
tary expectation of the outburst of the storm of war, the nearest
shelter from musketry is sought, whereat to establish the collecting or
dressing station for the wounded. When the same command is in
camp with no danger of immediate hostilities, the medical officer and
his men are in camp also, and ready at all times to render aid in
accidents and injuries. Again, when in times of peace the troops form
the garrison of a military post, the medical officer and his men are still
to be found in the immediate vicinity of the quarters of the soldiers,
the medical establishment being then known as the post hospital.
This hospital, however, is, from our present point of view, merely
the collecting station of the battlefield, so altered by the various additions and comforts that have crystallized around it during the unruffled

quietude of the times as to be scarcely recognized at first glance. Here is to be found all that contributes to first aid to the injured, and with it much more that is of high value; but with this surplus we are at present not concerned. Does an accident happen at this military post? Immediately a litter squad, equipped as for the field of battle, is on the ground to care for the injured man and bring him to the post hospital. Does the command participate in some military parade? The medical officer and his detachment, with litters, ambulances and field equipment, are there also, not for show, but for first aid. Where the command goes there goes the hospital corps; and when the former cuts loose entirely from the post, as frequently happens in our Western service, the latter does so likewise, and is as fully prepared to meet the emergencies of field service as it was to meet the accidents of garrison life. It carries with it its litters and other requisites of first aid, and its ambulances as the basis of a hospital system. When several such commands meet and are united into one force under the senior commander, the several hospital corps fragments coalesce into one whole under the senior medical officer. When hundreds of such commands are gathered together in time of war, the medical organization progresses step by step with the organization of the commands into an army, and when this is completed, no part of the column when on march, nor of the line when formed for defense or attack, is left without its medical officer and his orderly and his assignment of litter-bearers for first aid to the injured. If one part of the line suffers more severely in battle than another, the supervising authority of the medical corps on the field sees to it that a corresponding increase of force is placed on duty there; but the working elements of this force continue to be the medical officer, his orderly and his litter-bearers.

A provision of this kind is of immense value to an army irrespective of all considerations of first aid to the injured. The assurance that he will be taken care of should he fall exerts a steadying influence on the soldier, which improves the morale of the fighting line. In the progress of battle, however, the very integrity of this line is often dependent on the vigorous and efficient action of the hospital corps. Ranks are speedily depleted if men drop out to assist a wounded comrade to the rear, and the thinning of the ranks has a serious influence on the spirit of those who remain. So thorough a depressant is this depletion that military men have made calculations as to the percentage of loss which an organization can sustain without losing its identity and disappearing from its place in the line. An efficient hospital corps which comes to the front for the wounded deprives the men of all excuse for leaving their position. It is true our present Army Regulations provide for the education in first aid of four men from each company. These men are called company bearers, and their duty outside of the regular duties of a soldier is to assist the wounded from the field, until relieved by the members of the hospital corps, when they return to their places in the firing line. The company bearer system is now recognized as a mistake. It is a survival from the time when there was no hospital corps, and when the wounded had to find their way to the rear with such assistance as their friends could give them. It was embodied in our hospital corps law, as a source of recruits for the corps which was to be organized and sustained by transfers from the line of the army, and those who took kindly to the duties of company bearers were naturally the best men for transfer. Now the hospital corps can enlist its men from any source, and the only method of showing the need of company bearers is to show that the litter squads of the hospital corps are incapable of performing their duty.

The litter consists of a canvas bed 6 feet long and 22 inches wide, made fast to two poles 7½ feet long and stretched by two jointed braces. The ends of the poles form the handles, 9 inches long, by which the litter is carried. The fixed iron legs are loop-shaped, 4 inches high and 1¾ inches wide. A sling is used with it for long distance carriage. It is carried closed or strapped, and is opened only for purposes of drill or inspection, and for actual service in the transportation of the sick and wounded.

The bearers work in squads of four men, known individually as No. 1, 2, 3 and 4. The litter is carried by 2 and 3; 1 and 4 are on either side, and the former is chief of squad. All carry water and dressing packets, but No. 4 has in addition a pouch containing field surgical necessaries. These men march into the exposure of the field for their wounded. When a patient is discovered, 1 and 4 may run ahead to determine his condition. In the various accidents of civil life or of military garrison life this oftentimes requires much knowledge, with time and patient enquiry and investigation. On the battlefield the questions are simpler, being mainly reduced to a determination of the conditions that bear upon transportation on a litter for a short distance and a corresponding time. Do shock, hemorrhage or fractured bones have to be cared for? A draught of water, with or without a stimulant, a field tourniquet and intelligent care in handling, one or more are at hand as required ; and perhaps by the time Nos. 2 and 3 have arrived with the litter, No. 1 is ready to command : *At patient; right* (or *left*, as he may consider best), when the members of his squad, each at his post, kneel on one knee by the wounded man. *Prepare to lift; lift*, he commands, and the patient is immediately removed from the ground and resting on the knees of three of the bearers while the other places the litter along their front, *Lower patient*, and the injured man is laid gently on the litter and adjusted thereon according to the requirements of the condition or injury. Then, at the command, *Prepare to lift; Lift; Forward; March*, they are off with their burden, moving rapidly but without haste and without jolting or other unevenness of movement. All this is accomplished almost automatically. The orders are given and obeyed ; and the wounded man is on his way from the exposure of the field in less time than would have been lost by intelligent but undrilled men in determining how best to raise their patient from the ground. The best methods have been studied for them, and practised by them, so that when moments are precious and delays dangerous, there is no time lost by ignorance, awkwardness or indecision. Even in the adjustment on the litter, practice makes it a matter of course to support and comfortably raise the head by an overcoat, blanket, blanket-bag, knapsack or other suitable article picked up from the field, to raise the patient further if there is difficulty of breathing, but to keep him low if, from shock or loss of blood, there is danger of fainting ; to place him on his back or uninjured side if the abdomen is wounded, with a pillow under his knees to keep them bent; to place an injured arm over the body, and to bind a fractured leg to its fellow for the sake of its support.

The litter squad may not do any more for the wounded man than has been stated, but its members can do more if there is time, opportunity or necessity. They do no more if other wounded men are awaiting removal, if there is notable danger from the fire of the enemy, or if the collecting station be close at hand ; and, when required by the work on hand, the litter squads of four do not hesitate to break up into squads of two. What they are able to do may be understood from a glance at the contents of the hospital corps pouch which No. 4 carries slung from his right shoulder to his left hip. It contains a candle and matches, lest there should be need of artificial light, the tin case acting as a candlestick when required.

Then there are two field tourniquets and a vial of aromatic spirits of ammonia for dealing with internal hemorrhage and shock, as already instanced. Held together in a small leather book are a pair of scissors, dressing forceps, jack-knife, pins, needles and thread. Packed loosely in the pouch are three 5-yard rollers of 2½-inch antiseptic bandage, a strong metal box containing 15 yards of adhesive plaster 1 inch wide, another box containing ½ ounce of 2 per cent carbolated vaseline, a hard rubber iodoform sprinkler, two sponges in a waterproof bag, a first aid package, a 2-ounce packet of sublimated lint and another of boric wool, and lastly, two wire splints with six strong tapes and buckles. The first aid package, an extra one of which is carried by each of the members of the squad, requires to be opened to appreciate its possibilities. Its wrapper is strong rubber cloth, 9 inches square, and its contents 2 yards each of sublimated gauze and cambric, 4 inches wide, a triangular bandage and two safety pins. The bandage measures 50 inches along its base and half of that measurement to its apex; it is stamped with figures showing the method of its application to the various parts of the body either as a support or as merely retentive of dressings.

The intentions of first aid to a wound are to arrest hemorrhage, remove foreign bodies, prevent bacterial invasion, and protect from injury during transportation. The wound has to be laid bare, to effect which the scissors, if need be, are used along the seams of the clothing. Dried and clotted blood, fragments of cloth or other foreign bodies have to be removed, capillary, venous or slight arterial hemorrhage to be checked, and the whole thoroughly cleaned, dried with antiseptic gauze, dusted with iodoform and protected with a compress of gauze and a suitable bandage. Adhesive strips are used to secure apposition of the sides of incised or gaping wounds. If there is fracture of the bones of the arm or fore-arm, the splints have to be applied, with the triangular bandage as a sling. The splints may also be used in fracture of the leg and thigh; in the latter as aids to a long splint obtained by improvisation. The members of the litter squad can apply rifles, sword-blades and scabbards, telegraph wire, straw, strong grass or rushes as temporary supports in fractures; they can utilize all kinds of cardboard and other stiff materials, and with their heavy sheath-knives they can hew the splint that is required out of that which at first sight might look like most unpromising timber.

At the collecting or dressing station are gathered many wounded men who are able to reach this place of aid and comparative safety without assistance. The non-commissioned officers and men of the hospital corps attend to these cases, while the medical officer deals with those of greater severity. In many instances the first aid given by the latter differs in no way from that which would have been given by his litter squad, but in every case he is prepared by the higher grade of his knowledge to render more valuable services if such should be required. His orderly, who always accompanies him, carries his pouch of field necessaries, such as are found in that of the litter squad, but containing in addition an Esmarch's tourniquet, a 4-oz. bottle of chloroform, a hypodermic syringe with tablets of morphine, and a book of button-holed tags by which he may convey information to the hospital surgeons concerning a particular case, fastening the tag over a button to the patient's breast. This pouch is furnished also with a small leather case of six screw-top vials, containing tablet doses of acetanilid, sulphate of quinine, compound cathartic pill, of brown mixture and diarrhœal remedy, and lastly, tablets of corrosive sublimate and sal ammoniac, each equal to one pint of a .001 sublimate solution. Slung on his own shoulder, the medical officer carries his field case, which, if examined, will show to what extent he is prepared to aid the injured. In it there are a bistoury, scalpel and amputating knife, the blade of the last 4¾ inches long, a saw, scissors, artery, bone, bullet and dressing forceps, Nelaton's probe, director, aneurism needle, tenaculum and serrefines, needles, ligature silk and wire, and a catheter.

The wounded brought in by the litter squads are examined by the medical officer without disturbing the first dressings, except in those cases in which there are obvious reasons for so doing. If they have been carried off hurriedly undressed they receive immediate attention at the hands of the non-commissioned officers and men of the station, under the supervision of the medical officer, who gives his personal skill to special cases. The first aid dressings are of the simplest character in all cases in which it is evident that careful examination or operation will be needful at the field hospital. Hemorrhage is arrested by substituting the ligature for the tourniquet which was applied by the litter squad; bullets, fragments of shell or other missiles are extracted; fractured bones brought in unsecured are bound up in the best immovable dressings that are available, and tags are buttoned upon those for whom the prompt attention of the operating staff of the field hospital is desired. The wounded are then transferred to the ambulances, each of which starts for the hospital as soon as loaded, and returns as soon as unloaded for further service at the front. The ambulance carries two men inside lying down, and one, who is able to sit in front with the driver, or four or five inside seated and one lying. The change to the ambulance and thence to the interior of the field hospital does not involve any disturbance of a severely wounded man, for it is the litter, not the patient, that is moved. The litter on which he is first placed forms his mattress on the floor of the ambulance and his bed when in the field division hospital. Men with flesh wounds, not suffering from shock, accompany the ambulances on foot or start for the hospital with a non-commissioned officer of the hospital corps in charge.

It may be observed that the field surgical case of the medical officer is more elaborate than seems called for by the work above indicated. A pocket case containing a scalpel, bistoury and probe, tenaculum, dressing and artery forceps, silk, needles and scissors, would suffice, and it is probable that in the field medical equipment of large armies the medical officers assigned to duty at collecting stations would carry only such a case. In our present service, however, where small commands take the field, the medical officer may have not only to give first aid, but to do all that is needful for his wounded during the days that may elapse before he can transfer them to the post hospital of some permanent station. The light field case was provided for his necessities. Cavalry commands operating in regions impassable to ambulances carry their medical and surgical supplies on pack animals, and the *travois* is provided for the transportation of severely wounded men. The *travois* consists of two strong elastic shafts, each fastened by its front end to the side of the saddle of a mule or horse, the rear ends trailing on the ground nine or ten feet behind the animal. They are kept in proper position, apart from each other, by cross bars, and the litter is suspended between them. When there is no *travois* the men of the hospital corps can construct one by cutting suitable poles and lashing on the cross-pieces. This is the Indian method of transporting the disabled.

After a battle the field is searched by the hospital corps for those who have fallen and been obliged to remain on the ground either on account of their disabled condition or by reason of the danger attending any attempt to get away. The conditions under which this duty is performed are exceedingly various, differing perhaps in every engagement, but the first aid brought to the wounded soldier is always prompt and efficient as above described.

In times of peace the special education of the hospital corps soldier is carried so far as to enable him to act intelligently when confronted with various accidents and emergencies in the absence of medical supervision. He is thus qualified to enter on a more extensive field of duty than is offered to a litter-bearer on the battlefield. Even in times of peace and slow promotion he is on his way to an acting hospital stewardship, and there are few of our acting stewards who are not looking forward to a steward's position. In case of the expansion of our army for war service this educated body of sanitary soldiers would ·fill the non-commissioned positions in the corps and permit of its expansion by recruiting merely for the litter-bearer and ambulance companies. For the duties of field service in time of war the education of the litter-bearer in first aid need not be very extensive. The primary management of patients suffering from gunshot wounds is soon learned by intelligent men, and only such should be enlisted for the corps. Moreover, State troops mustered into the service of the United States would bring to the corps their proportion of men more or less trained in army methods. Drill and discipline would soon fit the new men for the work before them, and enable the medical department to meet its responsibilities with full assurance of satisfactory results.

Aid given by the hospital corps soldier on the field of battle or in the accidents of garrison life differs in no respect in its professional details from that furnished by civilians in injuries of a like character. A fractured femur requires the same treatment whether the patient is a soldier run over by a caisson or a laborer by a dray. The aid itself differs from that afforded by competent civilians only in the systematic manner in which it is brought to bear in a given case. The same knowledge of conditions and requirements is needful to the citizen Samaritan and to the sanitary soldier, but the efficiency of the latter is due to his drill and discipline. These, intended to support him in the discharge of his duties when exposed to personal danger, are naturally always sufficient for efficiency when there is no personal danger to distract attention from the care of the injured. When acting officially the efficiency of the soldier is also secured by a judiciously selected equipment which is always on hand for his use. In fact, drill, discipline and equipment form the tripod by which the efficiency of the hospital corps is sustained and first aid rendered to the injured soldier both in times of peace and in times of war.

Since the accidents of peace among soldiers are so satisfactorily met by these military methods, it might be well to enquire to what extent they are or ought to be employed in civil life. This enquiry must, however, be taken up at another time or by some other individual, as it lies beyond the lines prescribed for the present paper.

FIRST AID TO THE INJURED AND HOW IT SHOULD BE TAUGHT.

By HENRY G. BEYER, M. D., Ph. D., M. R. C. S.

Surgeon, U. S. Navy.

In the attempt to outline a method for teaching " First Aid to the Injured," we must be guided by the careful consideration of three very important items, namely: 1. The subject-matter in hand; 2. The class of people to whom it is to be taught; 3. The teacher.

I.

A careful selection of the topics intended to be taken up and a judicious division and classification of them are, under all conditions and circumstances, the most necessary and important preliminary steps to be taken. This is no less true for " First Aid " than for any other subject.

So far as the subject of first aid is concerned and, following the excellent example given us by Prof. von Esmarch, I have very successfully taught it in six consecutive lessons for several years past.

Inasmuch as the method used is a very good one, the arrangement of the subject-matter tolerably judicious, and the instruction graded and progressive, it will, perhaps, not be without advantage for those interested to hear a brief synopsis of it, notwithstanding the well acknowledged fact that no one single method will do in all cases, and that even the best may have to suffer some modification according to the circumstances of the case.

Thus in the course of instruction which we have given, each lesson began with a lecture explaining theoretically the particular part of the subject under immediate consideration ; then followed the practical demonstrations, during which the pupils and the teacher were working together, assisting one another in putting into practice and applying the theoretical notions and ideas that had been discussed in the lecture.

For example, the first lecture begins with some few introductory remarks concerning the reasons why the subject should be taught at all ; then follows a short resumé of our present ideas of the nature, causation and prevention of infectious diseases. An attempt is made to give the pupils as nearly as possible some correct notions of what germs or bacteria are, how they look under the microscope, how they are cultivated and grow. Special importance, of course, is attached to the discussion of the relation of bacteria to wounds, and the meaning of the terms antisepsis and asepsis is made plain to them.

In the practical part of this first lesson the teacher begins by demonstrating on himself the several methods at present in vogue for rendering the different regions of the body aseptic preliminary to an operation ; the pupils then do the same, paying strict attention to all the necessary details and under the critical eye of the teacher. In this part of the work the teacher will probably find the most startling differences in the power of application in the different pupils. While some need but little correction in their work, others seem to have failed entirely in appreciating the great importance of surgical cleanliness, and which it was nevertheless the object of the lecture to impress upon them, but at the same time proving more than anything else the necessity of the practice. Finally, a sham operation is performed and an antiseptic dressing put over the parts, some of the pupils assisting, being obliged to pay strict attention to all the customary rules of antiseptic surgery. During the operation the different methods of sterilizing instruments and of preparing antiseptic dressings are discussed and the first lesson is concluded.

In my experience, very few pupils, after attending this lesson, leave the room without a very fair idea of the necessity and importance of cleanliness in dealing with wounds, and the majority can be trusted for making no mistakes in dressing a wound, no matter under what circumstances they might be called upon to do so, with perfect safety to the injured party.

In the second lecture anatomy is taken up. A skeleton and manikin, of course, would be of great assistance and a very great advantage, but charts take their places very satisfactorily. By the aid of charts and a living subject for purposes of illustration, all the most important parts of anatomy that a first aid man needs to know can be gone over in an hour. The anatomy and physiology of the circulatory system must be illustrated especially well on account of its relation to the subject of the arrest of hemorrhage.

In the second or practical part of the second lesson the art of bandaging is practiced. Besides applying the ordinary roller bandage to different parts of the body, the triangular bandage of Esmarch is applied by every pupil in all the different ways. Two pupils can practice on one another; the teacher first showing how it is to be done and the class following him step by step until all the necessary details of bandaging are mastered. One of these triangular bandages for two pupils being sufficient, the number of bandages to be provided may, therefore, be easily calculated from the number of pupils present.

The class having by this time attained a fair knowledge of antiseptic principles and the necessary anatomy, and acquired furthermore a tolerably good knowledge of handling certain bandages, they are now prepared for the subject of injuries, which are therefore taken up in the following or third lesson. For purposes of classification the injuries are divided into those of the *soft parts* and those of the *hard parts* of the human body. In the third lesson injuries of the "soft parts" only are discussed, and these are again treated of under two heads, namely, *contusions* and *wounds*.

Contusions are defined, their nature and pathology made clear as far as that is possible, and the proper treatment to be applied explained. In connection with the subject of wounds, that of hemorrhage finds a convenient place for treatment, and the various manual and instrumental methods of compression are thoroughly looked into and illustrated; also the treatment of hemorrhage from internal organs is mentioned.

In the practical part of the third lesson some few hints are given in the different methods of applying massage, and the pupils are made to practice them on each other; the best part of the time, however, is devoted to the different methods of compression and the arrest of hemorrhage generally.

In the fourth lesson, injuries of the hard parts or fractures are taken up; the diagnosis, method of setting and the mode of healing are mentioned; but by far the greater share of the time is devoted to the manner of applying splints and of extemporizing them from all sorts of material.

The fifth lesson is devoted to a number of subjects, viz. burns and scalds, the general effects of extreme cold, death by freezing, foreign bodies, swimming and drowning, resuscitation, unconsciousness, sunstroke, and apparent death. The practical exercises in this lesson consist in each pupil practicing the several methods of resuscitation.

In the sixth or last lesson the class receives instruction in the different methods of transporting the wounded and in the stretcher drill as practiced in the army.

The number of subjects in the above-detailed programme may seem somewhat limited, but in my experience a strict line should be drawn between instruction for nurses and instruction for first aid men. A first aid man who has mastered all the practical work in this course will be found not only a useful but also a safe and trustworthy helpmate to his injured comrade. A thorough practical knowledge of a few things is at all times better than a great mass of undigested knowledge; moreover, a first aid man must know and be impressed with the fact that his knowledge and aid have their limits beyond which he has no right to go.

At any rate, the success which has attended this sort of instruction leaves, at least in my limited experience, nothing to be desired, and I can therefore most heartily recommend it. All that seems to be necessary for keeping the knowledge thus acquired fresh and alive is an occasional drill consisting in treating supposed injuries.

The course must of course be adapted to the class of people to whom it is to be taught, and this brings us to the second part of our discourse.

II.

The people to whom this knowledge is to be imparted may differ in many ways; they may happen to belong to the working-class of, comparatively speaking, limited education and intelligence, and yet be greatly in need of just such information. Indeed, it may be said that it is primarily for the benefit of just that class of people that the subject should be more generally taught than it is. The method of instructing this class of people must naturally be different from the one adopted to teach the student class of the community. Still, this difference is, in my experience, not as great as it might at first sight seem, and I have been much oftener greatly surprised at the readiness and intelligence with which my lessons were received and handled than I have had reasons to be surprised at their ignorance.

One thing, however, must be remembered, and that is, the more practical and demonstrative the method of instruction, the more conversational the oral instruction, the closer the contact between the teacher and the audience, the better will be the results of the method employed. Every little detail, no matter how simple ñ may seem, must be illustrated at once in more than one form. The blackboard, charts, apparatus and living subjects should always be freely used for the one end in view, and until every point is fully understood and every detail has been thoroughly mastered. While this is necessary in instructing most all classes of people, it is, according to my experience, particularly necessary with the class of people under consideration. Mere lectures produce little good beyond impressing upon the audience the dangers it is liable to meet with, and perhaps the necessity of knowing some little about the subject.

It is my firm belief that the time will come when first aid will be regularly taught in our high schools and colleges, and particularly in those schools that are intended to train teachers. Teachers are in a position to do a great deal of good with it in more than one way; they have the care of a large number of children during the greater part of the day, and many of them meet with slight accidents during play-time. The teachers of public schools especially have ample opportunity not only to render valuable assistance to an injured child, but at the same time whatever they do in such cases will be witnessed by a large number of children and thus be indelibly impressed on their little minds. It is therefore essential that whatever the teacher does should be the proper thing in all cases.

A large number of college boys are devoting themselves to athletic sports more and more every year all over the country and should be encouraged in doing so. Accidents of all sorts occur during a season's play, and therefore a knowledge on their part of the principles and practice of first aid is, to say the least, a very desirable accomplishment.

Clubs, no matter what their object, ought to be prevailed upon to set aside at least one evening a month for instruction and drill in first aid. If the instruction is well managed there will be no end of interest in the matter.

Women of all classes of society having their little parties and meetings for either one object or another, might easily be persuaded to receive instruction in this most charitable subject. Women as a class, and to their praise it must be said, are much more charitably inclined than are the men, and some of the foremost workers in this field have indeed been women. But when we reflect on the fact that the largest share in both the home and school education of our children is performed by the women, we may perhaps realize much better how many are the opportunities that they have of rendering valuable assistance in case of accidents, and of teaching the little ones what is the right thing to be done under certain circumstances and how to do it. While it may be impossible to teach one subject regularly to children under a certain age, they will probably be impressed by seeing their mothers and teachers do it. Certainly every child, no matter what its age, can at least be taught to be clean with regard to the wounds which it accidentally receives while playing, and let us not forget that cleanliness is after all the first and foremost of all the lessons to be impressed on the minds of first aid men. But this can be done by no other persons so effectually as by mothers and teachers. The old notions of dressing a bleeding wound with spider's webs and garden-earths, still very common among certain people, ought to be speedily discouraged, as being productive of blood poisoning and lockjaw. Not long ago a workingman in Norfolk, Va., having received a wound, and dressing it with garden-earth, died of lockjaw ; the germ was not only discovered in the earth from which the dressing came, but also in the blood of the dying man. A similar case occurred here in Annapolis, on board the Santee about two years ago.

Instruction of first aid to soldiers and sailors is now so general the world over that little need be said on that subject. Its usefulness in times of war is so generally recognized that it has become an integral part in the education of every soldier all over the civilized world. Our navy alone is behindhand in this respect, and there exists no regulation that makes the systematic instruction of our men-of-wars men in first aid obligatory.

Perhaps the most perfect system of instruction at the present day exists in Germany. The organization of the Red Cross Association in all its details, both in times of peace and war, is truly wonderful, and shows the earnestness with which this subject has been handled by German army surgeons. This association, which is almost gigantic in numbers and extent, actually becomes a part of the sanitary corps of the army in the event of a war, and thousands will no doubt reap the benefits and blessings of this truly grand and most charitable of all associations.

III.

As regards the third part of our theme, namely the teacher, it is our firm conviction that he should always be a physician, and a good one at that. It is, according to my experience, a fatal mistake to imagine that any one knowing a little about anatomy and physiology can also successfully teach first aid to the injured. The most excellent first aid men may yet be unfit for teaching the subject as it should be taught, and there is no such thing as a medical man too well informed to teach this branch; he must, on the contrary, be quite abreast with all the modern improvements and advancements concerning not only the practice but also the science of his profession, to do it successfully. To these qualities of a medical man he must furthermore unite the qualifications of the teacher, that is, the faculty of expressing himself clearly, and of being able to put the most scientific principles in the plainest and most intelligible language, so that even a child may grasp them.

Speaking more especially with regard to college instruction, three subjects might be taught there under one head, namely, anatomy, physiology and hygiene, physical training and first aid to the injured.

Anatomy, physiology and personal hygiene for a foundation might suffice and enable pupils to understand the laws of normal growth and development, and apply them to a certain extent as well as the principles of first aid to the injured. But in order to teach these subjects the person must have a thorough medical education besides the special one that he is intended to teach.

NOTE.—Accompanying this paper, Surgeon Beyer presented a little volume of 90 pages, with 100 illustrations, entitled " First Aid to the Injured and Transportation of the Wounded. Six Lectures delivered to the Naval Cadets of the First Class at the Naval Academy during the Winter of 1892."—[EDITORS.]

ON THE ORGANIZATION IN PARIS OF FIRST AID TO THE WOUNDED.

By Dr. Alan Herbert, D. M., and Dr. W. Douglas Hogg, D. M., Paris.

In this paper we propose to consider: 1. The nature and number of accidents which have been recorded as having taken place in the streets of Paris during the year 1890.

2. The different organizations, whether of a public nature or the result of private benevolence, which exist with a view to relieve the wounded or those suddenly taken ill in the streets of Paris.

3. We will rapidly describe the different means of instruction on this subject which are obtainable in Paris, and finally we shall offer some general considerations as to the result of this study.

" L'annuaire statistique de la ville de Paris " informs us that during 1890, 1022 persons have received assistance: 330 in the " Pavillons de Secours" for the drowned situated either on the banks of the Seine or the canals which pass through the town; 621 in the different police stations; 51 in the " Poste de Secours," situated in the outskirts of Paris. Of the 330 received in the " Pavillons de Secours," the lives of seventeen only have been lost by drowning.

Of the 621 wounded received at the police stations, 175 were for wounds of the head, 93 for wounds on different parts of the body, 3 for fractures of the upper limbs, 17 for fractures of the lower limbs, 2 for different fractures, 9 for dislocation of the upper limbs, 17 for dislocation of the lower limbs, 42 for contusions, 1 for burns, 1 for a wound by firearms, 53 for attacks of epilepsy, 166 for various ailments, 1 for drunkenness, 6 for confinements, 3 for wounds results of attempted suicide, 3 for submersion, 29 cases not mentioned, total 621.

The causes of these accidents were: 128 falls by accident, 127 the result of accidents from quarrels or fights, 81 accidents from professional causes, 33 falls during drunkenness, 19 carriage accidents, 16 falls results of professional causes, 4 accidents occasioned by dogs, 3 from pigs, 7 from bulls, total 418.

In the outskirts of Paris 31 persons received aid in the year 1890: 23 for different wounds, 15 different forms of illness, 2 attempts to commit suicide, 11 accidental submersion (5 were drowned).

Organization of First Aid.

With a view to the medical organization of first aid to the wounded, the municipality of Paris maintains posts in different quarters of the town.

These posts are kept open day and night; each is provided with a box containing surgical dressings, and a stretcher which is so constructed as to permit of its being rolled on wheels or carried.

The following is a list of the number of stretchers existing at the different posts in Paris:

	Ordinary Stretchers.	Stretchers on Wheels.
Police stations,	86	15
" Commissariat,"	76	1
Military posts,	31	0
" Pavillons de Secours,"	18	0
" Octrois,"	4	1
Night refuges,	2	0

In 1890, 785 persons were transported from these different posts. The causes were as follows: Suicide by firearms, 17; sudden death, 61; falls, fractures, 214; various contusions, 70; burns, 6; pleuropneumonia, 44; bronchitis, 28; gastro-intestinal affections, 14; confinements, 112; epilepsy, 29; paralysis, 30; rheumatism, 23; alcoholism, 2; hernia, 11; typhoid fever, 9; various indispositions, 115; hemorrhage, 3. Total, 785.

We must also refer to the system of ambulances instituted in 1888 by Dr. Nachtel, on the same system as in New York.

Lately (in 1889) the prefecture of the police and the municipal authorities of the town of Paris have organized a service of "horse ambulances" for the gratuitous transport of the sick and infectious cases. If we mention this here it is because these ambulances are frequently called into practice for street accidents.

The work done by the municipal station of the "rue de Staël" and that of the "rue de Chaligny" in the year 1890 amounted to 1273 transports of non-contagious cases.

Medical Night Service.

We think it right to mention this service here, as it is so intimately connected with that of first aid.

It was instituted in 1876, the object being to provide medical aid for all persons who may require it during the night.

A certain number of medical practitioners in each district are enrolled at the prefecture of police. These names are inscribed at every police station.

They are liable to be called on between the hours of 10 p. m. to 7 a. m. in winter, and 11 p. m. to 4 a. m. in summer. The person asking for medical help at night can choose the doctor he prefers on the list of his arrondissement. A policeman sent from the station accompanies the person asking for medical aid to the doctor's residence, and from thence to the sick person's house. After the visit, he escorts the doctor again to his own home. He then presents to the doctor the fee of 10 francs (or 20 francs if it be a case of confinement or surgical operation). Next day the municipal administration institutes an enquiry, and if the sick person be in a position to pay, the sum given to the doctor is reclaimed of him; or in case he is too poor to pay, the administration bears the expense itself. This institution has rendered great service, and the number of night visits paid during the year 1876 rose from 3616 to 9123 in the year 1890.

In 1890 there were on the lists 520 doctors, 526 pharmaciens, and 505 midwives.

Popular Instruction on Medical Matters.

Till within the last few years there was little or no popular teaching for the treatment of the sick or wounded. Some private societies had attempted to give instruction on these points, but their efforts met with little success.

Lately, however, the "Union des Femmes de France" took the matter in hand and has very successfully instituted popular instruction on these subjects. In fifteen out of twenty of the arrondissements (districts) of Paris they have organized lectures. The course consists of 17 lectures on the following subjects: Outlines of anatomy and physiology, minor surgery, nursing, hygiene, and pharmacy. Two other societies which form, with the "Union des Femmes de France," the "Croix Rouge Française," viz. the "Société Française des Secours aux Blessés" and the "Association des Dames Françaises" are doing their utmost to popularize the study of these branches of medicine.

The "Assistance Publique" has also instituted lectures for the instruction of male and female nurses. The courses are gratuitous and are held at the hospitals of "La Salpetrière, Bicêtre and La Pitié."

We may perhaps also be permitted to refer to the Paris Centre of the St. John's Ambulance, which was founded by one of the undersigned, in 1889, to supply similar means of education to the English-speaking colony of Paris.

It is not easy to give the exact result of the teaching. As regards results obtained by the Union des Femmes de France, of which association one of the undersigned was among the earliest promoters, and is still the Director, the following is an outline :

Between the years 1882 and 1891, 633 persons (of whom 555 were women and 78 men) were presented with primary certificates, obtained by examination, after having followed the course of lectures of which we have just spoken.

The diploma for women nurses can only be obtained by passing a second examination, after having received three months' practical teaching in a hospital. This diploma has been conferred on 139 women.

These figures may appear small when compared with those of certain other societies, such as St. John's Ambulance of England ; but it must be borne in mind that these institutions for teaching and examination are of much more recent date in France than in England.

In England 100,000 certificates have been given to policemen alone ; it is therefore easy to understand that this kind of study being novel in France, it is a question of time before they take it up as a regular branch of study.

The important society of the Union des Femmes de France, numbering over 30,000 members, has in every county (or department) a committee which organizes the local courses of instruction.

The number of doctors and pharmaciens attached to the work as professors amounts to nearly 1500.

Conclusions.

The statistics in this paper will enable to some extent the formation of an opinion on the requirements of Paris, and also of the resources which that city offers in case of accident.

Let us, however, examine the case a little closer and try to judge whether the existing organization meets all the wants of the population.

The official report states that in the year 1890, 1022 persons suffering from accidents received help, but it is impossible to say how many other cases have failed to attract any notice.

Let us consider what generally happens in such cases in Paris. If an accident happens in the street, the wounded person is almost always conveyed to the nearest pharmacy. The pharmacien sends for a doctor, but the wounded person is often obliged to wait for a long time before medical aid arrives. The pharmacien gives the best help in his power, and after this the wounded person is taken home in a carriage. The stretchers, already mentioned, are rarely used in such cases ; the reason is that so much time is lost in going to the police station to get the stretcher and in finding men capable of using it (for it is dangerous to allow persons unaccustomed to the work to act as bearers of the stretcher of a wounded man). These cases, which are very numerous, are naturally not included in any statistics. One of us presented to the prefect of the police, at his request, a report on this subject in 1885.

In that report he recommended that stretchers on wheels, such as used in England, should be deposited in all the police stations, district town-halls, pharmacies, etc.

These stretchers would serve to carry wounded persons either to a hospital, a "poste de secours," or to their own home.

It would be too long to enter into the details of this report, therefore we shall only add that the administration accepted the proposal in a limited and tentative manner. They placed 17 stretchers on wheels in different "postes de secours." Considering how many accidents occur in the streets of Paris, this number is very small.

The popular habit in Paris when an accident happens is to carry the injured person immediately to the nearest pharmacy. These pharmacies are to be found in all parts of the town, and the public suppose that, thanks to the long and varied studies through which pharmaciens have to pass in France before obtaining a diploma, they must necessarily have acquired sufficient knowledge to treat such cases ; and no doubt their belief is well founded.

In point of fact, if we except such accidents as those of hemorrhage, poisoning and some other exceptional cases, there are very few which require any immediate active intervention. In most cases all that is necessary is to place the wounded person in such a position as to prevent any aggravation of his condition. The most important thing is to take him where he can receive proper care—to a hospital or to his own home, and certainly the pharmacien is quite capable of rendering these services. No doubt it is a troublesome duty to impose on him and a heavy call on his time, but they have never complained, and in fact they look on it as a matter of honor to fulfil these duties.

In this report, one of the points on which we have insisted was to give suitable teaching in these matters to all members of the police force.

We went further and advanced that this teaching should be given not only to pharmaciens and police agents, but to all persons likely to come directly into contact with those suffering from accidents.

In a country like France, where the influence of the state is so great, its co-operation is necessary.

School-teachers, men or women, military servants and many others ought to be obliged to go through the teaching and hold the certificate. We must not, however, dilate too lengthily on this topic, but let us recall the conclusions presented by one of us to the Minister of the Interior, at his request, on the subject, which although written some years ago are true to-day.*

1. The interest of the sick or the injured on the public thoroughfare requires that there be instituted a regular service of stretchers on wheels in all police stations.

The administration should have charge of these stretchers, and a police agent should be attached to each of them.

Between each of these stations and the pharmacies there should be telephonic communication.

2. The police agent should receive instruction how to raise and transport sick or injured persons, and also how to give them first aid.

3. The course of instruction should be followed by all government servants who are likely, by the nature of their occupations, to be called to practice first aid to the wounded, or all those who by the nature of their occupations are in a position to extend and generalize this teaching. We refer particularly to masters or mistresses of schools.

* Étude sur les hôpitaux d'isolation. Paris, 1886. J. B. Baillière (editor).

THE AMBULANCE SYSTEM OF NEW YORK CITY.

BY MR. GEO. P. LUDLAM,

Superintendent of New York Hospital, New York.

The very thorough and exhaustive article by Geo. W. Leonard, M. D., of New York City, on " Ambulances and the Ambulance Service in Larger Cities," published in the Reference Handbook of the Medical Sciences, Vol. 1, edition of 1885, leaves very little in the way of original material for subsequent writers. It is to that article that the writer of this paper is chiefly indebted, and his aim has been to present briefly an outline sketch of the ambulance system in New York City, its origin, development, and present condition.

It cannot be doubted that the credit of originating the system, which has grown to its present efficiency, belongs to Dr. E. B. Dalton, of New York City. His model was the army ambulance, and his incentive the desire to alleviate suffering by bringing the patient under the surgeon's care as soon as possible after the accident. His views on this subject having attracted the attention of the Department of Public Charities and Correction in New York City, he was requested by the commissioners to formulate a plan for the establishment of an ambulance service. He at once complied with the request, and the first service was established at Bellevue Hospital, in New York City, in December, 1869.

The service thus established has grown rapidly, and long since came to be recognized as an essential part of a well equipped modern hospital. New York City is now fully covered by the ambulance service of the different hospitals, and every day it is set in operation to meet the medical and surgical emergencies occurring in that great city. The system has also been adopted in other American cities, so that now the passing of an ambulance through the streets is one of the most familiar sights.

The details of the growth of the service in New York City are interesting. From 1870 to 1876 Bellevue Hospital alone maintained an ambulance service. According to the published record, 1466 calls were received by that hospital in 1870 and 1610 calls in 1876. In the latter year (1876) the service was established in the New York Hospital House of Relief (known as the Chambers Street Hospital), and very soon after in most of the other city hospitals. Although the districts covered by those earlier in the field have been curtailed by the assignment of territory to others as they established the service, yet the volume of business has increased so enormously that there has been an almost uninterrupted annual increase for each hospital. The subjoined table will show this very clearly. The years are selected as showing the first full year of service in each case, and these are compared with the year just closed.

	1870.	1877.	1878.	1879.	1881.	1892.
Bellevue,	1466	1217	1606	1888	2282	4858
House of Relief,	...	1155	1253	1321	2293	3216
New York,	...	...	651	585	1154	1520
Roosevelt,	...	...	273	291	352	1675
St. Vincent's,	...	...	...	823	1387	2066
Presbyterian,	...	...	...	...	387	1730

Or, starting with the 1466 calls of Bellevue Hospital in 1870, the aggregate of calls of all the hospitals in 1883 was 10,413, in 1889 was 15,215, and in 1893 was upwards of 20,000.

In New York City the service has become a part of city hospital work. It is recognized and counted upon by the departments in the city government. The police department has direct telegraphic and telephonic communication with the different hospitals. The fire department has introduced ambulance calls into its code of signals, and these may be sent out from all the signal boxes throughout the city. The introduction and rapid growth of the telephone has also been a factor in the growth of the ambulance business, as now the calls are sent in promptly by any one who is a spectator at the scene of accident. So completely has the fact of its importance come to be recognized that a recent grand jury made the service the subject of official investigation, and while finding in it much to praise, declared that it had not even yet been developed to the extent that is possible and desirable, and urged such an expansion as would make it almost as easy to summon an ambulance as to hail a passing cab.

The ambulance of the present day is essentially the same as the original one. Certain minor changes have been made, adding to the efficiency of the vehicle, but there has been no material departure from the original plan. This plan, doubtless, is a familiar one, and yet a description may not be amiss here.

It would be difficult to improve on the description given by Dr. Leonard in the article already referred to, and which is substantially as follows: The ambulance is a covered, four-wheeled wagon, with an arch at the forward end, under which the front wheels may turn. The length of the body is sufficient to receive a patient and permit him to lie at length. The surgeon's seat is a padded cross-board at the rear, hinged to the wagon body at one end and fastened by a catch at the other. This arrangement permits the seat to be raised and held out of the way by a snap or catch in the roof, when the ambulance is being loaded. The driver's seat, over the arch, extends the entire width of the vehicle. The tail-board is hinged on the lower edge and is held in place by snaps or catches at both ends of the upper edge. When these snaps are withdrawn the tail-board drops down out of place. Below this is a broad wooden step, hanging low and near the ground. On either side of the rear pillars of the wagon frame, and directly over the surgeon's seat, are leather loops, or straps, by the aid of which the surgeon may swing himself from the step into his seat while the ambulance is in motion. On the floor of the wagon and filling the entire space is a rolling bed, consisting of a stout padded frame, with wheels on the under side, arranged to run on a track, and provided with clutches or clamps at the inner end which, when the bed is withdrawn, fits into the rings fixed in the rear end of the wagon body, to prevent its being drawn all the way out. At the sides of the bed frame are iron rods, or legs, fixed at one end by eye and staple, and simply held up out of the way by clamps, as the other. When these clamps are loosened the legs fall and assume a perpendicular position, thus supporting the drawn-out bed at a level. The patient is brought to the ambulance on a canvas stretcher, and is placed upon the bed, which has been drawn out in preparation, and which is then rolled back into the vehicle; the tail-board, which has been dropped, is shut up in its place, the surgeon's seat, which has been held up against the roof, is drawn down, and all is ready for the return trip.

The interior of the ambulance, sides and roof, is covered with wood paneling and may be washed down with hose or bucket, the bed being drawn entirely out for the purpose, so that thorough cleanliness is easily secured.

The space under the driver's seat is a box in which are placed splints of different lengths and kinds, cotton bandages of all kinds, unbleached muslin, and the material for different kinds of dressings. Long and short thigh splints are carried in leather straps close to the roof. The surgeon's lantern, for use at night, hangs within his reach at the side of the ambulance, upon a hook and kept in place by a spring clamp. There is also a satchel which the surgeon takes with him from the ambulance on arriving at the place of call. This satchel is in two compartments, one containing bandages and dressings sufficient for a single case, and the other such drugs as may be needed for immediate and emergency use. The surgeon also carries his pocket case of instruments.

The method of summoning the ambulance varies. Most of the calls, perhaps, come through the police. The officer whose attention is called to the need reports the fact to his station house. Word is telegraphed thence to police headquarters, where the telegraph operator receives the message and forwards it to the hospital in whose territory or district the patient has been found.

Or the signal may be sent out from any fire box. In this case the signal sounds on the bells in all hospitals maintaining the ambulance service and having connection with the fire lines. The hospitals respond to fire calls within such limits as each one has fixed for its own guidance.

Or any citizen may send the call over the public telephone.

The action at the hospital when a call is received is, probably, essentially the same at all. A signal is given by electric bell or otherwise, whereby the surgeon on duty, the driver and the gate-keeper are notified simultaneously. By ingenious and improved methods of harnessing, the time required by the driver for harnessing and driving out of the hospital premises into the street has been reduced to a minimum. There he is met by the surgeon, who in passing out has received a slip of paper on which is written the source of the call, the time and the place. He calls out the latter to the driver, who immediately starts. The whole process from reception of call to start requires from one to two minutes.

This is the ambulance service of the present day in our larger cities. It may vary in minor details in some places, but essentially it is everywhere as herein described. It is somewhat remarkable that a system so advantageous in every respect, and which so soon became a necessity in modern hospital management, should fail to find favor in European cities. Thus far, however, it is practically unknown there. Many intelligent visitors from abroad have often examined it and familiarized themselves with its details, but have as yet been unsuccessful in their attempts to introduce it into the cities and towns of their residence.

Even in New York City it has not yet reached its highest development. The public need and indeed the public expectation and demand, which found expression in the deliverance of the grand jury already referred to, will undoubtedly be responded to in the future by such an expansion and adaptation of the system as will meet the necessities of every case.

AN IMPROVED STRETCHER FOR HOSPITAL, AMBULANCE AND MILITARY USE.

By E. D. Worthington, M. D., F. R. C. S. Edin.,

Sherbrooke, Province of Quebec, Canada.

Some time ago I put together a rather primitive apparatus for use in a very troublesome case of fracture of the neck of the femur, and I was so satisfied with its great usefulness that since that time I have frequently called its aid into requisition. The following is copied from my notes from this first case:

"*Case of fracture of the neck of the femur.*—The patient is upwards of sixty years of age and weighs 165 pounds. At the time of the accident she received some abrasions of the skin behind the trochanter of the injured side and on the back, but, as she did not complain of them, they remained undiscovered. After a few days, however, these abrasions became so painful it was necessary to ascertain their exact locality and extent.

How to do this was a matter of some difficulty, as the slightest attempt at moving the patient was attended with excruciating agony. I therefore adopted the following simple plan, and not having seen any similar contrivance used for this specific purpose, beg to recommend it to the profession, even at the risk of repeating 'an old, old story.'

My apparatus was as follows: Eight pieces of pine, six of them being thirty inches in length, four in breadth and three-eighths of an inch thick. The other two were three inches in breadth, three-quarters of an inch thick, and the length of the patient's bedstead, inside measurement. The ends and edges of them were rounded and made perfectly smooth.

When everything was ready I passed the short pieces under the patient, from side to side, at regular intervals from the head to the

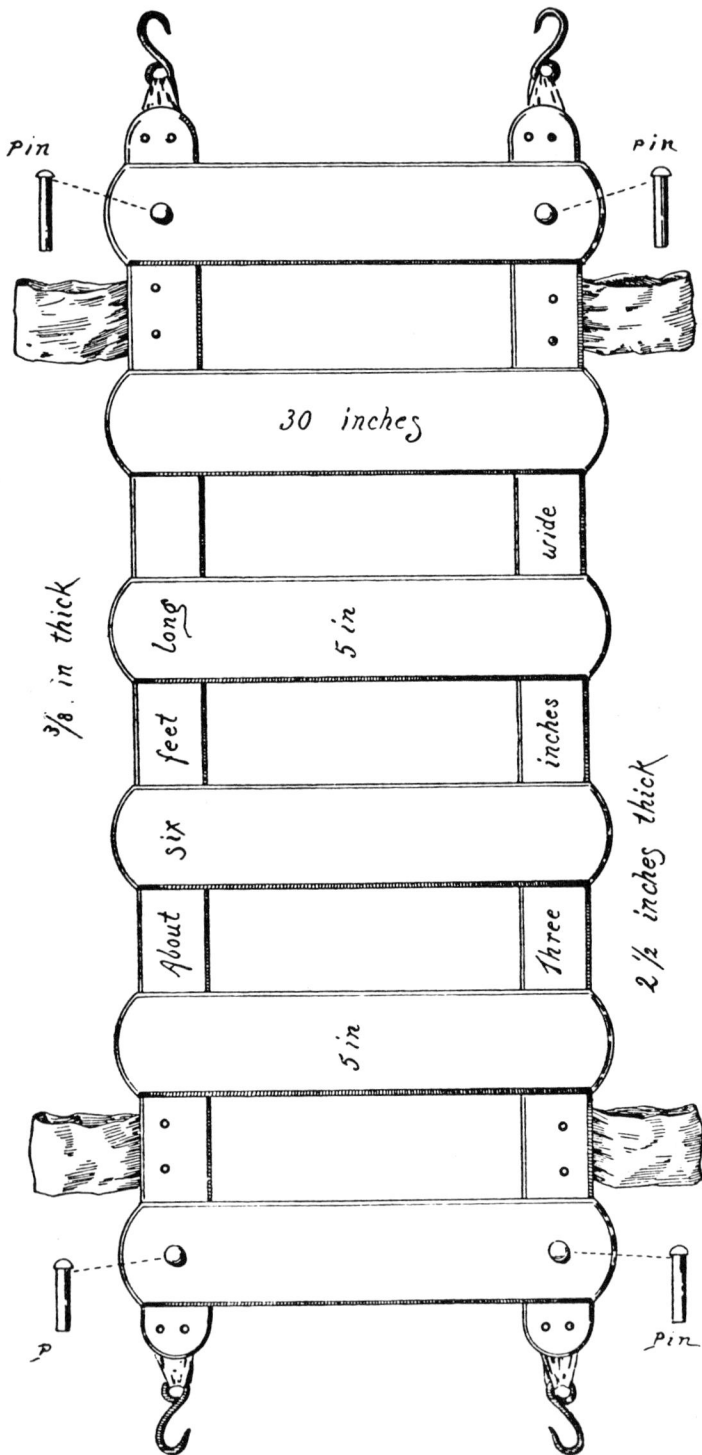

Pin

Pin

30 inches

wide

long

5 in

3/8. in thick

six feet

inches

About

Three

2 1/2 inches thick

5 in

P

Pin

feet—say one at the heel, the calf of the leg, the middle of the thigh, the hips, small of the back, and shoulders. The long pieces were then carefully inserted under the ends of the short ones. The apparatus was put together in a minute, and one person at each corner lifted the patient easily and steadily on this temporary stretcher. The bed underneath was then arranged without the least discomfort to the patient. In this way my patient has been moved two or three times a day. She likes it. As her bedstead is rather low, two ends of the long side pieces are lifted so as to rest on the headboard, and a couple of hassocks support the lower ends until the process of bedmaking is complete."

In all the stretchers I have seen the patient had to be lifted upon them, while in this plan the stretcher is made under the patient. As a matter of prudence the four corners may be secured, so as to prevent the possibility of their spreading, but the weight of the patient, and a little care on the part of the attendants, will render this unnecessary.

It is sometimes difficult for the nurse to pass the bed-pan well under a patient, but by adopting the above suggestion, either the bed-pan, or the ordinary "utensil," according to the peculiar notions of invalids on this delicate subject, may be used without risk of making the patient a victim of misplaced confidence.

In conclusion, I believe that for field use the above put together in sets, with a wooden pin to be dropped in a hole at each corner, would be more serviceable and in every respect better than the present army stretcher.

The patient, who was the wife of a judge, was proverbially sensitive, and accustomed to every luxury. At first she remonstrated against being asked to lie upon "these bare hard slats," but in a short time she was loud in their praise. She frequently said, " I cannot tell you what a comfort they are to me. The girls lift me up with the greatest ease six or eight inches above the level of the bed while they are changing the sheet. They have even carried me into another room while this one was being aired. I could lie on this temporary bed for an hour or more without inconvenience. You must write a description of it to the medical papers."

Second case.—A poor fellow had been fearfully mangled in a railroad accident. He was two miles away from his home, and to carry him that distance with as little suffering as possible was most desirable. Even if a canvas stretcher, the traditional barn-door, or a wide board could have been procured, the poor man would have to be lifted upon it, and when he got home be lifted from it, whereas an old picket fence by the side of the track supplied the short pieces as above described, and a couple of saplings the side pieces, and the man was carried home and laid on his bed, when the stretcher was removed.

Third case.—On October 1st a gentleman received a gunshot wound from the accidental discharge of a Winchester rifle. The bullet entered the thigh posteriorly, fractured the femur about its middle, and made its exit on the front of the thigh, exactly opposite the point of entrance. The accident occurred on a line of railway in construction between Montreal and Sherbrooke, so that he received all the attention necessary. My friend, Dr. Fenwick of Montreal, saw the patient with me, and though we urged him to go to the hospital in Montreal, he insisted on remaining in Sherbrooke. I had applied the long straight splint, to which I adjusted pulley and weight, and next morning put the whole leg up in a glue bandage with traps over both wounds. He had my stretcher in his private ward, the nurses being well drilled in its use, and it was used upon every occasion, freely, when using the bed-pan and making or changing his bed.

On the 14th of December, a few days over ten weeks from the injury, he sailed for Scotland in one of the Allan steamers. A few months later he returned to Canada with a scarcely perceptible limp, the shortening not being more than half an inch.

I do not pretend for one moment that the success of this case of gunshot wound of the thigh involving fracture of the femur was due to the use of the stretcher, but I claim it assisted materially in securing as much as is possible of absolute rest for the broken ends of the bone.

I hope the diagram with its explanatory notes will be understood. It is on a scale of one inch to a foot. The short pieces may be made of pine, bass-wood, maple, anything; they should be beautifully smooth and lightly beveled at each end. When wanted for use, the under sheet of the bed should be pulled smooth and the short pieces passed under the patient, beginning just above the heel, and up to the head at regular intervals, of course between the under sheet and the patient's shirt or chemise; the piece at the head should be passed under the pillow. The side pieces are then introduced, the mattress being gently depressed, if necessary, to pass them along, the wooden pins are dropped into the holes at the four corners, and the attendants lift the patient up, and drop the claws or hooks over the end bars of the iron bedstead. The patient will then be lying on a hammock from six to twelve inches above the mattress, high enough for any procedure. I have never found it necessary to use the pins at the corners, but using them will inspire confidence.

For a description of the stretcher I refer to the accompanying diagram. It will be noticed that at each corner of the diagram there is a loop and hook. The loop should be of rather stout webbing, and fastened on the under surface of the ends of the long side pieces with a couple of copper rivets. Each loop holds as a fixture a claw or a hook for suspending the stretcher on the cross bars of the bedstead at the head and foot.

In ordinary ambulance service, when the wagon reaches the scene of the accident, the tray or slide is run out, with its comfortable-looking mattress, upon which the injured person is lifted. When he reaches his home or the hospital he is lifted off, at a great expense of unnecessary suffering. All this time the mattress has been under him, and it will cost him as much pain to get it from under him as it cost originally to get him on it.

My stretcher, on the other hand, may be adjusted under the patient, the stretcher slung in the ambulance, and when the hospital is reached the stretcher may be run out, carried to the ward, and hung to the cross bars of the bedstead, the clothing of the patient removed, the stretcher lowered upon the sheet of the bed and the wooden frame removed. There is no lifting and pulling from one side of the bed to the other.

What I have here written will apply equally to civil and military ambulance service. The objection may be urged that in an apparatus composed of so many pieces some may be lost, but those in charge should see to that. The two side pieces and the six short ones with poles, constituting one set, when strapped together are not very cumbersome. They can be put together and taken apart in a minute, and any extra care required in adjustment is more than made up in usefulness.

All that is necessary to render this stretcher suitable for field use will be the addition of four loops of webbing of suitable strength, two on each side, fastened with copper rivets on the under surface of the long side pieces, the loops being large enough to allow a pole to pass on each side, to answer the double purpose of handles to lift by and sides for the stretcher.

In conclusion I have to say that it would be difficult to over-estimate the value of this very simple contrivance in post-partum hemorrhages, hemorrhage in typhoid, or in cases of accident, or extreme debility from whatever cause. Whenever a change of bed and raiment is desirable, but where the change cannot be made without risk, this apparatus affords an easy solution of the difficulty. In cases, too, where it is necessary to reduce the temperature by placing the patient in a cold bath, the move can be made without subjecting the patient to unnecessary loss of vital force.

VI

HOSPITAL SATURDAY AND SUNDAY.

HOSPITAL SATURDAY AND SUNDAY.

By Frederick F. Cook,

General Agent and Organizer of the Hospital Saturday and Sunday Association of New York City.

I have been asked to say a word to you on the topic of " Hospital Saturday and Sunday." The pleasure would be great were it not for a feeling that I shall be able to do the subject only scant justice. While the movement known by the rather infelicitous title of " Hospital Saturday and Sunday " stands in the minds of the many for the single object of collecting money for hospital purposes, with an incidental provision for a return of favors to donors in the form of free hospital service, it is singularly adapted, both by reason of the humanitarian promptings that underlie it, and its organic form, to allay social friction, and has likewise proved capacity for serving ends of administrative economy. It is inevitable that development should follow lines of local conditions, and what I may say, therefore, though expressed in terms of the subject in general, had best be received as a reflex of the state of things in New York, about which I may claim some familiarity.

The primary object of Hospital Saturday and Sunday may be regarded as the raising of money for hospital support, and this is done by methods so diversified as to reach every part of the community. Another is to develop and extend the work of hospitals on lines to benefit in largest measure the sick poor, and this is served by making *free work* the basis upon which the fund collected is distributed amongst associated institutions. A third object is to inform the charitable to ends of judicious discrimination, and this is in part accomplished through the medium of statistics. A fourth is the promotion of administrative economy in our institutions, and this is brought about by the same means that enable donors to

make a wise discrimination in their gifts, namely, the annual statements of hospitals made to the association, as a basis for the distribution of the general fund, wherein all important items of service, of
income, and of relative cost, are brought into direct comparison.
Finally, a most important object is to enlist the powerful stimulus
potential in suffering in the interest of social solidarity, and this is
furthered by making the movement so broad and elastic that all
classes and shades of opinion find it possible to unite under its ægis
for humanitarian ends.

Precedence is given to the money-getting side of the work, for
the reason that that is the most obvious, and was probably the only
aspect before the minds of its early promoters. But now that the
movement has assumed international dimensions, and it is seen that
other things important in many ways to this age are served by it, its
uses as a social conservator and promoter of fraternal relations
between diverging forces in the community come more and more
into prominence, and with not a few of its friends this is the
weightiest object in the balance. As a rule, however, it is the
totality of ends served by the movement that gives spur to its
supporters in the work at home, and incites them to spread the seed
over the widest possible field.

That the movement had a natural and spontaneous origin is
clearly shown by the difficulty to fix its beginnings. As in the case
of the great discoverer, many cities claim the honor of being its
birthplace. Historically the initiative is most distinctly traced to
Birmingham, England, and its contention for priority would seem to
derive some support (in addition to proofs less speculative) from the
biological theory which attaches greatest potency to primal cells,
inasmuch as Birmingham has steadily held the lead amongst the
larger cities, and stands to-day well to the front in the matter of
financial results.

In England there are now above fifty Hospital Saturday and
Sunday Associations, and so highly is the movement esteemed
that in several instances hospitals have been named for those most
prominently identified with its beginnings. In America there are at
present perhaps half a score of associations, counting large and
small, the leading ones being those of New York, Brooklyn, Baltimore, and Pittsburgh. Recently the New York association has
taken steps looking to the extension of the work to all the principal
cities of the country, with an ultimate hope of bringing about a

"National Hospital Saturday and Sunday," and it is my purpose while here to give what impetus I may to the founding of an association in Chicago, and with a like object in view I shall probably visit other western cities.

This seems hardly the place to give a detailed history of Hospital Saturday and Sunday. Suffice it to say that its beginnings must be looked for in instances where individual churches in one or another place adopted the plan of taking an annual collection for some particular hospital. The next step is indicated by a division of the collection between several hospitals. A third stage was reached when several churches made the work a common cause. Thus part was added to part, now in this place, then in that one, until in Birmingham (to which some earliest beginnings in the form indicated are also traceable), in the year 1860, the full-fledged Hospital Sunday was born. Finding that a collection in the churches did not meet the object of enlisting the entire population, Liverpool, in 1870, added Hospital Saturday for a secular collection, and other cites were not slow to follow the example. In most places Hospital Saturday and Hospital Sunday are under one management, but separated by an interval of weeks or months in time. In London, however, Hospital Saturday and Hospital Sunday are not only separated in point of time, but each is under a different management—a form of development not only unnecessarily expensive, but one prone to result in friction and discord, where it should be a means to social harmony.

In New York, as in most cities, Hospital Saturday and Hospital Sunday are promoted by a single association, but in some respects original connotations are somewhat departed from. In England, for example, Hospital Saturday is a purely secular institution, whereas in New York, in recognition of the interest taken in this movement by those who worship in the synagogue, it is made the symbol of the Jewish Sabbath, and of the collection in the synagogues on the Saturday preceding Hospital Sunday, which is fixed for the last Sunday of the year. However, to avoid any unnecessary complication of title, Hospital Saturday also retains its secular meaning, and is a general term to cover the secular branch of the work, and is applicable to the entire period devoted to collections in the trades, upon exchanges, in factories and public resorts. This secular activity generally antedates Hospital Sunday by several weeks, and often continues well beyond it, so that the day for church collection may be regarded as the pivot around which the work revolves.

In all essentials Hospital Saturday and Sunday in America is as indigenous and spontaneous as the English product. Early in the sixties several Episcopal churches in New York formed societies for the maintenance in St. Luke's Hospital of the sick poor of their respective parishes. A year or two later several Presbyterian churches adopted a similar plan with respect to the Presbyterian Hospital, the plan in a few instances being extended to the endowment of a bed. Early in the seventies the work had grown to such extent amongst Episcopal churches that a score or more took an annual collection for the benefit of St. Luke's, and a year or two later St. Mary's Free Hospital for Children was included as a beneficiary. And from these beginnings—the trustees of St. Luke's taking the initiative—the New York association came into existence, first in a tentative form in 1879, and on a permanent basis in 1880; beginning in 1879 with 13 hospitals, now represented by 33, and a collection of $26,000, now advanced to $63,000.

The differences that result from local conditions are often very marked, and illustrate alike tendencies and stable characteristics. Thus, in London, which is pre-eminently a city of churches and church-goers, Hospital Sunday outranks Hospital Saturday in its financial results in the proportion of three to one. In New York, on the other hand, because of its exceptionally large foreign-born population, little inclined to church-going, the comparison is almost reversed, and the secular contributions outrank the offerings in the churches in the proportion of three to two. This difference in mode in which the charity of the two chief English-speaking cities in the world expresses itself is to the student of sociology a significant fingerpost.

How collections are taken in churches you all know, and Hospital Sunday collections differ from other offerings only in their object. But a word about Hospital Saturday collections may not come amiss. For all the leading trades there are auxiliary associations. To these is left the task of thoroughly canvassing their respective trades by such means as are most effective. Similar auxiliaries are organized within the exchanges, and, when practicable, likewise amongst the professions. There is also a "Woman's Auxiliary." It is the fashion to make light of what is technically called "society," and it undoubtedly stands for a good deal that is purely frivolous. On the other hand, this very frivolity operates to turn a strong tide in the opposite direction—a reaction for counter-poise. If, therefore, "society" be frivolous in parts, it is also extremely serious in other parts, where social obligations are inter-preted more and more in terms of moral obligations. To-day, the success of all charitable work depends to a very large degree on the interest woman takes in it, and especially the woman of social influ-ence. The "Woman's Auxiliary of the Hospital Saturday and Sunday Association of New York," while it is as broad as woman-kind itself, has nevertheless an acknowledged social basis, and it is from this leverage that its work is mainly accomplished. Within the general scheme of the Woman's Auxiliary there is a place for a "Woman's Fund," made up exclusively of the gifts of women, and this holds a leading position amongst the association's contributions.

The results to administrative economy, arising from an annual comparison of work and relative cost can scarcely be overestimated, and it is the opinion of those who speak from the standpoint of expe-rience that it fairly equals the sum derived from the collections, while in a few notable instances it has led to a complete change of methods. Recently there has come into existence in New York an association of hospital superintendents, which meets frequently for conference upon administrative methods and economies, and this practical means to reform is the direct corollary and effect of Hospital Saturday and Sunday methods and influences.

The New York Association is constituted of one representative from each of its 33 component hospitals, and about an equal number from the public at large, so that those who give and those who receive are balanced in the administration. It is a union of many nationalities, and all shades of religious and social opinion work together to a common end. And the influences that are operative at the heart of the movement extend both in kind and in degree to its farthest extremities, into the busy marts of trade and to the toilers in the workshops. There is no place in the city so remote or isolated that the influence and operations of Hospital Saturday do not extend to it, and its catholic spirit makes appeal where anything less broad, less unselfish, less fraternal would pass unheeded. And it is this broad charity that has enlisted in its behalf a united press, ever ready to bring the merits of the movement home to the hearts of the people. For many reasons, therefore, the value of Hospital Satur-day and Sunday associations should not be estimated merely or solely by dollars and cents results. Indeed, when compared with the total amount of hospital expenditure, it may, as to individual institutions, be quite insignificant; and, in such circumstances, it is because of other good and beneficent results that flow from co-operation and the spirit of confraternity that it wins and holds support.

However, having regard only to the money-getting aspect, it is the judgment of those oldest in the work that the familiarity with hospitals as a humanitarian concern, brought about by the public and wide-spread methods of Hospital Saturday and Sunday associations, conduces to hospital support by gifts independent of these general collections. Certain it is that in cities where associations exist, special hospital support was never more free-handed than since the time the general collections were instituted.

Now and again some one makes the contention that the ingathering of relatively small gifts on Hospital Saturday or Sunday is a bar to the giving of larger sums on other occasions to particular institutions—in other words, that a person who gives $10 or $25 or $100 in a general collection will make that an excuse for refusing to make a subscription at another time to some particular hospital of the association, when, if he gave at all, he would put down his name for $50 or $100 or $500. It may be frankly admitted that such instances are possible, but, happily, none is within the knowledge of those who have taken special pains, under exceptional opportunities, to examine the matter. It is an unwritten law of this large-hearted charity that the Hospital Saturday or Sunday gift, being for the good of all, shall not be counted in any one's personal or particular scheme of hospital support. Hence few large gifts are received. The contributions are made up of the pennies of the poor, the dimes and quarters of mechanics, and in advancing proportions as there is rise in the scale of wealth, up to $100. A few, it is true, give in terms of thousands, but they are no more than a few in any collection, it being expected that those who give by four, five or six figures will do so for particular ends. Yet, though the sum that goes to any institution as its share of the general collection be not large, it seems to fill just the place where otherwise a deficit would be noted, and few would care to do without it. The London *Lancet*, probably the leading medical journal of the world, has issued a general challenge to show that Hospital Saturday and Sunday collections abate from special hospital support, but no proof is furnished. On the contrary, induction as well as deduction sustain the position of those who claim for the associative work precisely the opposite effect. Varying with local conditions, the cost of these collections ranges from 2 to 5 per cent., covering every form of an association's expense.

Hospital Saturday and Sunday is pre-eminently an educative influence in the field of charity. By combination, such as could probably be made for no other object, people are moved to give who have never before contributed towards any charity. Having given once, it is far easier to secure a contribution from them a second time, and at the third call the thing has become a matter of course. Again, it is a common experience that when a person has aided any object he comes to regard himself as part of it. He unconsciously makes it his own, and inevitably becomes its advocate, for no one likes to think he has given to an unworthy cause. If, therefore, a person has come to look with friendly eyes upon hospital work in general, he is fairly tractable material when approached to aid some particular institution at other times than Hospital Saturday or Sunday.

To what extent the giving to charitable objects is a matter of education only those can appreciate who are engaged in the charitable propaganda. Given wealth, if you succeed in breaking the ice for $50 one year, another year it is easier to get $100, and in time $500 or $1000 to any object will be less of a strain upon the donor than was the first $50. Man is a creature of custom. Psycho-physiologically our ordinary actions correspond to definite brain-tracts. It is making the first impression, however faint, that is hardest. Once a line is defined it is comparatively easy to follow it up, and as with each recurrence it grows deeper and wider, it becomes the symbol of a larger charity. It is thus we may regard the Hospital Saturday and Sunday association as a pioneer charity brain-tract maker, and from this follows the corollary that it benefits hospitals at other times than upon the occasions of its annual collections, and other and all worthy charitable objects as well.

Surely it is true that it is more blessed to give than to receive. Because of the many objects seeking support now before the public, the pressure upon the rich is undoubtedly great; but who that sees how wealth and luxury naturally tend to increase man's selfishness would care to see one feather's weight of this pressure lightened? It is in the nature of a public safety-valve. It helps the struggling poor surely somewhat, and it helps the rich in tenfold greater degree.

In the beginning I alluded to the potency of human suffering as a means of confraternity. I would close with this thought. When the dream of the social reformer shall be realized and all men shall stand equal in material estate, there will still remain the one supreme difference whose mark is pain and whose seal is death. To-day, because of conventional or adventitious distinctions, the inherent and fundamental disparity between health and disease is almost lost to view. But whenever there shall come a social development in which the mere externals shall be fairly equalized, the inherent and inexpugnable differences will be lifted into their proper rank in human eyes, and because of the leveling in other regards, it will appear to the sympathetic helper, as well as to the sufferer, that the distinctions between man and man are greater than ever; and because this will so appear, the humanities will be more and more cultivated, while sickness with its attendant afflictions will become more and more a humanizing agency, a spiritual and moral potency, a teacher of duty and the supreme bond of brotherhood. In the last analysis, it is the one impulse that underlies all our moral activity now, and it needs but open eyes, eyes trained to look beyond the conventional and accidental to the actual, to realize it. From sickness and its results none may escape. It is the angel with the flaming sword that keeps man out of his earthly paradise.

Addenda.

Favors to Donors.

An important aid to the work of the New York association is the return made to donors in the form of free hospital service for the benefit of any poor sick person recommended by them. The method is for donors to apply to some officer of the auxiliary through which they make their contribution, and for the officer to report the case to the general agent of the association, who forthwith proceeds to place the patient in the hospital best suited to the conditions of the case.

About Auxiliaries.

A Trade or Exchange is regarded as organized on an auxiliary basis when there is a nucleus of working members sufficient to fill the offices of president, secretary, treasurer, and executive committee of three. These auxiliaries are supplied with blank subscription lists by the parent association. Then the work is divided among the members with special reference to location or sphere of influence, and when the canvass is finished, the treasurer of the auxiliary turns the sum collected over to the general treasurer of the association.

The Distribution.

In New York the distributing committee of the undesignated fund is composed *ex officio* of the mayor, the postmaster, and the president of the Chamber of Commerce; in addition to which four members are annually elected, the present incumbents being Messrs. Morris K. Jesup, Jesse Seligman, Edward Cooper and Cornelius Vanderbilt.

Special Designations.

By the rules of the association, special designations of gifts to particular hospitals are received. These do not pass through the hands of the distributing committee, but are sent directly to the hospitals indicated by the donors. The amount designated to various institutions, some of which may be outside of the association, is generally about one-sixth of the total collection. The rule under which the undesignated fund is distributed reads as follows:

"The plan of distribution of undesignated funds by this committee in any year shall be to divide them among the institutions certified to it by this association as entitled to share in the distribution for such year, according to the number of hospital days *free* patients have been treated in the beds of each institution, for the year ending with the 30th day of September preceding such distribution.

"To entitle any hospital to share in the distribution of said undesignated funds in any year, it shall submit to this association and file with it, on or before November 1st each year, a report of its work, receipts and expenditures for the year ending September 30th next previous, and of its pecuniary resources and condition on such date, according to the schedule issued by this association for this purpose."

Modes of Collection.

In addition to the collections in churches on Hospital Sunday, and the work of the auxiliaries in the organized trades, all unorganized trades and manufactories are supplied by mail with subscription lists, accompanied by circulars setting forth the object of the movement and requesting that employers and employes make this work of succoring the sick poor a common cause. These lists number about 3000, and are usually sent out several weeks before Hospital Sunday, and returned to the general treasurer with the sums subscribed, about a month later. In some factories collection boxes are preferred and supplied. Similar boxes to the number of several hundred are placed in public resorts, restaurants, drug stores, and at the stations of the elevated railways. These boxes, in addition to the money secured through them, serve the purpose of keeping the movement before the public and, by advertising the needs of hospitals, contribute to their support in general.

DISCUSSION.

MR. HENRY C. BURDETT, of London.—Apart from the financial aspects of the Hospital Saturday and Sunday, their educational aspects are of far greater importance. It is certain we can never secure humane, active and efficient management of our hospitals unless we can quicken the public conscience.

In this country hospitals do not depend upon voluntary contributions, and therefore this quickening of the public conscience is relatively unimportant as compared to what it is in England. In Chicago there is a necessity for awakening the public conscience. I visited the Cook County Hospital yesterday and I find an absence of all conscience in the management of the institution, except among the nurses ; but the condition of nursing in the Cook County Hospital makes my heart bleed. I have never seen anything so appalling from the point of view of the humane work. Instead of being helped by the medical profession of this city and by those who have the responsibility of the charity, I venture to think, and I grieve to say it, that for some unaccountable reason their labor is made hideously difficult. The Cook County Hospital is only a workhouse hospital. I have never seen anything in the whole course of my experience, and I have visited hospitals in every country of the world, including Russia, which has gone so straight to my heart, which has been so appallingly awful as what I saw in my visit to the Cook County Hospital. In 1882 I visited this hospital and then sealed my lips because I hoped as the city grew things would improve. They have improved, but the old system prevails as harmfully as it did in 1882.

THE CHAIRMAN.—I will remind the gentleman that the subject under discussion is Hospital Saturday and Sunday.

Mr. Burdett.—The Chairman reminds me that the paper is Hospital Saturday and Sunday, but I venture to say that these remarks are in line ; as I have before said, the important thing to do is to arouse the public conscience in those who have anything to do in connection with the administration of charity. If Chicago had an active demonstration or organization for a Hospital Saturday and Sunday fund, it would be impossible for the Cook County Hospital administration to remain as I found it yesterday.

Now I should like to see this movement of a Hospital Saturday and Sunday largely extended. At present the Hospital Saturday collects one-third of the total amount received in London. That is about 65,000 pounds a year, of which 45,000 is raised by Hospital Sunday and 21,000 by Hospital Saturday. That is a tremendous growth in Hospital Saturday and Sunday fund. Last year we proposed to extend as far as possible this movement, and very much good has come from arousing public opinion on the subject. The Hospital Saturday fund has gone up and up, and the Hospital Sunday has steadily come down.

There have been various Hospital Saturday funds, one where 5200 pounds were raised in the workshops by six weeks' work, a thing that would have been impossible years ago. Since then workmen have been admitted to the administration of hospitals, and the result has been that workmen have come to feel that they have an interest and they like to contribute, and so the funds have gone up and up and up until they collected this year not less than 13,000 pounds from the workingmen alone. This Saturday fund or these contributors have organized a separate fund for the establishment of a large convalescent institution which has cost nearly 10,000 pounds, from the workingmen of Birmingham.

I think these facts should encourage everybody, because when Hospital Saturday was commenced in Birmingham the politicians—for we have politicians in England as you have in America—combined to stop it. The newspapers said it is a question for the people, and we believe our mission is to quicken the conscience of the people by representing to them the facts and speaking to them as man to man and woman to woman. We started out in Birmingham, and in those days it was difficult to get women to speak upon the subject, although that day has gone by now. We got three or four assistants, and they enlisted the sympathy of three or four large manufacturing works, and they left off a quarter of an hour before the dinner hour so that we might get them together in a big hall and speak to the men. The result was that in six weeks 5700 pounds were raised by the workingman for the support of hospitals. And Mr. G. F. Munce said that while the whole expense was only 700 pounds yet he wanted the entire amount raised to go to the hospitals, and he sent his check for 700 pounds, the cost of the work, so that every dollar went into the coffers of the hospital.

The success of Hospital Sunday depends upon the individual clergyman and his churchwardens and the personal interest which they have in it. There is one minister who sends out what he calls "The Golden Pheasant Circular," that is, a little letter written in burning words, and he invariably collects 700 or 800 pounds. The collections are much larger than where there is a simple announcement. This question of Hospital Sunday organization should be clearly presented to the congregation, and there should be an organization to which could be sent delegates of three members, and they should decide upon the constitution of the funds in each city, and the principles upon which it should be maintained and the fund distributed. In that way you get a representation of public opinion which is most useful. It is well also to interest the proprietors of the shops and the foremen of the shops as well as the ministers, churchwardens and elders. If you can secure the support of the foremen you can then organize the penny-a-week collections in the shops, and in this way I think you would raise a very large sum. Success depends upon thorough organization, and you cannot bring it before the people without a systematic organization on the part of those responsible for the fund.

I think we are immensely indebted to the gentleman who read this paper. The people in hundreds of cities can be interested, and by organizing a little nucleus, getting men and women together, you can make this or any other system properly organized the means for quickening public conscience and thus meet success. Unless it is well organized and you have the combined feeling that it is the privilege to do this work for Christ and enjoy it more than the luxuries of the world, it cannot attain its highest end. All money and power is useless except it can be turned to good account. That man is not doing his full duty who does not understand and appreciate and do something to meet the needs and requirements of his day. It is the duty of every one to return a portion of God's gifts, of which he is but a responsible trustee. None of us can take our money away with us. Some one has truly said here in these Congresses that "there was no wealth in shrouds." That man whose faith is pinned to shrouds is miserable indeed.

In conclusion, to do this work properly you must get to the hearts of the people, and give this great work personal service conscientiously done, and you will soon have more money than you know what to do with.

INDEX.

Titles in This Series

14   Annette Fiske. *First Fifty Years of the Waltham Training School for Nurses.* New York, 1984. BOUND WITH Alfred Worcester. "The Shortage of Nurses—Reminiscences of Alfred Worcester '83." *Harvard Medical Alumni Bulletin 23*, 1949.

15   Virginia Henderson et al. *Nursing Studies Index, 1900–1959.* Philadelphia, 1963, 1966, 1970, 1972.

16   Darlene Clark Hine, editor. *Black Women in Nursing: An Anthology of Historical Sources.*

17   Ellen N. LaMotte. *The Tuberculosis Nurse.* New York, 1915.

18   Barbara Melosh, editor. *American Nurses in Fiction: An Anthology of Short Stories.*

19   Mary Adelaide Nutting. *A Sound Economic Basis for Schools of Nursing.* New York, 1926.

20   Sara E. Parsons. *Nursing Problems and Obligations.* Boston, 1916.

21   Juanita Redmond. *I Served on Bataan.* Philadelphia, 1943.

22   Susan Reverby, editor. *The East Harlem Health Center Demonstration: An Anthology of Pamphlets.*

23   Isabel Hampton Robb. *Educational Standards for Nurses.* Cleveland, 1907.

24   Sister M. Theophane Shoemaker. *History of Nurse-Midwifery in the United States.* Washington, D.C., 1947.

25   Isabel M. Stewart. *Education of Nurses.* New York, 1943.

26   Virginia S. Thatcher. *History of Anesthesia with Emphasis on the Nurse Specialist.* Philadelphia, 1953.

27   Adah H. Thoms. *Pathfinders—A History of the Progress of Colored Graduate Nurses.* New York, 1929.

28   Clara S. Weeks-Shaw. *A Text-Book of Nursing for the Use of Training Schools, Families, and Private Students.* New York, 1885.

29   Writers Program of the WPA in Kansas, compilers. *Lamps on the Prairie: A History of Nursing in Kansas.* Topeka, 1942.

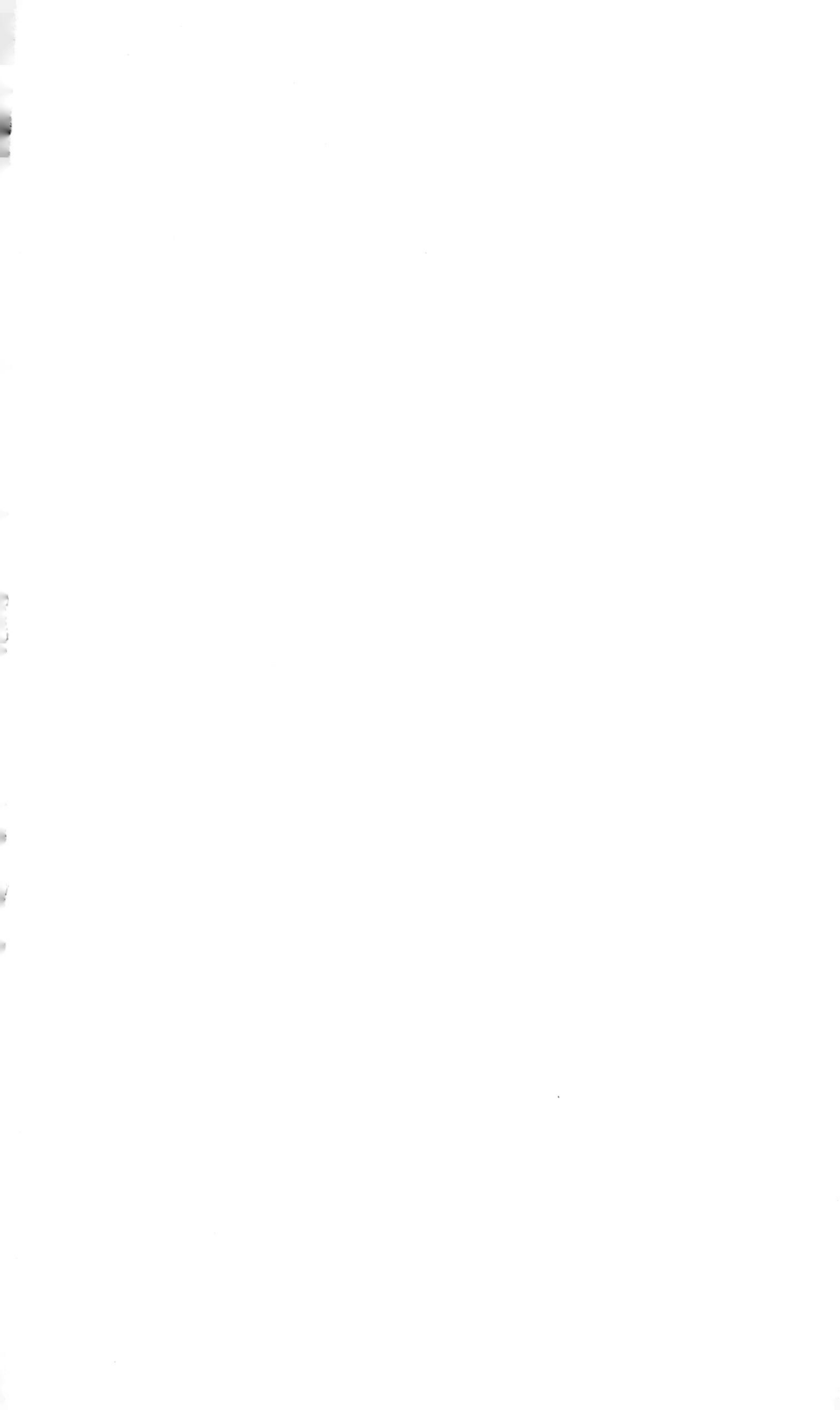